Symptoms, Pathophysiology and Treatment of Multiple Sclerosis

Symptoms, Pathophysiology and Treatment of Multiple Sclerosis

Editor: Steven Pitts

AMERICAN
MEDICAL PUBLISHERS
www.americanmedicalpublishers.com

AMERICAN
MEDICAL PUBLISHERS
www.americanmedicalpublishers.com

Cataloging-in-Publication Data

Symptoms, pathophysiology and treatment of multiple sclerosis / edited by Steven Pitts.
p. cm.
Includes bibliographical references and index.
ISBN 979-8-88740-282-6
1. Multiple sclerosis. 2. Multiple sclerosis--Diagnosis. 3. Multiple sclerosis--Pathophysiology.
4. Multiple sclerosis--Treatment. I. Pitts, Steven.
RC377 .S96 2023
616.834--dc23

American Medical Publishers,
41 Flatbush Avenue,
1st Floor, New York,
NY 11217, USA

ISBN 979-8-88740-282-6 (Hardback)

Contents

Preface

It is often said that books are a boon to mankind. They document every progress and pass on the knowledge from one generation to the other. They play a crucial role in our lives. Thus I was both excited and nervous while editing this book. I was pleased by the thought of being able to make a mark but I was also nervous to do it right because the future of students depends upon it. Hence, I took a few months to research further into the discipline, revise my knowledge and also explore some more aspects. Post this process, I begun with the editing of this book.

Multiple sclerosis (MS) is an autoimmune disease that causes damage to nerve fibers of the central nervous system (brain and the spinal cord). It can be categorized into four types namely, clinically isolated syndrome (CIS), relapsing-remitting MS (RRMS), primary progressive MS (PPMS), and secondary progressive MS (SPMS). Some common symptoms of multiple sclerosis are vision problems muscle weakness, fatigue, changes in gait, muscle spasms, loss of balance or coordination, etc. As of now, no cure has been found for multiple sclerosis. Some treatments can slow the disease progression and help relieve the symptoms. Its treatment plans include disease-modifying therapies (DMTs), physical rehabilitation, mental health counseling, and relapse management medications. There are some preventive measures such as regular exercise, stress management, healthy food intake, etc. that can improve this condition. This book outlines the symptoms, pathophysiology, and treatments of multiple sclerosis in detail. A number of latest researches have been included to keep the readers up-to-date with the latest concepts in this area of study. This book will serve as a valuable source of reference for graduate and post graduate students of medicine.

I thank my publisher with all my heart for considering me worthy of this unparalleled opportunity and for showing unwavering faith in my skills. I would also like to thank the editorial team who worked closely with me at every step and contributed immensely towards the successful completion of this book. Last but not the least, I wish to thank my friends and colleagues for their support.

Editor

1

The Role of B Cells and Antibodies in Multiple Sclerosis, Neuromyelitis Optica, and Related Disorders

Silke Häusser-Kinzel[1] *and Martin S. Weber*[1,2*]

[1] *Institute of Neuropathology, University Medical Center, Göttingen, Germany,* [2] *Department of Neurology, University Medical Center, Göttingen, Germany*

***Correspondence:**
Martin S. Weber
martin.weber@med.uni-goettingen.de

Our pathophysiological concept of the most common central nervous system demyelinating disease, multiple sclerosis, strikingly evolved by recent discoveries suggesting that B lymphocytes substantially contribute in its initiation and chronic propagation. In this regard, activated B cells are nowadays considered to act as important antigen-presenting cells for the activation of T cells and as essential source of pro-inflammatory cytokines. Hereby, they create a milieu in which other immune cells differentiate and join an orchestrated inflammatory infiltration of the CNS. Without a doubt, this scientific leap was critically pioneered by the empirical use of anti-CD20 antibodies in recent clinical MS trials, which revealed that the therapeutic removal of immature and mature B cells basically halted development of new inflammatory flares in otherwise relapsing MS patients. This stabilization occurred largely independent of any indirect effect on plasma cell-produced antibody levels. On the contrary, peripherally produced autoantibodies are probably the most important B cell component in two other CNS demyelinating diseases which are currently in the process of being delineated as separate disease entities. The first one is neuromyelitis optica in which an antibody response against aquaporin-4 targets and destroys astrocytes, the second, likely distinct entity embraces a group of patients containing antibodies against myelin oligodendrocyte glycoprotein. In this review, we will describe and summarize pro-inflammatory B cell properties in these three CNS demyelinating disorders; we will however also provide an overview on the emerging concept that B cells or B cell subsets may exert immunologically counterbalancing properties, which may be therapeutically desirable to maintain and foster in inflammatory CNS demyelination. In an outlook, we will discuss accordingly, how this potentially important aspect can be harnessed to advance future B cell-directed therapeutic approaches in multiple sclerosis and related diseases.

Keywords: B cells, multiple sclerosis, central nervous system, antigen-presenting cell, cytokine secretion, regulatory B cells, anti-CD20 therapy, neuromyelitis optica-spectrum disorders

INTRODUCTION

The fulminant clinical success of anti-CD20 antibodies in the treatment of multiple sclerosis (MS) and neuromyelitis optica-spectrum disorders (NMO-SD) raised awareness that beside T cells, B cells play a decisive role in their initiation, and propagation. Here, the rather immediate benefit of anti-CD20 therapy has been mainly attributed to the extinction of B cells from the blood, but even more so from immunological relevant organs, such as lymph nodes and spleen (1). In these peripheral compartments, B cells interact with other immune cells after encountering antigen, promote their differentiation and in turn undergo expansion and maturation themselves (2). In NMO-SD, this peripheral B cell activation results in a highly relevant antibody response against CNS antigen. Consequently, most investigations focused on elucidating mechanisms by which B cells contribute to the pathogenesis of MS and NMO-SD in the periphery. These studies revealed that beyond antibody production, cellular properties of B cells such as antigen presentation and cytokine production shape the response of other immune cells such as T cells and myeloid cells both in a pro-inflammatory, but also in a regulatory manner. Besides these properties in the periphery, B cells and their antibodies probably play an important role within the CNS, which may however substantially differ between MS and NMO-SD.

B CELLS CONTRIBUTE AS ANTIGEN-PRESENTING CELLS TO THE ACTIVATION OF T CELLS

B cells are professional antigen-presenting cells (APC): they recognize even low concentrations of antigens specifically and constitutively express major histocompatibility complex (MHC) class II and co-stimulatory molecules. This enables B cells to prime T cells and in turn induces their own differentiation into memory cells and antibody-producing plasma cells (**Figure 1A**). In contrast to myeloid APC, which randomly ingest peptides, B cells are capable of specifically recognizing, and internalizing natively folded "conformational" protein antigens via their B cell receptor. Subsequently, B cells process these structures to short linearized peptides and present it to antigen-specific T cells via MHC class II molecules. Thus, B cells are most efficient APC when they share antigen recognition with responding T cells (3). In genetically-altered mice containing myelin specific B and T cells, the mere coexistence of these cells induces a spontaneous form of experimental autoimmune encephalomyelitis (EAE) (4, 5), a commonly used murine model for human inflammatory CNS demyelinating disorders. In the very same model, the selective ablation of MHC class II on B cells renders mice resistant to disease induction (6), showing their substantial contribution as APC to this model. However, efficient priming of naïve T cells does not only rely on peptide presentation via MHC class II, but furthermore requires the ligation of co-stimulatory molecules, such as CD40, CD80, and CD86. The quality of these signals in conjunction with soluble factors shapes the emerging effector T cell type. While for instance a strong cell-cell contact via CD40 on B cells and CD40 ligand (CD40L) on T cells is necessary for the generation of pro-inflammatory T cells, a weaker molecular contact induces rather regulatory T cell functions and a complete block of CD40-CD40L interaction even prevents EAE (7, 8). In line with these findings, B cells of active MS patients compared to controls express increased amounts of CD40 together with higher level of MHC class II and CD80 (9, 10) suggesting that they harbor an enhanced APC capacity. Furthermore, peripheral as well as CNS B cells exhibit signs of chronic activation with a shift toward antigen-experienced memory B cells (11, 12) pointing toward an active involvement of B cells in MS pathogenesis. This assumption is further corroborated by functional studies which revealed that in a subgroup of relapsing-remitting MS patients, B cells were capable of initiating proliferation, and interferon-gamma (IFN-γ) secretion of potentially pathogenic $CD4^+$ T helper (Th)1 cells *ex vivo* (13). In summary, these findings point toward an active involvement of B cells in the pathogenesis of MS, potentially by activating CNS-infiltrating T cells that in turn drive inflammation in brain and spinal cord.

B CELLS SECRETE PATHOGENIC, BUT ALSO REGULATORY CYTOKINES, WHICH CONTROL OTHER IMMUNE CELLS

Besides being equipped with molecules required for direct cell-cell contact, B cells provide a variety of cytokines for inter-cell signaling. This is important as T cell activation does not only rely on the strength of co-stimulatory signals, but furthermore the cytokine milieu provided by the presenting cell (**Figure 1B**). For instance, interleukin (IL)-6 secreted by B cells fosters the differentiation of Th17 cells, while it prevents the generation of regulatory T cells (14, 15). Thus, in a B cell dependent EAE setting, B cell-restricted IL-6 deficiency diminished the Th17 response and ameliorated the disease severity (6, 16). B cells isolated from the blood of MS patients though exhibit an abnormal pro-inflammatory cytokine profile when compared to healthy controls. They secrete elevated amounts of IL-6, lymphotoxin alpha and tumor necrosis factor alpha (TNF-α), and produce less anti-inflammatory IL-10 (11, 16). The observation that these abnormalities were apparent upon polyclonal stimulation suggests that not only autoreactive B cells but rather the B cell pool at large is deregulated in individuals with MS (11, 17). Moreover, MS patients showed an increased frequency of memory B cells that co-express the pro-inflammatory cytokines granulocyte-macrophage colony-stimulating factor (GM-CSF), IL-6, and TNF-α. In the small MS cohort investigated, therapeutic removal of B cells including the latter memory B cell subpopulation resulted in a diminished pro-inflammatory IL-6 response by macrophages in a GM-CSF-dependent manner (18). An observation that points toward an inflammation-promoting potential of B cells in MS. However, a similar investigation aiming to assess the activation of myeloid APC in blood before and after therapeutic B cell removal in MS and NMO patients did not reveal such uniform results. Here, the macrophages of the study participant showed similar TNF-α secretion before treatment initiation, but varied widely after anti-CD20 therapy (19). This suggests that B cell depletion had a differential effect on the activation of myeloid cells in individual patients, with either pro-inflammatory, or anti-inflammatory outcomes (**Figure 1C**). Moreover, it indicates that in a subgroup of MS patients, B cells may exert immune regulatory functions prior to their therapeutic removal. Indeed, B cells are not only a relevant source of pro-inflammatory, but moreover of

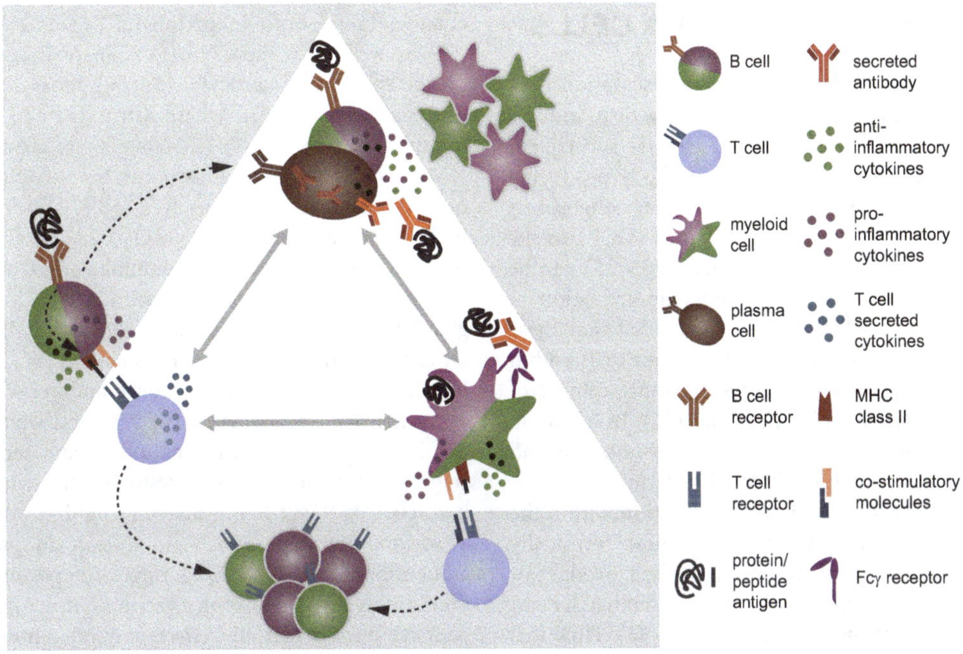

FIGURE 1 | B cells, T cells, and myeloid cells shape each other's immune response via direct interaction and/or secretion of cytokines. **(A)** B cells encounter protein antigens specifically via their B cell receptor and present linearized peptides bound to the major histocompatibility complex (MHC) class II to T cells. Thereby, they act as efficient antigen presenting cells and control the differentiation of T cells by the density of co-stimulatory molecules on their cell surface and the cytokine milieu they provide. In turn, this interaction fosters **(B)** the differentiation of B cells into antibody-producing plasma cells and memory B cells. B and plasma cells secrete pro- and anti-inflammatory cytokines, which affect the expression of co-stimulatory molecules and the production of chemokines/cytokines by myeloid antigen-presenting cells. Vice versa, myeloid cells have an impact on B cell activity through the secretion of distinct cytokines and chemokines. **(C)** Myeloid antigen-presenting cells, such as monocytes, macrophages, and dendritic cells internalize antigen randomly or opsonized antigen specifically via Fcγ receptors, process them, and present the linearized peptides via MHC class II to T cells. They are able to induce both pro- and anti-inflammatory T cells, controlled by the expression density of co-stimulatory molecules on myeloid APC and their distinct secretion of cytokines.

anti-inflammatory cytokines: while antigen-activated B cells mostly secrete pro-inflammatory ones, antigen-naïve B cells, plasmablasts, and plasma cells produce relevant amounts of anti-inflammatory IL-10, IL-35, and transforming growth factor beta (TGF-β). In the context of EAE, adoptive transfer of IL-10-secreting B cells for instance suppressed disease (20), while B cell-restricted abrogation of IL-10 or IL-35 augmented its severity. Moreover, both B cell-derived IL-10 and IL-35 were required for physiological recovery from an acute disease flare (21, 22), and the presence of B cell-secreted TGF-β limited the induction phase of EAE (23). In all of these studies, augmented EAE severity went along with an increased number of differentiated, pro-inflammatory Th1, and Th17 cells, suggesting that anti-inflammatory cytokines secreted by B cells were required to limit the pathogenic T cell response during EAE. In humans, similar regulatory B cell properties have been described (24) and are assumed to be impaired in MS patients (11). However, further research is required to validate this assumption and to ascertain whether regulatory B cells are equally relevant in MS as they are in EAE. If this proves true however, future therapies should aim to maintain or restore regulatory B cell functions, while targeting pro-inflammatory properties selectively; an issue that currently available therapies cannot address (25, 26). In this context, a promising approach may be the inhibition of Bruton's tyrosine kinase (Btk), an enzyme that is present in B cells, and innate immune cells, such as myeloid APC, but not in T cells. B cells require Btk for proper B cell receptor signaling, where it rather modulates the signal responsiveness, than turning it on or off (27). Thus, its inhibition does not deplete B cells, but presumably lowers their response to B cell receptor stimuli (28). In this way, Btk inhibition is assumed to foster the induction and maintenance of tolerogenic B cells, while it counteracts their antigen-mediated pro-inflammatory activation (29–31). In mice with collagen-induced arthritis and in a murine lupus model, both autoimmune disorders with pathogenic B cells involvement, an orally applied Btk inhibitor reduced the amount of circulating autoantibodies and inhibited the development of disease (32), showing its ability to limit a pathogenic B cell response. In MS, first phase II clinical trials testing evobrutinib (ClinicalTrials.gov Identifier: NCT02975349), an orally applied, highly selective Btk inhibitor, significantly reduced the number of new enhancing T1, and new or enlarging T2 lesions when compared to placebo (ECTRIMS Online Library. Montalban X. Oct 12, 2018; 232075). These preliminary results suggest that a monotherapy aiming to inhibit Btk can be promising in MS. Moreover, Btk inhibition may be suitable as maintenance therapy after initial anti-CD20-mediated B cell depletion to avoid recurrence of pathogenic B cells.

B CELLS DIFFERENTIATE INTO ANTIBODY-PRODUCING PLASMA CELLS

As mentioned before, the process of antigen presentation does not only activate the responding T cell but in turn induces the proliferation of the presenting B cell and its subsequent differentiation into memory cells and antibody-producing plasma cells. Hence, the presence of persisting oligoclonal immunoglobulins (Ig) termed oligoclonal bands (OCB) in the cerebrospinal fluid (CSF) of most MS patients (33–35) can be construed as a first evidence of the pathogenic activation of B cells in MS. More detailed investigation revealed that these intrathecal Ig were most likely produced by plasma cells within the CSF as the CSF Ig proteome and the Ig transcriptome of CSF-located B cells matched with each other (36). In addition, intrathecal B cells show signs of somatic hypermutation and clonal expansion (37, 38) pointing toward a germinal center-like reaction with antigen-driven affinity maturation within the CNS. However, there is new evidence that these terminally differentiated B cells in the CSF were not solely a product of intrathecal maturation, but can cross the blood-brain barrier and interact with the peripheral immune system (39–42). How this migration though influences the maturation of intrathecal B cells in detail and whether it affects the peripheral B cell response is not yet fully understood. Up to now, the expression pattern of OCB in the CSF do not have an apparent correlate in the blood, indicating that despite the ability of B cells to exchange, antibody-secreting plasma cells mainly accumulate within the CNS of MS patients. However, the pathogenic relevance of these CNS-located B cells and their products for the pathogenesis of MS is still controversially discussed. The presence of co-localizing Ig and complement depositions in ongoing MS lesions (43) suggests that autoantibodies are involved in CNS injury. A assumption that has been further fueled by studies demonstrating that antibodies isolated from the CSF of MS patients induce axonal damage and complement-mediated demyelination when applied to human CNS tissue *ex vivo* or *in vitro* (44, 45). Nevertheless, the particular antigen(s) recognized by these antibodies are still unclear (46). Reiber et al. (47) for instance claimed that OCB of MS patients were mostly directed against CNS-unrelated antigens, such as rubella, measles, and varicella zoster virus indicating an unspecific "bystander" activation of B cells. Others however proposed autoantibodies against CNS structures, such as myelin, astrocytes, and neuroglial cells to be part of this intrathecal humoral immune response. They report that OCB of MS patients contain autoantibodies against myelin basic protein (48), myelin-associated lipids (49), contactin-2 (50), and KIR4.1 (51). However, the variety of proposed antibody specificities and the fact that some of the aforementioned findings were not easily reproducible by other laboratories (52–54) possibly reflect the complexity of MS pathogenesis. Alternatively, it suggests that MS may consist of multiple disease entities with distinct disease driving mechanisms. In fact, the first clinical variant of MS, which has been separated from the "core disorder" was NMO based on the discovery of anti-aquaporin (AQP)4 autoantibodies in the patients' blood (55, 56). AQP4 is a water channel found both in peripheral organs such as the kidney (57) as well as in the CNS (58). There it is mainly expressed on the end feet of astrocytes (59, 60), most densely in the optic nerve and spinal cord where astrocytes and oligodendrocytes are in close proximity (61). Hence, these are the regions where NMO lesions predominantly occur. Since AQP4 is not expressed on oligodendrocytes themselves (58), astrocytes are suggested to be the main target in NMO (62, 63). Corroborating this notion, active NMO lesions contain areas of co-localizing Ig and complement depositions with a vast loss of AQP4 and glial fibrillary acid protein immunoreactivity that points toward an antibody-mediated destruction of astrocytes. Older lesions however show in addition a reduced number of oligodendrocytes and extensive demyelination of gray and white matter (56, 64, 65) indicating that demyelination occurs secondarily in later stages of the disease as a result of the preceding astrocyte loss. Hence, NMO is nowadays recognized as an autoimmune astrocytopathy (66) which is, at least in part, mediated by autoantibodies against AQP4. Interestingly, anti-AQP4 antibody titer are relatively low or even absent in the CSF of NMO patients even when the corresponding antibody titer in the blood are high (67). Furthermore, only 15–30% of NMO patients have OCB in the CSF, which in addition mostly disappear with disease progression (68). These findings together suggest that in NMO, B cells are in the first place activated outside the CNS resulting in a pronounced humoral immune response against AQP4 in the periphery. However, new data indicate that also in NMO patients, similar to MS, B cells exchange across the blood-brain barrier resulting in the presence of AQP4-specific B and plasma cells both in the blood and the CSF (69). Nevertheless, the particular trigger(s) of these astrocyte-directed attacks and the exact sequence of B cell activation including the circumstances under which AQP4-directed B cells and/or antibodies gain access to the CNS to induce lesion formation are not fully understood. Despite these pending mechanistic issues, the diagnosis of NMO is nowadays closely tied to the presence of antibodies against AQP4. However, some patients with clinical features suggestive for NMO do not have detectable anti-AQP4 antibody titers. Instead, about a third of them produce antibodies against myelin oligodendrocyte glycoprotein (MOG) in the blood (70–72). MOG is a transmembrane protein expressed on the outermost lamella of the myelin sheath and the surface of oligodendrocytes (73). Its extracellular localization and its lack of expression in the thymus renders MOG a plausible target for autoimmune responses (74, 75). Patients with autoantibodies against MOG have a severe disease course with high relapse rates, strong brainstem, and spinal cord involvement and do hardly respond to several disease-modifying treatments (54). Evaluation of their CSF and histological analysis of biopsy/autopsy tissue revealed no astrocytopathy, but myelin damage as primary injury in the CNS (1, 54, 76–78). Similar to classical NMO, OCB occur only occasionally (79), and anti-MOG antibodies can be found in the serum, but not in the CSF (80, 81).

PATHOGENIC INVOLVEMENT OF B CELLS AND THEIR PRODUCTS IN THE PERIPHERY AND WITHIN THE CNS

The occurrence of a peripheral humoral immune response against CNS antigen is the most striking similarity between patients with anti-AQP4 and anti-MOG antibodies. It delineates them distinctly from MS patients, which show an accumulation of Ig in the CSF, but have no apparent reflection of these antibody patterns in the blood. However, the pathogenic role of these autoantibodies outside the CNS is still elusive. In mice, it has been demonstrated that peripheral anti-MOG antibodies foster the activation of encephalitogenic T cells in the periphery by opsonization of otherwise unrecognized traces of CNS antigen, which results in the induction of EAE (82, 83). How these endogenous CNS antigens though reach the periphery is uncertain, but presumably by being drained from the CNS to peripheral lymph nodes along lymphatic vessels (84). Even though it is not yet proven that this mechanism is of relevance for the human condition, it is conceivable as antibodies isolated from anti-MOG antibody positive patients were capable of opsonizing human MOG (83). Furthermore, traces of myelin have been found in cervical lymph nodes of MS patients as well as healthy controls (85, 86) indicating that also in humans, CNS structures can be made accessible to the peripheral immune system by this route. Consequently, it includes the possibility that CNS antigens are recognized and opsonized by CNS-directed autoantibodies in the periphery. Overall, these findings suggest that anti-AQP4 antibody positive NMO as well as MOG antibody-associated disease is primarily driven by a pathogenic B cell activation in the periphery resulting in the generation of antibody-producing plasma cells, again in the first place in the periphery. In contrast, in MS, B cells probably exert their pathogenic properties both in the periphery as well as within the chronically inflamed CNS itself, but most probably independent of CNS-specific peripheral antibodies. After activation, B cells migrate through blood or lymph vessels into peripheral lymphoid organs, where they undergo full activation and maturation. Currently available immune-modulating MS therapies are very efficient in targeting these peripheral immune cells, but have only little or no access to the CNS-compartmentalized cells (87, 88). New concepts though suggest that two, probably independent, inflammatory processes drive CNS injury in MS, and potentially involve B cells: on the one hand, *de novo* infiltration of immune cells from the periphery into the CNS that correspond with focal inflammation, MRI-detectable lesions, and relapses. On the other hand, chronic progression supposedly driven by CNS-intrinsic inflammation that is promoted by CNS-resident immune cells in conjunction with CNS-trapped leukocytes (89). The first mechanism is premised on abnormally activated immune cells that migrate from lymphatic tissue, the location of their priming, across the blood-brain barrier into the CNS. There, these leukocytes are assumed to reactivate and contribute to the injury of axons and glial cells (90–92) forming focal lesions. These lesions are typically located perivascular and contain T cells, monocytes, B, and plasma cells (93). Since anti-CD20-mediated B cell depletion is highly efficient in preventing the formation of such focal CNS lesions, its assumed therapeutic efficiency is mainly based on the abrogation of the aforementioned cellular B cell properties in the periphery, and within the perivascular space (94). Chronic progression in contrast is characterized by gradual expansion of consisting lesions with myelin-containing macrophages at the lesion border, gray, and white matter atrophy as well as diffuse aberrant inflammation of the normal-appearing white matter (95, 96). In progressive MS, this cortical demyelination has been further associated with B cell-rich structures in the meninges (97, 98) as well as with plasma cell accumulation in experimental CNS inflammation (99). These findings point toward a gradual shift of disease-driving B cell functions from the periphery to the CNS with disease progression. Furthermore, they indicate that B cells may be involved—directly or indirectly—in cortical injury. An observation that is further corroborated by the findings of Lisak et al. (100) demonstrating that secretory products independent of antibodies and multiple cytokines produced by B cells of progressive MS patients are cytotoxic to oligodendrocytes and neurons (101). In line with these results, it is not surprising that even though anti-CD20 is highly efficient in limiting the formation of new CNS lesions, it does not entirely stop chronic progression. This further strengthens the assumption that chronic CNS injury in MS is not primarily caused by *de novo* infiltrating immune cells, but by an established CNS-compartmentalized inflammation, which results in a CNS-autonomous immune response over time.

CONCLUSION

Current research indicates that in MS, B cells contribute to the formation of relapses as well as to the progression of the disease independent of *de novo* CNS infiltration. In contrast, in NMO and anti-MOG antibody-associated demyelination, a peripherally generated CNS-targeting antibody response is suggested to be the main disease driver. Accordingly, these delineating disease entities may require MS-independent therapeutic strategies, a concept that is currently evolving. Thus, therapies targeting distinct aspects of NMO-relevant B cell functions such as plasma cell differentiation and complement fixation are currently under evaluation. First trials showed promising results for the treatment with tocilizumab, an therapeutic antibodies against IL-6 receptor (102, 103), and eculizumab, an complement component 5-specific antibody (104). Besides these pathogenic B cell properties, B cells, or B cells subsets likely exert a therapeutically desirable regulatory function in either disease, limiting tissue inflammation as well as pro-inflammatory activation of other immune cells. Accordingly, one of the prime challenges for the long-term targeting of B cells in MS and related demyelinating diseases will be to delineate and specifically target pathogenic B cell properties by novel strategic concepts, such as the selective depletion of differentiated B cells, interference with their activation or ablation of a disease-driving antibody response.

AUTHOR CONTRIBUTIONS

SH-K drafted the manuscript and prepared the figure. MW drafted, wrote, and finalized the manuscript.

ACKNOWLEDGMENTS

We acknowledge publication support by the German Research Foundation (Deutsche Forschungsgemeinschaft; DFG) and the Open Access Publication Funds of the Göttingen University. MW is supported by the DFG (WE 3547/5-1), as well as the ProFutura Program of the Universitätsmedizin Göttingen.

REFERENCES

1. Kinzel S, Weber MS. B cell-directed therapeutics in multiple sclerosis: rationale and clinical evidence. *CNS Drugs* (2016) 30:1137–48. doi: 10.1007/s40263-016-0396-6
2. Weber MS, Prod'homme T, Patarroyo JC, Molnarfi N, Karnezis T, Lehmann-Horn K, et al. B-cell activation influences T-cell polarization and outcome of anti-CD20 B-cell depletion in central nervous system autoimmunity. *Ann Neurol.* (2010) 68:369–83. doi: 10.1002/ana.22081
3. Weber MS, Hemmer B. Cooperation of B cells and T cells in the pathogenesis of multiple sclerosis. *Results Probl Cell Differ.* (2010) 51:115–26. doi: 10.1007/400_2009_21
4. Krishnamoorthy G, Lassmann H, Wekerle H, Holz A. Spontaneous opticospinal encephalomyelitis in a double-transgenic mouse model of autoimmune T cell/B cell cooperation. *J Clin Invest.* (2006) 116:2385–92. doi: 10.1172/JCI28330
5. Pollinger B, Krishnamoorthy G, Berer K, Lassmann H, Bosl MR, Dunn R, et al. Spontaneous relapsing-remitting EAE in the SJL/J mouse: MOG-reactive transgenic T cells recruit endogenous MOG-specific B cells. *J Exp Med.* (2009) 206:1303–16. doi: 10.1084/jem.20090299
6. Molnarfi N, Schulze-Topphoff U, Weber MS, Patarroyo JC, Prod'homme T, Varrin-Doyer M, et al. MHC class II-dependent B cell APC function is required for induction of CNS autoimmunity independent of myelin-specific antibodies. *J Exp Med.* (2013) 210:2921–37. doi: 10.1084/jem.20130699
7. Grewal IS, Flavell RA. The role of CD40 ligand in costimulation and T-cell activation. *Immunol Rev.* (1996) 153:85–106. doi: 10.1111/j.1600-065X.1996.tb00921.x
8. Martin S, Agarwal R, Murugaiyan G, Saha B. CD40 expression levels modulate regulatory T cells in Leishmania donovani infection. *J Immunol.* (2010) 185:551–9. doi: 10.4049/jimmunol.0902206
9. Genc K, Dona DL, Reder AT. Increased CD80(+) B cells in active multiple sclerosis and reversal by interferon beta-1b therapy. *J Clin Invest.* (1997) 99:2664–71. doi: 10.1172/JCI119455
10. Mathias A, Perriard G, Canales M, Soneson C, Delorenzi M, Schluep M, et al. Increased *ex vivo* antigen presentation profile of B cells in multiple sclerosis. *Mult Scler.* (2016) 23:802–9. doi: 10.1177/1352458516664210
11. Duddy M, Niino M, Adatia F, Hebert S, Freedman M, Atkins H, et al. Distinct effector cytokine profiles of memory and naive human B cell subsets and implication in multiple sclerosis. *J Immunol.* (2007) 178:6092–9. doi: 10.4049/jimmunol.178.10.6092
12. Harp C, Lee J, Lambracht-Washington D, Cameron E, Olsen G, Frohman E, et al. Cerebrospinal fluid B cells from multiple sclerosis patients are subject to normal germinal center selection. *J Neuroimmunol.* (2007) 183:189–99. doi: 10.1016/j.jneuroim.2006.10.020
13. Harp CT, Ireland S, Davis LS, Remington G, Cassidy B, Cravens PD, et al. Memory B cells from a subset of treatment-naive relapsing-remitting multiple sclerosis patients elicit CD4(+) T-cell proliferation and IFN-gamma production in response to myelin basic protein and myelin oligodendrocyte glycoprotein. *Eur J Immunol.* (2010) 40:2942–56. doi: 10.1002/eji.201040516
14. Bettelli E, Carrier Y, Gao W, Korn T, Strom TB, Oukka M, et al. Reciprocal developmental pathways for the generation of pathogenic effector TH17 and regulatory T cells. *Nature* (2006) 441:235–8. doi: 10.1038/nature04753
15. Korn T, Mitsdoerffer M, Croxford AL, Awasthi A, Dardalhon VA, Galileos G, et al. IL-6 controls Th17 immunity *in vivo* by inhibiting the conversion of conventional T cells into Foxp3+ regulatory T cells. *Proc Natl Acad Sci USA.* (2008) 105:18460–5. doi: 10.1073/pnas.0809850105
16. Barr TA, Shen P, Brown S, Lampropoulou V, Roch T, Lawrie S, et al. B cell depletion therapy ameliorates autoimmune disease through ablation of IL-6-producing B cells. *J Exp Med.* (2012) 209:1001–10. doi: 10.1084/jem.20111675
17. Miyazaki Y, Li R, Rezk A, Misirliyan H, Moore C, Farooqi N, et al. A novel MicroRNA-132-Surtuin-1 axis underlies aberrant B-cell cytokine regulation in patients with relapsing-remitting multiple sclerosis. *PLoS ONE* (2014) 9:e105421. doi: 10.1371/journal.pone.0105421
18. Li R, Rezk A, Miyazaki Y, Hilgenberg E, Touil H, Shen P, et al. Proinflammatory GM-CSF-producing B cells in multiple sclerosis and B cell depletion therapy. *Sci Transl Med.* (2015) 7:310ra166. doi: 10.1126/scitranslmed.aab4176
19. Lehmann-Horn K, Schleich E, Hertzenberg D, Hapfelmeier A, Kumpfel T, von Bubnoff N, et al. Anti-CD20 B-cell depletion enhances monocyte reactivity in neuroimmunological disorders. *J Neuroinflammation* (2011) 8:146. doi: 10.1186/1742-2094-8-146
20. Matsushita T, Yanaba K, Bouaziz J-D, Fujimoto M, Tedder TF. Regulatory B cells inhibit EAE initiation in mice while other B cells promote disease progression. *J Clin Invest.* (2008) 118:3420–30. doi: 10.1172/JCI36030
21. Fillatreau S, Sweenie CH, Mcgeachy MJ, Gray D, Anderton SM. B cells regulate autoimmunity by provision of IL-10. *Nat Immunol.* (2002) 3:944–50. doi: 10.1038/ni833
22. Shen P, Roch T, Lampropoulou V, O'connor RA, Stervbo U, Hilgenberg E, et al. IL-35-producing B cells are critical regulators of immunity during autoimmune and infectious diseases. *Nature* (2014) 507:366–370. doi: 10.1038/nature12979
23. Bjarnadottir K, Benkhoucha M, Merkler D, Weber MS, Payne NL, Bernard CC, et al. B cell-derived transforming growth factor-beta1 expression limits the induction phase of autoimmune neuroinflammation. *Sci Rep.* (2016) 6:34594. doi: 10.1038/srep34594
24. Iwata Y, Matsushita T, Horikawa M, Dilillo DJ, Yanaba K, Venturi GM, et al. Characterization of a rare IL-10-competent B-cell subset in humans that parallels mouse regulatory B10 cells. *Blood* (2011) 117:530–41. doi: 10.1182/blood-2010-07-294249
25. Lehmann-Horn K, Kronsbein HC, Weber MS. Targeting B cells in the treatment of multiple sclerosis: recent advances and remaining challenges. *Ther Adv Neurol Disord.* (2013) 6:161–73. doi: 10.1177/17562856124 74333
26. Lehmann-Horn K, Kinzel S, Weber M. Deciphering the role of B cells in multiple sclerosis—towards specific targeting of pathogenic function. *Int J Mol Sci.* (2017) 18:2048. doi: 10.3390/ijms18102048
27. Crofford LJ, Nyhoff LE, Sheehan JH, Kendall PL. The role of Bruton's tyrosine kinase in autoimmunity and implications for therapy. *Exp Rev Clin Immunol.* (2016) 12:763–73. doi: 10.1586/1744666X.2016.1152888
28. Menzfeld C, John M, Van Rossum D, Regen T, Scheffel J, Janova H, et al. Tyrphostin AG126 exerts neuroprotection in CNS inflammation by a dual mechanism. *Glia* (2015) 63:1083–99. doi: 10.1002/glia.22803
29. Satterthwaite AB, Cheroutre H, Khan WN, Sideras P, Witte ON. Btk dosage determines sensitivity to B cell antigen receptor cross-linking. *Proc Natl Acad Sci USA.* (1997) 94:13152–7. doi: 10.1073/pnas.94.24.13152
30. Whyburn LR, Halcomb KE, Contreras CM, Lowell CA, Witte ON, Satterthwaite AB. Reduced dosage of Bruton's Tyrosine Kinase Uncouples B Cell hyperresponsiveness from autoimmunity in *lyn*$^{-/-}$ mice. *J Immunol.* (2003) 171:1850–8. doi: 10.4049/jimmunol.171.4.1850
31. Kil LP, De Bruijn MJW, Van Nimwegen M, Corneth OBJ, Van Hamburg JP, Dingjan GM, et al. Btk levels set the threshold for B-cell activation and negative selection of autoreactive B cells in mice. *Blood* (2012) 119:3744–56. doi: 10.1182/blood-2011-12-397919
32. Honigberg LA, Smith AM, Sirisawad M, Verner E, Loury D, Chang B, et al. The Bruton tyrosine kinase inhibitor PCI-32765 blocks B-cell activation and is efficacious in models of autoimmune disease and B-cell malignancy. *Proc Natl Acad Sci.* (2010) 107:13075–80. doi: 10.1073/pnas.10045 94107

33. Kabat EA and Freedman DA. A study of the crystalline albumin, gamma globulin and total protein in the cerebrospinal fluid of 100 cases of multiple sclerosis and in other diseases. *Am J Med Sci.* (1950) 219:55–64. doi: 10.1097/00000441-195001000-00009
34. Link H, Huang Y-M. Oligoclonal bands in multiple sclerosis cerebrospinal fluid: an update on methodology and clinical usefulness. *J Neuroimmunol.* (2006) 180:17–28. doi: 10.1016/j.jneuroim.2006.07.006
35. Siritho S, Freedman MS. The prognostic significance of cerebrospinal fluid in multiple sclerosis. *J Neurolog Sci.* (2009) 279:21–5. doi: 10.1016/j.jns.2008.12.029
36. Obermeier B, Mentele R, Malotka J, Kellermann J, Kumpfel T, Wekerle H, et al. Matching of oligoclonal immunoglobulin transcriptomes and proteomes of cerebrospinal fluid in multiple sclerosis. *Nat Med.* (2008) 14:688–93. doi: 10.1038/nm1714
37. Qin Y, Duquette P, Zhang Y, Talbot P, Poole R, Antel J. Clonal expansion and somatic hypermutation of V(H) genes of B cells from cerebrospinal fluid in multiple sclerosis. *J Clin Invest.* (1998) 102:1045–50. doi: 10.1172/JCI3568
38. Beltrán E, Obermeier B, Moser M, Coret F, Simó-Castelló M, Boscá I, et al. Intrathecal somatic hypermutation of IgM in multiple sclerosis and neuroinflammation. *Brain* (2014) 137:2703–14. doi: 10.1093/brain/awu205
39. Von Büdingen HC, Kuo TC, Sirota M, Van Belle CJ, Apeltsin L, Glanville J, et al. B cell exchange across the blood-brain barrier in multiple sclerosis. *J Clin Invest.* (2012) 122:4533–43. doi: 10.1172/JCI63842
40. Bankoti J, Apeltsin L, Hauser SL, Allen S, Albertolle ME, Witkowska HE, et al. In multiple sclerosis, oligoclonal bands connect to peripheral B-cell responses. *Ann Neurol.* (2014) 75:266–76. doi: 10.1002/ana.24088
41. Palanichamy A, Apeltsin L, Kuo TC, Sirota M, Wang S, Pitts SJ, et al. Immunoglobulin class-switched B cells form an active immune axis between CNS and periphery in multiple sclerosis. *Sci Transl Med.* (2014) 6:248ra106. doi: 10.1126/scitranslmed.3008930
42. Stern JNH, Yaari G, Vander Heiden JA, Church G, Donahue WF, Hintzen RQ, et al. B cells populating the multiple sclerosis brain mature in the draining cervical lymph nodes. *Sci Transl Med.* (2014) 6:248ra107. doi: 10.1126/scitranslmed.3008879
43. Genain CP, Cannella B, Hauser SL, Raine CS. Identification of autoantibodies associated with myelin damage in multiple sclerosis. *Nat Med.* (1999) 5:170–5. doi: 10.1038/5532
44. Elliott C, Lindner M, Arthur A, Brennan K, Jarius S, Hussey J, et al. Functional identification of pathogenic autoantibody responses in patients with multiple sclerosis. *Brain* (2012) 135:1819–33. doi: 10.1093/brain/aws105
45. Blauth K, Soltys J, Matschulat A, Reiter CR, Ritchie A, Baird NL, et al. Antibodies produced by clonally expanded plasma cells in multiple sclerosis cerebrospinal fluid cause demyelination of spinal cord explants. *Acta Neuropathol.* (2015) 130:765–81. doi: 10.1007/s00401-015-1500-6
46. Weber MS, Hemmer B, Cepok S. The role of antibodies in multiple sclerosis. *Biochim Biophys Acta* (2011) 1812:239–45. doi: 10.1016/j.bbadis.2010.06.009
47. Reiber H, Ungefehr S, Jacobi C. The intrathecal, polyspecific and oligoclonal immune response in multiple sclerosis. *Mult Scler.* (1998) 4:111–7. doi: 10.1177/135245859800400304
48. Warren KG, Catz I. Relative frequency of autoantibodies to myelin basic protein and proteolipid protein in optic neuritis and multiple sclerosis cerebrospinal fluid. *J Neurol Sci.* (1994) 121:66–73. doi: 10.1016/0022-510X(94)90158-9
49. Brennan KM, Galban-Horcajo F, Rinaldi S, O'leary CP, Goodyear CS, Kalna G, et al. Lipid arrays identify myelin-derived lipids and lipid complexes as prominent targets for oligoclonal band antibodies in multiple sclerosis. *J Neuroimmunol.* (2011) 238:87–95. doi: 10.1016/j.jneuroim.2011.08.002
50. Derfuss T, Parikh K, Velhin S, Braun M, Mathey E, Krumbholz M, et al. Contactin-2/TAG-1-directed autoimmunity is identified in multiple sclerosis patients and mediates gray matter pathology in animals. *Proc Natl Acad Sci USA.* (2009) 106:8302–7. doi: 10.1073/pnas.0901496106
51. Srivastava R, Aslam M, Kalluri SR, Schirmer L, Buck D, Tackenberg B, et al. Potassium channel KIR4.1 as an immune target in multiple sclerosis. *N Engl J Med.* (2012) 367:115–23. doi: 10.1056/NEJMoa1110740
52. Ketelslegers IA, Van Pelt DE, Bryde S, Neuteboom RF, Catsman-Berrevoets CE, Hamann D, et al. Anti-MOG antibodies plead against MS diagnosis in an acquired demyelinating syndromes cohort. *Mult Scler J.* (2015) 21:1513–20. doi: 10.1177/1352458514566666
53. Pröbstel A-K, Kuhle J, Lecourt A-C, Vock I, Sanderson NSR, Kappos L, et al. Multiple sclerosis and antibodies against KIR4.1. *N Engl J Med.* (2016) 374:1496–8. doi: 10.1056/NEJMc1507131
54. Spadaro M, Gerdes LA, Krumbholz M, Ertl-Wagner B, Thaler FS, Schuh E, et al. Autoantibodies to MOG in a distinct subgroup of adult multiple sclerosis. *Neurol Neuroimmunol Neuroinflamm.* (2016) 3:e257. doi: 10.1212/NXI.0000000000000257
55. Lennon VA, Kryzer TJ, Pittock SJ, Verkman AS, Hinson SR. IgG marker of optic-spinal multiple sclerosis binds to the aquaporin-4 water channel. *J Exp Med.* (2005) 202:473–7. doi: 10.1084/jem.20050304
56. Misu T, Fujihara K, Kakita A, Konno H, Nakamura M, Watanabe S, et al. Loss of aquaporin 4 in lesions of neuromyelitis optica: distinction from multiple sclerosis. *Brain* (2007) 130:1224–34. doi: 10.1093/brain/awm047
57. Agre P, Nielsen S. The aquaporin family of water channels in kidney. *Nephrologie* (1996) 17:409–15.
58. Nagelhus EA, Ottersen OP. Physiological roles of aquaporin-4 in brain. *Physiol Rev.* (2013) 93:1543–62. doi: 10.1152/physrev.00011.2013
59. Frigeri A, Gropper MA, Umenishi F, Kawashima M, Brown D, Verkman AS. Localization of MIWC and GLIP water channel homologs in neuromuscular, epithelial and glandular tissues. *J Cell Sci.* (1995) 108:2993–3002.
60. Nielsen S, Arnulf Nagelhus E, Amiry-Moghaddam M, Bourque C, Agre P, Petter Ottersen O. Specialized membrane domains for water transport in glial cells: high-resolution immunogold cytochemistry of aquaporin-4 in rat brain. *J Neurosci.* (1997) 17:171–80. doi: 10.1523/JNEUROSCI.17-01-00171.1997
61. Matiello M, Schaefer-Klein J, Sun D, Weinshenker BG. Aquaporin 4 expression and tissue susceptibility to neuromyelitis optica. *JAMA Neurol.* (2013) 70:1118–25. doi: 10.1001/jamaneurol.2013.3124
62. Marignier R, Nicolle A, Watrin C, Touret M, Cavagna S, Varrin-Doyer M, et al. Oligodendrocytes are damaged by neuromyelitis optica immunoglobulin G via astrocyte injury. *Brain* (2010) 133:2578–91. doi: 10.1093/brain/awq177
63. Lucchinetti CF, Guo Y, Popescu BF, Fujihara K, Itoyama Y, Misu T. The pathology of an autoimmune astrocytopathy: lessons learned from neuromyelitis optica. *Brain Pathol.* (2014) 24:83–97. doi: 10.1111/bpa.12099
64. Lucchinetti CF, Mandler RN, Mcgavern D, Bruck W, Gleich G, Ransohoff RM, et al. A role for humoral mechanisms in the pathogenesis of Devic's neuromyelitis optica. *Brain* (2002) 125:1450–61. doi: 10.1093/brain/awf151
65. Wrzos C, Winkler A, Metz I, Kayser DM, Thal DR, Wegner C, et al. Early loss of oligodendrocytes in human and experimental neuromyelitis optica lesions. *Acta Neuropathol.* (2014) 127:523–38. doi: 10.1007/s00401-013-1220-8
66. Levy M, Wildemann B, Jarius S, Orellano B, Sasidharan S, Weber MS, et al. Immunopathogenesis of neuromyelitis optica. *Adv Immunol.* (2014) 121:213–42. doi: 10.1016/B978-0-12-800100-4.00006-4
67. Takahashi T, Fujihara K, Nakashima I, Misu T, Miyazawa I, Nakamura M, et al. Anti-aquaporin-4 antibody is involved in the pathogenesis of NMO: a study on antibody titre. *Brain* (2007) 130:1235–43. doi: 10.1093/brain/awm062
68. Jarius S, Franciotta D, Paul F, Ruprecht K, Bergamaschi R, Rommer PS, et al. Cerebrospinal fluid antibodies to aquaporin-4 in neuromyelitis optica and related disorders: frequency, origin, and diagnostic relevance. *J Neuroinflamm.* (2010) 7:52. doi: 10.1186/1742-2094-7-52
69. Kowarik MC, Astling D, Gasperi C, Wemlinger S, Schumann H, Dzieciatkowska M, et al. CNS Aquaporin-4-specific B cells connect with multiple B-cell compartments in neuromyelitis optica spectrum disorder. *Ann Clin Transl Neurol.* (2017) 4:369–80. doi: 10.1002/acn3.418
70. Kitley J, Woodhall M, Waters P, Leite MI, Devenney E, Craig J, et al. Myelin-oligodendrocyte glycoprotein antibodies in adults with a neuromyelitis optica phenotype. *Neurology* (2012) 79:1273–7. doi: 10.1212/WNL.0b013e31826aac4e
71. Probstel AK, Rudolf G, Dornmair K, Collongues N, Chanson JB, Sanderson NS, et al. Anti-MOG antibodies are present in a subgroup of patients with a neuromyelitis optica phenotype. *J Neuroinflamm.* (2015) 12:46. doi: 10.1186/s12974-015-0256-1

72. Sepulveda M, Armangue T, Martinez-Hernandez E, Arrambide G, Sola-Valls N, Sabater L, et al. Clinical spectrum associated with MOG autoimmunity in adults: significance of sharing rodent MOG epitopes. *J Neurol.* (2016) 263:1349–60. doi: 10.1007/s00415-016-8147-7
73. Varrin-Doyer M, Shetty A, Spencer CM, Schulze-Topphoff U, Weber MS, Bernard CC, et al. MOG transmembrane and cytoplasmic domains contain highly stimulatory T-cell epitopes in MS. *Neurol Neuroimmunol Neuroinflamm.* (2014) 1:e20. doi: 10.1212/NXI.0000000000000020
74. Bruno R, Sabater L, Sospedra M, Ferrer-Francesch X, Escudero D, Martinez-Caceres E, et al. Multiple sclerosis candidate autoantigens except myelin oligodendrocyte glycoprotein are transcribed in human thymus. *Eur J Immunol.* (2002) 32:2737–47. doi: 10.1002/1521-4141(2002010)32:10<2737::AID-IMMU2737>3.0.CO;2-0
75. Shetty A, Gupta SG, Varrin-Doyer M, Weber MS, Prod'homme T, Molnarfi N, et al. Immunodominant T-cell epitopes of MOG reside in its transmembrane and cytoplasmic domains in EAE. *Neurol Neuroimmunol Neuroinflamm.* (2014) 1:e22. doi: 10.1212/NXI.0000000000000022
76. Ikeda K, Kiyota N, Kuroda H, Sato DK, Nishiyama S, Takahashi T, et al. Severe demyelination but no astrocytopathy in clinically definite neuromyelitis optica with anti-myelin-oligodendrocyte glycoprotein antibody. *Mult Scler.* (2015) 21:656–9. doi: 10.1177/1352458514551455
77. Kaneko K, Sato DK, Nakashima I, Nishiyama S, Tanaka S, Marignier R, et al. Myelin injury without astrocytopathy in neuroinflammatory disorders with MOG antibodies. *J Neurol Neurosurg Psychiatry* (2016) 87:1257–9. doi: 10.1136/jnnp-2015-312676
78. Wang JJ, Jaunmuktane Z, Mummery C, Brandner S, Leary S, Trip SA. Inflammatory demyelination without astrocyte loss in MOG antibody-positive NMOSD. *Neurology* (2016) 87:229–31. doi: 10.1212/WNL.0000000000002844
79. Jurynczyk M, Messina S, Woodhall MR, Raza N, Everett R, Roca-Fernandez A, et al. Clinical presentation and prognosis in MOG-antibody disease: a UK study. *Brain* (2017) 140:3128–38. doi: 10.1093/brain/awx276
80. Jarius S, Ruprecht K, Kleiter I, Borisow N, Asgari N, Pitarokoili K, et al. MOG-IgG in NMO and related disorders: a multicenter study of 50 patients. Part 1: frequency, syndrome specificity, influence of disease activity, long-term course, association with AQP4-IgG, and origin. *J Neuroinflamm.* (2016) 13:279. doi: 10.1186/s12974-016-0717-1
81. Weber MS, Derfuss T, Bruck W. Anti-myelin oligodendrocyte glycoprotein antibody-associated central nervous system demyelination-a novel disease entity? *JAMA Neurol.* (2018) 75:909–10. doi: 10.1001/jamaneurol.2018.1055
82. Flach AC, Litke T, Strauss J, Haberl M, Gomez CC, Reindl M, et al. Autoantibody-boosted T-cell reactivation in the target organ triggers manifestation of autoimmune CNS disease. *Proc Natl Acad Sci USA.* (2016) 113:3323–8. doi: 10.1073/pnas.1519608113
83. Kinzel S, Lehmann-Horn K, Torke S, Hausler D, Winkler A, Stadelmann C, et al. Myelin-reactive antibodies initiate T cell-mediated CNS autoimmune disease by opsonization of endogenous antigen. *Acta Neuropathol.* (2016) 132:43–58. doi: 10.1007/s00401-016-1559-8
84. Louveau A, Smirnov I, Keyes TJ, Eccles JD, Rouhani SJ, Peske JD, et al. Structural and functional features of central nervous system lymphatic vessels. *Nature* (2015) 523:337–41. doi: 10.1038/nature14432
85. De Vos AF, Van Meurs M, Brok HP, Boven LA, Hintzen RQ, Van Der Valk P, et al. Transfer of central nervous system autoantigens and presentation in secondary lymphoid organs. *J Immunol.* (2002) 169:5415–23. doi: 10.4049/jimmunol.169.10.5415
86. Fabriek BO, Zwemmer JN, Teunissen CE, Dijkstra CD, Polman CH, Laman JD, et al. *In vivo* detection of myelin proteins in cervical lymph nodes of MS patients using ultrasound-guided fine-needle aspiration cytology. *J Neuroimmunol.* (2005) 161:190–4. doi: 10.1016/j.jneuroim.2004.12.018
87. Weber MS, Menge T, Lehmann-Horn K, Kronsbein HC, Zettl U, Sellner J, et al. Current treatment strategies for multiple sclerosis - efficacy versus neurological adverse effects. *Curr Pharm Des.* (2012) 18:209–19. doi: 10.2174/138161212799040501
88. Bruck W, Gold R, Lund BT, Oreja-Guevara C, Prat A, Spencer CM, et al. Therapeutic decisions in multiple sclerosis: moving beyond efficacy. *JAMA Neurol.* (2013) 70:1315–24. doi: 10.1001/jamaneurol.2013.3510
89. Kowarik MC, Cepok S, Sellner J, Grummel V, Weber MS, Korn T, et al. CXCL13 is the major determinant for B cell recruitment to the CSF during neuroinflammation. *J Neuroinflamm.* (2012) 9:93. doi: 10.1186/1742-2094-9-93
90. Kebir H, Kreymborg K, Ifergan I, Dodelet-Devillers A, Cayrol R, Bernard M, et al. Human TH17 lymphocytes promote blood-brain barrier disruption and central nervous system inflammation. *Nat Med.* (2007) 13:1173–5. doi: 10.1038/nm1651
91. Friese MA, Fugger L. Pathogenic CD8(+) T cells in multiple sclerosis. *Ann Neurol.* (2009) 66:132–41. doi: 10.1002/ana.21744
92. Kasper LH, Shoemaker J. Multiple sclerosis immunology: the healthy immune system vs the MS immune system. *Neurology* (2010) 74 (Suppl. 1):S2–8. doi: 10.1212/WNL.0b013e3181c97c8f
93. Prineas JW, Wright RG. Macrophages, lymphocytes, and plasma cells in the perivascular compartment in chronic multiple sclerosis. *Lab Invest.* (1978) 38:409–21.
94. Martin Mdel P, Cravens PD, Winger R, Kieseier BC, Cepok S, Eagar TN, et al. Depletion of B lymphocytes from cerebral perivascular spaces by rituximab. *Arch Neurol.* (2009) 66:1016–20. doi: 10.1001/archneurol.2009.157
95. Lassmann H. New concepts on progressive multiple sclerosis. *Curr Neurol Neurosci Rep.* (2007) 7:239–44. doi: 10.1007/s11910-007-0036-0
96. Nylander A, Hafler DA. Multiple sclerosis. *J Clin Invest.* (2012) 122:1180–8. doi: 10.1172/JCI58649
97. Serafini B, Rosicarelli B, Magliozzi R, Stigliano E, Aloisi F. Detection of ectopic B-cell follicles with germinal centers in the meninges of patients with secondary progressive multiple sclerosis. *Brain Pathol.* (2004) 14:164–74. doi: 10.1111/j.1750-3639.2004.tb00049.x
98. Magliozzi R, Howell O, Vora A, Serafini B, Nicholas R, Puopolo M, et al. Meningeal B-cell follicles in secondary progressive multiple sclerosis associate with early onset of disease and severe cortical pathology. *Brain* (2007) 130:1089–104. doi: 10.1093/brain/awm038
99. Kramann N, Neid K, Menken L, Schlumbohm C, Stadelmann C, Fuchs E, et al. Increased Meningeal T and plasma cell infiltration is associated with early subpial cortical demyelination in common marmosets with experimental autoimmune encephalomyelitis. *Brain Pathol.* (2015) 25:276–86. doi: 10.1111/bpa.12180
100. Lisak RP, Benjamins JA, Nedelkoska L, Barger JL, Ragheb S, Fan B, et al. Secretory products of multiple sclerosis B cells are cytotoxic to oligodendroglia *in vitro*. *J Neuroimmunol.* (2012) 246:85–95. doi: 10.1016/j.jneuroim.2012.02.015
101. Lisak RP, Nedelkoska L, Benjamins JA, Schalk D, Bealmear B, Touil H, et al. B cells from patients with multiple sclerosis induce cell death via apoptosis in neurons *in vitro*. *J Neuroimmunol.* (2017) 309:88–99. doi: 10.1016/j.jneuroim.2017.05.004
102. Araki M, Matsuoka T, Miyamoto K, Kusunoki S, Okamoto T, Murata M, et al. Efficacy of the anti–IL-6 receptor antibody tocilizumab in neuromyelitis optica. A pilot study. *Neurology* (2014) 82:1302–6. doi: 10.1212/WNL.0000000000000317
103. Ringelstein M, Ayzenberg I, Harmel J, Lauenstein AS, Lensch E, Stögbauer F, et al. Long-term therapy with interleukin 6 receptor blockade in highly active neuromyelitis optica spectrum disorder. *JAMA Neurol.* (2015) 72:756–63. doi: 10.1001/jamaneurol.2015.0533
104. Pittock SJ, Lennon VA, Mckeon A, Mandrekar J, Weinshenker BG, Lucchinetti CF, et al. Eculizumab in AQP4-IgG-positive relapsing neuromyelitis optica spectrum disorders: an open-label pilot study. *Lancet Neurol.* (2013) 12:554–62. doi: 10.1016/S1474-4422(13)70076-0

2

The Cerebrospinal Fluid in Multiple Sclerosis

Florian Deisenhammer[1], Henrik Zetterberg[2,3,4,5], Brit Fitzner[6] and Uwe K. Zettl[6]*

[1] Department of Neurology, Innsbruck Medical University, Innsbruck, Austria, [2] Department of Psychiatry and Neurochemistry, Institute of Neuroscience and Physiology, The Sahlgrenska Academy at the University of Gothenburg, Mölndal, Sweden, [3] Clinical Neurochemistry Laboratory, Sahlgrenska University Hospital, Mölndal, Sweden, [4] Department of Neurodegenerative Disease, UCL Institute of Neurology, London, United Kingdom, [5] The Fluid Biomarker Laboratory, UK Dementia Research Institute at UCL, London, United Kingdom, [6] Division of Neuroimmunology, Department of Neurology, University Medicine Rostock, Rostock, Germany

***Correspondence:**
Florian Deisenhammer
florian.deisenhammer@tirol-kliniken.at

Investigation of cerebrospinal fluid (CSF) in the diagnostic work-up in suspected multiple sclerosis (MS) patients has regained attention in the latest version of the diagnostic criteria due to its good diagnostic accuracy and increasing issues with misdiagnosis of MS based on over interpretation of neuroimaging results. The hallmark of MS-specific changes in CSF is the detection of oligoclonal bands (OCB) which occur in the vast majority of MS patients. Lack of OCB has a very high negative predictive value indicating a red flag during the diagnostic work-up, and alternative diagnoses should be considered in such patients. Additional molecules of CSF can help to support the diagnosis of MS, improve the differential diagnosis of MS subtypes and predict the course of the disease, thus selecting the optimal therapy for each patient.

Keywords: CSF (cerebrospinal fluid), biomarker, multiple sclerosis, oligoclonal band (OCB), neurofilament light (NfL)

INTRODUCTION

Oligoclonal bands (OCB) of the cerebrospinal fluid (CSF) have been important in the diagnosis of multiple sclerosis (MS) for many years. The further search for biomarkers is of great importance in order to improve the diagnosis and therapy of MS. This review is divided into 2 parts. The first part focuses on OCB as diagnostic biomarker for MS and briefly describes other diagnostic markers such as aquaporin4 (AQP4) and biomarkers that are about to enter clinical routine, such as anti-myelin oligodendrocyte glycoprotein (MOG). The second part is about CSF molecules, which have been described in research as potential biomarkers.

PART I: THE CLINICAL LABORATORY

Cerebrospinal Fluid—General Considerations

Whenever investigations are required either to make or rule out a particular disease, it is of utmost importance to know what one would normally expect from such an investigation, i.e., to have access to normal or reference values. This goes of course also for clinical chemistry tests performed in CSF. As a prerequisite for making reference values global and assay-independent, it is important to standardize the field through the certification of reference methods and materials that can be used as external calibrators for assay manufacturers. It is also important to establish external quality control programmes to make sure laboratories are both accurate and precise. Internal stability of the measurements also has to be monitored using internal control samples each time a test is performed.

It is surprising how little progress has been made in the field of reference values for CSF analytes since the first systematic assessment of CSF normal values by Meritt and Fremont-Smith (1). For one of the most basic CSF variables, i.e., total protein and albumin, normal values based on modern quality standards have been evaluated and published only recently (2). Most labs adopt historical reference values without validating their own (3). Even if normal values have been established in some labs the methods of evaluation suffer from methodological shortcomings, such as selection bias, poor definition of normal cohorts, and statistical errors (2). Because upper reference limits for total CSF protein are mostly too low it has been estimated that approximately in 15% of normal CSFs total protein values are falsely reported as pathologically elevated. Similar issues have been found with CSF glucose measurements and formulas for intrathecal immunoglobulin synthesis (4, 5). Glucose measurements must be done in CSF and serum simultaneously and a ratio needs to be calculated. The glucose ratio cut-off values depend on serum glucose levels because the transporter systems across the blood-brain-barrier (BBB) have limited capacities. This fact is often not considered by CSF labs. For intrathecal synthesis of immunoglobulins it is well-known that the widespread Reiber-formula overestimates particularly intrathecal IgM and IgA synthesis rates (4, 6).

How Is All This Related to the Diagnosis of MS?

Because the etiology and specific pathogenesis of MS are unknown, there is no specific test, be it lab-based or otherwise, available. In diseases with a known cause, e.g., infections, a specific test detecting the infectious agent or antibodies against it is most frequently available. Even in entities in which the cause is not fully elucidated but the pathomechanism is evident, such as autoimmune encephalitides, a specific test detecting the auto-antibody can be used to make the diagnosis (7). In MS there is no such specific test available which is why one needs to rely on "circumstantial evidence." The diagnosis is based on typical, yet not limited to, clinical findings, magnetic resonance imaging (MRI), and CSF as well as other investigations (8). Doctors are well-advised to use all these tools in order to optimize the diagnostic accuracy.

In the past two decades the diagnostic criteria for MS have been updated 4 times (8–11). Starting with the revision in 2001 (9) CSF was less and less required to confirm the diagnosis in the subsequent updates until 2010 (11). As some authors suspected (12), ignorance of diagnostic tools might have led to insufficient diagnostic performance, in that the rate of MS misdiagnosis increased, even though there is no formal proof that this phenomenon occurred due to the decrease in CSF examinations (13). Mostly, misdiagnosis was due to overinterpretation and misinterpretation of MRI findings (13). Moreover, the true diagnoses were most often migraine, fibromyalgia, unspecific symptoms, or psychogenic disorders (14). In these diagnoses, CSF findings are usually normal, including markers of intrathecal immune-activation such as quantitative elevation of immunoglobulins (e.g., IgG-index) or detection of OCB. One must keep in mind that the negative predictive value of OCB in neurological patients who had undergone LP was 90% (15), and even in patients with clinically isolated syndromes (CIS—a clinical syndrome highly suspicious of a first manifestation of MS) the negative predictive value of OCB was 88% (16). So, the lack of OCB in CSF must be considered a red flag in the differential diagnostic work-up. In this context, it should be remembered that the first reported case of natalizumab-associated progressive multifocal leukoencephalopathy occurred in a very likely misdiagnosed patient, who had no detectable OCB in CSF in two consecutive occasions (17). In fact, the vast majority of misdiagnosed patients get actually treated with MS drugs (14).

Oligoclonal Bands in CSF—How Likely Is It MS?

It is well-known that OCB in CSF are not exclusively found in MS. OCB are thought to indicate chronic immune-activation in the CNS and therefore, can be found in a variety of chronic inflammatory diseases. The positive predictive value (PPV) of OCB for MS depends on the control or reference population—an inherent issue with PPV—and on the integration of other CSF findings, such as cell counts or albumin/protein concentrations. E.g., in neuroborreliosis, OCB are frequently encountered, in contrast to MS, however, total protein concentration and CSF cell counts are substantially higher (18). Several authors found OCB in CSF highly sensitive and specific for MS (19), which is likely due to the fact that other diseases with OCB in CSF occur relatively seldom. However, when inflammatory diseases are particularly considered, the specificity of OCB for MS drops substantially from 94 to 61%, as shown in a meta-analysis (20). This highlights again that the diagnostic tools for MS are not uni-dimensional.

Apart from MS, there is a long list of diagnoses with CSF OCBs reported: systemic lupus erythematosus, neurosyphilis, neurological paraneoplastic disorders, Behcet's disease neuroborreliosis, aseptic meningitis, neurosarcoidosis, HIV infection, cerebral tumors including lymphomas, Sjögren's syndrome, herpes encephalitis, Morvan syndrome, Anti-NMDA and other autoimmune encephalitis, neurotuberculosis, anticardiolipin syndrome, HTLV myelopathy, prion disease, schistosomiasis, stiff-person syndrome, cerebral cysticercosis, GBS, CNS vasculitis (20). One must be careful however, in our experience running a clinical CSF lab for decades, we rarely detected OCB in solid cerebral tumors, prion disease, or GBS for instance.

Abbreviations: AQP4, aquaporin 4; C1inh, Complement component 1-inhibitor; CAM, cell adhesion molecule; CDMS, clinical definite MS; CSF, cerebrospinal fluid; CHI3L, protein chitinase 3-like; CIS, clinically isolated syndrome; CXCL, chemokine (c-x-c motif) ligand; GFAP, glial fibrillary acidic protein; HC, healthy control; IL, interleukin; JCV, John Cunningham virus; MOG, myelin oligodendrocyte glycoprotein; MS, multiple sclerosis; Nf, neurofilament; NfH, Nf heavy; NfL, Nf light; NIND, non-inflammatory neurological disease; NMOSD, neuromyelitis optica spectrum disorders; OCB, oligoclonal bands; OCGB, oligoclonal immunoglobulin G bands; OCMB, oligoclonal immunoglobulin M bands; OIND, other inflammatory neurological disease; OND, other neurological disease; RRMS, relapsing-remitting MS; sCD, soluble cluster of differentiation; sICAM, soluble intercellular CAM; sVCAM, soluble vascular CAM.

Some Methodological Considerations

As outlined above, a proper assessment of normal and reference values should be done in each CSF lab rather than adopting such values from the literature. Also, validation in case of in-house developed assays must be done, or at least verification in case of commercially available, externally validated tests (21). One of the key CSF tests in query MS including differentials is the method of isoelectric focusing (IEF) (22). This method has been developed in the 70ies and has since then undergone several refinements. Today, IEF followed by IgG specific immunoblot is the recommended standard for detection of OCB (19). These guidelines developed some essential rules for CSF IgG detection as shown in **Table 1**. Importantly, intrathekal IgG synthesis can only be assessed if compared to serum. OCB in CSF can only be considered intrathecally synthesized if the bands selectively occur in CSF or if there are more bands in CSF than in serum, referred to as pattern 2 and 3 according to Freedman et al. (19). Depending on the IgG separation method, serum bands should be outnumbered by 1–3 bands in CSF (23). Identical bands in CSF and serum do not reflect pathological immunoglobulin synthesis in the CNS because the CSF bands have their origin in the systemic circulation. These findings are referred to as pattern 4 (identical oligoclonal) and 5 (identical monoclonal) according to Freedman et al. (19).

More recent developments regarding measurements of intrathecal immune activation include detection of free light chains (FLC). There are several reports that, particularly, kappa FLC are equally sensitive and specific for clonal expansion as detection of OCB in MS (24). The advantages of FLC measurements are its methodological simplicity and its objective read-out by instrumental measurements of concentrations rather than visual inspection of OCB. However, before general implementation of FLC detection or even replacement of IEF there is more work needed including independent confirmation by different labs and validation of specificity using broader ranges of control groups, particularly other inflammatory diseases.

A comprehensive overview regarding methodological aspects of CSF investigations in general can be found in recent publication (23).

TABLE 1 | Guidelines for IgG detection in CSF according to Freedman et al. (19).

CSF immunoglobulins must be separated by IEF
CSF immunoglobulins must not be separated by electrophoresis
CSF must not be concentrated
CSF immunoglobulins should be immunofixed/blotted
CSF and parallel serum must have similar amounts of immunoglobulin on the same analytical run
IEF is always more sensitive than any quantitative formula for immunoglobulins in CSF/serum
To use "only" a quantitative formula is not recommended
Non-linear formulations are recommended over linear formulations
A quantitative formula may be more useful in treatment/prognosis than in diagnosis
Light chain immunofixation can extend the value of IgG immunofixation

Expected CSF Changes in MS

As MS is considered an inflammatory CNS disease with focal breakdown of the BBB one could expect markers of these events in CSF to be altered (**Figure 1**). Markers of these changes are CSF leukocyte counts as an indicator of inflammation (apart from elevated immunoglobulin levels), and total protein or albumin concentrations as an indicator of BBB disruption (23) (**Table 2**).

In about one half of MS patients CSF leukocyte counts will be elevated up to 50 cells per uL (22). Higher leukocyte counts occur in only 1–2% of patients and should give raise to consider alternative diagnoses, particularly infectious CNS diseases. On differential cell count lymphocytes dominate by far, accounting for more than 90% of cells, 90% of which are T-cells and 10% B-cells, which excludes lymphocyte subtyping as a distinctive feature of MS (25). The remainder is constituted by monocytes although other leukocyte types may be encountered such as plasma cells, macrophages, and very rarely granulocytes. Again, a substantial deviation from this pattern should be regarded as red flag regarding the correctness of the diagnosis.

Glucose CSF to serum ratios are normal in MS (26).

Total protein or albumin quotient is normal in the vast majority of patients (22, 27), which is in line with the very focal and transient BBB leakage in MS.

The hallmark of typical CSF changes in MS however, is the increased production of intrathekal immunoglobulins (28). To demonstrate this, the MS diagnostic guidelines refer to two different methods: first, quantitatively elevated IgG as shown by e.g., the IgG index, and second, detection of OCB by IEF (9). It must be kept in mind that any quantitative formula is less sensitive than OCB detection with elevated IgG being found in ~60% of MS patients compared to 95% being OCB positive (i.e., diagnostic sensitivity) (19, 29). Even though it is not an MS specific test, the diagnostic specificity lies between 61 and 93% depending on the reference group (30). The lowest specificity rates occur if other inflammatory CNS diseases are exclusively included in the comparator group. In a mixed reference population, one would expect the diagnostic specificity to be probably in the middle of these values, which means that OCB have a very acceptable diagnostic performance comparable to, e.g., amyloid-beta and tau proteins in Alzheimer's disease (30).

Apart from a diagnostic role OCB are of prognostic value in CIS patients with a hazard ratio of 2.18 (95% confidence interval: 1.71–2.77) for the prediction to convert to clinically definite MS (31). A fact that has been described for conversion to MS after optic neuritis 20 years ago (32).

Given the inflammatory process, MS patients also have increased concentrations of a number of cytokines, chemokines, and interleukins in their CSF, e.g., CXCL13, IL6, IL8, and IL10 (33).

CSF Findings in Other Inflammatory Demyelinating Diseases

At first onset some symptoms are similar between MS and other inflammatory demyelinating diseases, particularly neuromyelitis optica (NMO) spectrum diseases. These syndromes can be diagnosed by IgG antibodies against AQP4 or MOG (34). In

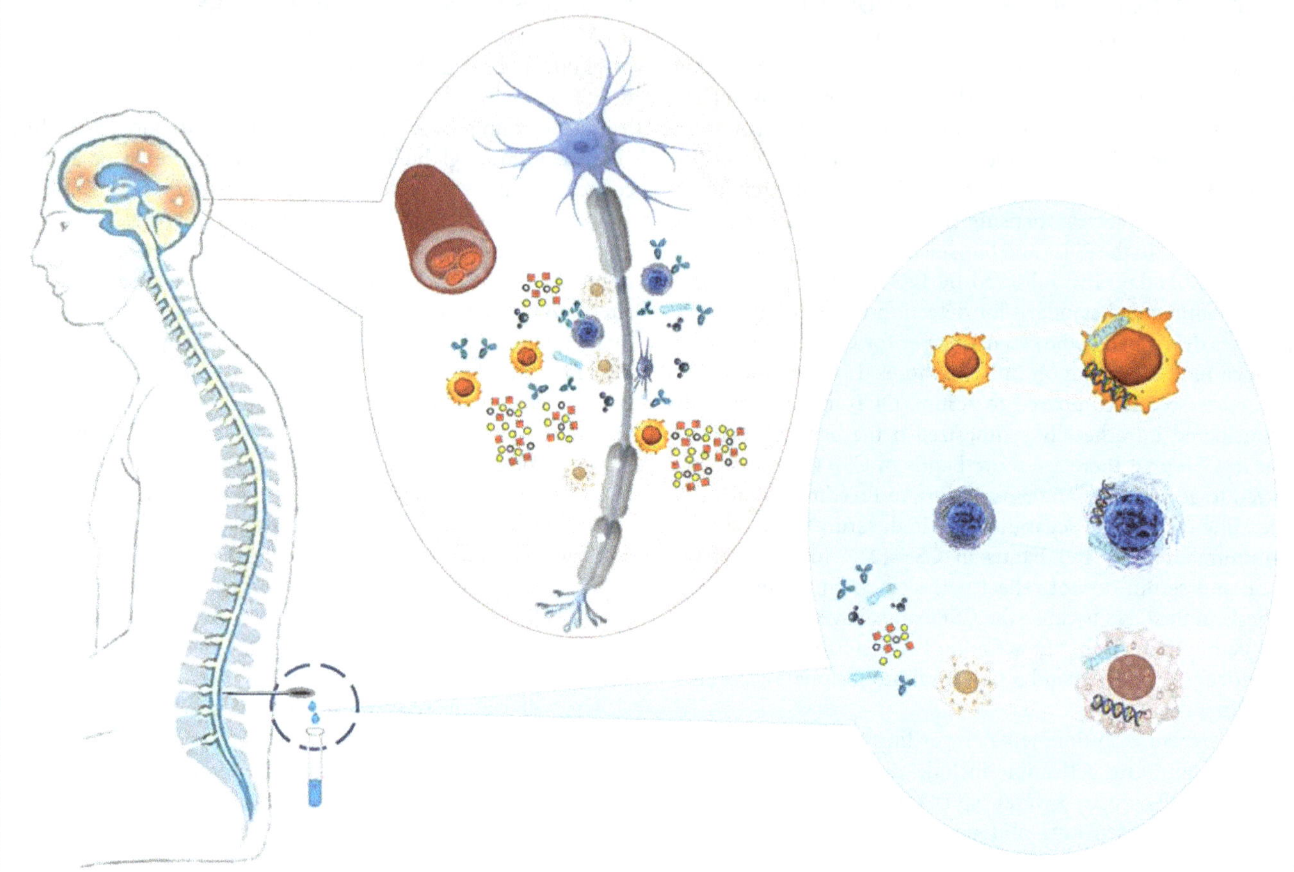

FIGURE 1 | MS causes neuronal damage (demyelination, axon degeneration, synaptic loss) to the brain and spinal cord. Immune cells, pathological antibodies, adhesion molecules, cytokines, chemokines, and nucleic acids, which reflect inflammations in the CNS, are present in the CSF of the patients and can serve as biomarkers to support MS diagnosis and therapy.

TABLE 2 | CSF changes in MS.

CSF variable	Expected finding
Total protein/albumin quotient	Normal, rarely slightly elevated
CSF:serum glucose ratio	Normal
CSF leukocyte count	Mild pleocytosis in 50% of patients Less than 50 cells/uL in 98%
Cytology	Dominated by lymphocytes (90%), some monocytes. Rarely macrophages, plasma cells, granulocytes
Immunoglobulins quantitative	IgG concentration by linear or non-linear formulae elevated in 60–70% of patients, IgA and IgM synthesis may be found less frequently
Immunoglobulins qualitative	Oligoclonal bands in 95% of definitive MS cases, 85% in CIS

general CSF work-up there is a distinct feature, which is a lack of CSF OCB in NMO spectrum diseases in 80–90% of patients (35). Total leukocyte counts in NMO spectrum disorders are similar to MS with pleocytosis being found in around 50% of patients, exceeding rarely 100 cells per uL (36). However, on differential cell counts granulocytes occur somewhat more frequently in NMO spectrum disorders compared to MS (36).

In MOG-IgG antibody associated syndromes the frequency of OCB of 13% is similarly low as in NMO spectrum disorders (37). It seems however, that CSF pleocytosis occurs more frequently, i.e., in almost two thirds of patients with a relatively high proportion of neutrophils making up 22% of all leukocytes (37). Also, an elevated albumin quotient can be found in roughly one third of patients with MOG IgG antibodies, particularly if spinal symptoms occur.

Altogether, the main distinctive feature between these syndromes and MS is the frequency of OCB, whereas general CSF changes (i.e., cell counts, cytology, protein) differ slightly but do not provide compelling evidence for or against one of the entities.

PART II: THE RESEARCH LABORATORY

Spectrum of Biomarkers in CSF

MS is an inflammatory disease characterized by damage and repair processes. The search for biomarkers focuses not only on cells and molecules of the immune response, but also on molecules reflecting the heterogeneity of mechanisms involved in the disease. Many findings on potential biomarkers have been published, including antibodies, cytokines, and chemokines molecules involved in damage and repair processes, proteins of the complement system as well as nucleic acids, that could help in MS diagnosis, differential diagnosis, prognosis, and in disease or therapy monitoring. In **Table 3** we listed information on various biomarkers mentioned in this article. Of these biomarkers, neurofilament light (NfL) is currently one of the most promising.

CSF and Serum NfL as a Biomarker of Disease Intensity in MS

Research over the past three decades have revealed that increased CSF concentration of the axonal injury marker NfL reflects disease activity and progression in all forms of MS (81). It has also become clear the concentrations dynamically change in response to relapses and treatment; MS patients starting natalizumab, a disease-modifying therapy (DMT) with high efficacy, experienced a normalization of their CSF NfL levels down to those seen in healthy controls within 6–12 months (82), suggesting that NfL can be used to monitor therapeutic efficacy. Similar observations have been made for fingolimod in patients with relapsing remitting (RR) MS and for mitoxantrone or rituximab and natalizumab in progressive MS (81). Recent ultrasensitive assays have made it possible to measure the biomarker in blood (serum or plasma; either matrix works fine), showing excellent correlation with CSF (99). Blood NfL behaves similar to CSF, also in response to DMTs, making it a promising blood biomarker for monitoring of treatment efficacy (100, 101). Ongoing studies are now also exploring it as a potential biomarker to detect side effects and suboptimal treatment efficacy. A limitation of CSF and blood NfL is that the marker is not specific to any diagnosis; it is a general marker of axonal injury and increases in all neurological disorders that involve such a process (81).

Areas of Application for CSF Biomarkers

Diagnosis

For a more reliable diagnosis of MS, many studies focus on changes in CSF composition to find markers that distinguish between MS and neuronal diseases with similar symptoms. Recently, antibodies against aquaporin 4 (AQP4) were identified in CSF of NMO, but not in MS patients (38, 39) (**Table 3**). Since these antibodies are not present in every NMO patient, additional markers are needed. Another newly discovered biomarker is the anti-MOG antibody found in the CSF of patients with demyelinating diseases such as optic neuritis (usually recurrent), myelitis encephalitis, brainstem encephalitis, and acute disseminated encephalomyelitis (ADEM)-like presentations. Today, MOG-IgG-associated encephalomyelitis (MOG-EM) is considered a separate disease entity (34).Other candidates of potential biomarkers are described in the group of cytokines [e.g., interleukin (IL)-6] (39), adhesion molecules [such as soluble intracellular and vascular cell adhesion molecule (sICAM and sVCAM) (89)], damage and repair associated molecules [like glial fibrillary acidic protein (GFAP) and haptoglobin] (39) and complement components [e.g. Complement component 1-inhibitor (C1inh), C1s, C5 and factor H] (94) (**Table 3**). Further studies need to evaluate the benefit of these molecules in diagnosis.

Prognosis

Prognostic CSF markers may influence the choice of therapy for MS, for example, when it is possible to distinguish between a very active disease course and a mild progression. Protein chitinase 3-like1 (CHI3L1) and NfL are today the most promising prognostic CSF markers to predict conversion of MS on the one hand and disability on the other (58). Other markers that have been shown to have prognostic potential for predicting the conversion of CIS to clinical definite (CD) MS, from RRMS to secondary progressive (SP) MS and a worse disease progression include oligoclonal IgM bands (OCMB) and protein 14-3-3 (39).

Monitoring of Therapy Response and Side Effects

For MS various DMTs are approved by EMA and FDA. Different CSF markers are described in particular molecules of neuronal damage, pro- and anti-inflammatory cytokines and chemokines, as well as damage and repair molecules that are influenced by DMTs and that may reflect the efficacy of therapy (**Table 3**). Treatment with Natalizumab, for which most data on CSF molecules are available, leads, besides a decrease of NfL, to a downregulation of CHI3L1, neurofilament heavy (NfH), IL-6, IL-8, and chemokine (c-x-c motif) ligand CXCL13 (33, 39, 82, 102) in CSF (**Table 3**). CXCL13 is also downregulated in CSF of MS patients treated with steroids, B-cell depletion therapy or fingolimod (39, 59). CHI3L1 is down-regulated in CSF of MS patients not only by natalizumab but also by treatment with fingolimod and mitoxantrone (39, 59). Thus, both molecules could serve as markers for therapy-response, CXCL13 as marker of anti-inflammatory drugs and CHI3L1 for monitoring the decrease in cell damage. Recently, elevated levels of soluble cluster of differentiation (sCD) 27 and sCD21 have been found in the CSF of MS patients (95) and, in particular, sCD27 has been highlighted as a therapeutically responsive (natalizumab and methylprednisolone) potent and sensitive marker for intrathecal inflammation in progressive MS (96).

DMTs have been available for MS treatment for over 20 years and new DMTs with higher efficacy have been continuously developed since then. Depending on the mode of action of individual drugs, the risk of bacterial, viral, parasitic and/or fungal infection may increase (103). Existing latent viral infections can become active and trigger a severe infection under DMT, as the modulation of the immune system can lead to a decreased anti-viral immune response. Best known is the development of progressive multifocal leukoencephalopathy (PML) in MS patients infected with John Cunningham Virus (JCV) as a severe side effect of natalizumab therapy. Natalizumab is associated with the highest risk of PML (incidence: one in 250) of all approved MS therapies to our current knowledge (104–106). The frequency of PML increases with the duration of natalizumab and former JCV-negative patients may change to JCV-positive ones. Several cases of PML have also been reported in MS patients treated

TABLE 3 | Selection of molecular and cellular markers and their potential utility in MS diagnosis, prognosis and monitoring.

	Diagnosis		Prognosis (risk factor for)		Monitoring		
	CDMS	**NMOSD**	**CDMS**	**Worse disease course**	**Therapy effects**	**Therapy side effects**	**References**
ANTIBODIES							
Anti-AQP4		↑[4,6,8*]					(38, 39)
Anti-JCV						↑[a]	(40, 41)
Anti-MOG					↓[f]		(42–44)
OCB	↑[4]	↓[6]	x				(31, 32, 35, 39, 45, 46)
OCGB	↑[1]		x	x	↓[a]		(39, 47–51)
OCMB	↑[4,3,5]		x	x			(39, 51–57)
CYTOKINES/CHEMOKINES							
CXCL13 (SDF-1α)	↑[9]		x	x	↓[a,b,c,g]		(33, 39, 51, 58–66)
IL-6		↑[4,6]			↓[a]		(33, 39, 60, 67, 68)
IL-8					↓[a]		(33, 60)
DAMAGE AND REPAIR MOLECULES							
14-3-3	↑[2]		x	x			(39, 69, 70)
CHI3L1	↑[1,4,7]		x	x	↓[a,d,g]		(39, 58, 59, 61, 71–74)
GFAP	↑[1]	↑[6]		x			(39, 59, 61, 64, 75–77)
Haptoglobin		↑[6]					(39)
NfH	↑		x		↓[a]		(39, 58, 59, 78–80)
NfL	↑[1,2]		x	x	↓[a,c,d,g]		(39, 58, 59, 61, 64, 75, 77, 79–88)
ADHESION MOLECULES							
sICAM-1		↑[1,2,6]					(89–92)
sVCAM-1		↑[1,2,6]					(65, 89, 90, 93)
COMPLEMENT COMPONENTS							
C1inh		↑[6,9]					(94)
C1s		↑[6,9]					(94)
C5		↑[6,9]					(94)
Factor H		↑[6,9]					(94)
OTHER MOLECULES							
sCD21	↑[2]				↓[a,b]		(95, 96)
sCD27	↑[1,2]				↓[a,b]		(95, 96)
NUCLEIC ACIDS							
JCV DNA						↑[a,c,e,g]	(97, 98)

*Findings of molecular markers in MS-specific clinical contexts are listed in the table. An arrow pointing upwards indicates an elevation and an arrow pointing downwards a decrease in the amount of the respective molecule in CSF. NMOSD data were only considered when a difference to MS was described. (1) compared to HC; (2) compared to NIND; (3) compared to OIND; (4) compared to OND; (5) compared to distinct disease groups or mixtures of control groups; (6) compared to MS; (7) compared to CIS; (8) compared to RRMS (*in remission); (9) compared to control whose composition was not mentioned; (a) natalizumab; (b) steroids; (c) B-cell depletion therapy; (d) mitoxantrone; (e) dimethylfumarate; (f) DNA plasmid vaccine BHT-3009; (g) fingolimod.*

with fingolimod or dimethylfumarate (104–106). Although there are no known cases of PML from alemtuzumab, mitoxantrone, B-cell depletion or teriflunomide in MS patients, a risk cannot be dismissed because these drugs or closely related compounds have been associated with PML in other diseases (105). The detection of JCV infection by anti-JCV indices can be prevented by B-cell depletion therapies such as Rituximab (107), since antibody production decreases with decreasing B-cell numbers. Therefore, careful monitoring of anti-JCV antibodies and/or JCV DNA in the blood and CSF is necessary, in particular for natalizumab treatment and suspected PML (108).

Not only JCV, but also other viral infections, which can even lead to encephalitis, can occur under DMTs. The risk of severe viral infections increases with cladribine (mainly herpes zoster), ocrelizumab and natalizumab (herpes), and fingolimod (herpes and varicella). Two deaths from herpes and varicella encephalitis have been reported for fingolimod (106). For this reason, careful monitoring of MS patients treated with DMTs is recommended. If virus-induced encephalitis is suspected, DNA analyses in the CSF may be useful for diagnosis.

CONCLUSIONS

OCB are important biomarkers that can support MRI diagnostics and help to avoid false-positive MS diagnoses. Therefore, the revised McDonalds criteria have increased the importance of the OCB.

New biomarkers such as AQP4 have now established themselves in clinical practice, and others such as Anti-MOG and NfL are about to enter clinical routine.

An important focus in the search for new biomarkers is the monitoring of therapy efficacy and the prediction of severe side effects.

Many other CSF molecules such as CHI3L1, IL-6, or CXCL13 show potential as markers for clinical practice, but further research is needed to prove their importance.

AUTHOR CONTRIBUTIONS

All authors listed have made a substantial, direct and intellectual contribution to the work, and approved it for publication.

REFERENCES

1. Meritt HH, Fremont-Smith F, Meritt HH, Fremont-Smith F. *The Cerebrospinal Fluid.* Philadelphia, PA: W. B. Saunders Company (1937).
2. Hegen H, Auer M, Zeileis A, Deisenhammer F. Upper reference limits for cerebrospinal fluid total protein and albumin quotient based on a large cohort of control patients: implications for increased clinical specificity. *Clin Chem Lab Med.* (2016) 54:285–92. doi: 10.1515/cclm-2015-0253
3. McCudden CR, Brooks J, Figurado P, Bourque PR. Cerebrospinal fluid total protein reference intervals derived from 20 years of patient data. *Clin Chem.* (2017) 63:1856–65. doi: 10.1373/clinchem.2017.278267
4. Auer M, Hegen H, Zeileis A, Deisenhammer F. Quantitation of intrathecal immunoglobulin synthesis - a new empirical formula. *Eur J Neurol.* (2016) 23:713–21. doi: 10.1111/ene.12924
5. Hegen H, Auer M, Deisenhammer F. Serum glucose adjusted cut-off values for normal cerebrospinal fluid/serum glucose ratio: implications for clinical practice. *Clin Chem Lab Med.* (2014) 52:1335–40. doi: 10.1515/cclm-2014-0077
6. Reiber H. Flow rate of cerebrospinal fluid (CSF)–a concept common to normal blood-CSF barrier function and to dysfunction in neurological diseases. *J Neurol Sci.* (1994) 122:189–203. doi: 10.1016/0022-510X(94)90298-4
7. Bechter K, Deisenhammer F. Psychiatric syndromes other than dementia. *Handb Clin Neurol.* (2017) 146:285–96. doi: 10.1016/B978-0-12-804279-3.00017-4
8. Thompson AJ, Banwell BL, Barkhof F, Carroll WM, Coetzee T, Comi G, et al. Diagnosis of multiple sclerosis: 2017 revisions of the McDonald criteria. *Lancet Neurol.* (2018) 17:162–73. doi: 10.1016/S1474-4422(17)30470-2
9. McDonald WI, Compston A, Edan G, Goodkin D, Hartung HP, Lublin FD, et al. Recommended diagnostic criteria for multiple sclerosis: guidelines from the International Panel on the diagnosis of multiple sclerosis. *Ann Neurol.* (2001) 50:121–7. doi: 10.1002/ana.1032
10. Polman CH, Reingold SC, Edan G, Filippi M, Hartung HP, Kappos L, et al. Diagnostic criteria for multiple sclerosis: 2005 revisions to the "McDonald Criteria." *Ann Neurol.* (2005) 58:840–6. doi: 10.1002/ana.20703
11. Polman CH, Reingold SC, Banwell B, Clanet M, Cohen JA, Filippi M, et al. Diagnostic criteria for multiple sclerosis: 2010 revisions to the McDonald criteria. *Ann Neurol.* (2011) 69:292–302. doi: 10.1002/ana.22366
12. Tumani H, Deisenhammer F, Giovannoni G, Gold R, Hartung HP, Hemmer B, et al. Revised McDonald criteria: the persisting importance of cerebrospinal fluid analysis. *Ann Neurol.* (2011) 70:520. doi: 10.1002/ana.22508
13. Solomon AJ, Klein EP, Bourdette D. "Undiagnosing" multiple sclerosis: the challenge of misdiagnosis in MS. *Neurology.* (2012) 78:1986–91. doi: 10.1212/WNL.0b013e318259e1b2
14. Solomon AJ, Bourdette DN, Cross AH, Applebee A, Skidd PM, Howard DB, et al. The contemporary spectrum of multiple sclerosis misdiagnosis: a multicenter study. *Neurology.* (2016) 87:1393–99. doi: 10.1212/WNL.0000000000003152
15. Bourahoui A, de Seze J, Guttierez R, Onraed B, Hennache B, Ferriby D, et al. CSF isoelectrofocusing in a large cohort of MS and other neurological diseases. *Eur J Neurol.* (2004) 11:525–9. doi: 10.1111/j.1468-1331.2004.00822.x
16. Tintore M, Rovira A, Brieva L, Grive E, Jardi R, Borras C, et al. Isolated demyelinating syndromes: comparison of CSF oligoclonal bands and different MR imaging criteria to predict conversion to CDMS. *Mult Scler.* (2001) 7:359–63. doi: 10.1177/135245850100700603
17. Kleinschmidt-DeMasters BK, Tyler KL. Progressive multifocal leukoencephalopathy complicating treatment with natalizumab and interferon beta-1a for multiple sclerosis. *N Engl J Med.* (2005) 353:369–74. doi: 10.1056/NEJMoa051782
18. Kaiser R. Variable CSF findings in early and late Lyme neuroborreliosis: a follow-up study in 47 patients. *J Neurol.* (1994) 242:26–36. doi: 10.1007/BF00920571
19. Freedman MS, Thompson EJ, Deisenhammer F, Giovannoni G, Grimsley G, Keir G, et al. Recommended standard of cerebrospinal fluid analysis in the diagnosis of multiple sclerosis: a consensus statement. *Arch Neurol.* (2005) 62:865–70. doi: 10.1001/archneur.62.6.865
20. Petzold A. Intrathecal oligoclonal IgG synthesis in multiple sclerosis. *J Neuroimmunol.* (2013) 262:1–10. doi: 10.1016/j.jneuroim.2013.06.014
21. Standardization IO for. ISO 15189:2012 Medical laboratories – Requirements for quality and competence. (2012) 3:1–53.
22. Andersson M, Alvarez-Cermeno J, Bernardi G, Cogato I, Fredman P, Frederiksen J, et al. Cerebrospinal fluid in the diagnosis of multiple sclerosis: a consensus report. *J Neurol Neurosurg Psychiatry.* (1994) 57:897–902. doi: 10.1136/jnnp.57.8.897
23. Deisenhammer F, Sellebjerg F, Teunissen CE, Tumani H, Deisenhammer F, Sellebjerg F, et al. *Cerebrospinal Fluid in Clinical Neurology.* 1st ed. Cham; New York, NY; Dordrecht; London: Springer (2015). doi: 10.1007/978-3-319-01225-4
24. Presslauer S, Milosavljevic D, Huebl W, boulenein-Djamshidian F, Krugluger W, Deisenhammer F, et al. Validation of kappa free light chains as a diagnostic biomarker in multiple sclerosis and clinically isolated syndrome: a multicenter study. *Mult Scler.* (2016) 22:502–10. doi: 10.1177/1352458515594044
25. Polman CH, de Groot CJ, Koetsier JC, Sminia T, Veerman AJ. Cerebrospinal fluid cells in multiple sclerosis and other neurological diseases: an immunocytochemical study. *J Neurol.* (1987) 234:19–22. doi: 10.1007/BF00314003
26. Osenbruck M, Rao ML, Quednau HD. Pattern of albumin, immunoglobulins, and glucose in cerebrospinal fluid and serum of patients with disorders of the central nervous system. *Eur Neurol.* (1985) 24:16–22. doi: 10.1159/000115756
27. Hayward RA, Shapiro MF, Oye RK. Laboratory testing on cerebrospinal fluid. A reappraisal. *Lancet.* (1987) 1:1–4. doi: 10.1016/S0140-6736(87)92845-5
28. Link H. Immunoglobulin G and low molecular weight proteins in human cerebrospinal fluid. Chemical and immunological characterisation with special reference to multiple sclerosis. *Acta Neurol Scand.* (1967) 43:1–136.

29. Mayringer I, Timeltaler B, Deisenhammer F. Correlation between the IgG index, oligoclonal bands in CSF, and the diagnosis of demyelinating diseases. *Eur J Neurol.* (2005) 12:527–30. doi: 10.1111/j.1468-1331.2005.00997.x
30. Olsson B, Lautner R, Andreasson U, Ohrfelt A, Portelius E, Bjerke M, et al. CSF and blood biomarkers for the diagnosis of Alzheimer's disease: a systematic review and meta-analysis. *Lancet Neurol.* (2016) 15:673–84. doi: 10.1016/S1474-4422(16)00070-3
31. Kuhle J, Disanto G, Dobson R, Adiutori R, Bianchi L, Topping J, et al. Conversion from clinically isolated syndrome to multiple sclerosis: a large multicentre study. *Mult Scler.* (2015) 21:1013–24. doi: 10.1177/1352458514568827
32. Soderstrom M, Ya-Ping J, Hillert J, Link H. Optic neuritis: prognosis for multiple sclerosis from MRI, CSF, and HLA findings. *Neurology.* (1998) 50:708–14. doi: 10.1212/WNL.50.3.708
33. Magliozzi R, Howell OW, Nicholas R, Cruciani C, Castellaro M, Romualdi C, et al. Inflammatory intrathecal profiles and cortical damage in multiple sclerosis. *Ann Neurol.* (2018) 83:739–55. doi: 10.1002/ana.25197
34. Jarius S, Paul F, Aktas O, Asgari N, Dale RC, de SJ, et al. MOG encephalomyelitis: international recommendations on diagnosis and antibody testing. *J Neuroinflammation.* (2018) 15:134. doi: 10.1186/s12974-018-1144-2
35. Aboul-Enein F, Seifert-Held T, Mader S, Kuenz B, Lutterotti A, Rauschka H, et al. Neuromyelitis optica in Austria in 2011: to bridge the gap between neuroepidemiological research and practice in a study population of 8.4 million people. *PLoS ONE.* (2013) 8:e79649. doi: 10.1371/journal.pone.0079649
36. Jarius S, Paul F, Franciotta D, Ruprecht K, Ringelstein M, Bergamaschi R, et al. Cerebrospinal fluid findings in aquaporin-4 antibody positive neuromyelitis optica: results from 211 lumbar punctures. *J Neurol Sci.* (2011) 306:82–90. doi: 10.1016/j.jns.2011.03.038
37. Jarius S, Ruprecht K, Kleiter I, Borisow N, Asgari N, Pitarokoili K, et al. MOG-IgG in NMO and related disorders: a multicenter study of 50 patients. Part 2: epidemiology, clinical presentation, radiological and laboratory features, treatment responses, and long-term outcome. *J Neuroinflamm.* (2016) 13:280. doi: 10.1186/s12974-016-0718-0
38. Long Y, Qiu W, Lu Z, Bao J, Wu A, Wang Y, et al. Aquaporin 4 antibodies in the cerebrospinal fluid are helpful in diagnosing chinese patients with neuromyelitis optica. *Neuroimmunomodulation.* (2012) 19:96–102. doi: 10.1159/000330240
39. Matute-Blanch C, Montalban X, Comabella M. *Multiple Sclerosis, and Other Demyelinating and Autoimmune Inflammatory Diseases of the Central Nervous System.* 1st ed. Amsterdam: Elsevier B.V (2017).
40. Cepok S, Zhou D, Srivastava R, Nessler S, Stei S, Büssow K, et al. Identification of Epstein-Barr virus proteins as putative targets of the immune response in multiple sclerosis. *J Clin Invest.* (2005) 115:1352–60. doi: 10.1172/JCI23661
41. Lindsey JW, Khan U, Ansari W, Powell T, Wang YH, Guirguis MS. The antibody response to Epstein-Barr virions is altered in multiple sclerosis. *J Neuroimmunol.* (2013) 254:146–53. doi: 10.1016/j.jneuroim.2012.09.007
42. Guggenmos J, Schubart AS, Ogg S, Andersson M, Olsson T, Mather IH, et al. Antibody cross-reactivity between myelin oligodendrocyte glycoprotein and the milk protein butyrophilin in multiple sclerosis. *J Immunol.* (2004) 172:661–8. doi: 10.4049/jimmunol.172.1.661
43. Hecker M, Fitzner B, Lorenz P, Flechtner K, Steinbeck F, Schröder I, et al. High-density peptide microarray analysis of igg autoantibody reactivities in serum and cerebrospinal fluid of multiple sclerosis patients. *Mol Cell Proteomics.* (2016) 15:1360–80. doi: 10.1074/mcp.M115.051664
44. Bar-Or A, Vollmer T, Antel J, Arnold DL, Bodner CA, Campagnolo D, et al. Induction of antigen-specific tolerance in multiple sclerosis after immunization with DNA encoding myelin basic protein in a randomized, placebo-controlled phase 1/2 trial. *Arch Neurol.* (2007) 64:1407–15. doi: 10.1001/archneur.64.10.nct70002
45. Link H, Huang Y-MM. Oligoclonal bands in multiple sclerosis cerebrospinal fluid: an update on methodology and clinical usefulness. *J Neuroimmunol.* (2006) 180:17–28. doi: 10.1016/j.jneuroim.2006.07.006
46. Dobson R, Ramagopalan S, Davis A, Giovannoni G. Cerebrospinal fluid oligoclonal bands in multiple sclerosis and clinically isolated syndromes: a meta-analysis of prevalence, prognosis and effect of latitude. *J Neurol Neurosurg Psychiatry.* (2013) 84:909–14. doi: 10.1136/jnnp-2012-304695
47. Sellebjerg F, Jensen CV, Christiansen M. Intrathecal IgG synthesis and autoantibody-secreting cells in multiple sclerosis. *J Neuroimmunol.* (2000) 108:207–15. doi: 10.1016/S0165-5728(00)00292-7
48. Kasai N, Pachner AR, Yu RK. Anti-glycolipid antibodies and their immune complexes in multiple sclerosis. *J Neurol Sci.* (1986) 75:33–42. doi: 10.1016/0022-510X(86)90048-1
49. Nilsson P, Larsson E-M, Maly-Sundgren P, Perfekt R, Sandberg-Wollheim M. Predicting the outcome of optic neuritis: evaluation of risk factors after 30 years of follow-up. *J Neurol.* (2005) 252:396–402. doi: 10.1007/s00415-005-0655-9
50. Menéndez-Valladares P, García-Sánchez MI, Martínez MA, De Veas Silva JLG, Guitarte CB, Ayuso GI. VALIDATION and meta-analysis of kappa index biomarker in multiple sclerosis diagnosis. *Autoimmun Rev.* (2018) 18:43–9. doi: 10.1016/j.autrev.2018.07.010
51. Gastaldi M, Zardini E, Franciotta D. An update on the use of cerebrospinal fluid analysis as a diagnostic tool in multiple sclerosis. *Expert Rev Mol Diagn.* (2017) 17:31–46. doi: 10.1080/14737159.2017.1262260
52. Perini P, Ranzato F, Calabrese M, Battistin L, Gallo P. Intrathecal IgM production at clinical onset correlates with a more severe disease course in multiple sclerosis. *J Neurol Neurosurg Psychiatry.* (2006) 77:953–5. doi: 10.1136/jnnp.2005.086116
53. Villar LM, Masjuan J, González-Porqué P, Plaza J, Sádaba MC, Roldán E, et al. Intrathecal IgM synthesis in neurologic diseases: relationship with disability in MS. *Neurology.* (2002) 58:824–6. doi: 10.1212/WNL.58.5.824
54. Mandrioli J, Sola P, Bedin R, Gambini M, Merelli E. A multifactorial prognostic index in multiple sclerosis: cerebrospinal fluid IgM oligoclonal bands and clinical features to predict the evolution of the disease. *J Neurol.* (2008) 255:1023–31. doi: 10.1007/s00415-008-0827-5
55. Villar LMM, Masjuan J, González-Porqué P, Plaza J, Sádaba MCC, Roldán E, et al. Intrathecal IgM synthesis predicts the onset of new relapses and a worse disease course in MS. *Neurology.* (2002) 59:555–9. doi: 10.1212/WNL.59.4.555
56. Villar LM, Masjuan J, González-Porqué P, Plaza J, Sádaba MC, Roldán E, et al. Intrathecal IgM synthesis is a prognostic factor in multiple sclerosis. *Ann Neurol.* (2003) 53:222–6. doi: 10.1002/ana.10441
57. Schneider R, Euler B, Rauer S. Intrathecal IgM-synthesis does not correlate with the risk of relapse in patients with a primary demyelinating event. *Eur J Neurol.* (2007) 14:907–11. doi: 10.1111/j.1468-1331.2007.01871.x
58. Comabella M, Sastre-Garriga J, Montalban X. Precision medicine in multiple sclerosis: biomarkers for diagnosis, prognosis, and treatment response. *Curr Opin Neurol.* (2016) 29:254–62. doi: 10.1097/WCO.0000000000000336
59. Lycke J, Zetterberg H. The role of blood and CSF biomarkers in the evaluation of new treatments against multiple sclerosis. *Expert Rev Clin Immunol.* (2017) 13:1143–53. doi: 10.1080/1744666X.2017.1400380
60. Pranzatelli MR. Advances in biomarker-guided therapy for pediatric- and adult-onset neuroinflammatory disorders: targeting chemokines/cytokines. *Front Immunol.* (2018) 9:557. doi: 10.3389/fimmu.2018.00557
61. Barro C, Leocani L, Leppert D, Comi G, Kappos L, Kuhle J. Fluid biomarker and electrophysiological outcome measures for progressive MS trials. *Mult Scler.* (2017) 23:1600–13. doi: 10.1177/1352458517732844
62. Khademi M, Kockum I, Andersson ML, Iacobaeus E, Brundin L, Sellebjerg F, et al. Cerebrospinal fluid CXCL13 in multiple sclerosis: a suggestive prognostic marker for the disease course. *Mult Scler.* (2011) 17:335–43. doi: 10.1177/1352458510389102
63. Harris VK, Sadiq SA. Biomarkers of therapeutic response in multiple sclerosis: current status. *Mol Diagn Ther.* (2014) 18:605–17. doi: 10.1007/s40291-014-0117-0
64. Axelsson M, Malmeström C, Gunnarsson M, Zetterberg H, Sundström P, Lycke J, et al. Immunosuppressive therapy reduces axonal damage in progressive multiple sclerosis. *Mult Scler.* (2014) 20:43–50. doi: 10.1177/1352458513490544
65. Graber JJ, Dhib-Jalbut S. Biomarkers of disease activity in multiple sclerosis. *J Neurol Sci.* (2011) 305:1–10. doi: 10.1016/j.jns.2011.03.026
66. Krumbholz M, Theil D, Cepok S, Hemmer B, Kivisäkk P, Ransohoff RM, et al. Chemokines in multiple sclerosis: CXCL12 and CXCL13 up-regulation is

differentially linked to CNS immune cell recruitment. *Brain.* (2006) 129:200–11. doi: 10.1093/brain/awh680

67. Baraczka K, Nékám K, Pozsonyi T, Szüts I, Ormos G. Investigation of cytokine (tumor necrosis factor-alpha, interleukin-6, interleukin-10) concentrations in the cerebrospinal fluid of female patients with multiple sclerosis and systemic lupus erythematosus. *Eur J Neurol.* (2004) 11:37–42. doi: 10.1046/j.1351-5101.2003.00706.x
68. Malmeström C, Andersson BAA, Haghighi S, Lycke J. IL-6 and CCL2 levels in CSF are associated with the clinical course of MS: implications for their possible immunopathogenic roles. *J Neuroimmunol.* (2006) 175:176–82. doi: 10.1016/j.jneuroim.2006.03.004
69. Bartosik-Psujek H, Archelos JJ. Tau protein and 14-3-3 are elevated in the cerebrospinal fluid of patients with multiple sclerosis and correlate with intrathecal synthesis of IgG. *J Neurol.* (2004) 251:414–20. doi: 10.1007/s00415-004-0336-0
70. Martínez-Yélamos A, Rovira A, Sánchez-Valle R, Martínez-Yélamos S, Tintoré M, Blanco Y, et al. CSF 14-3-3 protein assay and MRI as prognostic markers in patients with a clinically isolated syndrome suggestive of MS. *J Neurol.* (2004) 251:1278–9. doi: 10.1007/s00415-004-0524-y
71. Correale J, Fiol M. Chitinase effects on immune cell response in neuromyelitis optica and multiple sclerosis. *Mult Scler.* (2011) 17:521–31. doi: 10.1177/1352458510392619
72. Malmeström C, Axelsson M, Lycke J, Zetterberg H, Blennow K, Olsson B. CSF levels of YKL-40 are increased in MS and replaces with immunosuppressive treatment. *J Neuroimmunol.* (2014) 269:87–9. doi: 10.1016/j.jneuroim.2014.02.004
73. Comabella M, Fernández M, Martin R, Rivera-Vallvé S, Borrás E, Chiva C, et al. Cerebrospinal fluid chitinase 3-like 1 levels are associated with conversion to multiple sclerosis. *Brain.* (2010) 133:1082–93. doi: 10.1093/brain/awq035
74. Stoop MP, Singh V, Stingl C, Martin R, Khademi M, Olsson T, et al. Effects of natalizumab treatment on the cerebrospinal fluid proteome of multiple sclerosis patients. *J Proteome Res.* (2013) 12:1101–7. doi: 10.1021/pr3012107
75. Malmeström C, Haghighi S, Rosengren L, Andersen O, Lycke J. Neurofilament light protein and glial fibrillary acidic protein as biological markers in MS. *Neurology.* (2003) 61:1720–5. doi: 10.1212/01.WNL.0000098880.19793.B6
76. Axelsson M, Malmeström C, Nilsson S, Haghighi S, Rosengren L, Lycke J. Glial fibrillary acidic protein: a potential biomarker for progression in multiple sclerosis. *J Neurol.* (2011) 258:882–8. doi: 10.1007/s00415-010-5863-2
77. Avsar T, Korkmaz D, Tütüncü M, Demirci NO, Saip S, Kamasak M, et al. Protein biomarkers for multiple sclerosis: semi-quantitative analysis of cerebrospinal fluid candidate protein biomarkers in different forms of multiple sclerosis. *Mult Scler.* (2012) 18:1081–91. doi: 10.1177/1352458511433303
78. Brettschneider J, Petzold A, Junker A, Tumani H. Axonal damage markers in the cerebrospinal fluid of patients with clinically isolated syndrome improve predicting conversion to definite multiple sclerosis. *Mult Scler.* (2006) 12:143–8. doi: 10.1191/135248506ms1263oa
79. Teunissen CE, Iacobaeus E, Khademi M, Brundin L, Norgren N, Koel-Simmelink MJA, et al. Combination of CSF N-acetylaspartate and neurofilaments in multiple sclerosis. *Neurology.* (2009) 72:1322–9. doi: 10.1212/WNL.0b013e3181a0fe3f
80. Trentini A, Comabella M, Tintoré M, Koel-Simmelink MJA, Killestein J, Roos B, et al. N-Acetylaspartate and neurofilaments as biomarkers of axonal damage in patients with progressive forms of multiple sclerosis. *J Neurol.* (2014) 261:2338–43. doi: 10.1007/s00415-014-7507-4
81. Khalil M, Teunissen CE, Otto M, Piehl F, Sormani MP, Gattringer T, et al. Neurofilaments as biomarkers in neurological disorders. *Nat Rev Neurol.* (2018) 14:577–89. doi: 10.1038/s41582-018-0058-z
82. Gunnarsson M, Malmestrom C, Axelsson M, Sundstrom P, Dahle C, Vrethem M, et al. Axonal damage in relapsing multiple sclerosis is markedly reduced by natalizumab. *Ann Neurol.* (2011) 69:83–9. doi: 10.1002/ana.22247
83. Salzer J, Svenningsson A, Sundström P. Neurofilament light as a prognostic marker in multiple sclerosis. *Mult Scler.* (2010) 16:287–92. doi: 10.1177/1352458509359725
84. Kuhle J, Malmeström C, Axelsson M, Plattner K, Yaldizli Ö, Derfuss T, et al. Neurofilament light and heavy subunits compared as therapeutic biomarkers in multiple sclerosis. *Acta Neurol Scand.* (2013) 128:e33–6. doi: 10.1111/ane.12151
85. Kuhle J, Disanto G, Lorscheider J, Stites T, Chen Y, Dahlke F, et al. Fingolimod and CSF neurofilament light chain levels in relapsing-remitting multiple sclerosis. *Neurology.* (2015) 84:1639–43. doi: 10.1212/WNL.0000000000001491
86. Fialová L, Bartos A, Švarcová J, Zimova D, Kotoucova J, Malbohan I. Serum and cerebrospinal fluid light neurofilaments and antibodies against them in clinically isolated syndrome and multiple sclerosis. *J Neuroimmunol.* (2013) 262:113–20. doi: 10.1016/j.jneuroim.2013.06.010
87. Romme Christensen J, Börnsen L, Hesse D, Krakauer M, Sørensen PS, Søndergaard HB, et al. Cellular sources of dysregulated cytokines in relapsing-remitting multiple sclerosis. *J Neuroinflammation.* (2012) 9:215. doi: 10.1186/1742-2094-9-215
88. Cai L, Huang J. Neurofilament light chain as a biological marker for multiple sclerosis: a meta-analysis study. *Neuropsychiatr Dis Treat.* (2018) 14:2241–54. doi: 10.2147/NDT.S173280
89. Uzawa A, Mori M, Masuda S, Kuwabara S. Markedly elevated soluble intercellular adhesion molecule 1, soluble vascular cell adhesion molecule 1 levels, and blood-brain barrier breakdown in neuromyelitis optica. *Arch Neurol.* (2011) 68:913–7. doi: 10.1001/archneurol.2011.148
90. Rieckmann P, Altenhofen B, Riegel A, Baudewig J, Felgenhauer K. Soluble adhesion molecules (sVCAM-1 and sICAM-1) in cerebrospinal fluid and serum correlate with MRI activity in multiple sclerosis. *Ann Neurol.* (1997) 41:326–33. doi: 10.1002/ana.410410307
91. Acar G, Idiman F, Kirkali G, Özakbaş S, Oktay G, Çakmakçi H, et al. Intrathecal sICAM-1 production in multiple sclerosis Correlation with triple dose Gd-DTPA MRI enhancement and IgG index. *J Neurol.* (2005) 252:146–50. doi: 10.1007/s00415-005-0618-1
92. Mitosek-Szewczyk K, Stelmasiak Z, Bartosik-Psujek H, Belniak E. Impact of cladribine on soluble adhesion molecules in multiple sclerosis. *Acta Neurol Scand.* (2010) 122:409–13. doi: 10.1111/j.1600-0404.2010.01330.x
93. Correale J, de los Milagros Bassani Molinas M, Bassani Molinas MDLM. Temporal variations of adhesion molecules and matrix metalloproteinases in the course of MS. *J Neuroimmunol.* (2003) 140:198–209. doi: 10.1016/S0165-5728(03)00204-2
94. Tatomir A, Talpos-Caia A, Anselmo F, Kruszewski AM, Boodhoo D, Rus V, et al. The complement system as a biomarker of disease activity and response to treatment in multiple sclerosis. *Immunol Res.* (2017) 65:1103–9. doi: 10.1007/s12026-017-8961-8
95. Komori M, Blake A, Greenwood M, Lin YC, Kosa P, Ghazali D, et al. Cerebrospinal fluid markers reveal intrathecal inflammation in progressive multiple sclerosis. *Ann Neurol.* (2015) 78:3–20. doi: 10.1002/ana.24408
96. Christensen JR, Komori M, Von Essen MR, Ratzer R, Börnsen L, Bielekova B, et al. CSF inflammatory biomarkers responsive to treatment in progressive multiple sclerosis capture residual inflammation associated with axonal damage. *Mult Scler.* (2018) 1–10. doi: 10.1177/1352458518774880
97. Kappos L, Bates D, Edan G, Eraksoy M, Garcia-Merino A, Grigoriadis N, et al. Natalizumab treatment for multiple sclerosis: updated recommendations for patient selection and monitoring. *Lancet Neurol.* (2011) 10:745–58. doi: 10.1016/S1474-4422(11)70149-1
98. Warnke C, Wattjes MP, Adams O, Hartung HP, Martin R, Weber T, et al. Progressive multifokale Leukenzephalopathie. *Nervenarzt.* (2016) 87:1–5. doi: 10.1007/s00115-016-0225-7
99. Gisslen M, Price RW, Andreasson U, Norgren N, Nilsson S, Hagberg L, et al. Plasma concentration of the Neurofilament Light protein (NFL) is a biomarker of CNS injury in HIV infection: a cross-sectional study. *EBio Med.* (2016) 3:135–40. doi: 10.1016/j.ebiom.2015.11.036

100. Disanto G, Barro C, Benkert P, Naegelin Y, Schadelin S, Giardiello A, et al. Serum neurofilament light: a biomarker of neuronal damage in multiple sclerosis. *Ann Neurol.* (2017) 81:857–70. doi: 10.1002/ana.24954
101. Novakova L, Zetterberg H, Sundstrom P, Axelsson M, Khademi M, Gunnarsson M, et al. Monitoring disease activity in multiple sclerosis using serum neurofilament light protein. *Neurology.* (2017) 89:2230–7. doi: 10.1212/WNL.0000000000004683
102. Axelsson M, Dubuisson N, Novakova-Nyren L, Malmeström C, Giovannoni G, Lycke J, et al. Cerebrospinal fluid NCAM levels are modulated by disease modifying therapies. *Acta Neurol Scand.* (2019). doi: 10.1111/ane.13069.
103. Celius EG. Infections in patients with multiple sclerosis: implications for disease-modifying therapy. *Acta Neurol Scand.* (2017) 136:34–6. doi: 10.1111/ane.12835
104. Bartsch T, Rempe T, Leypoldt F, Riedel C, Jansen O, Berg D, et al. The spectrum of progressive multifocal leukoencephalopathy: a practical approach. *Eur J Neurol.* (2019) 26:566-e41. doi: 10.1111/ene.13906
105. Berger JR. Classifying PML risk with disease modifying therapies. *Mult Scler Relat Disord.* (2017) 12:59–63. doi: 10.1016/j.msard.2017.01.006
106. Sedal L. Current concepts in multiple sclerosis therapy. *Degener Neurol Neuromuscul Dis.* (2017)7:109–25. doi: 10.2147/DNND.S109251
107. Baber U, Bouley A, Egnor E, Sloane JA. Anti-JC virus antibody index changes in rituximab-treated multiple sclerosis patients. *J Neurol.* (2018)265:2342–5. doi: 10.1007/s00415-018-8996-3
108. Warnke C, Von Geldern G, Markwerth P, Dehmel T, Hoepner R, Gold R, et al. Cerebrospinal fluid JC virus antibody index for diagnosis of natalizumab-associated progressive multifocal leukoencephalopathy. *Ann Neurol.* (2014) 76:792–801. doi: 10.1002/ana.24153

3

Carnosol Modulates Th17 Cell Differentiation and Microglial Switch in Experimental Autoimmune Encephalomyelitis

Xing Li[1,2†], Li Zhao[1†], Juan-Juan Han[1†], Fei Zhang[1], Shuai Liu[1], Lin Zhu[3], Zhe-Zhi Wang[1], Guang-Xian Zhang[2] and Yuan Zhang[1,2]**

[1] National Engineering Laboratory for Resource Development of Endangered Crude Drugs in Northwest China, Key Laboratory of the Ministry of Education for Medicinal Resources and Natural Pharmaceutical Chemistry, College of Life Sciences, Shaanxi Normal University, Xi'an, China, [2] Department of Neurology, Thomas Jefferson University, Philadelphia, PA, United States, [3] Department of Pharmacy, Zhengzhou University, Zhengzhou, China

***Correspondence:**
Guang-Xian Zhang
guang-xian.zhang@jefferson.edu;
Yuan Zhang
yuanzhang_bio@126.com

†These authors have contributed equally to this work.

Medicinal plants as a rich pool for developing novel small molecule therapeutic medicine have been used for thousands of years. Carnosol as a bioactive diterpene compound originated from *Rosmarinus officinalis* (Rosemary) and *Salvia officinalis*, herbs extensively applied in traditional medicine for the treatment of multiple autoimmune diseases (1). In this study, we investigated the therapeutic effects and molecule mechanism of carnosol in experimental autoimmune encephalomyelitis (EAE), an animal model of multiple sclerosis (MS). Carnosol treatment significantly alleviated clinical development in the myelin oligodendrocyte glycoprotein (MOG_{35-55}) peptide-induced EAE model, markedly decreased inflammatory cell infiltration into the central nervous system and reduced demyelination. Further, carnosol inhibited Th17 cell differentiation and signal transducer and activator of transcription 3 phosphorylation, and blocked transcription factor NF-κB nuclear translocation. In the passive-EAE model, carnosol treatment also significantly prevented Th17 cell pathogenicity. Moreover, carnosol exerted its therapeutic effects in the chronic stage of EAE, and, remarkably, switched the phenotypes of infiltrated macrophage/microglia. Taken together, our results show that carnosol has enormous potential for development as a therapeutic agent for autoimmune diseases such as MS.

Keywords: Carnosol, multiple sclerosis, experimental autoimmune encephalomyelitis, Th17 cell, macrophage/microglia

INTRODUCTION

Multiple sclerosis (MS) and its animal model, experimental autoimmune encephalomyelitis (EAE), are chronic immune-mediated demyelinating diseases of the central nervous system (CNS), characterized by infiltrated inflammatory cells, demyelination, and damage to neurons (2). Although the underlying mechanism of MS has not been well defined, a growing body of evidence supports its being an autoimmune disease (3). While Th1 cells have been considered pathogenic for MS/EAE, Th17 cells, a subpopulation of pro-inflammatory T helper cells defined by their secretion of IL-17 (4), have recently emerged as an important player in inflammatory and autoimmune diseases *via* the secretion of pro-inflammatory cytokines, such as IL-17A, IL-17F, GM-CSF, and IL-22

(5, 6). Polarization of Th17 populations and the related cytokine production are directly regulated by RORγt (7), and the signals that cause Th17 cells to differentiate actually inhibit regulatory T cell (Treg) differentiation (8). Therefore, targeted inhibition of RORγt transcription or a Th17 differentiation-related signaling pathway such as NF-κB and signal transducer and activator of transcription 3 (STAT3) represents an encouraging therapeutic strategy in treatment of Th17-related diseases (4, 9, 10).

Current MS therapies either have limited efficacy or important safety issues (11, 12). A great deal of research effort has gone into developing novel therapies that specifically target Th17 cells, while sparing other immune cells. Recently, several new anti-inflammatory or immunomodulatory drugs derived from medicinal plants have been explored and are considered to have great potential for treatment of autoimmune diseases (4, 13–15). These natural compounds represent a rich source for the identification of effective and safe candidate medicines with innovative targets and/or mechanisms of action in the therapy of MS and other autoimmune diseases.

Rosmarinus officinalis (rosemary) and *Salvia officinalis* are common household plants that grow all over the world and have been used as medicinal herbs due to their powerful antioxidant and anti-inflammatory effects (16, 17). Carnosol, a major diterpene present in *R. officinalis* (rosemary) and *S. officinalis*, has been reported to possess strong antioxidant, anti-tumor, anti-viral, and especially anti-inflammatory properties (18–20). Carnosol treatment also induced T-cell leukemia/lymphoma apoptosis and decreased IL-6 and TNF-α levels in serum (21, 22). These studies indicate that carnosol may be effective in the treatment of autoimmune diseases; however, this possibility has not been tested. To elucidate this question, in the present work, we studied the potential therapeutic anti-inflammatory abilities of carnosol on actively induced and adoptively transferred EAE models and the mechanism of its action.

MATERIALS AND METHODS

EAE Induction and Treatment

Female C57BL/6 mice (purchased from the Fourth Military University (Xi'an, China)) were used at the age of 8 weeks. All animal experiments were performed with the approval of the Institutional Animal Care and Use Committee of Shaanxi Normal University and according to the approved institutional guidelines and regulations. For acute and chronic EAE, a previously described method was followed (23). Briefly, mice were subcutaneously injected with 200 μg of myelin oligodendrocyte glycoprotein (MOG) peptide 35–55 (Genescript, Piscataway, NJ, USA) in 200 μl of emulsified complete Freund's adjuvant with 5 mg/ml *Mycobacterium tuberculosis* H37Ra (Difco, Lawrence, KS, USA). For adoptive transfer EAE, mice were sacrificed 10 days after MOG_{35-55} immunization, and splenocytes and draining lymph nodes were provided as previously described (4). Cells were cultured for 3 days in the presence of 25 μg/ml MOG_{35-55}, 10 ng/ml rmIL-23, and 2 ng/ml rmIL-2 (R&D Systems, Minneapolis, MN, USA) at 1×10^7 cell/ml. $CD4^+$ T cells were purified by $CD4^+$ T cell isolation kit and 4×10^6 cells per mouse were transferred *via* intravenous (i.v.) injection. Pertussis toxin (200 ng/mouse) was injected intraperitoneally (i.p.) on days 0 and 2. Clinical EAE was assessed by daily scoring using a 0–5 scale as described previously (24). Carnosol was obtained from Sigma-Aldrich (St. Louis, MO, USA) and was injected (50 mg/kg/day) i.p. daily starting at day 0 p.i.

Histological and Immunofluorescence Staining

Mice were euthanized at different time points after drug administration, and transcardially perfused with PBS. Tissues (brains and spinal cords) were collected for pathological assessment. Spinal cords were fixed with 4% paraformaldehyde overnight, cut into 5 μm sections and stained with H&E (hematoxylin and eosin) for inflammation and Luxol fast blue (LFB) for demyelination. Slides were examined and assessed following a previously described method (23).

For immunofluorescence, brain and spinal cord were cryopreserved in OCT compound (Tissue-Tek, Sakura Finetek, Japan) for frozen sections and cut into 12 μm sections (25). Immunofluorescence staining was performed using general methods and the appropriate dilutions of primary antibodies were applied. Immunofluorescence controls were routinely performed with incubations in which primary antibodies were omitted. Images were acquired by Nikon Eclipse E600 fluorescent microscopy (Nikon, Melville, NY, USA). For quantification of $CD45^+$, MOG^+, MBP^+, $iNOS^+$, $Arg1^+$, and $CD68^+$, 10 areas of the sections were selected and analyzed as previously described (23).

Cytokine Measurement by ELISA

Splenocytes from EAE mice were prepared and cultured in triplicates in RPMI 1640 supplemented with 10% fetal bovine serum (Thermo Fisher Scientific) and stimulated with 25 μg/ml MOG_{35-55} for 3 days. Cell-free supernatants were harvested and analyzed for IFN-γ, IL-17, GM-CSF, IL-5, and IL-10 by ELISA Kits (R&D Systems).

Mononuclear Cell (MNC) Preparation

Splenocytes of EAE mice were mechanically pushing spleen tissue through a 70 μm strainer (Falcon, Tewksbury, MA, USA) and treated with red blood cell (RBC) lysis buffer (Biolegend, San Diego, CA, USA) for 60 s. Collected cells were flushed with pre-cold PBS before stimulation. To collect MNC from CNS tissue, brain and spinal cords were administered with Liberase (Roche, Nutley, NJ, USA) for half hour and dissociated through a 70 μm strainer and flushed with pre-cold PBS. Cells were then separated by 70/30% percoll (Sigma-Aldrich) gradient method following previously described (26).

In Vitro T Cell Polarization

Polarization of Th1, Th17, and Treg cells was induced *in vitro* following a previously described method (4). Naive 8-week-old female C57BL/6 mice were sacrificed and spleen tissue was dissociated to single cell. Mouse CD4 microbeads (Miltenyi Biotech Inc.) were used to purify the $CD4^+$ T cells. Then, cells were cultured for 3 days under their respective polarizing conditions (27). Cells were stimulated for 3 days and examined on FACSAria (BD Biosciences).

Flow Cytometry Analysis

For cell surface staining, fluorochrome-conjugated Abs to CD4 (BD Biosciences, San Jose, CA, USA) or isotype control Abs were added to cells for 30 min. For all intracellular staining, CNS-infiltrating MNCs or splenocytes were stimulated for 5 h with phorbol 12-myristate 13 acetate (50 ng/ml), ionomycin (500 ng/ml) (Sigma-Aldrich), and GolgiPlug (BD Biosciences). The staining procedure was performed following a previously described protocol (4). Data were analyzed with FlowJo software (Treestar, Ashland, OR, USA).

Quantitative PCR

Total RNA from T cells or microglia cells was extracted by RNeasy Plus Mini Kit (QIAGEN, Valencia, CA, USA). cDNA was synthesized with QuantiTect Reverse Transcription Kit (QIAGEN). Quantitative PCR was performed in ABI Prism 7500 Sequence Detection System (Applied Biosystems, Foster City, CA, USA) using QuantiFast SYBR Green PCR Kit (QIAGEN). All experiments involving mRNA levels were normalized to glyceraldehyde 3-phosphate dehydrogenase and primers that were based on published cDNA sequences are listed in Table S2 in Supplementary Material.

Western Blot

T cells were activated on 24-well plate under Th17 differentiation condition w/o carnosol 10 μg/ml for 18 h and were then collected. Cells were lysed by cell lysis buffer (Cell Signaling Technology, Danvers, MA, USA) supplemented with 1 mM phenylmethylsulfonyl fluoride (Cell Signaling Technology). All samples containing 15 μg total proteins were separated by 10% SDS-PAGE and transferred to polyvinylidene difluoride membrane (Pierce Chemical, Rockford, IL, USA). Membranes were blocked with 5% (w/v) nonfat dry milk powder in Tris-buffered saline (TBS) for 2 h at room temperature. This was followed by incubation at 4°C overnight with primary antibodies. Afterward, the membrane was washed three times in TBS plus Tween and incubated with the corresponding secondary antibodies (Cell Signaling Technology). The protein band was detected using Pierce ECL Western Blotting Substrate (Thermo Fisher Scientific, Waltham, MA, USA).

Statistical Analysis

Data were analyzed using GraphPad Prism 6 software (GraphPad, La Jolla, CA, USA), and are presented as the mean ± SD. Significant differences in comparing multiple groups, data were analyzed by Tukey's multiple comparisons test. All other statistical comparisons were done using nonparametric statistical tests. Differences with p values of less than 0.05 were considered significant.

RESULTS

Carnosol Treatment Remarkably Alleviated Acute Clinical EAE

We first tested whether carnosol was effective in ameliorating the clinical severity of MOG-induced EAE by scoring disease signs daily on a 0–5 scale. The PBS-treated group of mice showed the first signs of EAE on day 10 p.i., while the carnosol-treated mice did so on day 12 p.i. Further, daily carnosol administration apparently led to decreased disease severity compared to the PBS-treated control group ($p < 0.01$; **Figure 1A**).

We then evaluated pathological changes by histologic analyses in lumbar spinal cords to examine CNS inflammatory infiltration and demyelination at day 30 p.i. As shown in **Figure 1B**, massive inflammatory infiltration and demyelination was observed in the spinal cord of PBS-treated EAE mice; by contrast, the carnosol-treated group displayed mild to moderate signs ($p < 0.0001$; **Figures 1B–D**). These results indicated that carnosol had a significantly suppressive effect in acute EAE.

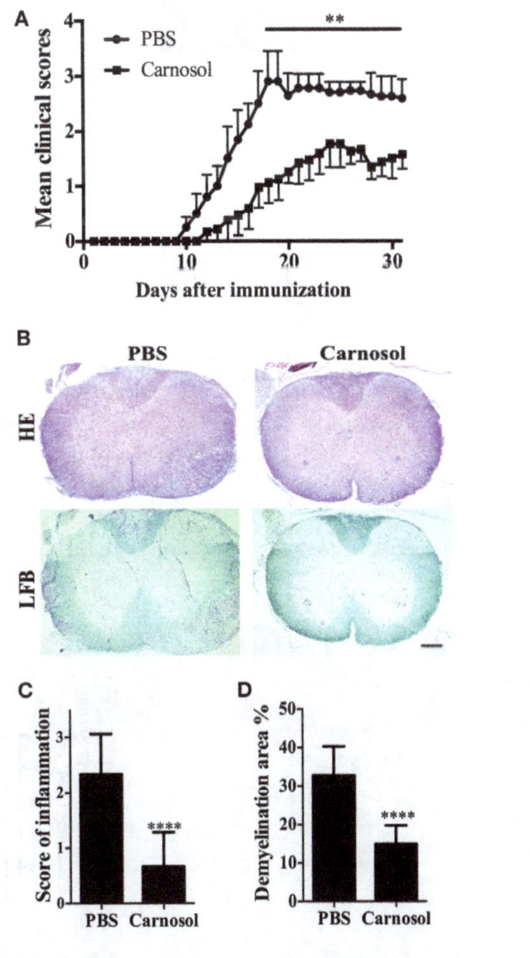

FIGURE 1 | Carnosol ameliorated clinical severity of experimental autoimmune encephalomyelitis (EAE). C57BL/6 mice were injected i.p. with PBS or carnosol (50 mg/kg) daily starting on the day of EAE induction, and scored daily following a 0–5 scale **(A)**. **(B)** Mice were sacrificed at day 30 p.i. and spinal cords were harvested. Sections at lumbar level (L3) were analyzed by H&E and Luxol fast blue (LFB) (scale bar = 1 mm), and pathology scores of inflammation **(C)** and percentage of demyelination area **(D)** were evaluated. Data are mean ± SD (n = 5 each group). $^{**}p < 0.01$ and $^{****}p < 0.0001$, determined by two-way ANOVA **(A)**, or nonparametric test **(C,D)**. One representative of three independent experiments is shown.

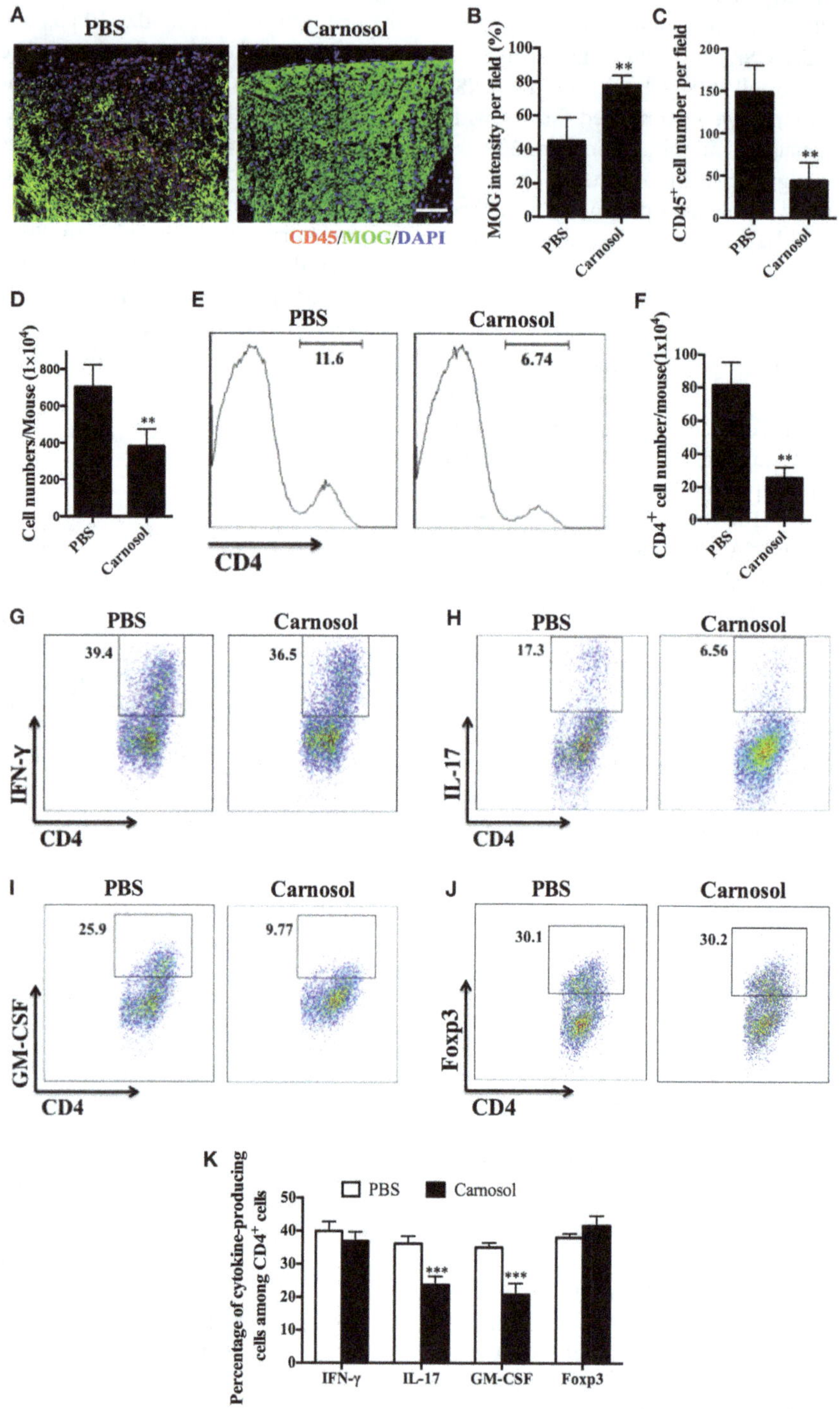

FIGURE 2 | Carnosol treatment suppressed inflammatory infiltration in the central nervous system (CNS). Mice were treated with PBS or carnosol at the day of experimental autoimmune encephalomyelitis induction and sacrificed at day 30 p.i. **(A)** Spinal cords were subjected to immunostaining analysis. **(A)** Representative sections of thoracic spinal cord from PBS- and carnosol-treated mice were stained with CD45 and MOG (scale bar = 100 µm), and the number of $CD45^+$ cells **(B)** and the intensity of MOG staining **(C)** were statistically analyzed. **(D)** Spinal cords and brains were harvested and mononuclear cells (MNCs) isolated (n = 10 each group). Total MNC numbers in CNS were counted under light microscopy. **(E)** The percentage of $CD4^+$ T cells was measured by flow cytometry. **(F)** Absolute numbers of infiltrated $CD4^+$ T were calculated by multiplying the percentages of these cells with total numbers of MNCs in each spinal cord and brain tissue. **(G–J)** Frequencies of IFN-γ^+, IL-17^+, GM-CSF^+, and $Foxp3^+$ cells among $CD4^+$ cells were assessed by flow cytometry, and **(K)** the percentages of these cells in total $CD4^+$ cell numbers in each CNS are shown. Symbols represent mean ± SD (n = 5 each group). $^{**}p < 0.01$ and $^{***}p < 0.001$. Student's t-test. One representative of three independent experiments is shown.

Carnosol Suppressed CNS Inflammation and Modulated Peripheral Immune Response in Acute EAE

To evaluate the therapeutic effects of carnosol on CNS pathology, spinal cords were obtained from carnosol- and PBS-treated EAE mice. Analysis of spinal cord tissue sections showed abundant CD45$^+$ inflammatory cells in the lesion area in the PBS-treated group, while these cells could barely be detected in the spinal cord tissue sections of carnosol-treated mice ($p < 0.01$; **Figures 2A,B**). Correspondingly, there was significantly reduced demyelination (MOG$^-$ area) in carnosol-treated mice compared with the PBS-treated group ($p < 0.01$; **Figures 2A,C**). These results were consistent with the HE and LFB staining, indicating that carnosol inhibited inflammatory cell infiltration and demyelination in the CNS.

To further evaluate the effects of carnosol on the infiltrated inflammatory T cells into the CNS, MNCs were separated from the CNS and analyzed by flow cytometry. The total number of MNCs was 703.8 ± 119.0 × 10^4 per mouse in the PBS-treated group vs. 382.6 ± 93.59 × 10^4 in the carnosol-treated group ($p < 0.01$; **Figure 2D**). In addition, carnosol treatment significantly decreased the percentage and absolute numbers of CD4$^+$ cells in the CNS compared to the PBS-treated control (**Figures 2E,F**). Furthermore, while the percentages of CD4$^+$IFN-γ^+ (Th1) and CD4$^+$Foxp3$^+$ (Treg) cells remained unchanged, percentages of CD4$^+$IL17$^+$, CD4$^+$GM-CSF$^+$, and IFN γ^+IL-17$^+$ cells decreased dramatically after carnosol treatment ($p < 0.001$; **Figures 2G–K**; Figure S1 in Supplementary Material). These results indicate that carnosol may play a significant role in the inhibition of CNS inflammatory infiltration, especially in the pathogenic Th17 cell population.

To study the autoantigen-induced cytokine production in the peripheral immune system of carnosol-treated mice, spleen cells were collected at day 30 p.i. and pulsed with MOG$_{35-55}$. As shown in **Figure 3**, the protein levels of IL-17 and GM-CSF in cell culture supernatants were significantly decreased in the carnosol-treated group, which was consistent with the findings in the CNS infiltrated cells, as shown in **Figures 2G–K**. Overall, our data show that carnosol specifically inhibited the cytokine production of pathogenic Th17 cells.

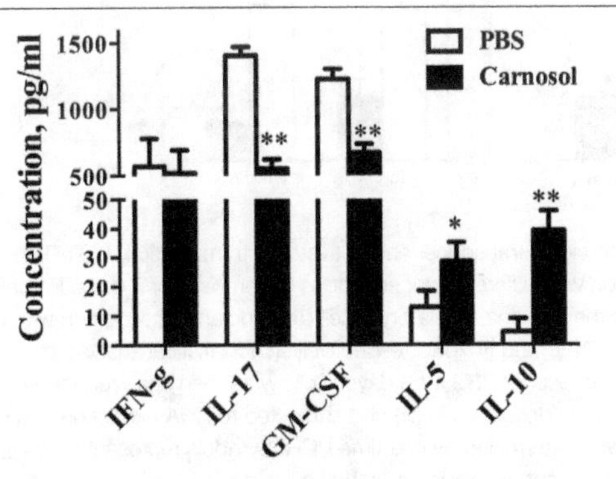

FIGURE 3 | Carnosol treatment decreased inflammation and cytokine production. Mice were treated with PBS or carnosol at the day of experimental autoimmune encephalomyelitis induction and sacrificed at day 30 p.i. as described in **Figure 1A**. Splenocytes were harvested and stimulated with 25 μg/ml MOG$_{35-55}$ for 3 days. Cytokine concentrations in culture supernatants were measured by ELISA. $n = 5$. Symbols represent mean ± SD ($n = 5$ each group). $^*p < 0.05$ and $^{**}p < 0.01$. Nonparametric test. One representative of three independent experiments is shown.

Carnosol Mediated Its Immunomodulation Function by Inhibiting Th17 Cell Differentiation

To clarify the mechanism underlying the effects of carnosol on CD4$^+$ T cell subsets, we defined its function in Th1, Th17, and Treg cell polarization *in vitro*. Under Th17-differentiation condition, about 25% of CD4$^+$ cells were IL-17$^+$ in the PBS group, while carnosol treatment at a dose of 10 μM significantly reduced Th17-polarized (IL-17-producing) CD4$^+$ T cells (25.06 ± 2.13 vs. 4.47 ± 0.52%, $p < 0.01$) (**Figures 4A,D**). In addition, carnosol treatment suppressed Th17 differentiation in a dose-dependent manner. We then investigated the effects of carnosol on Th1 and Treg cell differentiation. In contrast to the findings for Th17 cells, IFN-γ or Foxp3 expression under Th1 or Treg polarizing condition was not significantly affected under carnosol treatment (**Figures 4B–D**). Taken together, these data suggest that carnosol selectively inhibits Th17 polarization.

Carnosol Suppressed STAT3 and NF-κB Phosphorylation, Which Is Required for Th17 Differentiation

Inflammatory cytokine production depends on early events in the NF-κB signaling pathway (28). In order to study the mode of action of carnosol in T cell differentiation, the phosphorylation status of NF-κB was determined by Western blot. p65 phosphorylation at Ser536 regulates its activation and nuclear translocation (29). Results showed that carnosol suppressed cell response by a shift of NF-κBp65 to the cell nucleus, which was demonstrated by the proper shift in the ratio of phosphorylation NF-κB/total NF-κB (**Figures 4E,F**). Further, the pro-inflammatory cytokines in the downstream of NF-κB signal pathway, including IL-2 and TNF-α, were also significantly decreased (**Figure 4H**).

Signal transducer and activator of transcription 3 activities play an important role in the differentiation of Th17 cells. We determined that the basal STAT3 phosphorylation level was significantly decreased. The phosphorylation status at Tyr705 induced nuclear translocation and DNA binding, which promotes IL-17 production (30). Our results showed that carnosol treatment significantly suppressed STAT3 activation (**Figures 4E,G**) and IL-17A and IL-17F production of Th17 cells (**Figure 4I**) compared with the PBS-treated cells. In contrast, similar expression levels were observed for NF-κB and STAT4 phosphorylation in carnosol- and PBS-treated Th1 cells (Figure S2 in Supplementary Material). Together, these results indicate that carnosol may specifically inhibit differentiation of Th17 cells but not Th1 cells.

Carnosol Suppressed Pathogenicity of Th17 Cells in Passive EAE

To assess the effect of carnosol on the encephalitogenicity of Th17 cells, at day 10 p.i., MNCs were collected from lymph

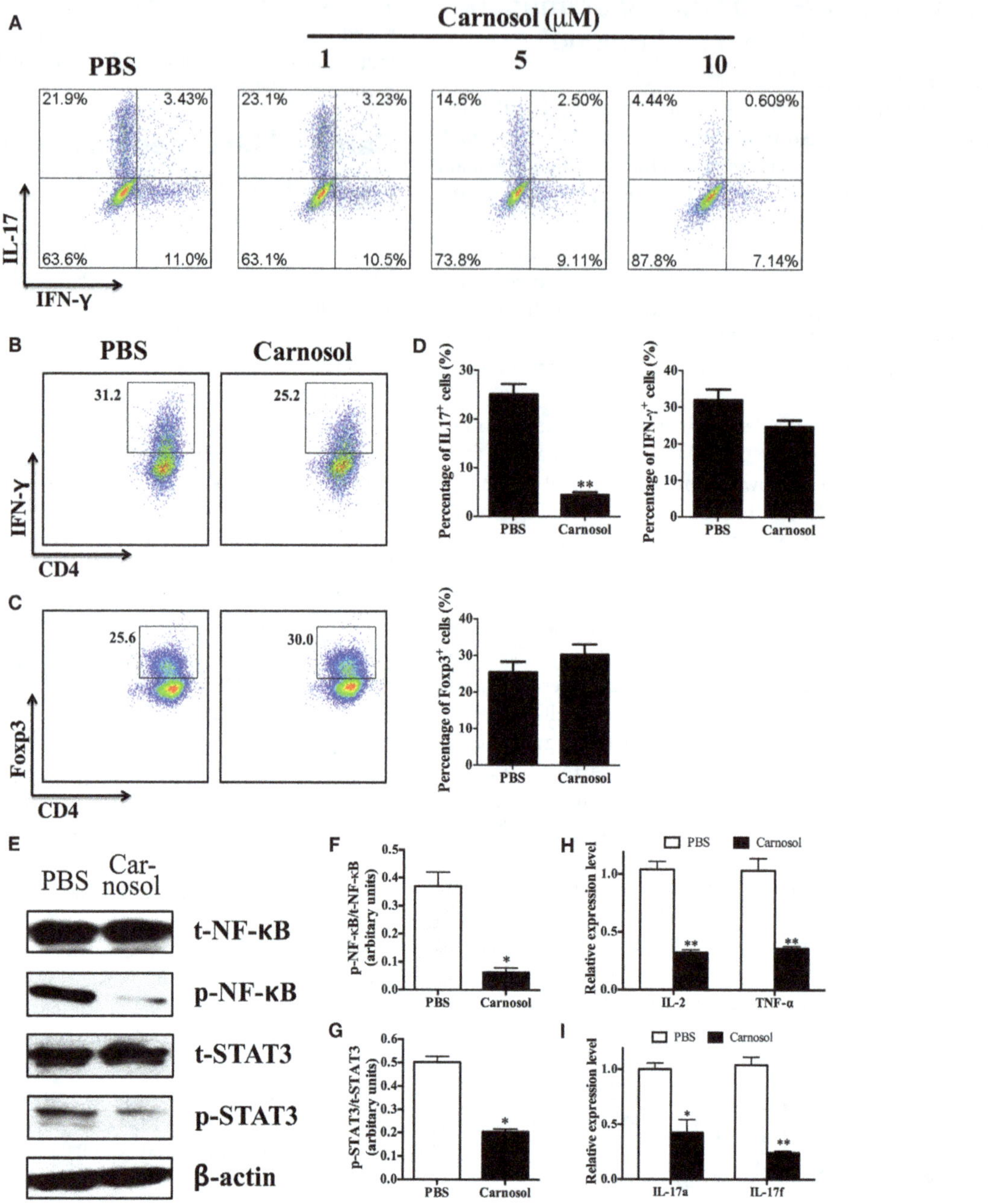

FIGURE 4 | Carnosol suppressed Th17 cell differentiation by blocking the function of NF-κB and signal transducer and activator of transcription 3 (STAT3). **(A)** CD4+ cells were isolated from C57Bl/6 mice and cultured under the Th17 polarizing condition with different concentrations of carnosol for 3 days. Percentage of Th17 cells was analyzed by intracellular staining of IL-17. **(B,C)** CD4+ cells were cultured under the Th1 and regulatory T cell (Treg) polarizing condition with carnosol (10 μM) for 3 days. Percentages of Th1 and Treg cells were analyzed by intracellular staining of IFN-γ+ and Foxp3+, respectively. **(D)** Statistical analysis of **(A–C)**. **(E)** CD4+ T cells were cultured under Th17 polarizing condition and treated with 10 μM carnosol or PBS for 3 days. Cells were then analyzed for NF-κB and STAT3 expression by Western blot. **(F,G)** Statistical analysis of **(E)**. **(H,I)** Cells were harvested as described in **(E)** and subjected to RNA extraction and cDNA production. Expression of pro-inflammation cytokines and IL-17 members (IL-17a and IL-17f) was determined by real-time PCR. Symbols represent mean ± SD (n = 3 each group). *$p < 0.05$ and **$p < 0.01$. Student's t-test. One representative of three independent experiments is shown.

nodes and spleen of IL-17A-IRES-GFP mice (C57BL/6 background), of which IL-17A-producing cells are GFP+ (The Jackson Laboratory, Stock # 018472). Cells were cultured under Th17-polarizing conditions with PBS or carnosol, and stimulated by MOG_{35-55} (20 μg/ml). After 3 days of culture, CD4+ T cells were separated and i.v. injected into naïve C57BL/6 recipient mice. As shown in **Figure 5A**, carnosol-treated T cells transferred significantly reduced clinical disease compared to the PBS-treated group ($p < 0.01$). Mice were sacrificed after 20 days, and brain tissues from different groups were collected

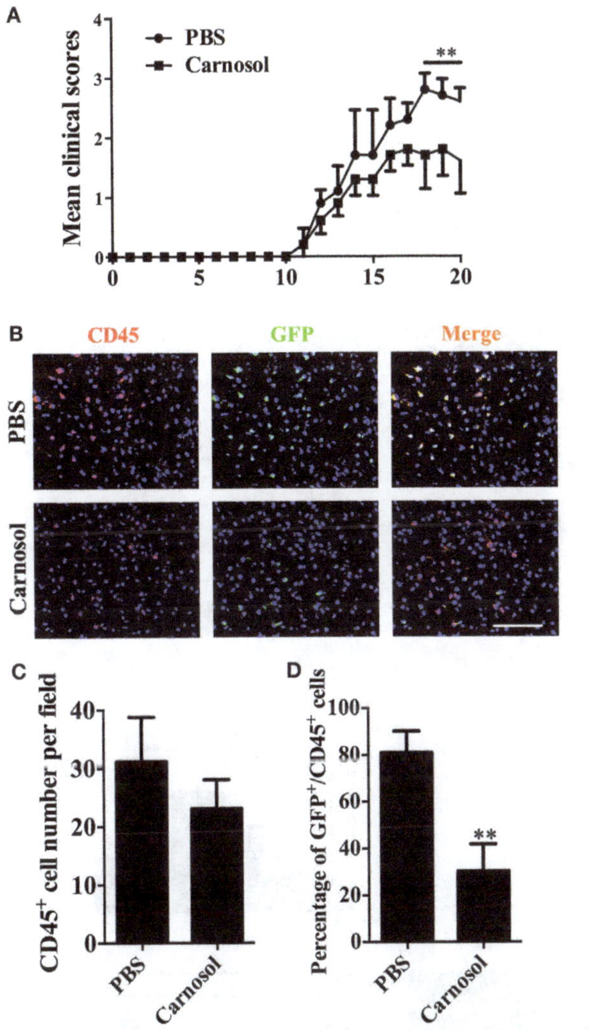

FIGURE 5 | Carnosol decreased clinical severity in an adoptive transfer model of experimental autoimmune encephalomyelitis (EAE). For adoptive transfer EAE, single-cell suspensions were derived from spleen and lymph nodes of IL-17A-IRES-GFP EAE mice at day 10 p.i. MOG (25 μg/ml) plus IL-23 (10 ng/ml) and IL-2 (2 ng/ml) were added to cultures in the presence or absence of carnosol (10 μM) for 3 days. 1×10^6 CD4 T cells were i.v. injected to the recipient mice. **(A)** Mean clinical score of adoptive transfer EAE (mean ± SD; $n = 5$ each group). **$p < 0.01$, Two-way ANOVA with Sidak test. **(B)** Mice were sacrificed at day 20 after cell transfer, and brains were subjected to immunostaining analysis of $CD45^+$ and GFP^+ cells (marker for Th17 cells). Statistical analyses of total $CD45^+$ cell numbers **(C)** and the percentage of GFP^+CD45^+ cell **(D)** for staining in **(B)** are shown. Scale bar = 100 μm. Symbols represent mean ± SD ($n = 5$ each group) **$p < 0.01$, determined by two-way ANOVA **(A)**, or nonparametric test **(C,D)**. One representative of two independent experiments is shown.

for immunohistochemistry. Results showed similar $CD45^+$ cell numbers in the tissue; however, in the CNS, the percentages of $GFP^+/CD45^+$ cells in the carnosol-treated group were markedly reduced compared with the PBS-treated group ($p < 0.01$; **Figures 5B–D**). These *in vivo* results further demonstrated a suppression function of carnosol on the encephalitogenicity of MOG-reactive Th17 cells.

Carnosol Alleviated Clinical Disease When Treatment Started at Chronic Stage of EAE

To further explore the therapeutic effects of carnosol, the chronic EAE model was used in this study. Mice were treated starting from day 25 p.i., when CNS demyelination and chronic tissue damage were already established. While clinical scores in the PBS-injected mice remained at 2.5–3.0, the disease was significantly alleviated in the carnosol-treated group after 10 days of treatment ($p < 0.01$–0.001; **Figure 6A**). The results indicate that, compared to the PBS-treated mice, carnosol showed potential for blockade of demyelination and recovery from neurological damage in the CNS, even when treatment was started after the peak of disease.

Compared to acute EAE (e.g., day 25 p.i.), in chronic EAE (e.g., day 60 p.i.; **Figures 6B,C**), rare infiltration inflammation cells were observed in the white matter of both PBS- and carnosol-treated mice, suggesting that neuroinflammation is no longer the major pathogenesis in the chronic stage (23). On the other hand, while PBS-treated EAE mice tended to have more severe demyelination, as shown by LFB and MBP staining, the demyelination area was obviously decreased in carnosol-treated mice compared to PBS-treated control mice. Increased MBP expression after carnosol treatment compared to that before treatment (day 25 p.i.) suggests that carnosol might induce myelin protein regeneration (**Figures 6D–G**).

Carnosol Promoted an M1/M2 Phenotype Shift of Macrophage/Microglia

Given that microglia/infiltrating macrophages with the activated type 1 phenotype (M1) have a significant role in CNS inflammation during EAE chronicity, whereas type 2 phenotype (M2) cells are immunomodulatory and promyelinating (31, 32), we determined the effects of carnosol on these cells in the CNS tissues of EAE mice that were euthanized after 60 days p.i. The number of M1 microglia/infiltrating macrophages ($iNOS^+CD68^+$) was decreased and an increase in M2 ($Arg1^+CD68^+$) phenotype was observed in carnosol-treated mice compared to PBS-treated control (**Figures 7A–D**). These results indicated that, at least partially, carnosol inhibited demyelination and promoted myelin recovery through inhibiting M1 microglia and switching them to M2. To further confirm this hypothesis, primary microglia were cultured with or without carnosol. Carnosol effectively inhibited production of important mediators of microglia activation, e.g., TNF-α (**Figure 7E**), and expression levels of IL-1β, NOSII, and TNF-α were also significantly decreased (**Figure 7F**). These results indicated that carnosol inhibits the infiltration of M1 phenotype microglia and switches it to a promyelinating and immunoregulatory M2 phenotype that promotes the process of myelin regeneration (32).

DISCUSSION

This work for the first time shows the beneficial effect of carnosol on both acute and chronic stages of EAE. Carnosol significantly decreased inflammatory infiltration into the CNS and the demyelination process, thus halting disease development. The role of

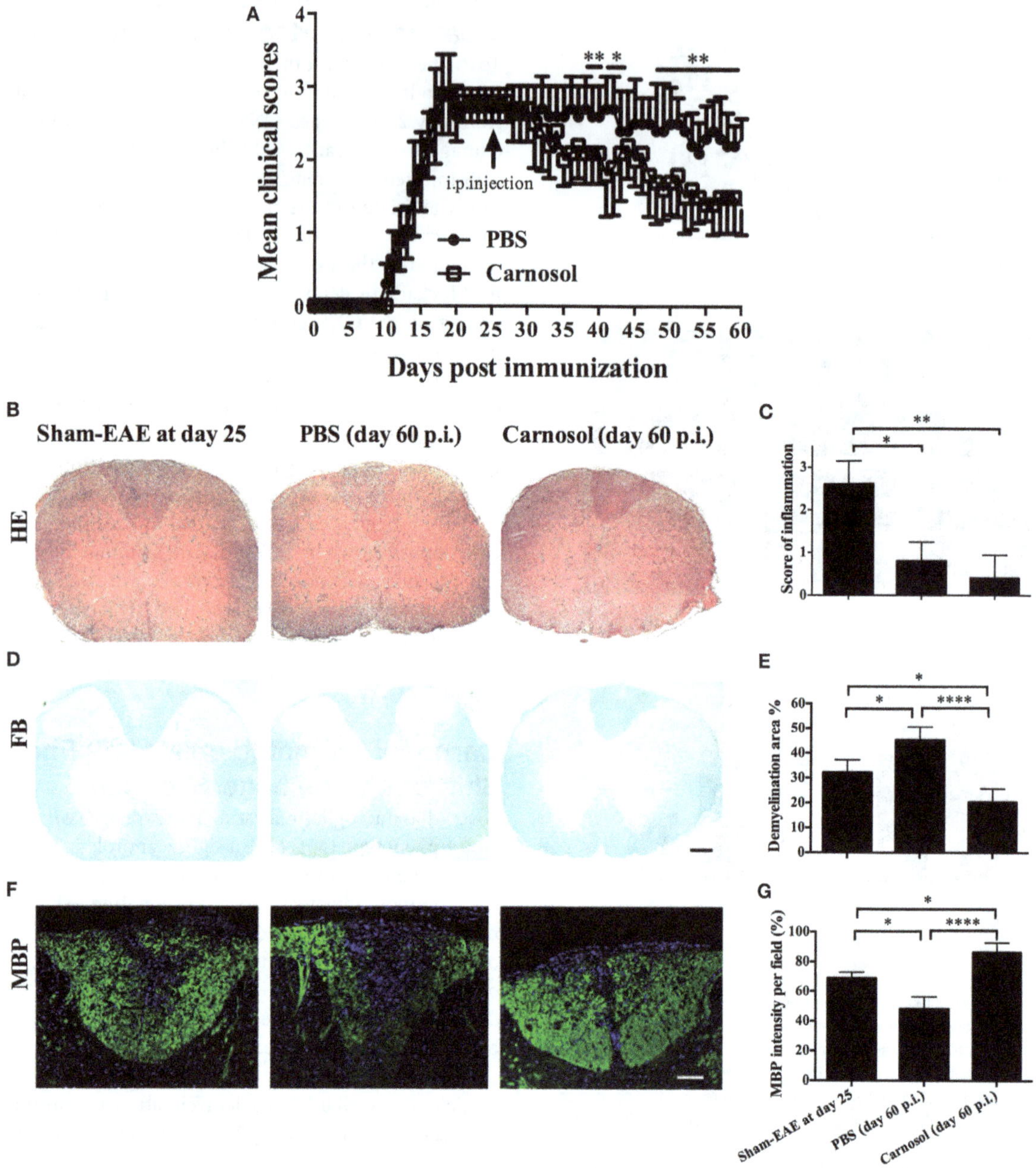

FIGURE 6 | Carnosol treatment alleviated the clinical severity of chronic experimental autoimmune encephalomyelitis (EAE) mice. **(A)** Clinical scores of carnosol- and PBS-treated mice at the chronic stage (treatment starting from day 25 p.i.) of EAE. Mice were sacrificed at day 60 p.i. ($n = 5$ each group), and spinal cords were harvested and evaluated for cell infiltration by H&E staining **(B)**, which was scored on a 0–3 scale **(C)**, and for demyelination by Luxol fast blue **(D)**. **(E)** Demyelination area was measured using Image-Pro Plus software. **(F)** Sections of lumbar spinal cord from **(A)** were assayed for demyelination by MBP staining. **(G)** Quantitative analysis of MBP expression. MBP intensity was measured in the lesion areas in the lumbar spinal cord using Image-Pro. Data represent mean ± SD ($n = 10$ each group). Scale bar = 1 mm **(B,D)** or 100 µm **(F)**. $^*p < 0.05$, $^{**}p < 0.01$, and $^{****}p < 0.0001$. Student's *t*-test. One representative of three independent experiments is shown.

carnosol in acute EAE is primarily due to its inhibitory effect on Th17 cell differentiation, CNS infiltration, and encephalitogenicity, in which the STAT3 signaling pathway plays an important role. Further, the shift of microglia/infiltrated macrophage phenotype from a pro-inflammatory (M1) to an immunoregulatory one (M2) may be an important mechanism underlying the therapeutic effect of carnosol on the chronic stage of EAE.

Carnosol, an ortho-diphenolic of abietane-type diterpene-lactone, consists of an abietane carbon skeleton with hydroxyl groups at positions C-11 and C-12 and a lactone moiety across the B ring (18). Carnosol showed a broad range of physiological benefits and bio-pharmacological effects, as well as exerted strong anti-oxidant, anti-cancer, and neuroprotection effects (17, 20). Furthermore, carnosol was reported to exert anti-inflammatory

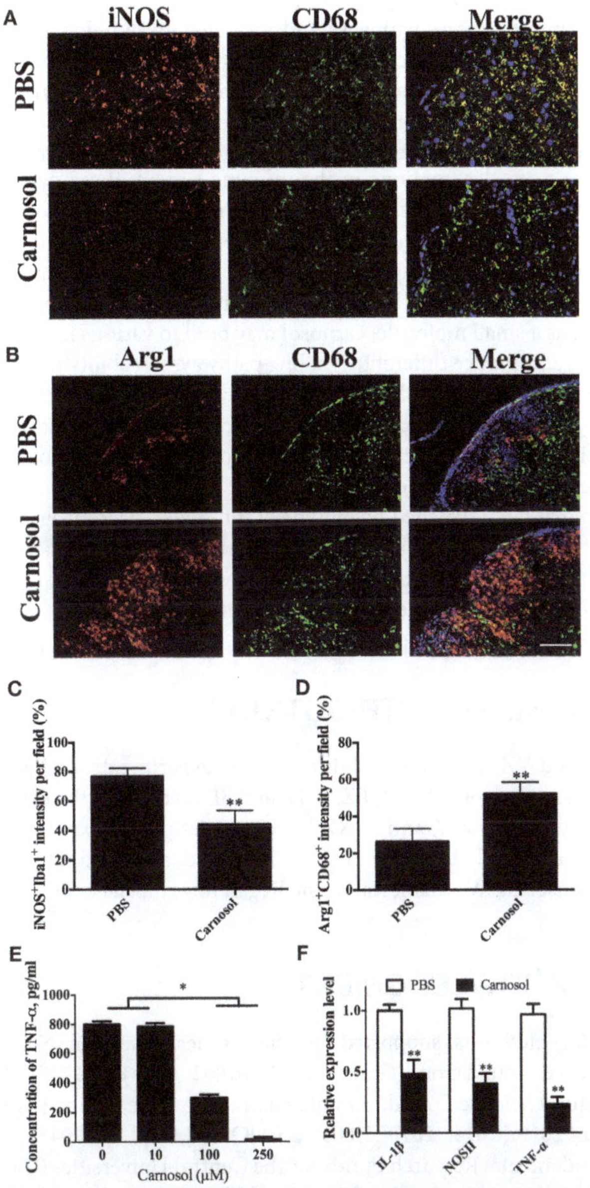

FIGURE 7 | Carnosol promoted an M2 phenotype in macrophages/microglia. Spinal cords of mice described in **Figure 6** were stained for markers for M1 [iNOS; **(A)**] and M2 [Arg-1; **(B)**] on microglia/infiltrating macrophages ($CD68^+$ cells). **(C,D)** Quantitative analysis of the percentages of double positive cells. **(E,F)** Primary microglia were prepared from newborn B6 mice, stimulated with LPS (100 ng/ml), and treated with carnosol at different concentrations for 2 days and **(E)** supernatants were harvested for TNF-α production and **(F)** cells were collected for expression levels of IL-1β, NOSII, and TNF-α by real-time PCR. Glyceraldehyde 3-phosphate dehydrogenase was used as an internal control. Scale bar = 100 μm. Data are shown as mean values ± SD ($n = 5$ each group). ANOVA with Tukey's multiple comparisons test was used. $^*p < 0.05$ and $^{**}p < 0.01$. One representative of three independent experiments is shown.

effects by reducing cytokine release (e.g., IL-1, IL-6) and iNOS formation (18). Also, carnosol, as an anti-inflammatory and anti-oxidant agent, has been considered as a potentially promising therapeutic drug for many incurable diseases, such as neurodegeneration, cancer, and cardiovascular disorders (33, 34). However, the mechanism underlying these functions has not been completely elucidated. Although it has already been shown that carnosol stimulates the MAPKs signaling pathway and down-regulates multiple transcription factors, including NF-κB as well as pro-inflammation protein such as COX-2 level (35–37), to our knowledge, this is the first study to show that carnosol treatment leads to an inhibition in Th17 differentiation and that it modulates microglial switch.

The major challenge for the clinical application of natural compounds is determining their detailed molecular mechanism (4). Indeed, the mechanism of carnosol's action on T helper cell differentiation in autoimmune disease remains largely unknown. It has been suggested that carnosol suppresses inflammation by targeting NF-κB signaling (37, 38), whose activation has been found in MS brain lesions (39, 40) and peripheral blood (41), as well as in the development of EAE (42, 43). Further, IL-17 plays a key role in the pathogenesis of MS and EAE (9, 44). Specifically, activated STAT3 is considered to be necessary for IL-17 production in mouse and human Th17 cells (45, 46). STAT3 controls various genes that contribute to the Th17 population cells including the IL-17 locus itself (47), and binds to genes encoding transcription factors that are critical for Th17 polarization, including Rorc, Irf4, and Batf (48). In our study, carnosol altered the level of Th17 lineage-associated cytokine IL-17. This finding suggests that carnosol inhibits polarization of T cells into Th17 cells, which may be due to carnosol's ability to diminish Th17-associated cytokines by targeting the NF-κB signaling pathway. In response to cytokines, STAT3 is phosphorylated by receptor-associated Janus kinases and forms homo- or heterodimers that translocate to the cell nucleus, where they act as transcription activators. Here, we show that carnosol suppressed STAT3 phosphorylation at the site of tyrosine 705, in response to the ligand IL-6. These findings further identified the mechanism of carnosol through suppressed NF-κB and STAT3 phosphorylation to block Th17 differentiation.

We have further identified the therapeutic effects of carnosol on chronic stage of EAE, and investigated the involvement of M1/M2 microglia shift as a potential mechanism of its action. Persistent CNS inflammation, particularly the activation of infiltrated macrophage/microglia, is recognized to be a crucial mechanism underlying EAE chronicity (49). Pro-inflammatory cytokines, including IL-1β, IL-6, and TNF-α, were secreted by these inflammatory cells, which, together with the accumulation of neurodegeneration inhibitors, form a hostile microenvironment against remyelination and neural repair (24). Therefore, diminishing the inflammatory cytokines of the CNS niche and promoting its change to a supportive environment for neural repair and remyelination will be helpful for treatment. Here, we showed that carnosol suppressed infiltrated macrophage/microglia activation both in EAE mice *in vivo* and microglia culture *in vitro*. A shift from M1 to M2 phenotype was observed following carnosol treatment. Previous studies indicated that carnosol reduced LPS-induced iNOS mRNA and protein expression. Administration of carnosol resulted in a reduction of nuclear factor-kappa B (NF-κB) subunit translocation and

NF-κB DNA binding activity in activated macrophages (50). Further experimental data added proof that carnosol blockades the IL-1β induced nuclear translocation of NF-κBp65, indicating that it mainly regulates through the NF-κB signaling (38). These findings were consistent with our results and indicated that carnosol could switch infiltrated macrophages/microglia from M1 to M2 phenotype and may play an essential role in myelin protein recovery.

One of the major mechanisms contributing to the chronic progression in MS is loss of neurotrophic factor support for both oligodendrocytes and neurons, resulting in persistent damage to CNS tissue damage, i.e., demyelination, axonal degeneration, and neuronal dysfunction (23). Exploring a novel medicine that both targets neuroinflammation and promotes neuroregeneration will, therefore, be of great value. Recently, Wang et al. showed the protective role of carnosol against spinal cord injury (37). This study led us to determine whether carnosol has a neuroprotective function in demyelinating disease. In the present study, we observed that carnosol blocks demyelination by means of the M1/M2 switch. However, no significant differences were observed in OPC differentiation *in vitro* or in the cuprizone-induced demyelination model (data not shown). This finding may illustrate that the underlying mechanism of carnosol-induced recovery in EAE mice is not due to its direct effect on oligodendrocyte differentiation/maturation, but rather an indirect effect through immunomodulation and reduced CNS inflammation and the M1/M2 switch, thus providing a supportive microenvironment for neural cells.

Although we demonstrated the efficacy of carnosol treatment of EAE, the immunomodulatory mechanism is not clear. We showed that carnosol could suppress IL-17 and GM-CSF production of splenocytes, but we also found that carnosol exerts its anti-inflammatory effect on microglia. Increasing evidence shows that carnosol can cross the blood–brain barrier (BBB) as a neuroprotective agent. We, therefore, provide compelling evidence supporting an effective role of carnosol in inhibiting Th17 cell differentiation in the periphery and modulating microglia phenotype by penetrating the BBB in the CNS.

In addition, a previous study showed that carnosol has antitumor capacity through prevention of Treg cell differentiation, decreasing IL-4 and IL-10 production, and enhancing IFN-γ secretion in tumor-associated lymphocyte populations (51). Tumor Tregs are a highly heterogeneous population that arises through disparate pathways and mediates immunologic effects by various means including soluble cytokines (52). An explanation of the principal mechanism of their increase would include a reaction to autoimmunity, tumor-specific factors, and control of inflammation. Although autoimmune disease and cancer both arise from dysfunctions in the immune system, these dysfunctions are extremely different. This phenomenon depends on the complex *in vivo* process and is also due to the different molecule target. Although it appears paradoxical that carnosol has antitumor capacity and the ability to suppress EAE, we hypothesize that as a small molecule, carnosol may bind to various molecular sites and induce different signaling pathways, an ability that may be determined by different microenvironments.

In summary, the present study demonstrates that carnosol ameliorated clinical severity of acute and chronic EAE. We propose that these effects are due to the inhibition of Th17 cell polarization and a remarkably switched phenotype of infiltrated macrophages and activated microglia. Taken together, our data indicate that carnosol is a natural molecule that has potential for the treatment of MS, and likely for autoimmune diseases in general.

AUTHOR CONTRIBUTIONS

XL and YZ conceived and designed the experiments, and wrote the manuscript. XL, LZ, FZ, J-JH, and SL carried out the experiments. LZ, Z-ZW, and G-XZ helped to design the experiments and analyzed data. All authors read and approved the final manuscript. We thank Katherine Regan for editorial assistance.

ACKNOWLEDGMENTS

This study was supported by the Chinese National Natural Science Foundation (Grant no. 81501062 and 81771345), the Natural Science Foundation of Shaanxi Province, China (Grant No. 2019ZC014, 2018JZ3001, 2018JQ8033, and 2017043), the Fundamental Research Funds for the Central Universities (Grant No. GK201802010, GK201703079, GK201701009, 2017CSZ007, and 2017CSY021). We thank Katherine Regan for editorial assistance.

REFERENCES

1. Yang CL, Or TC, Ho MH, Lau AS. Scientific basis of botanical medicine as alternative remedies for rheumatoid arthritis. *Clin Rev Allergy Immunol* (2013) 44(3):284–300. doi:10.1007/s12016-012-8329-8
2. Lassmann H, Bradl M. Multiple sclerosis: experimental models and reality. *Acta Neuropathol* (2017) 133(2):223–44. doi:10.1007/s00401-016-1631-4
3. Yshii LM, Hohlfeld R, Liblau RS. Inflammatory CNS disease caused by immune checkpoint inhibitors: status and perspectives. *Nat Rev Neurol* (2017) 13(12):755–63. doi:10.1038/nrneurol.2017.144
4. Zhang Y, Li X, Ciric B, Ma CG, Gran B, Rostami A, et al. Therapeutic effect of baicalin on experimental autoimmune encephalomyelitis is mediated by SOCS3 regulatory pathway. *Sci Rep* (2015) 5:17407. doi:10.1038/srep17407
5. El-Behi M, Ciric B, Dai H, Yan Y, Cullimore M, Safavi F, et al. The encephalitogenicity of T(H)17 cells is dependent on IL-1- and IL-23-induced production of the cytokine GM-CSF. *Nat Immunol* (2011) 12(6):568–75. doi:10.1038/ni.2031
6. Annunziato F, Romagnani C, Romagnani S. The 3 major types of innate and adaptive cell-mediated effector immunity. *J Allergy Clin Immunol* (2015) 135(3):626–35. doi:10.1016/j.jaci.2014.11.001
7. Sutton CE, Lalor SJ, Sweeney CM, Brereton CF, Lavelle EC, Mills KH. Interleukin-1 and IL-23 induce innate IL-17 production from gammadelta T cells, amplifying Th17 responses and autoimmunity. *Immunity* (2009) 31(2):331–41. doi:10.1016/j.immuni.2009.08.001
8. Oukka M. Interplay between pathogenic Th17 and regulatory T cells. *Ann Rheum Dis* (2007) 66(Suppl 3):iii87–90. doi:10.1136/ard.2007.078527
9. Xiao X, Shi X, Fan Y, Wu C, Zhang X, Minze L, et al. The costimulatory receptor OX40 inhibits interleukin-17 expression through activation of repressive chromatin remodeling pathways. *Immunity* (2016) 44(6):1271–83. doi:10.1016/j.immuni.2016.05.013

10. Zhao M, Tan Y, Peng Q, Huang C, Guo Y, Liang G, et al. IL-6/STAT3 pathway induced deficiency of RFX1 contributes to Th17-dependent autoimmune diseases via epigenetic regulation. *Nat Commun* (2018) 9(1):583. doi:10.1038/s41467-018-02890-0
11. Filippini G, Del Giovane C, Clerico M, Beiki O, Mattoscio M, Piazza F, et al. Treatment with disease-modifying drugs for people with a first clinical attack suggestive of multiple sclerosis. *Cochrane Database Syst Rev* (2017) 4:Cd012200. doi:10.1002/14651858.CD012200.pub2
12. Hemmer B, Muhlau M. Multiple sclerosis in 2016: immune-directed therapies in MS – efficacy and limitations. *Nat Rev Neurol* (2017) 13(2):72–4. doi:10.1038/nrneurol.2017.2
13. Wei CB, Tao K, Jiang R, Zhou LD, Zhang QH, Yuan CS. Quercetin protects mouse liver against triptolide-induced hepatic injury by restoring Th17/Treg balance through Tim-3 and TLR4-MyD88-NF-kappaB pathway. *Int Immunopharmacol* (2017) 53:73–82. doi:10.1016/j.intimp.2017.09.026
14. Thome R, de Carvalho AC, Alves da Costa T, Ishikawa LL, Fraga-Silva TF, Sartori A, et al. Artesunate ameliorates experimental autoimmune encephalomyelitis by inhibiting leukocyte migration to the central nervous system. *CNS Neurosci Ther* (2016) 22(8):707–14. doi:10.1111/cns.12561
15. Kan QC, Zhang HJ, Zhang Y, Li X, Xu YM, Thome R, et al. Matrine treatment blocks NogoA-induced neural inhibitory signaling pathway in ongoing experimental autoimmune encephalomyelitis. *Mol Neurobiol* (2017) 54(10):8404–18. doi:10.1007/s12035-016-0333-1
16. Liu M, Zhou X, Zhou L, Liu Z, Yuan J, Cheng J, et al. Carnosic acid inhibits inflammation response and joint destruction on osteoclasts, fibroblast-like synoviocytes, and collagen-induced arthritis rats. *J Cell Physiol* (2018) 233(8):6291–303. doi:10.1002/jcp.26517
17. Bendif H, Boudjeniba M, Djamel Miara M, Biqiku L, Bramucci M, Caprioli G, et al. *Rosmarinus eriocalyx*: an alternative to *Rosmarinus officinalis* as a source of antioxidant compounds. *Food Chem* (2017) 218:78–88. doi:10.1016/j.foodchem.2016.09.063
18. Kashyap D, Kumar G, Sharma A, Sak K, Tuli HS, Mukherjee TK. Mechanistic insight into carnosol-mediated pharmacological effects: recent trends and advancements. *Life Sci* (2017) 169:27–36. doi:10.1016/j.lfs.2016.11.013
19. Oliviero F, Scanu A, Zamudio-Cuevas Y, Punzi L, Spinella P. Anti-inflammatory effects of polyphenols in arthritis. *J Sci Food Agri* (2017) 98(5):1653–9. doi:10.1002/jsfa.8664
20. de Oliveira MR. The dietary components carnosic acid and carnosol as neuroprotective agents: a mechanistic view. *Mol Neurobiol* (2016) 53(9):6155–68. doi:10.1007/s12035-015-9519-1
21. Samarghandian S, Borji A, Farkhondeh T. Evaluation of antidiabetic activity of carnosol (phenolic diterpene in Rosemary) in streptozotocin-induced diabetic rats. *Cardiovasc Hematol Disord Drug Targets* (2017) 17(1):11–7. doi:10.2174/1871529X16666161229154910
22. Ishida Y, Yamasaki M, Yukizaki C, Nishiyama K, Tsubouchi H, Okayama A, et al. Carnosol, rosemary ingredient, induces apoptosis in adult T-cell leukemia/lymphoma cells via glutathione depletion: proteomic approach using fluorescent two-dimensional differential gel electrophoresis. *Human Cell* (2014) 27(2):68–77. doi:10.1007/s13577-013-0083-6
23. Li X, Zhang Y, Yan Y, Ciric B, Ma CG, Gran B, et al. Neural stem cells engineered to express three therapeutic factors mediate recovery from chronic stage CNS autoimmunity. *Mol Ther* (2016) 24(8):1456–69. doi:10.1038/mt.2016.104
24. Li X, Zhang Y, Yan Y, Ciric B, Ma CG, Chin J, et al. LINGO-1-Fc-transduced neural stem cells are effective therapy for chronic stage experimental autoimmune encephalomyelitis. *Mol Neurobiol* (2017) 54(6):4365–78. doi:10.1007/s12035-016-9994-z
25. Zhang Y, Han JJ, Liang XY, Zhao L, Zhang F, Rasouli J, et al. miR-23b suppresses leukocyte migration and pathogenesis of experimental autoimmune encephalomyelitis by targeting CCL7. *Mol Ther* (2018) 26(2):582–92. doi:10.1016/j.ymthe.2017.11.013
26. Zhao L, Li X, Ye ZQ, Zhang F, Han JJ, Yang T, et al. Nutshell extracts of *Xanthoceras sorbifolia*: a new potential source of bioactive phenolic compounds as a natural antioxidant and immunomodulator. *J Agric Food Chem* (2018) 66(15):3783–92. doi:10.1021/acs.jafc.7b05590
27. Wang LM, Zhang Y, Li X, Zhang ML, Zhu L, Zhang GX, et al. Nr4a1 plays a crucial modulatory role in Th1/Th17 cell responses and CNS autoimmunity. *Brain Behav Immun* (2018) 68:44–55. doi:10.1016/j.bbi.2017.09.015
28. Visekruna A, Volkov A, Steinhoff U. A key role for NF-kappaB transcription factor c-Rel in T-lymphocyte-differentiation and effector functions. *Clin Dev Immunol* (2012) 2012:239368. doi:10.1155/2012/239368
29. Sasaki CY, Barberi TJ, Ghosh P, Longo DL. Phosphorylation of RelA/p65 on serine 536 defines an I{kappa}B{alpha}-independent NF-{kappa}B pathway. *J Biol Chem* (2005) 280(41):34538–47. doi:10.1074/jbc.M504943200
30. Chaudhry A, Rudra D, Treuting P, Samstein RM, Liang Y, Kas A, et al. CD4+ regulatory T cells control TH17 responses in a Stat3-dependent manner. *Science* (2009) 326(5955):986–91. doi:10.1126/science.1172702
31. Pluchino S, Muzio L, Imitola J, Deleidi M, Alfaro-Cervello C, Salani G, et al. Persistent inflammation alters the function of the endogenous brain stem cell compartment. *Brain* (2008) 131(Pt 10):2564–78. doi:10.1093/brain/awn198
32. Miron VE, Boyd A, Zhao JW, Yuen TJ, Ruckh JM, Shadrach JL, et al. M2 microglia and macrophages drive oligodendrocyte differentiation during CNS remyelination. *Nat Neurosci* (2013) 16(9):1211–8. doi:10.1038/nn.3469
33. Foresti R, Bains SK, Pitchumony TS, de Castro Bras LE, Drago F, Dubois-Rande JL, et al. Small molecule activators of the Nrf2-HO-1 antioxidant axis modulate heme metabolism and inflammation in BV2 microglia cells. *Pharmacol Res* (2013) 76:132–48. doi:10.1016/j.phrs.2013.07.010
34. Giacomelli C, Daniele S, Natali L, Iofrida C, Flamini G. Carnosol controls the human glioblastoma stemness features through the epithelial-mesenchymal transition modulation and the induction of cancer stem cell apoptosis. *Sci Rep* (2017) 7(1):15174. doi:10.1038/s41598-017-15360-2
35. Chen CC, Chen HL, Hsieh CW, Yang YL, Wung BS. Upregulation of NF-E2-related factor-2-dependent glutathione by carnosol provokes a cytoprotective response and enhances cell survival. *Acta Pharmacol Sin* (2011) 32(1):62–9. doi:10.1038/aps.2010.181
36. Martin D, Rojo AI, Salinas M, Diaz R, Gallardo G, Alam J, et al. Regulation of heme oxygenase-1 expression through the phosphatidylinositol 3-kinase/Akt pathway and the Nrf2 transcription factor in response to the antioxidant phytochemical carnosol. *J Biol Chem* (2004) 279(10):8919–29. doi:10.1074/jbc.M309660200
37. Wang ZH, Xie YX, Zhang JW, Qiu XH, Cheng AB, Tian L, et al. Carnosol protects against spinal cord injury through Nrf-2 upregulation. *J Recept Signal Transduct Res* (2016) 36(1):72–8. doi:10.3109/10799893.2015.1049358
38. Schwager J, Richard N, Fowler A, Seifert N, Raederstorff D. Carnosol and related substances modulate chemokine and cytokine production in macrophages and chondrocytes. *Molecules* (2016) 21(4):465. doi:10.3390/molecules21040465
39. Gveric D, Kaltschmidt C, Cuzner ML, Newcombe J. Transcription factor NF-kappaB and inhibitor I kappaBalpha are localized in macrophages in active multiple sclerosis lesions. *J Neuropathol Exp Neurol* (1998) 57(2):168–78. doi:10.1097/00005072-199802000-00008
40. Bonetti B, Stegagno C, Cannella B, Rizzuto N, Moretto G, Raine CS. Activation of NF-kappaB and c-jun transcription factors in multiple sclerosis lesions. Implications for oligodendrocyte pathology. *Am J Pathol* (1999) 155(5):1433–8. doi:10.1016/S0002-9440(10)65456-9
41. Miterski B, Bohringer S, Klein W, Sindern E, Haupts M, Schimrigk S, et al. Inhibitors in the NFkappaB cascade comprise prime candidate genes predisposing to multiple sclerosis, especially in selected combinations. *Genes Immun* (2002) 3(4):211–9. doi:10.1038/sj.gene.6363846
42. Hucke S, Eschborn M, Liebmann M, Herold M, Freise N, Engbers A, et al. Sodium chloride promotes pro-inflammatory macrophage polarization thereby aggravating CNS autoimmunity. *J Autoimmun* (2016) 67:90–101. doi:10.1016/j.jaut.2015.11.001
43. Zhu S, Pan W, Song X, Liu Y, Shao X, Tang Y, et al. The microRNA miR-23b suppresses IL-17-associated autoimmune inflammation by targeting TAB 2, TAB 3 and IKK-alpha. *Nat Med* (2012) 18(7):1077–86. doi:10.1038/nm.2815
44. Patel DD, Kuchroo VK. Th17 cell pathway in human immunity: lessons from genetics and therapeutic interventions. *Immunity* (2015) 43(6):1040–51. doi:10.1016/j.immuni.2015.12.003
45. Chen Z, Laurence A, Kanno Y, Pacher-Zavisin M, Zhu BM, Tato C, et al. Selective regulatory function of Socs3 in the formation of IL-17-secreting T cells. *Proc Natl Acad Sci U S A* (2006) 103(21):8137–42. doi:10.1073/pnas.0600666103
46. Mathur AN, Chang HC, Zisoulis DG, Stritesky GL, Yu Q, O'Malley JT, et al. Stat3 and Stat4 direct development of IL-17-secreting Th cells. *J Immunol*

(2007) 178(8):4901–7. doi:10.4049/jimmunol.178.8.4901

47. Yang XP, Ghoreschi K, Steward-Tharp SM, Rodriguez-Canales J, Zhu J, Grainger JR, et al. Opposing regulation of the locus encoding IL-17 through direct, reciprocal actions of STAT3 and STAT5. *Nat Immunol* (2011) 12(3):247–54. doi:10.1038/ni.1995
48. Durant L, Watford WT, Ramos HL, Laurence A, Vahedi G, Wei L, et al. Diverse targets of the transcription factor STAT3 contribute to T cell pathogenicity and homeostasis. *Immunity* (2010) 32(5):605–15. doi:10.1016/j.immuni.2010.05.003
49. Rasmussen S, Wang Y, Kivisakk P, Bronson RT, Meyer M, Imitola J, et al. Persistent activation of microglia is associated with neuronal dysfunction of callosal projecting pathways and multiple sclerosis-like lesions in relapsing – remitting experimental autoimmune encephalomyelitis. *Brain* (2007) 130(Pt 11): 2816–29. doi:10.1093/brain/awm219
50. Lo AH, Liang YC, Lin-Shiau SY, Ho CT, Lin JK. Carnosol, an antioxidant in rosemary, suppresses inducible nitric oxide synthase through down-regulating nuclear factor-kappaB in mouse macrophages. *Carcinogenesis* (2002) 23(6):983–91. doi:10.1093/carcin/23.6.983
51. Rahnama M, Mahmoudi M, Zamani Taghizadeh Rabe S, Balali-Mood M, Karimi G, Tabasi N, et al. Evaluation of anti-cancer and immunomodulatory effects of carnosol in a Balb/c WEHI-164 fibrosarcoma model. *J Immunotoxicol* (2015) 12(3):231–8. doi:10.3109/1547691X.2014.934975
52. Curiel TJ. Regulatory T cells and treatment of cancer. *Curr Opin Immunol* (2008) 20(2):241–6. doi:10.1016/j.coi.2008.04.008

4

Brain Citrullination Patterns and T Cell Reactivity of Cerebrospinal Fluid-Derived CD4+ T Cells in Multiple Sclerosis

Wolfgang Faigle[1], Carolina Cruciani[1], Witold Wolski[2], Bernd Roschitzki[2], Marco Puthenparampil[1], Paula Tomas-Ojer[1], Carla Sellés-Moreno[1], Thomas Zeis[3], Ivan Jelcic[1], Nicole Schaeren-Wiemers[3], Mireia Sospedra[1†] and Roland Martin[1*†]

[1] Neuroimmunology and MS Research Section, Neurology Clinic, University Zurich, University Hospital Zurich, Zurich, Switzerland, [2] Functional Genomics Center Zurich, ETH Zurich & University of Zurich, Zurich, Switzerland, [3] Neurobiology, Department of Biomedicine, University Hospital Basel, University of Basel, Basel, Switzerland

***Correspondence:**
Roland Martin
roland.martin@usz.ch

† These authors have contributed equally to this work

Immune responses to citrullinated peptides have been described in autoimmune diseases like rheumatoid arthritis (RA) and multiple sclerosis (MS). We investigated the post-translational modification (PTM), arginine to citrulline, in brain tissue of MS patients and controls (C) by proteomics and subsequently the cellular immune response of cerebrospinal fluid (CSF)-infiltrating T cells to citrullinated and unmodified peptides of myelin basic protein (MBP). Using specifically adapted tissue extraction- and combined data interpretation protocols we could establish a map of citrullinated proteins by identifying more than 80 proteins with two or more citrullinated peptides in human brain tissue. We report many of them for the first time. For the already described citrullinated proteins MBP, GFAP, and vimentin, we could identify additional citrullinated sites. The number of modified proteins in MS white matter was higher than control tissue. Citrullinated peptides are considered neoepitopes that may trigger autoreactivity. We used newly identified epitopes and previously reported immunodominant myelin peptides in their citrullinated and non-citrullinated form to address the recognition of CSF-infiltrating CD4+ T cells from 22 MS patients by measuring proliferation and IFN-γ secretion. We did not detect marked responses to citrullinated peptides, but slightly more strongly to the non-modified version. Based on these data, we conclude that citrullination does not appear to be an important activating factor of a T cell response, but could be the consequence of an immune- or inflammatory response. Our approach allowed us to perform a deep proteome analysis and opens new technical possibilities to analyze complex PTM patterns on minute quantities of rare tissue samples.

Keywords: human brain, multiple sclerosis, citrullination, T cell reactivity, autoimmune, proteomics

INTRODUCTION

Citrullination is one of more than 400 known PTMs in human proteins. The enzyme, peptidylarginine deiminase (PADI), is responsible for modifying the amino acid arginine to the amino acid citrulline. PADI is part of an enzyme family with five known members (1), and each of these shows a distinct tissue and substrate specificity. The enzymatic reaction results in the loss of a positive charge of the peptide fragment and a mass increase by 1 Da. The process of deimination is considered irreversible since no citrulline-iminase is known so far (2). Gudman and colleagues described citrullination in the context of diseases and reported and postulated an increase of citrullinated proteins in all inflammatory diseases (3). The effects of citrullination on protein function depend on the location of the protein and the position of the amino acid arginine. Since it removes a positive charge from arginine, it may loosen protein interactions and render them more prone to denaturation and degradation (4, 5). Citrullination plays a role in several physiological mechanisms like skin keratinization, myelin formation/remyelination, gene regulation and immune functions. In specialized cells like neutrophils, histone hypercitrullination is an essential process in the formation of highly decondensed chromatin structures termed neutrophil extracellular traps (NETs), which enable these cells to trap and kill bacteria. During the last 10 years, great attention has been paid to citrullination because of its role in inducing anti-citrullinated proteins/peptide antibodies (ACPA) (6). Involvement of citrullination in various diseases like rheumatoid arthritis (RA), multiple sclerosis (MS), psoriasis, chronic obstructive pulmonary disease (COPD), and Alzheimer has been reported (7). In RA, immune reactivity toward various citrullinated self-proteins and self-peptides like fibrinogen, vimentin, fibrin, collagen type II, α-enolase and its involvement in the disease pathogenesis have been well-established (8).

In MS, a chronic inflammatory demyelinating autoimmune disease of the central nervous system (CNS), the amount of the citrullinated myelin sheath protein myelin basic protein (MBP) is increased in white matter as compared to control brains (9), although these findings remain controversial (10, 11). In MBP that has been purified from MS brain tissue, citrullination of six of the nineteen arginines has been found. Among the myelin components, MBP has been studied in greatest detail due to its importance for inducing experimental autoimmune encephalomyelitis (EAE), a rodent model for MS (12). The identification of $CD4^+$ T cells reactive against epitopes of several myelin proteins has been a consistent finding (12). We had previously described reactivity of peripheral blood T cells against post-translational modifications of autoantigens, specifically against citrullinated peptides, in MS patients (13). These preliminary studies hinted at elevated T cell reactivity against citrullinated MBP and indicated that T cells specific for citrullinated epitopes could escape central immune tolerance (13, 14).

In the last years the focus has shifted from peripheral blood-derived T cells to those that are found within the CNS compartment, i.e. in the brain and cerebrospinal fluid (CSF) (15, 16), since CNS-infiltrating T cells are considered more likely to be relevant than those from the peripheral blood due to their infiltration of the target tissue. Besides MBP, few other proteins including glial fibrillary acidic protein (GFAP), neurogranin, and histone H3 have been described to be citrullinated in MS brain (10, 17).

MATERIAL AND METHODS

Human Brain Tissue Preparation

Tissue Collection

The UK Multiple Sclerosis Tissue Bank (UK Multicenter Research Ethics Committee, MREC/02/2/39 and KEK-ZH-Nr. 2014-0243), funded by the Multiple Sclerosis Society of Great Britain and Northern Ireland (registered charity 207495) supplied all the tissue samples. Tissue samples from white- and gray matter were isolated from 9 control and 15 MS cases. Gray matter samples were from 6 controls and 6 MS cases, white matter samples from 3 controls and 9 MS cases. All brains have been screened by a neuropathologist to confirm the diagnosis of MS and to exclude other confounding pathologies (UK MS Tissue Bank).

Immunohistochemistry

All tissues were analyzed by immunohistochemistry. In order to differentiate between white and gray matter, we stained the tissue with anti-myelin oligodendrocyte glycoprotein antibodies (MOG) and Luxol fast blue (LFB) for myelin as well as anti-HLA-DR for macrophages/microglia. Regions of gray matter, white matter, as well as lesions with active inflammation, areas of remyelination, and demyelinated lesions without active inflammation, could be identified. For LFB staining, LN3 (anti-HLA-DR), and MOG cryostat sections (12 μm) were fixed for 10 min in 4% para-formaldehyde (PFA). Endogenous peroxidase was blocked with 0.6% hydrogen peroxide in PBS or 80% methanol for MOG staining. MOG staining was further delipidated in 100% methanol at −20°C for 8 min. Tissues were blocked with blocking buffer 1% normal donkey serum (NDS), 0.1% Triton, 0.05% Tween in PBS, LN3: 5% NDS, 1% fish skin gelatin 0.3 M glycine in PBS) and incubated with the primary antibodies at 4°C overnight. Secondary biotinylated antibodies were applied for 2 h at room temperature followed by the ABC complex reagent (Vector Labs, Burlingame, California, USA) for 1 h. The color reaction was performed with 3-Amino-9-ethylcarbazole (18). For some sections, counterstaining in hematoxylin was applied for 1 min followed by rinsing the slide in running tap water. For citrulline staining fresh frozen tissue sections were first air-dried for 20 min. before fixing them in methanol at −20°C. Incubation of sections with PBS before and blocking in PBS/10%BSA for 1 h at RT. Incubation with antibody F95 was performed overnight at 4°C. Secondary biotinylated antibody was applied for 1 h at RT followed by the ABC complex reagent (VectorLabs) for 1 h. The color reaction was performed with "ImpactDAB" (VectorLabs) and counterstaining with hematoxylin as described above. Antibodies: LN3 (Abcam, ab190298, 1:250), anti-MOG (Clone Z12, 1:100), anti-citrulline F95 (Millipore, Burlington, Massachusetts, USA). LFB staining was done with cryostat sections (12 μm), fixed for 10 min in 4%

PFA. Sections were washed in PBS (3 × 5 min) and ddH_2O (2 × 1 min), then incubated in 50% ethanol (5 min), 70% ethanol (5 min), 80% ethanol (5 min), and 96% ethanol (5 min). Sections were incubated in 0.1% LFB solution for 20 h at 56°C. Sections were washed in ethanol and ddH_2O and developed in lithium carbonate (0.05% in ddH_2O) for 15 s and 70% ethanol for 1 min at RT. After cresyl violet staining (4 min, RT) sections were differentiated in 96% ethanol (30 s), dehydrated in ethanol and xylol and finally mounted with "Entellan" (Merck Millipore).

Protein Extraction Protocol

We analyzed gray and white matter tissue from post-mortem human brains (control and MS patients) in order to establish a spectral library and protein database of the main protein constituents of the CNS. The characterization of the tissue used for the analysis is illustrated in **Figure 1A**. An overview of samples that were used in the analysis together with medical records is listed in **Supplementary Table 1**. For protein extraction, a barocycler (Barocycler 2320EXT, Pressure BioSciences, Inc, South Easton, MA, USA) was used. Tissue samples of the size of a needle-head (2–3 mg) were put into barocycler 150 μl micro tubes. The tubes were filled with 30 μl of lysis buffer (8 M urea and 0.1 M ammonium-bicarbonate) and complete protease inhibitor cocktail (Roche, Basel, Switzerland) and closed with 150 μl microcaps. After pre-heating the barocycler for 30 min at 33°C, run cycles were performed at 45 kpsi for 60 cycles and 1 min each. Each cycle lasted 50 s at high pressure and 10 s at ambient pressure.

Reduction and alkylation were carried out as follows: Mixing of TCEP [tris (2-carboxyethyl) phosphine] 2.5 mg and IAA (iodoacetamide) 3.7 mg in 50 μl of lysis buffer. A volume of 4.9 μl of this buffer was added to each tube, incubated at 25°C in a thermomixer while shaking at 1,000 rpm and protected from light. By adding lysis buffer, the urea concentration was diluted from 8 to 6 M. Lys-C enzyme digestion was applied to an enzyme to substrate ratio of 1:40. Lys-C (mass spectrometry grade, Wako, Richmond, VA, USA 20 μg/μl) was dissolved in "Milli-Q-water" to a final concentration 4 μg/μl. Digestion was performed in barocycler with 20 kpsi for 45 min. and cycles of 50 s duration at high pressure and 10 s ambient pressure.

A further dilution of urea from 6 to 1.6 M with 0.1 M ammonium-bicarbonate buffer was necessary to achieve trypsin digestion conditions. Trypsin (sequencing grade modified, Promega, Madison, WI, USA) was added to an enzyme to substrate ratio 1:20. The digestion took place for 90 min at 37°C in a barocycler at 20 kpsi and cycle periods of 50 s at high pressure and 10 s at ambient pressure (19). Finally, the solution was transferred to a 1.5 ml Eppendorf tube. The volume was adjusted to 1 ml by adding a 0.1%TFA/3%ACN solution and the reaction was stopped by adding 10% TFA and pH adjusted to a value between pH 2 and 3. The peptides were desalted on solid phase extraction columns (C18/Finisterre, Wicom, Heppenheim, Germany) according to manufacturer protocol. The samples were vacuum concentrated in a "SpeedVac" and the peptides re-dissolved in 3% ACN/0.1% formic acid in a volume of 20–50 μl to a final concentration of 1 μg/μl. Peptide concentration was measured with Nanodrop instrument (Nanodrop 1000,

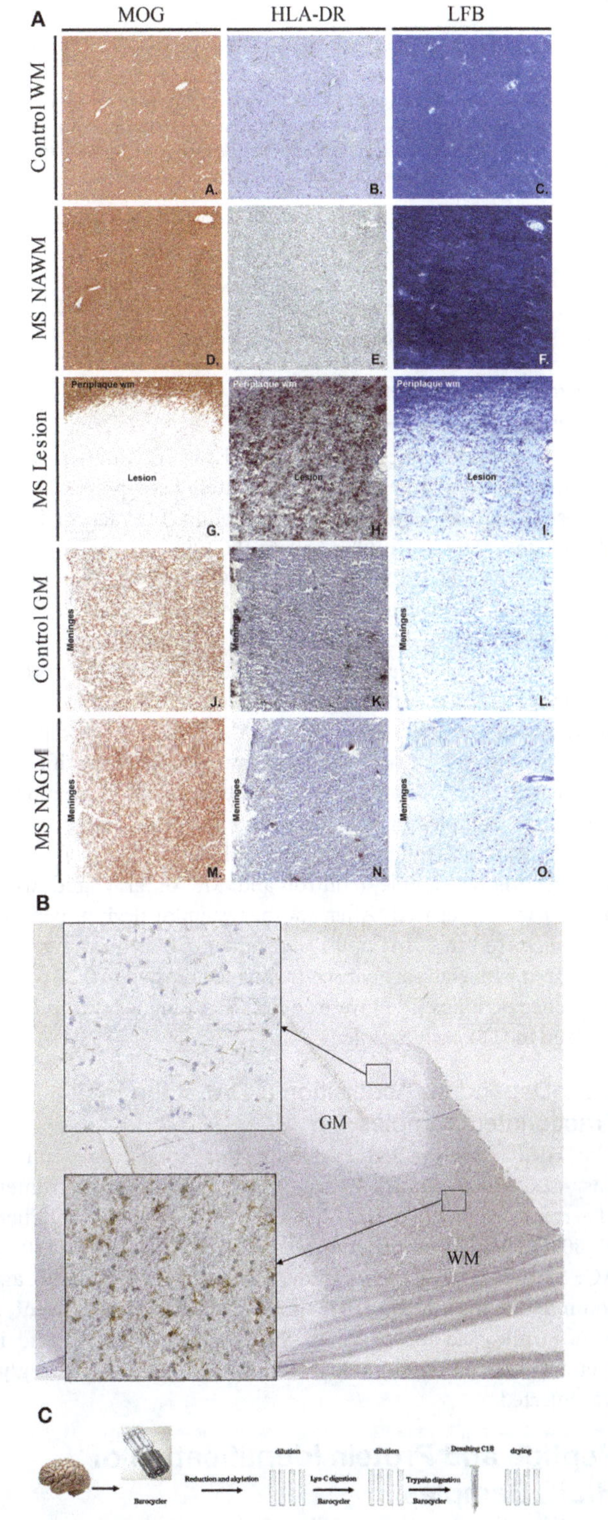

FIGURE 1 | (A) Histopathological examination of control and MS tissue. To identify normal as well as lesioned tissue, tissue blocks containing white as well as gray matter tissue were stained for MOG, HLA-DR, and Luxol Fast-Blue. White and gray Matter control tissue showed no sign of demyelination and inflammation (A–C and J–L). Also, NAWM and NAGM did not show any signs *(Continued)*

FIGURE 1 | of demyelination or inflammation (D–F and M–O). However, MOG as well as LFB staining clearly show demyelination in lesional areas (G and I). Further, a strong HLA-DR staining was visible in lesion tissue (H). **(B)** Citrullination pattern in WM and GM of MS brain (staining with anti-citrulline antibody F95). Inserts showing detail view of corresponding tissue. **(C)** 2–3 mg of brain tissue was disrupted in barocycler and digested by Lys-C and trypsin. All treatments were performed in barocycler instrument. Finally, peptides were desalted and dried.

spectrophotometer (Thermo Scientific, Wilmington, DE, USA) and a solution of a concentration of 0.5 μg/μl prepared.

Hydrophilic Interaction Liquid Chromatography (HILIC)

Pools of peptide samples of control tissue (C), as well as the MS tissues from gray and white matter were prepared (300 μg each) and separated using Hydrophilic Interaction Liquid Chromatography (HILIC) (Agilent LC1200 equipped with a column Polyamin II 250 × 3.0 mm 120 Å, 5 μm). The applied gradient was formed of the two solvents: **A**: 75% ACN, 8 mM KH_2PO_4 and **B**: 5% ACN, 100 mM KH_2PO_4 (pH4.0) for 60 min. Fractions of 1 ml were collected in 27 tubes (detailed protocol as **Figure S2**). To reduce the number of the samples to be analyzed on the mass spectrometer the fractions were pooled from two tubes. Before injection, samples were purified on "Finisterre SPE" columns (Wicom International, Heppenheim, Germany). Samples of 1 ml were vacuum dried and dissolved in an appropriate buffer, 3%ACN/0.1%TFA. In total 11 fractions for each tissue sample (control and MS of gray and white matter) were prepared. After another vacuum drying, peptides were dissolved in 3%ACN/0.1%FA buffer. Concentrations were measured with Nanodrop instrument and adjusted to 0.25 μg/μl. Reference peptides (iRT) were added (iRT, Biognosys, Schlieren, Switzerland) to each sample.

Data-Dependent Acquisition (DDA) of the HILIC Fractionated Samples

The HILIC fractionated samples, 44 in total, were run on Easy-nLC 1000 linked to an Orbitrap Fusion instrument (Thermo Fisher, Waltham, Massachusetts, USA) on a gradient of 80 min. Column material was ReproSil-Pur, C18, 120 Å, AQ, 1.9 μm (Dr. Maisch GmbH, Ammerbuch Germany) and column dimensions ID 0.075 mm/length 150 mm. Solvent A 0.1% formic acid in water and Solvent B 0.15 formic acid in acetonitrile. 4 μl of the sample at a concentration of 0.25 μg/μl was injected.

Peptide and Protein Identification of HILIC Samples

Identification by "Mascot"

We converted "Raw" files converted into "mgf" (20) files and analyzed them on MASCOT software with a human UniProtKB/Swiss-Prot protein database (date: March 22, 2016 with 40,912 entries): Search parameters were 0.05 Da fragment mass tolerance and 10 ppm precursor mass, minimal number of peptides 2, and FDR (false discovery rate) of 0.1%, allowing 2 mis-cleavages on trypsin fragments. We set carbamidomethyl at cysteine as a static modification and oxidation of methionine, deamidation on arginine (R) (with or without neutral loss), glutamine (Q) and asparagine (N) as variable modification. To estimate FDRs separately for deamidated and all the other proteins the mascot.dat files were converted to the bibliospec file format (Skyline).

Peptide Identification With "Ursgal"

The universal python module combining bottom-up proteomics tools for large-scale analysis (Ursgal) was used to perform a search with multiple search engines (xtandem vengeance, msgfplus_v9979 and MyriMatch 2 2 140) (21). Evaluation and post-processing of the search results were performed using percolator_2_08. We adjusted the do_it_all_folder_wide.py "Ursgal" example script (https://ursgal.readthedocs.io/en/latest/example_scripts.html#do-it-all-folder-wide) to our input data. We set the variable and fixed modifications in the same as for "Mascot." For instrument settings, we used the Q-Exactive+ Ursgal profile. We used the "unified_percolator_validated.u_merged_accepted.u_merged.csv" tables (PRIDE), generated by "Ursgal" for further analysis.

Post-translational Modifications, Citrullination and Local False Discovery Rate (FDR) Determination

For each peptide, we selected the best peptide-spectrum match (PSM) according to the lowest PEP- (percolator) or Mascot Ion score. We computed the peptide FDR using the target-decoy approach (22) implemented in the R-package TargetDecoyFDR prozor (https://github.com/protViz/TargetDecoyFDR; https://github.com/protViz/prozor). The FDR was estimated separately for the deamidated and citrullinated peptide sequences and all other sequences. The FDR for deamidated and citrullinated peptide sequences increased much faster than for all other sequences (see **Figure S1**) resulting in a more demanding cutoff score for those sequences. We deposited the mass spectrometry proteomics data in the ProteomeXchange Consortium via the PRIDE (23) partner repository with the dataset identifier PXD008344.

Isolation, Expansion, and Proliferative Testing of T Cells

Peripheral Blood Mononuclear Cell Isolation

Allogeneic peripheral blood mononuclear cells (PBMCs) where isolated freshly from anonymized buffy coats obtained from the Blood Bank of the University Hospital in Zurich. Buffy coats were first diluted 1:1 in PBS, and later PBMCs extracted using a Ficoll gradient. Irradiated (45 Gray) allogeneic PBMCs were used during the freezing procedure of the CSF cells and again during the expansion of CSF-infiltrating $CD4^+$ T cells where they functioned as feeder cells. Fresh blood was obtained in EDTA-containing tubes from all patients, from whom CSF samples were available. PBMCs were isolated from fresh blood using Ficoll density gradient centrifugation (PAA, Pasching, Austria) and cryopreserved in 90% FCS (Eurobio) and 10% DMSO (Applichem, Darmstadt, Germany).

Isolation and Expansion of CSF-Infiltrating CD4$^+$ T Cells

Fresh bulk CSF-derived mononuclear cells from the 22 CIS/RRMS patients were mixed with 5 × 10^6 allogeneic irradiated PBMCs, and CD4$^+$ T cells were subsequently positively selected with anti-CD4 magnetic beads according to the manufacturer's instructions (Miltenyi, Bergisch-Gladbach, Germany). CD4$^+$ cell fractions were seeded at 1,500 cells per well in 96-well U-bottom microtiter plates together with 1.5 × 10^5 allogeneic irradiated PBMCs, 1 μg/ml of PHA-L (Remel, Thermo Fisher, USA) and IL-2 supernatant, derived from the IL-2t6 (myeloma cells IL-2t6, a human lT cell leukemia line; kindly provided by Federica Sallusto, Institute for Research in Biomedicine, Bellinzona). The cell culture was cultivated in RPMI 1640 medium (Pan-Biotech, Aidenbach, Germany) supplemented with 2 mM glutamine (Pan-Biotech), 1% (vol/vol) non-essential amino acids (Gibco), 1% (vol/vol) sodium pyruvate (Gibco, Carlsbad, California, USA), 50 μg/ml penicillin-streptomycin (Corning, NY, USA), 0.00001% β-Mercaptoethanol (Gibco) and 5% inactivated human AB positive serum (Blood Bank Basel). Additional IL-2 was added every 4 days. Growing wells were transferred to 48/24 well plates and finally to 75 cm^3 cell culture flasks until cells were fully rested (20–25 days). Cells were highly expanded in a single round of stimulation.

Peptide Stimulation

Peptides were synthesized by Peptides and Elephants GmbH (Henningsdorf, Germany) and dissolved in DMSO at a stock concentration of 5 mM. The peptides and their sequences which we used are listed in **Supplementary Table 2**. The response of PHA-expanded CSF-infiltrating CD4$^+$ T cells to citrullinated or non-citrullinated myelin and the CEF (CMV, EBV, influenza virus, tetanus toxoid) (Peptides and Elephants GmbH), peptide pool was tested by seeding 6 × 10^4 of expanded CSF-infiltrating CD4$^+$ T cells and 2 × 10^5 irradiated autologous PBMCs in quadruplicates per each condition of peptide stimulation or in the absence of peptides. Stimulation with anti-CD2/CD3/CD28 beads (Miltenyi) was used as additional positive control.

Proliferation Assay

The above described peptide stimulations of bulk CD4$^+$ T cells from CSF of oligoclonal band (OCB) positive relapsing-remitting (RRMS) patients were then used to test T cell reactivity with autologous irradiated PBMCs as antigen-presenting cells. Proliferation of T cells was measured by ^{3}H-thymidine incorporation. At day 2, the cells were pulsed with 1 μCi of methyl-^{3}H-thymidine per well (Hartmann Analytic, Braunschweig, Germany) and harvested after 16 h onto a membrane (Filtermat A, GF/C, Perkin-Elmer, Waltham, Massachusetts, USA) using a semi-automated harvester (Tomtec, Hamden, Connecticut, USA). Incorporation was measured by β-scintillation counting (Wallac 1450, Perkin-Elmer). Proliferative responses were given as counts per min (cpm) and the stimulatory index (SI) was calculated as follows: SI = Mean (replicates cpm peptide)/Mean (replicates cpm without peptide).

Cytokine Measurement

After 48 h of incubation and before adding thymidine, 100 μl of cell culture supernatant were removed in order to test the cytokine secretion. Here, CD4$^+$ T cell reactivity to peptides was analyzed in supernatants for IFN-γ using an IFN-γ ELISA (Biolegend, San Diego, California, USA) according to manufacturer's instructions. Cytokine production higher than 100 pg/ml was considered as a strong positive response.

HLA Typing

Individuals were typed for HLA class I and -II alleles at Histogenetics LLC, NY, USA. Isolation of DNA from whole blood was performed with a standard DNA isolation protocol using a Triton lysis buffer and Proteinase K treatment. Purified genomic DNA with a final concentration of 15 ng/μl was used to type for HLA class I (A* and B*) and HLA class II (DRB1*, DRB3*, DRB4*, DRB5*, DQA1*, and DQB1*) using high-resolution HLA sequence-based typing (SBT). The patients' information is summarized in **Supplementary Table 3**.

Statistical Analysis

Pearson correlation analysis was performed between responses obtained from proliferation assay (thymidine incorporation) and cytokine secretion (IFN-γ) for MOG and CEF peptides.

RESULTS

Characterization of Brain Tissue

To identify the different tissue types, e.g. normal appearing white matter (NAWM) or lesion tissue, sections from tissue blocks were immunohistochemically stained and analyzed (**Figure 1A**). Stainings were performed for MOG (A, D, G, J, M), and HLA-DR (LN3; B, E, H, K, N), as a marker for microglia and macrophages and luxol fast blue (C, F, I, L, O), as markers for myelin and oligodendrocytes (**Figure 1A**). **Figure 1** shows representative staining for control- (C) and MS tissue. LFB and anti-MOG antibody staining identified sites of demyelination (**Figures 1A:G,I**). Staining with anti-HLA-DR antibody shows inflammatory cells (**Figure 1A:H**). Based on the staining, tissue types were defined and then cut for protein isolation. Tissue was taken from normal appearing gray matter (NAGM), normal appearing white matter (NAWM) as well as from active lesions from the diseased tissue. From control tissue, parts of gray (GMC)- and white matter (WMC) were excised. **Figure 1B** shows an immunohistochemistry staining of citrulline in a section of MS brain to illustrate the distribution of citrullination. We observed substantially higher citrullination staining in white compared to gray matter tissue.

Identification of Specific Post-translationally Modified Peptides and Proteins in Pre-fractionated Brain Tissue Samples

For proteomic analysis we decided to extract proteins from the brain tissue by barocycler. This technique allows to extract proteins efficiently from small sample sizes. It has the advantage of using a single test tube from tissue disruption until the tryptic digestion, thereby reducing the introduction of technical variations in the samples (**Figure 1C**). To be able to achieve a higher resolution of the brain proteome we decided to render the samples less complex and therefore easier to analyze. We first separated our peptide digests by hydrophilic interaction chromatography (HILIC), and then two fractions were pooled and injected into liquid chromatography coupled to a mass spectrometer (see illustration in **Figure S2**). The pre-fractionation process allowed us to identify 10,343 proteins in gray matter and 8,730 proteins in white matter tissue. These numbers correspond to combined data from control and MS patients (**Figure 2**). The higher number of proteins in gray matter tissue is not surprising since gray matter tissue is more densely packed with cells than white matter tissue. Overall, 7,950 proteins were common in both groups, white and gray matter. In gray matter 2,393 proteins could be uniquely identified compared with 780 in white matter (**Figure 2A**). Since we were interested in the fraction of proteins involved in processes of inflammation and the immune system an analysis with "STRING-DB" (https://string-db.org/) was performed. We submitted the entire protein list that we had obtained from MS white matter and control tissue. The MS white matter showed a network of proteins involved in immune reactions, which were completely absent in WM control. Control tissue showed an enrichment of a protein network of the nervous system (data not shown).

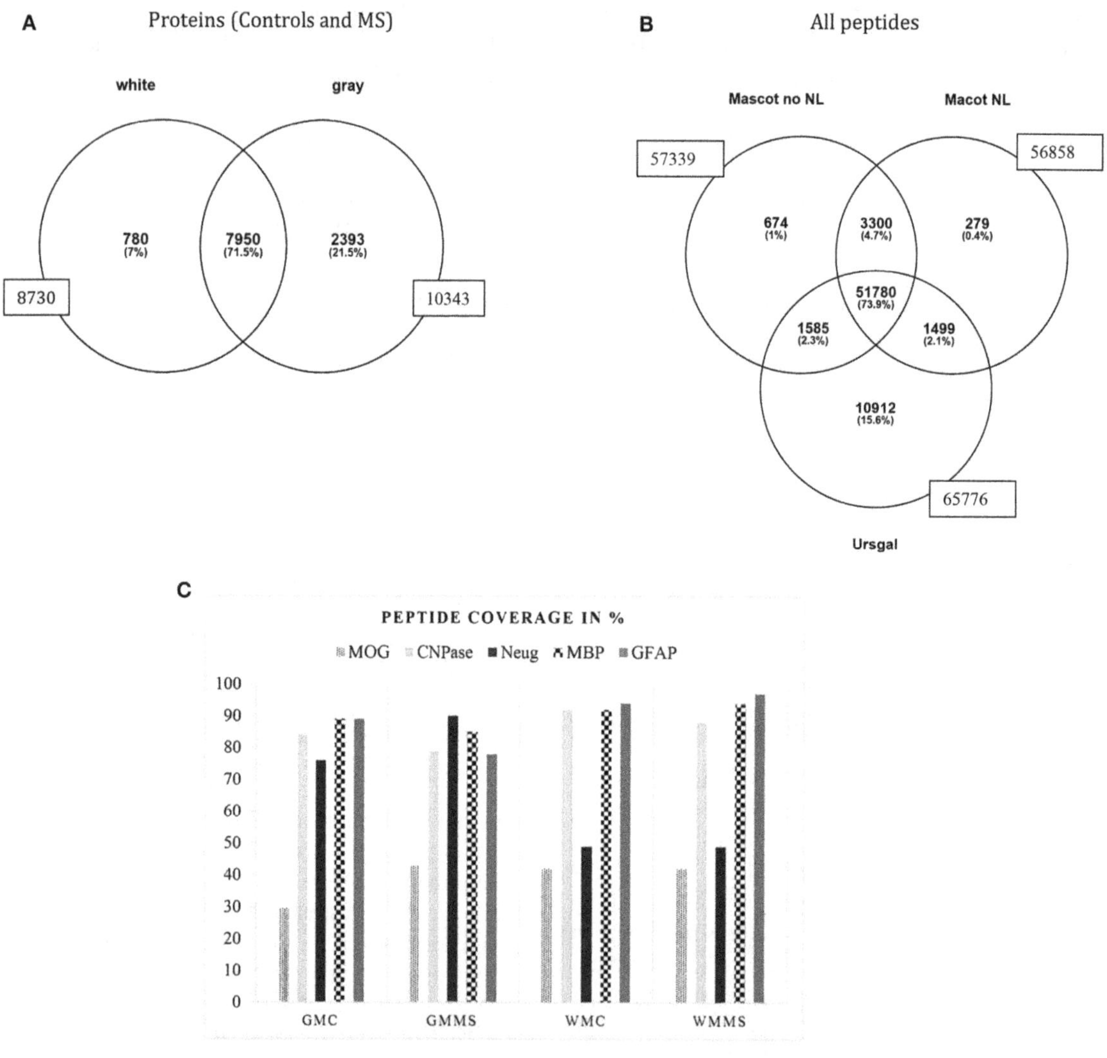

FIGURE 2 | Overall distribution of proteins identified in white and gray matter (control and MS combined). A total number 10,343 proteins was identified in gray matter and 8,730 proteins in white matter with an overlap of 7,950 proteins in both tissues **(A)**. A number of 780 proteins were uniquely attributed to white matter and 2,393 proteins to gray matter. **(B)** Shows all peptide counts in the different search engines from white matter tissue (representative for all tissues analyzed). **(C)** This graph presents the percentage of tryptic peptide sequence coverage of the whole protein, MOG, CNP, Neurogranin, MBP, and GFAP and their identification in the four tissues analyzed, gray matter control (GMC), gray matter MS (GMMS), white matter control (WMC), and white matter MS (WMMS).

Identification of Myelin Sheath- and Other CNS Proteins

An important first step for the comparison of different brain tissue samples is to assure that the protein extraction steps worked with equal efficiency for the different samples. For that reason, we analyzed "representative proteins" from the myelin sheath and considered their presence as quality control for the extraction efficiency. For myelin proteins, myelin basic protein (MBP), myelin oligodendrocyte protein (MOG), myelin-associated glycoprotein (MAG), myelin proteolipid protein (PLP), and 2′,3′-cyclic nucleotide 3′-phosphodiesterase (CNPase), for astrocytes, glial fibrillary acidic protein (GFAP), and neurogranin as neuronal marker, we identified a high number of peptides covering a major part of the respective protein sequences. **Figure 2C** shows the peptide coverage (in %) of these proteins. For MBP the coverage is optimal with more than 90%. The sequence coverage of MOG was between 30 and 40% and for CNPase around 80%. Peptide sequence coverage of GFAP was more than 90% and for neurogranin more than 45%. These numbers indicate a comparable efficiency of peptide extraction from the tissues analyzed.

Identification of "*in vivo*" Citrullinated Proteins

Our main goal was to analyze as detailed as possible, which proteins are citrullinated in MS- and control brain tissue and also for the main regions of the brain, i.e., gray and white matter.. In **Figure 2B**, we show the identification of all peptides from white matter from control and MS. The search with "Mascot no NL" (without neutral loss) identified 57,339 peptides, "MascotNL" (Mascot, with neutral loss) revealed 56,858 peptides and "Ursgal" identified 65,776 peptides. The majority of peptides was common to all three algorithms; 51,780 peptides. Unique to the individual search engines were 674 peptides for "Mascot no NL," 279 to "MascotNL" and 10,912 peptides for "Ursgal" (**Figure 2B**). Similar distributions were observed for gray matter tissue (data not shown).

We based the further analysis on combined identification from the software searches in Mascot (no NL), Mascot (NL) and "Ursgal." For most of the following analysis, we used peptides, which had been identified by at least 2 of the search engines since not all of them could be identified with all three. The distribution of all spectral peptide matches and citrullinated spectral peptide matches and their corresponding proteins numbers from the different tissues are illustrated in **Figure 3** and **Supplementary Data 1**. The highest number of citrullinated spectral matches peptides was found in WM tissue (**Figure 3A**). The lower part of the panel labeled with NO_Citr., represents the overall number of spectral matches from the four different tissues and shows a higher number in GM tissue. Further, very similar numbers were found for gray matter of controls and MS (179,299 and 172,620), and similarly also for white matter tissue (146,867 in controls and 145,040 in MS). In **Figure 3A** (Citr., upper part of the panel) the peptide spectral matches show a strong increase of the citrullinated fraction in the white matter tissue of MS (1,612) vs. control (1,013). In contrast, in gray matter tissue, the numbers were slightly lower in MS tissue (470) compared to control (500).

With respect to overall peptide numbers, there is little difference between MS and control tissue (lower panel). The elevated numbers of citrullinated peptides in white matter therefore indicate a specific enrichment of modified peptides. The diagram in **Figure 3B** shows the number of citrullinated proteins. Here we only show white matter proteins in control and MS. From the 179 proteins in MS white matter (WMMS) and 145 in control white matter (WMC), we found 36 citrullinated proteins to be unique to white matter tissue and 70 unique to gray matter with an overlap of 109 in both tissues. A more detailed analysis of these citrullinated proteins (>80) is shown in **Table 1** as a non-exhaustive list. It represents a selection of citrullinated proteins, for which we identified at least two citrullinated peptides. We grouped the proteins into functional or cellular processes,

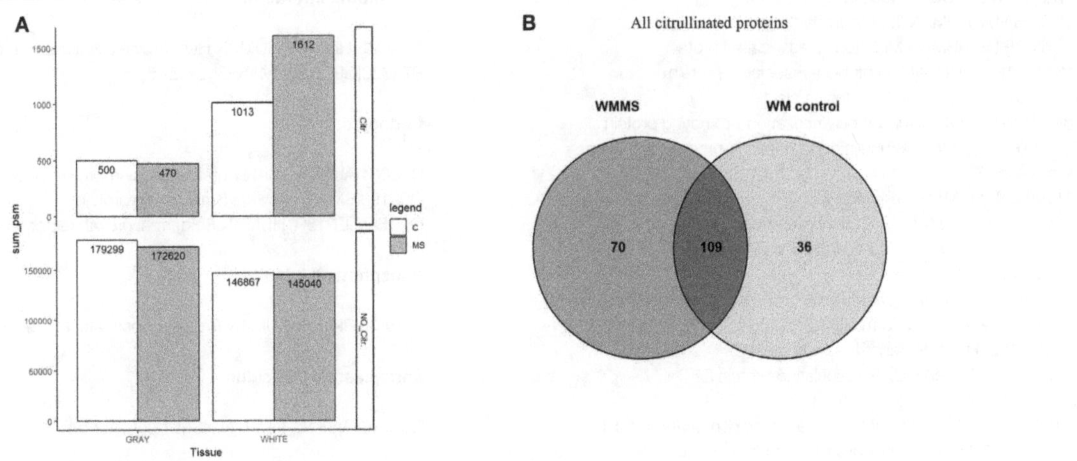

FIGURE 3 | (A) The number of spectrum matched peptide of citrullinated peptides in all tissues are shown in upper panel (Citr.). All peptide spectrum matches found in all four types of tissue gray (GM) and white matter are shown (WM) in lower panel (NO_Citr.). **(B)** Number of citrullinated proteins that were identified in white matter tissue. From the total amount of 179 proteins in MS tissue and 145 in controls 70 proteins were unique in MS tissue and 36 proteins in control tissue with an overlap of 109 proteins in both tissues.

TABLE 1 | List of proteins with at least two citrullinated peptides identified in classified in functional groups.

Myelin associated proteins

P02686-5 MBP_HUMAN Myelin basic protein
P20916|MAG_HUMAN Myelin-associated glycoprotein
P09543|CN37_HUMAN 2′,3′-cyclic-nucleotide 3′-phosphodiesterase
Q92597|NDRG1_HUMAN Protein NDRG1
Q8TAM6|ERMIN_HUMAN Ermin
Q13875|MOBP_HUMAN Myelin-associated oligodendrocyte basic protein

Neuronal development

Q09666|AHNK_HUMAN Neuroblast differentiation-associated protein AHNAK
O15075|DCLK1_HUMAN Serine/threonine-protein kinase DCLK1
P78324|SHPS1_HUMAN Tyrosine-protein phosphatase non-receptor type substrate 1
Q16555|DPYL2_HUMAN Dihydropyrimidinase-related protein 2
Q14195|DPYL3_HUMAN Dihydropyrimidinase-related protein
3P21291|CSRP1_HUMAN Cysteine and glycine-rich protein 1

Neuronal skeleton

P10636|TAU_HUMAN Microtubule-associated protein tau
P07196|NFL_HUMAN Neurofilament light polypeptide
P12036|NFH_HUMAN Neurofilament heavy polypeptide
Q16352|AINX_HUMAN Alpha-internexin

Astrocyte specific

P14136|GFAP_HUMAN Glial fibrillary acidic protein

Membrane signaling

Q8N7J2|AMER2_HUMAN APC membrane recruitment protein 2
Q9NZH0|GPC5B_HUMAN G-protein coupled receptor family C group 5 member B

Cytoskeleton

Q13885|TBB2A_HUMAN Tubulin beta-2A chain
Q9UEY8|ADDG_HUMAN Gamma-adducin
P04350|TBB4A_HUMAN Tubulin beta-4A chain
P07437|TBB5_HUMAN Tubulin beta chain
Q9BQE3|TBA1C_HUMAN Tubulin alpha
Q71U36|TBA1A_HUMAN Tubulin alpha-1A
P46821|MAP1B_HUMAN Microtubule-associated protein
P11137|MTAP2_HUMAN Microtubule-associated protein
P60709|ACTB_HUMAN Actin, cytoplasmic 1
O94811|TPPP_HUMAN Tubulin polymerization-promoting protein
Q9BW30|TPPP3_HUMAN Tubulin polymerization-promoting protein family member 3
P35611|ADDA_HUMAN Alpha-adducin
Q8N7J2|AMER2_HUMAN APC membrane recruitment protein 2
Q14847|LASP1_HUMAN LIM and SH3 domain protein 1
P06396|GELS_HUMAN Gelsolin
O01082|SPTB2_HUMAN Spectrin beta chain, non-erythrocytic 1
Q96PY5|FMNL2_HUMAN Formin-like protein 2
O43491|E41L2_HUMAN Band 4.1-like protein 2
O75122|CLAP2_HUMAN CLIP-associating protein 2
O75781|PALM_HUMAN Paralemmin-1
Q13813|SPTN1_HUMAN Spectrin alpha chain, non-erythrocytic 1
Q92614|MY18A_HUMAN Unconventional myosin-XVIIIa
Q16181|SEPT7_HUMAN Septin
Q15149|PLEC_HUMAN Plectin
Q14244|MAP7_HUMAN Ensconsin
Q9H3Q1|BORG4_HUMAN Cdc42 effector protein 4

Synapse

Q92686|NEUG_HUMAN Neurogranin
P61764|STXB1_HUMAN Syntaxin-binding protein 1
Q8N3V7|SYNPO_HUMAN Synaptopodin
Q9C0H9|SRCN1_HUMAN SRC kinase signaling inhibitor 1
Q13424|SNTA1_HUMAN Alpha-1-syntrophin

Membrane trafficking

Q9NRW1|RAB6B_HUMAN Ras-related protein rab6B
P63027|VAMP2_HUMAN Vesicle-associated membrane protein 2

Chaperonine like activity

P02511|CRYAB_HUMAN Alpha-crystallin B chain
P07900|HS90A_HUMAN Heat shock protein HSP 90-alpha
O95817|BAG3_HUMAN BAG family molecular chaperone regulator 3

RNA binding proteins

P61978|HNRPK_HUMAN Heterogeneous nuclear ribonucleoprotein K
P22626|ROA2_HUMAN Heterogeneous nuclear ribonucleoproteins A2/B1
P38159|AUXI_HUMAN RNA-binding motif protein, X chromosome
P23588|IF4B_HUMAN
Q14011|CIRBP_HUMAN Cold-inducible RNA-binding protein
P68104|EF1A1_HUMAN Elongation factor 1-alpha 1
P38159|RBMX_HUMAN RNA-binding motif protein, X chromosome

Histone

P62807|H2B1C_HUMAN Histone H2B type 1-C/E/F/G/I

Cell adhesion

Q07157|ZO1_HUMAN Tight junction protein ZO-1
Q9UDY2|ZO2_HUMAN Tight junction protein ZO-2
P26232|CTNA2_HUMAN Catenin alpha-2

Cell matrix interaction

Q14CZ8|HECAM_HUMAN Hepatocyte cell adhesion molecule
P78333|GPC5_HUMAN Glypican-5

Endocytosis

O75061|AUXI_HUMAN Putative tyrosine-protein phosphatase auxilin
O00193|SMAP_HUMAN Small acidic protein
Q9UBC2|EP15R_HUMAN Epidermal growth factor receptor substrate 15-like 1

Phosphatase inhibitor

Q96A00|PP14A_HUMAN Protein phosphatase 1 regulatory subunit 14A

Endoplasmic Reticulum

Q9UNZ2|NSF1C_HUMAN NSFL1 cofactor p47

Energy transduction

P12277|KCRB_HUMAN Creatine kinase B-type
P11216|PYGB_HUMAN Glycogen phosphorylase, brain form

(Continued)

TABLE 1 | Continued

Q765P7|MTSSL_HUMAN MTSS1-likEprotein
P35241|RADI_HUMAN Radixin
Q9H9H5|MA6D1_HUMAN MAP6 domain-containing protein 1

Nuclear membrane

P20700|LMNB1_HUMAN Lamin-B1
P02545|LMNA_HUMAN Prelamin-A/C
Q9H910|HN1L_HUMAN Hematological and neurological expressed 1-like protein

Immune response

P43243|MATR3_HUMAN Matrin-3
P17858|PFKAL_HUMAN ATP-dependent 6-phosphofructokinase

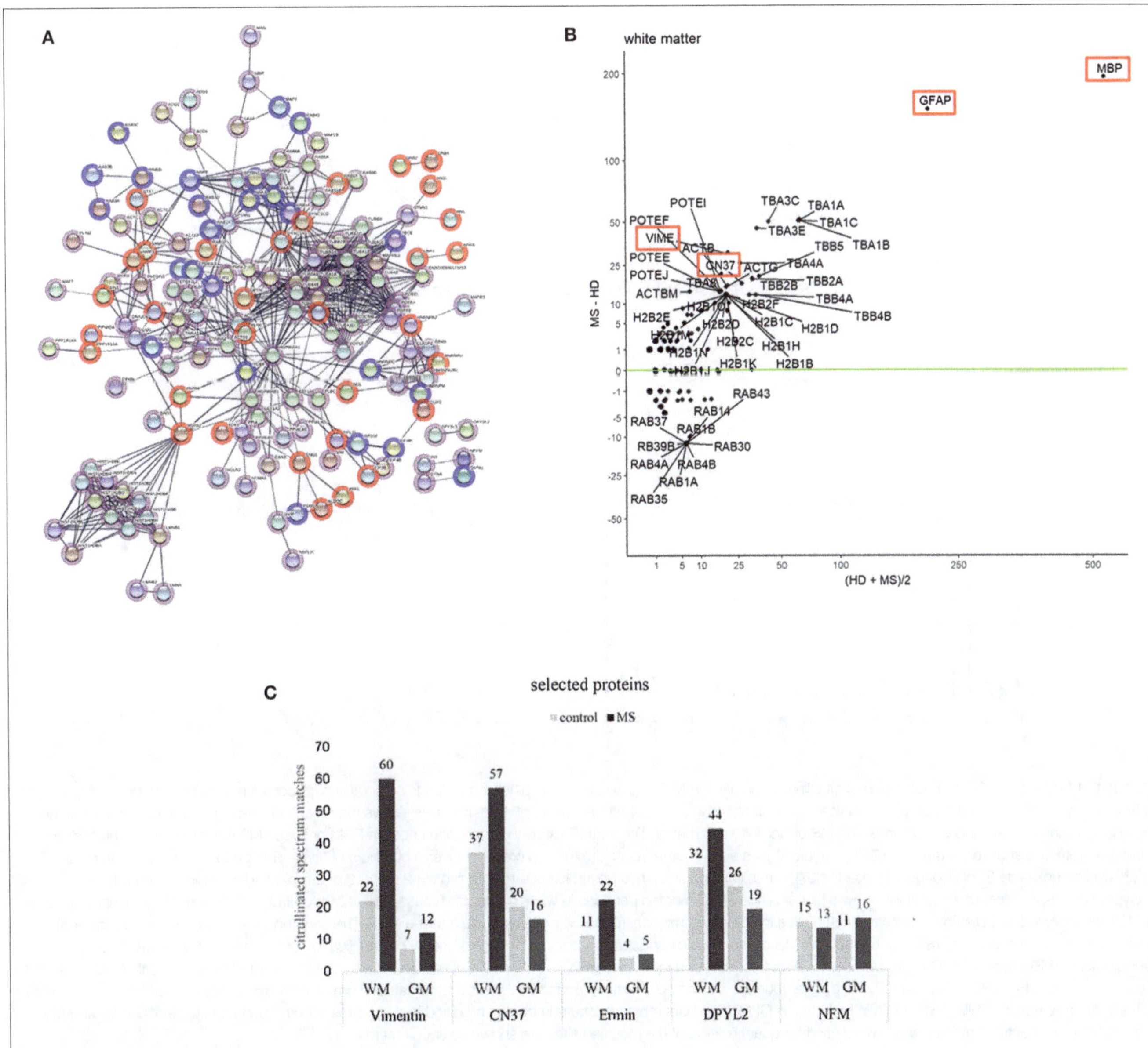

FIGURE 4 | Continued

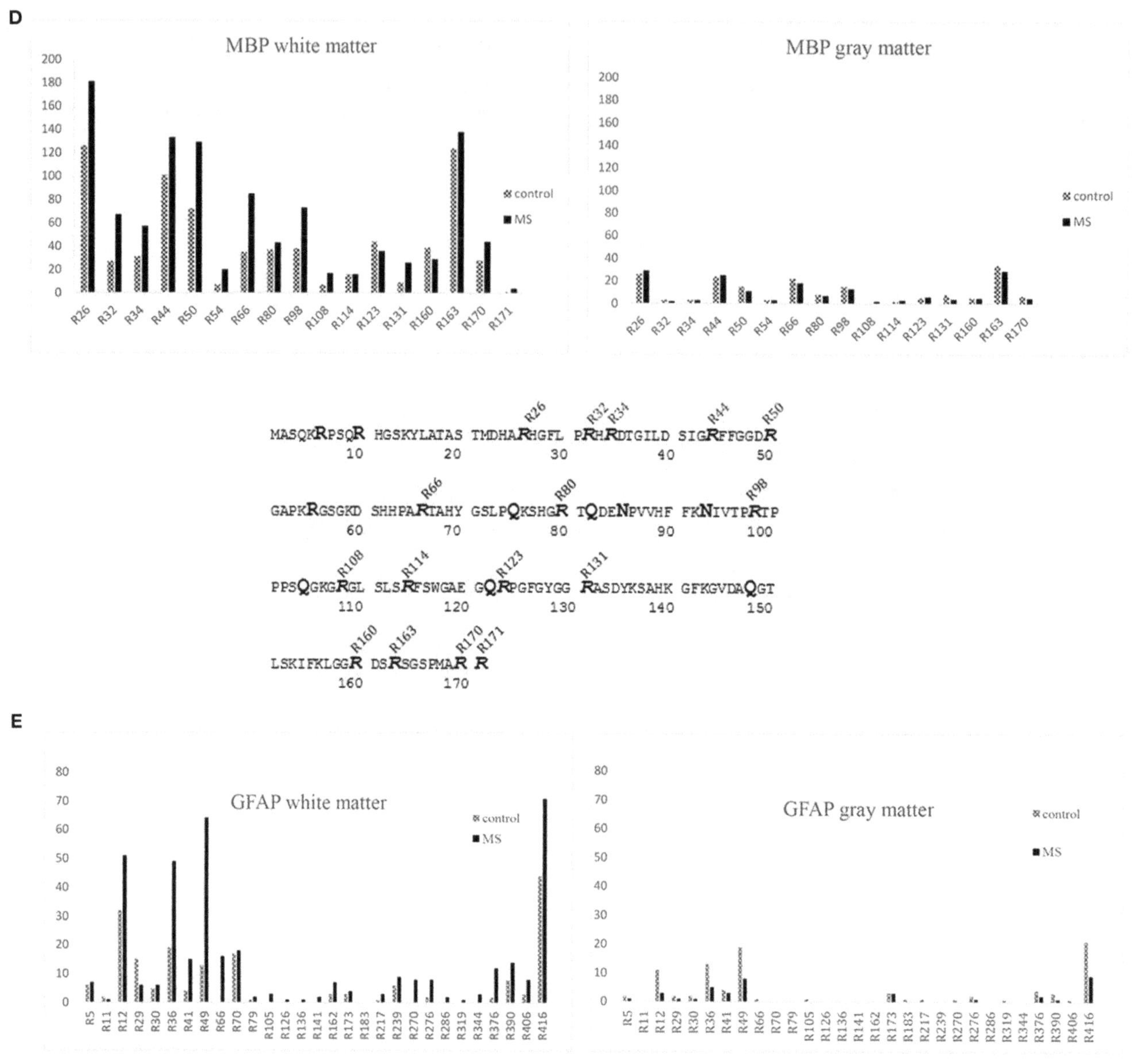

FIGURE 4 | (A) A StringDB representation of citrullinated proteins in MS (red) and controls (blue) tissue. Edge settings is high-confidence (minimum required interaction score 0.700). Overlapping in both tissues are depicted in pink. **(B)** Altman Bland plot. Vertical axis shows the mean number of peptide spectrum matches against citrullinated sequences in controls and MS donor for white matter. The vertical axis shows the differences in PSM between MS and controls. Highlighted in Red are proteins discussed in the text. **(C)** This figure shows a list of other most citrullinated proteins. Overall numbers of tissue distributions are shown: Vimentin, 2′,3′-cyclic-nucleotide 3′-phosphodiesterase (CN37), ermin (juxtanodin), dihydropyrimidinase-related protein 2 (DPYL2 or crmp2) and neurofilament medium polypeptide (NFM). Most of the proteins show a higher range of citrullinated peptides in white matter of diseased tissue. Only NFM is citrullinated in a similar manner in all tissues analyzed. **(D)** Distribution of citrullinated sites in one of the major citrullinated proteins in brain tissue MBP. The bars represent the numbers of modified arginine sites in corresponding tissue of control and MS cases. Peptide spectral matches, which were used for quantification of the modified sites are shown as supplements. MBP sequence (P02686-5) with modified arginine found in our analysis. 16 out of 19 arginine sites were found to be citrullinated in control and diseased brain (MS) tissue. Sites R6, R10, and R55 were never found to be altered. We never found R171 to be citrullinated in gray matter tissue. **(E)** Distribution of citrullinated sites in another major citrullinated protein in brain tissue GFAP. The bars represent the numbers of modified arginine sites in corresponding tissue of control and MS cases. Peptide spectral matches, which were used for quantification of the modified sites are shown as supplements.

such as myelin-associated proteins, neuronal development, neuronal skeleton, astrocytes, synapse, energy transduction, membrane trafficking, cytoskeleton in general immune response and anti-apoptotic activity. The distribution and the possible interactions of the citrullinated proteins are illustrated in **Figure 4A** in the protein interaction network generated by String (24). **Figure 4B** shows the differences regarding citrullination as numbers of peptide-spectrum matches between MS and controls. For GFAP and MBP much higher numbers of spectra matching citrullinated sequences were detected in MS than in controls.

Other proteins worth mentioning are vimentin (VIME) and CNPase (CN37). Proteins with strong citrullination pattern, i.e. more than three citrullination sites, are represented in **Figure 4C**.

Vimentin, an intermediate filament protein, is important for maintaining the structure of a cell. It had already been described in AD (25) and is one of the most citrullinated proteins besides MBP and GFAP in WMMS. We found an increased number of modifications in both tissues of MS in comparison to controls.

CNPase is an oligodendrocyte-specific protein and one of the most abundant proteins in CNS myelin. Its function remains unknown. CN37 has been described as an autoantigen in MS (26) and had been identified to be citrullinated in a mouse model (27). We identified a higher number of citrullinated CN37 peptides in human brain white matter tissue as compared to published data (28). In gray matter, we noticed slightly more citrullinated spectral matches in controls.

We describe for the first time citrullinated sites of members of neurofilament protein family (NFL, NFM and NFH), DPYL2 (dihydropyrimidase-related protein 2, CRMP2), a protein involved in neuronal development and polarity (29), and human ermin, a protein playing a role in myelin development and maintenance and stability of myelin sheath (30). Among the three members of neurofilament proteins, there was no difference with regard to citrullination across tissues and donors. We show neurofilament medium chain (NFM) as a representative member of that group.

The protein DPYL2 showed a particularly increased number of modified peptides in WMMS tissue and a slight increase in GMC.

The protein with the highest number of modified/citrullinated peptides in all tissues was MBP followed by GFAP, which will be described in more detail. The analysis of total spectral counts showed that overall comparable amounts of spectra were observed in control and MS tissue of gray matter, and in white matter citrullinated spectral counts were strongly increased in MS white matter whereas the number of citrullinated spectral counts in gray matter was slightly reduced in MS tissue.

Citrullination and Other Modifications of Myelin Basic Protein

We examined in more detail MBP as one of the import proteins of the myelin sheath and due to its role as target in autoimmune responses. MBP can undergo post-translational modifications at various sites. Those modifications are phosphorylation, methylation, oxidation, citrullination and deamidation/isomerization. So far, very little is known about the implication of these modifications in disease processes in MS (31–33). In our study, we found 16 out of the 19 arginine sites to be modified into citrulline (**Figure 4D**). Earlier studies described 6–9 arginine sites in MBP to be citrullinated in MS "*in vivo*" (32, 34). In these studies, MBP was purified prior to analysis, while we analyzed whole tissue extracts from histologically characterized sites. We observed various modifications on different amino acids and will describe some of them in more detail. The peptide MBP (77–92) "(K)SHG**RTQ**DE**N**PVVHFFK(N)" was modified at multiple sites. Modifications occurred at asparagine (N-85), arginine (R-80), and glutamine (Q-82); DENP, HGRT, and RTQD. The peptide "(K)GVDA**Q**GTLS(K)" (144–154) was deamidated at DAQG (Q-148). We mention these deamidations since these modifications have been analyzed previously in MS patients and healthy donors (32, 35). These two reports show that deamidation of the latter peptide (MBP 144–154) can increase with age in MS patients and others in animals (32). The deamidation of glutamine (Q) in the peptide sequence (82–90) (QDENP) has been shown to block its degradation by the protease cathepsin-D in Alzheimer's Disease (36). In our analysis, we found that 15 (16) identified citrullination sites were present in control as well as in MS tissue, in gray—and in white matter. A 16th position could only be found in WMMS.

To see if there is any specific citrullination pattern of MBP, we counted the number of peptides and the respective citrullinated sites and plotted them over the whole protein sequence (**Figure 4D**). Citrullination is not unique to MS tissue and neither in GM nor WM tissue. Some citrullinated sites were strongly over-represented in MS tissue, i.e., R26, R32, R34, R44, R50, R66, and R98. In GM, only the sites R26 and R44 were slightly more citrullinated in MS tissue compared to control.

The situation for the structural protein GFAP looked similar. GFAP protein was found to be much more modified in WM as compared to GM from MS tissue. Highly modified sites among others were positions R12, R36, R41, R49, and R390 and R416. Similar to MBP, GM tissue generally shows a much lower state of citrullination and a relatively higher rate in control tissue (**Figure 4E**; **Supplementary Data 1**). Since citrullination depends on the activity of PADI, we looked for the presence of PADI in the tissues. We could identify a substantial number of peptides from the isoform PADI2 (between 18 and 20 peptides across all tissue representing between 32 and 45% of protein sequence, data not shown). No peptide of PADI4, the other isoform described to be present in CNS (17), could be found.

Immunological Reactivity Against Citrullinated MBP Peptides

In order to find out if the citrullinated MBP peptides are targeted by the immune system we examined CSF-infiltrating CD4$^+$ T cells from 22 MS patients. We analyzed CSF-derived T cells under the assumption that they are more likely to be biologically relevant in MS than peripheral blood lymphocytes, since the T cells have already infiltrated the CNS compartment. For that purpose, CD4 T cells were freshly isolated and expanded as described (16) from CSF of 19 relapsing remitting MS, 2 primary progressive MS and 1 clinically isolated syndrome patients (**Table 2** and **Supplementary Table 3**), and, subsequently tested in quadruplicates for eight newly identified citrullinated MBP peptides together with the non-modified peptides. Furthermore, seven immunodominant myelin peptides were examined, and, only for MBP, the most abundant citrullinated epitopes were included in the assay (**Supplementary Table 2**). Proliferation and IFN-γ production were used as functional readouts. Positive responses to CEF, a peptide pool of CMV, EBV, influenza virus

TABLE 2 | Main clinical information and CSF findings of MS patients.

	MS patients (22 subjects)
Age (y)	37.3 ± 12.6 (17–58)
Gender (F/M)	15/7
Disease duration (y)	1.6 ± 4.4
Patients with disease duration < 12 months (%)	16 (73%)
Time from last relapse (m)	1.3 ± 2.2 (0–8)
Patients with MRI-LP delay < 1 month (%)	20 (91%)
MRI active patients (%)	11 (50%)
CSF-restricted IgGOCB	21 (95.5%)
Patients with IgG Index > 0.70 (%)	15 (68.2%)
Blood-brain barrier damage (%)	5 (22.7%)
CSF cell count (/μL)	7 ± 3

Disease duration was defined as the time-span between disease onset and lumbar puncture (median value and range are reported). The "time from last relapse" value did not include Primary Progressive MS data. As indicated by the narrow interval between MRI and LP (MRI-LP delay), the great majority of MS patients received MRI the day before LP. Blood Brain Barrier (BBB) damage was considered when the albumin quotient (Q_{Alb}) exceeded the normal value for patient's age (i.e., age/15 + 4). y, years; m, months.

and tetanus toxoid, and global T cell stimulation by anti-CD2/CD3/CD28 beads were tested in parallel as positive controls. Four patients (1444ME, 1479CR, 1453AN, 1489HE) showed responses to CEF peptides with a stimulation index (SI) > 2, but we did not observe specific recognition of citrullinated- and non-citrullinated MBP peptides in proliferation assays (**Figure 5A**). When we analyzed the IFN-γ secretion in the culture supernatant of the same wells tested for proliferation, we did also not find strong IFN-γ release upon exposure to citrullinated MBP peptides, but weak responses in only a few patients and one of the four replicate wells (**Figure 5B**). On the other hand, in two patients (1673UR, 1283RO), IFN-γ secretion (~50 pg/ml) in response to several non-modified epitopes of the MBP protein was seen (**Figure 5B**). Given these results, we conclude that the non-modified peptides are more frequently recognized by CSF-infiltrating $CD4^+$ T cells compared to the citrullinated version and that the reactivity to the latter is overall very low.

Global T cell stimulation resulted in clear responses in all donors, whereas responses to CEF peptides were less frequent. The reactivity observed in proliferation assays to CEF positive control peptides was partially paralleled by IFN-γ release. Only two out of the four patients (1453AN, 1489HE) responding in thymidine incorporation assay, produced also IFN-γ at high concentrations (~400 pg/ml). However, additional patients (1460ML, 1188ZA) responded to these antigens (**Figure 5B**).

When examining other immunodominant myelin peptides (9, 37) we observed in most cases IFN-γ secretion. Several patients reacted clearly to MOG2 (35–55) peptide (**Figure 6A**). 1444ME showed proliferation with a stimulatory index (SI) of 5 (data not shown), 1673UR, 1283RO, and 1560RO release of IFN-γ (~300 pg/ml). 1283RO responded with high IFN-γ release to other non-citrullinated, immunodominant MBP peptides (**Figure 6A**) in comparison to the citrullinated version (**Figure 6A**). These data show that bulk CSF-infiltrating $CD4^+$ T cells of MS patients are able to recognize at the same time different epitopes of the same protein but also different antigens. No significant association between peptide recognition and the MS risk-associated HLA-DRB1 alleles, i.e., DRB1*15:01, DRB1*13:01, and DRB1*03:01, was observed (reported below the graphs).

Since we observed substantial differences in the results obtained from the two response readouts, i.e., thymidine incorporation vs. IFN-γ release, we wanted to assess a correlation between the two measures and applied Pearson Correlation testing on CEF- and MOG peptides responses. We observed (**Figure 6B**) a strong positive correlation ($r = 0.7671$) for CEF peptides ($p < 0.0001$), but only a weak correlation for MOG ($r = 0.1857$), where the majority of responses were detected by ELISA. These results show that IFN-γ secretion appeared to be more sensitive than proliferation as readout.

DISCUSSION

We investigated the composition of citrullinated proteins from human post-mortem brain tissue. Tissues were characterized by immunohistochemistry staining with antibodies against MOG and HLA-DR and LFB. These markers allowed to distinguish tissue with lesions from NAWM. Some of the tissue sections showed increased staining for citrullination in white matter compared to gray matter tissue, an observation that correlated well with our proteomic findings. Based on mass-spectrometry, we could identify a high number of citrullinated proteins, which far exceeded the numbers already published in human CNS (9, 38). By establishing a "spectral peptide library" from different disease-relevant brain tissues and controls, we provide a basis for further, more extensive investigation of the MS brain proteome. We combined an optimized protein extraction technique based on PCT (pressure cycle technology) with chromatographic pre-fractionation, HILIC, to obtain high proteome coverage. We searched our mass spectrometry data with various search engines to distinguish post-translational modifications and identify citrullination. The difficulty of correctly identifying minute mass changes, i.e., an increase of 1 Da per citrullinated site, made it necessary to apply complementary bioinformatics approaches to validate the results, since another post-translational modification, deamidation, which also increases the molecular mass by 1 Da, occurs in aging tissue on asparagine (N) and glutamine (Q) and can be a source of misinterpretation. Therefore, we used different algorithms to interpret the spectra and features, which are inherent of citrullinated proteins, i.e., resistance to tryptic digestion and the neutral loss of 43 Da inside the mass spectrometer instrument (39). Most of the citrullinated proteins we identified, as well as new citrullinated sites of MBP had not been described in MS tissue before. So far, citrullinated myelin proteins had been analyzed from excised bands (SDS-PAGE) or after "*in vitro*" citrullination, but not from entire tissue. We used two software "Mascot" and "Ursgal" to identify citrullination. Depending on the search parameters and software the number of identified peptides varied as illustrated in **Figure 2B**. We could not detect any of the N-terminal arginines to be citrullinated. This

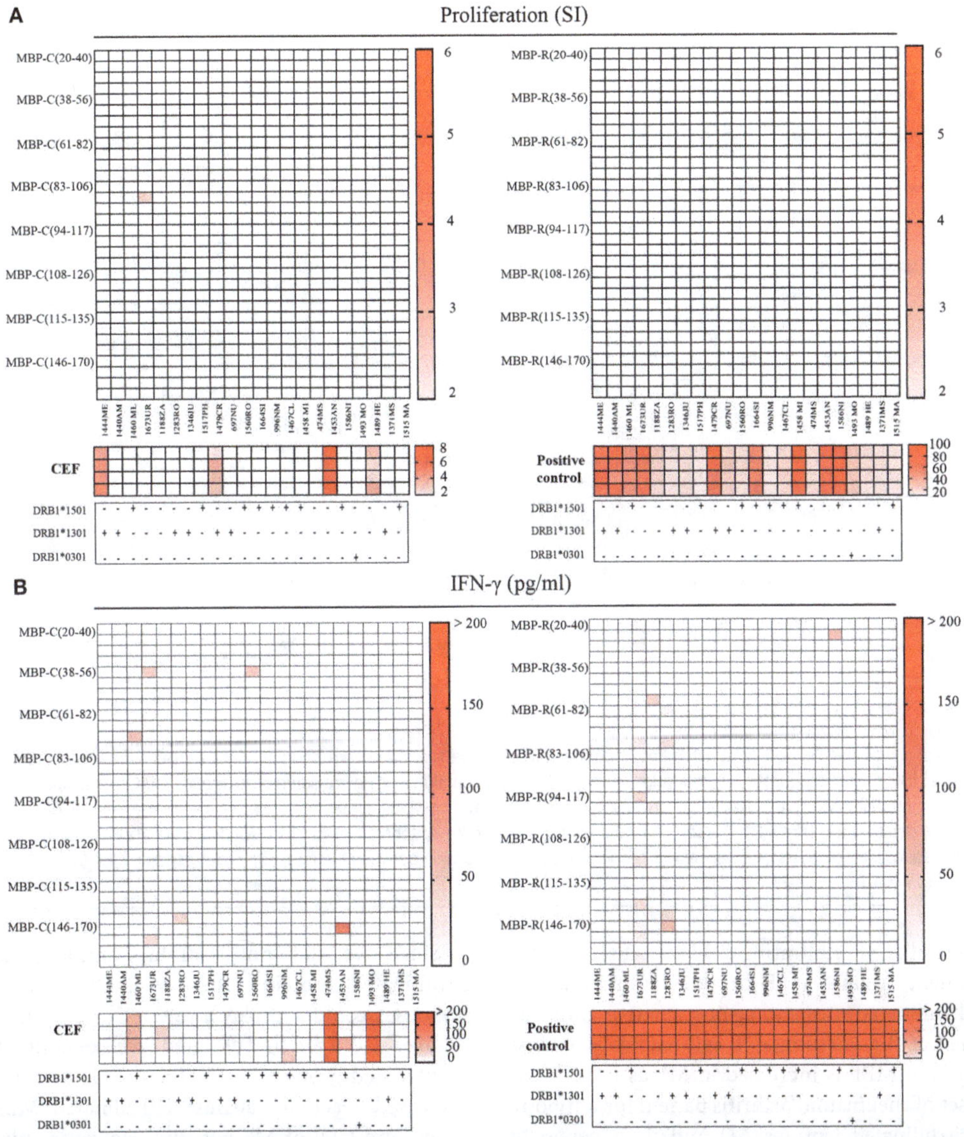

FIGURE 5 | Recognition of citrullinated vs. non-citrullinated MBP in CSF-infiltrating T helper cells of MS patients. **(A,B)** Reactivity of CSF-infiltrating CD4+ T cells from untreated MS patients to citrullinated MBP (left) and non-citrullinated MBP peptides (right), using irradiated autologous PBMCs as antigen-presenting cells. Each square represents one well. MS risk-associated HLA-DRB1 alleles are reported for each individual under the respective graph. **(A)** Proliferative responses to MBP peptides, CEF peptides or anti-CD2/CD3/CD28 stimulation as positive control are given as stimulatory index (SI). The strength of the response is depicted by color coding. A SI > 2 is considered as positive response. **(B)** Responses detected by IFN-γ secretion against to MBP peptides or CEF peptides in the same wells that have been tested in the proliferation assay. The IFN-γ concentration in culture supernatants is depicted as pg/ml.

phenomenon had been reported earlier concluding that "N-termini" are less prone to be citrullinated (38).

Citrullination facilitates enzymatic degradation of MBP but in the situation of increased citrullination, especially of myelin proteins, scavenger cells like macrophages might have difficulties coping with a high amount of proteins to degrade. It could also be that the presence/absence or activity of specific proteases like cathepsins play a role.

Citrullinated residues can be considered "neo-antigens" since they are not necessarily available during thymic selection of T cells and since citrulline is not one of the naturally occurring L-amino acids. Hence, T cells with high avidity T cell receptors against citrullinated peptides, which are presented via MHCII molecules, might escape negative selection in the thymus and target citrullinated peptides in the CNS. Earlier data from testing PBMCs and PBMC-derived T cell lines with proteolytic fragments (13) and 6 modified arginines in MBP, which had been known at that time (40), had indicated increased reactivity against citrullinated MBP epitopes. However, these data were preliminary due to incomplete knowledge of the citrullinated sites and other limitations. After analyzing in detail the possible citrullination sites in the present study, we wanted to expand the

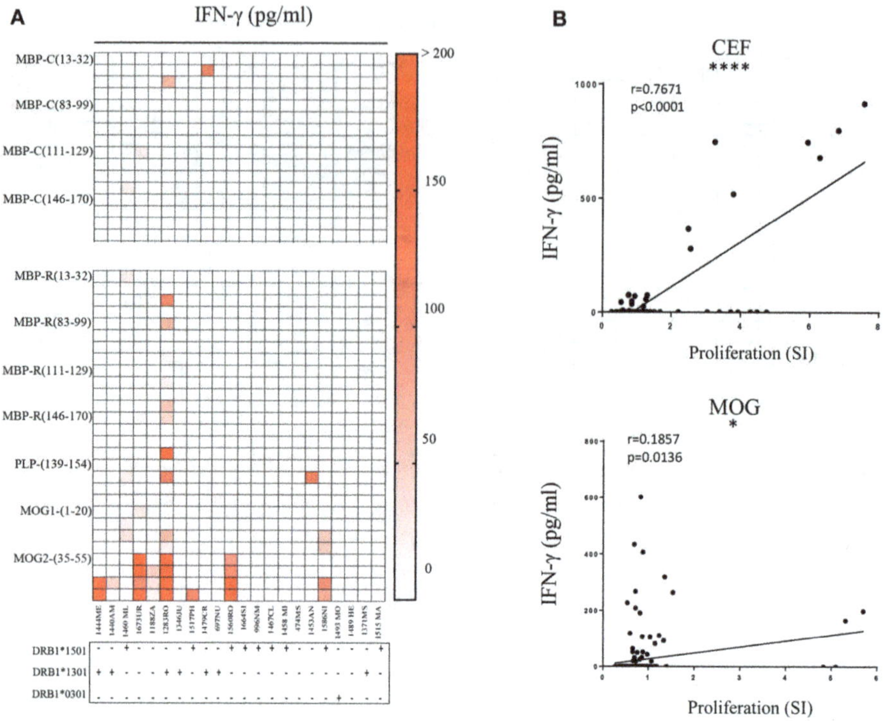

FIGURE 6 | Recognition of citrullinated vs. non-citrullinated immunodominant myelin peptides and correlation of readouts. **(A)** Reactivity of CSF-infiltrating CD4+ T cells to immunodominant MBP citrullinated (up) and immunodominant myelin (down) peptides, using irradiated autologous PBMCs as antigen-presenting cells. Each square represents one well. MS risk-associated HLA-DRB1 alleles are reported for each individual under the respective graph. Responses detected by IFN-γ secretion in culture supernatants are depicted as pg/ml. **(B)** Pearson correlation analysis is performed for MOG and CEF peptides. Data obtained from ELISA and proliferation assay are compared and each dot represents one well-tested. Significant strong correlation between the readouts is detected for CEF ($p < 0.0001$) while for MOG a mild correlation is shown ($p = 0.0136$).

prior data by testing bulk CSF-infiltrating CD4+ T cells, i.e., from the CNS compartment, against MBP peptides containing the newly identified citrullinated sites and against control antigens. These studies aimed at the question if T cell reactivity against citrullinated epitopes of MBP is increased in MS as it has been described in a subset of rheumatoid arthritis patient for antibody reactivity against citrullinated peptides (41), and, if not generally increased in MS, whether it is found in a subset of patients. Our findings show that there is very little reactivity again citrullinated MBP epitopes and that it is thus unlikely to play a role in the autoimmune response in MS. When comparing the present study with previous data (12, 13), the testing of CSF-infiltrating T cells, which are more likely to be disease-relevant than PBMC-derived T cells, and of a larger number of individuals are the most important differences. The fact that we observed reactivity against MOG- and CEF peptides in a number of individuals, indicate that the lack of reactivity against citrullinated MBP peptides was not a technical problem. The observation that some wells were only positive when testing for IFN-γ, is likely explained by the fact that individual functions of T cells require different strengths of stimulation (42). Modified/citrullinated peptides may be less potent ligands compared to native peptides and, since only one antigen concentration was tested, it is possible that responsiveness was only observed for one functional readout instead of both (42).

Since we did not examine antibody reactivity against citrullinated proteins, the possibility remains that humoral responses could still play a role in MS as is the case in RA (42). Bodil et al. did not find elevated levels of antibodies either against citrullinated proteins or PAD in MS patients (43). Furthermore, decreased reactivity against citrullinated MBP was found in serum and CSF of MS patients. However, this study examined only two citrullinated MBP peptides (44).

Besides myelin proteins, we also identified additional citrullinated sites in vimentin and CN37 from WMMS, whereas numbers of CN37 and DPYL2 citrullinated peptides were slightly increased in GMC tissue (**Figure 4C**). Some of the newly identified citrullinated proteins like ermin (juxtanodin) and DPYL2 (crmp-2) are of particular interest. Little is known about ermin. It appears to be expressed only by oligodendrocytes and involved in the compaction of myelin (45) and the formation of axonal microtubules (46). It is interesting to note that citrullinated ermin is present in tissue were compaction of myelin is lost. Moscarello et al. were the first to hypothesize that damage of white matter in MS results from a failure to maintain compact myelin sheaths due to an increased citrullination of MBP (47). Citrullination of ermin may occur as "collateral damage." MBP like ermin belongs to a group of proteins, which are characterized as "intrinsically disordered proteins" that adopt tertiary structure depending on the molecular environment (48).

DPYL2 or (CRMP2) is a protein, which has been linked to neurodegenerative disorders (49) and shown to be involved in synaptic function. It appears in an interactome with proteins involved in B cell differentiation (49) and in T cells in the context of neuroinflammation in an animal model (50). Further, it has been shown to have multiple PTMs and potentially many interactors, among them structural proteins as tubulin (51).

Our list of citrullinated proteins shows a large number of molecules involved in cytoskeleton formation, especially vimentin, GFAP, tubulin and actin. The picture we obtained from our MS tissues indicates that structural proteins are the main targets of this particular post-translational modification. Citrullination is considered to result from insult and damage, leading to molecular and cellular breakdown. In addition, recent publications show that post-translational modifications as citrullination and deamidation also occur in the aging brain (32, 34, 36). Therefore, it is possible that the citrullination patterns we obtained from control brain reflect the natural aging of brain tissue. Nevertheless, citrullination occurred with a much higher frequency in MS tissue as compared to control. This could be due to inflammation, even if tissue is not overtly inflamed and considered "normal-appearing," and support the argument that citrullination is not an initiator of the disease but the result. Other PTM, such as phosphorylation occur also on MBP, but their possible influence on disease course is currently not clear.

In summary, our study provides a comprehensive analysis of citrullinated peptides in white- and gray matter of MS patients and controls. We combined efficient protein extraction- and separation techniques to analyze very small samples. Thorough data mining with the support of complementary software allowed us to establish a map of citrullinated peptides and proteins. This proteomic approach in principle provides the basis for multiple other studies on the role of citrullination in MS brain tissue, but more broadly also with respect to analyzing other post-translational modifications in small tissue samples and identifying potential neo-antigens. This information, i.e., whether structural proteins and or those involved in inflammatory processes are citrullinated, should improve the understanding whether citrullination is implicated in distinct pathomechanisms in MS. Altered myelin, either via structural alterations, during the processes of de- and remyelination, neuronal/axonal loss or autoimmune inflammation could result in neoantigens and thereby induce an autoimmune reaction or increase demyelination (5).

The immunological testing in the present study focussed on citrullinated MBP epitopes based on previous reports, and, even though we examined CSF-infiltrating $CD4^+$ T cells, we did not find a marked response, which argues against a major pathogenetic involvement of autoimmune T cells directed against citrullinated MBP epitopes in MS.

AUTHOR CONTRIBUTIONS

WF designed and performed brain tissue experiments and wrote the manuscript. CC performed all the cellular assays and participated in writing the manuscript. WW performed data extraction and bioinformatics analysis, and contributed to discussions and writing of the manuscript. BR ran the mass spectrometers and contributed to the progress in experimental setups. PT-O and CS-M helped with $CD4^+$ T cell expansion. TZ performed immunohistochemistry and excision of brain tissue samples. MP analyzed MRI images and clinical data. IJ helped with analyzing the data and revised the manuscript. NS-W provided the characterized brain tissue samples. MS and RM were responsible for designing the questions of the study, acquisition of grants, and contributed to writing the manuscript.

FUNDING

The project was supported by the Clinical Research Priority Program Multiple Sclerosis $CRPP^{MS}$ of the University of Zürich, the European Research Council (ERC; ERC-2013-ADG 340733), the Swiss National Science Foundation Sinergia grant Unmet-MS (grant number CRSII3_54483) and Highly Specialized Medicine II (HSMII) Targeted and interdisciplinary treatment of severe immune-mediated diseases.

ACKNOWLEDGMENTS

We thank Richard Reynolds and the UK MS Tissue Bank for the brain tissue. We acknowledge the histology laboratory at the Department of Neuropathology, University Hospital Zürich for their support, Christian Kempf for initial brain storming, Tiannan Guo for introduction to PCT.

SUPPLEMENTARY MATERIAL

Figure S1 | FDR (vertical axis) vs. score (horizontal axis). Green line FDR for deamidated and citrullinated peptides. Yellow line. FDR for all the other peptides.

Figure S2 | Schematic picture of peptide fractionation and tissue sampling on HILIC.

Supplementary Table 1 | Patient information: List of all patient tissues used in the study including tissue block numbers for proteomics studies.

Supplementary Table 2 | List of peptides and quantification in control and MS brain tissues. The table includes the complete list of peptides used in the assays and the number of equivalent tryptic peptides found in the brain tissues of controls (C) and MS cases using LC-mass spectrometry (LC-MS) technique.

Supplementary Table 3 | Extended clinical, including demographic and HLA-DRB1 haplotypes of MS patients. Gender, age, disease duration at LP, interval between last relapse and LP (Last relapse-LP delay), presence of ongoing clinical relapse (Clinically Active), the delay between MRI and LP (MRI-LP delay), presence of gadolinium-enhancing lesion at T1-MRI sequence (Radiologically active), IgG index, IgGOB Pattern, IgM Index, IgA index, and CSF cells count (/uL) and HLA-DRB1 typing are reported for each individual. CIS, clinical isolated syndrome; RRMS, relapsing remitting MS; OCB, oligoclonal bands.

Supplementary Data 1 | All peptides identified with Mascot and Ursgal. PSM of each peptides with reference to search engines used and their tissue distribution.

REFERENCES

1. Hensen SMM, Pruijn GJM. Methods for the detection of peptidylarginine deiminase (PAD) activity and protein citrullination. *Mol Cell Proteomics.* (2014) 13:388–96. doi: 10.1074/mcp.R113.033746
2. György B, Tóth E, Tarcsa E, Falus A, Buzás EI. Citrullination: a posttranslational modification in health and disease. *Int J Biochem Cell Biol.* (2006) 38:1662–77. doi: 10.1016/j.biocel.2006.03.008
3. Gudmann NS, Hansen NUB, Jensen ACB, Karsdal MA, Siebuhr AS. Biological relevance of citrullinations: diagnostic, prognostic and therapeutic options. *Autoimmunity.* (2015) 48:73–9. doi: 10.3109/08916934.2014.962024
4. Tarcsa E, Marekov LN, Mei G, Melino G, Lee S-C, Steinert PM. Protein unfolding by peptidylarginine deiminase Substrate specificity and structural relationships of the natural substrates trichohyalin and filaggrin. *J Biol Chem.* (1996) 271:30709–16.
5. Cao L, Goodin R, Wood D, Moscarello MA, Whitaker JN. Rapid release and unusual stability of immunodominant peptide 45–89 from citrullinated myelin basic protein. *Biochemistry (Mosc).* (1999) 38:6157–63. doi: 10.1021/bi982960s
6. Catrina AI, Ytterberg AJ, Reynisdottir G, Malmström V, Klareskog L. Lungs, joints and immunity against citrullinated proteins in rheumatoid arthritis. *Nat Rev Rheumatol.* (2014) 10:645–53. doi: 10.1038/nrrheum.2014.115
7. GS Chirivi R. Citrullination: a target for disease intervention in multiple sclerosis and other inflammatory diseases? *J Clin Cell Immunol.* (2013) 4:146. doi: 10.4172/2155-9899.1000146
8. Pieper J, Dubnovitsky A, Gerstner C, James EA, Rieck M, Kozhukh G, et al. Memory T cells specific to citrullinated α-enolase are enriched in the rheumatic joint. *J Autoimmun.* (2018) 92:47–56. doi: 10.1016/j.jaut.2018.04.004
9. Moscarello MA, Mastronardi FG, Wood DD. The role of citrullinated proteins suggests a novel mechanism in the pathogenesis of multiple sclerosis. *Neurochem Res.* (2006) 32:251–6. doi: 10.1007/s11064-006-9144-5
10. Bradford CM, Ramos I, Cross AK, Haddock G, McQuaid S, Nicholas AP, et al. Localisation of citrullinated proteins in normal appearing white matter and lesions in the central nervous system in multiple sclerosis. *J Neuroimmunol.* (2014) 273:85–95. doi: 10.1016/j.jneuroim.2014.05.007
11. Nicholas AP, Sambandam T, Echols JD, Tourtellotte WW. Increased citrullinated glial fibrillary acidic protein in secondary progressive multiple sclerosis. *J Comp Neurol.* (2004) 473:128–36. doi: 10.1002/cne.20102/abstract
12. Sospedra M, Martin R. Immunology of multiple sclerosis. *Annu Rev Immunol.* (2005) 23:683–747. doi: 10.1146/annurev.immunol.23.021704.115707
13. Martin R, Whitaker JN, Rhame L, Goodin RR, McFarland HF. Citrulline-containing myelin basic protein is recognized by T-cell lines derived from multiple sclerosis patients and healthy individuals. *Neurology.* (1994) 44:123.
14. Apostolopoulos V, Deraos G, Matsoukas M-T, Day S, Stojanovska L, Tselios T, et al. Cyclic citrullinated MBP87–99 peptide stimulates T cell responses: implications in triggering disease. *Bioorg Med Chem.* (2016) 25:528–38. doi: 10.1016/j.bmc.2016.11.029
15. Jelcic I, Al Nimer F, Wang J, Lentsch V, Planas R, Jelcic I, et al. Memory B cells activate brain-homing, autoreactive CD4$^+$ T cells in multiple sclerosis. *Cell.* (2018) 175:85–100.e23. doi: 10.1016/j.cell.2018.08.011
16. Planas R, Santos R, Tomas-Ojer P, Cruciani C, Lutterotti A, Faigle W, et al. GDP-l-fucose synthase is a CD4$^+$ T cell-specific autoantigen in DRB3*02:02 patients with multiple sclerosis. *Sci Transl Med.* (2018) 10:eaat4301. doi: 10.1126/scitranslmed.aat4301
17. Mastronardi FG, Wood DD, Mei J, Raijmakers R, Tseveleki V, Dosch HM, et al. Increased citrullination of histone H3 in multiple sclerosis brain and animal models of demyelination: a role for tumor necrosis factor-induced peptidylarginine deiminase 4 translocation. *J Neurosci.* (2006) 26:11387–96. doi: 10.1523/JNEUROSCI.3349-06.2006
18. Erne B, Sansano S, Frank M, Schaeren-Wiemers N. Rafts in adult peripheral nerve myelin contain major structural myelin proteins and myelin and lymphocyte protein (MAL) and CD59 as specific markers. *J Neurochem.* (2002) 82:550–62. doi: 10.1046/j.1471-4159.2002.00987.x/full
19. Guo T, Kouvonen P, Koh CC, Gillet LC, Wolski WE, Röst HL, et al. Rapid mass spectrometric conversion of tissue biopsy samples into permanent quantitative digital proteome maps. *Nat Med.* (2015) 21:407–13. doi: 10.1038/nm.3807
20. Barkow-Oesterreicher S, Türker C, Panse C. FCC – an automated rule-based processing tool for life science data. *Source Code Biol Med.* (2013) 8:1–7. doi: 10.1186/1751-0473-8-3
21. Kremer LPM, Leufken J, Oyunchimeg P, Schulze S, Fufezan C. Ursgal, universal python module combining common bottom-up proteomics tools for large-scale analysis. *J Proteome Res.* (2016) 15:788–94. doi: 10.1021/acs.jproteome.5b00860
22. Käll L, Storey JD, MacCoss MJ, Noble WS. Assigning significance to peptides identified by tandem mass spectrometry using decoy databases. *J Proteome Res.* (2008) 7:29–34. doi: 10.1021/pr700600n
23. Vizcaíno JA, Csordas A, del-Toro N, Dianes JA, Griss J, Lavidas I, et al. 2016 update of the PRIDE database and its related tools. *Nucleic Acids Res.* (2016) 44:D447–56. doi: 10.1093/nar/gkv1145
24. Szklarczyk D, Franceschini A, Wyder S, Forslund K, Heller D, Huerta-Cepas J, et al. STRING v10: protein–protein interaction networks, integrated over the tree of life. *Nucleic Acids Res.* (2015) 43:D447–52. doi: 10.1093/nar/gku1003
25. Ishigami A, Ohsawa T, Hiratsuka M, Taguchi H, Kobayashi S, Saito Y, et al. Abnormal accumulation of citrullinated proteins catalyzed by peptidylarginine deiminase in hippocampal extracts from patients with Alzheimer's disease. *J Neurosci Res.* (2005) 80:120–8. doi: 10.1002/jnr.20431/abstract
26. Muraro PA, Kalbus M, Afshar G, McFarland HF, Martin R. T cell response to 2′,3′-cyclic nucleotide 3′-phosphodiesterase (CNPase) in multiple sclerosis patients. *J Neuroimmunol.* (2002) 130:233–42. doi: 10.1016/S0165-5728(02)00229-1
27. Moscarello MA, Lei H, Mastronardi FG, Winer S, Tsui H, Li Z, et al. Inhibition of peptidyl-arginine deiminases reverses protein-hypercitrullination and disease in mouse models of multiple sclerosis. *Dis Model Mech.* (2013) 6:467–78. doi: 10.1242/dmm.010520
28. Lee C-Y, Wang D, Wilhelm M, Zolg DP, Schmidt T, Schnatbaum K, et al. Mining the human tissue proteome for protein citrullination. *Mol Cell Proteomics.* (2018) 17:1378–91. doi: 10.1074/mcp.RA118.000696
29. Arimura N, Menager C, Fukata Y, Kaibuchi K. Role of CRMP-2 in neuronal polarity. *J Neurobiol.* (2004) 58:34–47. doi: 10.1002/neu.10269
30. Brockschnieder D. Ermin, a myelinating oligodendrocyte-specific protein that regulates cell morphology. *J Neurosci.* (2006) 26:757–62. doi: 10.1523/JNEUROSCI.4317-05.2006
31. Kim JK, Mastronardi FG, Wood DD, Lubman DM, Zand R, Moscarello MA. Multiple sclerosis an important role for post-translational modifications of myelin basic protein in pathogenesis. *Mol Cell Proteomics.* (2003) 2:453–62. doi: 10.1074/mcp.M200050-MCP200
32. Sarg B, Faserl K, Lindner HH. Identification of novel site-specific alterations in the modification level of myelin basic protein isolated from mouse brain at different ages using capillary electrophoresis–mass spectrometry. *Proteomics.* (2017) 17:1700269. doi: 10.1002/pmic.201700269
33. Opdenakker G, Proost P, Van Damme J. Microbiomic and posttranslational modifications as preludes to autoimmune diseases. *Trends Mol Med.* (2016) 22:746–57. doi: 10.1016/j.molmed.2016.07.002
34. Friedrich MG, Hancock SE, Raftery MJ, Truscott RJW. Isoaspartic acid is present at specific sites in myelin basic protein from multiple sclerosis patients: could this represent a trigger for disease onset? *Acta Neuropathol Commun.* (2016) 4:83. doi: 10.1186/s40478-016-0348-x
35. Bielekova B, Sung MH, Kadom N, Simon R, McFarland H, Martin R. Expansion and functional relevance of high-avidity myelin-specific CD4$^+$ T cells in multiple sclerosis. *J Immunol.* (2004) 172:3893–904. doi: 10.4049/jimmunol.172.6.3893
36. Gallart-Palau X, Lee BST, Adav SS, Qian J, Serra A, Park JE, et al. Gender differences in white matter pathology and mitochondrial dysfunction in Alzheimer's disease with cerebrovascular disease. *Mol Brain.* (2016) 9:27. doi: 10.1186/s13041-016-0205-7
37. Lutterotti A, Yousef S, Sputtek A, Sturner KH, Stellmann J-P, Breiden P, et al. Antigen-specific tolerance by autologous myelin peptide-coupled cells: a phase 1 trial in multiple sclerosis. *Sci Transl Med.* (2013) 5:188ra75. doi: 10.1126/scitranslmed.3006168
38. Nomura K. Specificity and mode of action of the muscle-type protein-arginine deiminase. *Arch Biochem Biophys.* (1992) 293:362–9.
39. Hao G, Wang D, Gu J, Shen Q, Gross SS, Wang Y. Neutral loss of isocyanic acid in peptide CID spectra: a novel diagnostic marker for mass spectrometric

identification of protein citrullination. *J Am Soc Mass Spectrom.* (2009) 20:723–7. doi: 10.1016/j.jasms.2008.12.012

40. Tranquill LR, Cao L, Ling NC, Kalbacher H, Martin RM, Whitaker JN. Enhanced T cell responsiveness to citrulline-containing myelin basic protein in multiple sclerosis patients. *Mult Scler.* (2000) 6:220–5. doi: 10.1177/135245850000600402
41. Ge C, Xu B, Liang B, Lönnblom E, Lundström SL, Zubarev RA, et al. Structural basis of cross-reactivity of anti-citrullinated protein antibodies. *Arthritis Rheumatol.* (2018) 71:210–21. doi: 10.1002/art.40698
42. Hemmer B, Stefanova I, Vergelli M, Germain RN, Martin R. Relationships among TCR ligand potency, thresholds for effector function elicitation, and the quality of early signaling events in human T cells. *J Immunol.* (1998) 160:5807–14.
43. Bodil Roth E, Theander E, Londos E, Sandberg-Wollheim M, Larsson Å, Sjöberg K, et al. Pathogenesis of autoimmune diseases: antibodies against transglutaminase, peptidylarginine deiminase and protein-bound citrulline in primary Sjögren's syndrome, multiple sclerosis and Alzheimer's disease. *Scand J Immunol.* (2008) 67:626–31. doi: 10.1111/j.1365-3083.2008.02115.x
44. de Seze J, Dubucquoi S, Lefranc D, Virecoulon F, Nuez I, Dutoit V, et al. IgG reactivity against citrullinated myelin basic protein in multiple sclerosis. *J Neuroimmunol.* (2001) 117:149–55. doi: 10.1016/S0165-5728(01)00312-5
45. Liang F, Hwang JH, Tang NW, Hunziker W. Juxtanodin in retinal pigment epithelial cells: expression and biological activities in regulating cell morphology and actin cytoskeleton organization: LIANG et al. *J Comp Neurol.* (2018) 526:205–15. doi: 10.1002/cne.24301
46. Niwa S, Nakamura F, Tomabechi Y, Aoki M, Shigematsu H, Matsumoto T, et al. Structural basis for CRMP2-induced axonal microtubule formation. *Sci Rep.* (2017) 7:10681. doi: 10.1038/s41598-017-11031-4
47. Moscarello MA, Wood DD, Ackerley C, Boulias C. Myelin in multiple sclerosis is developmentally immature. *J Clin Invest.* (1994) 94:146–54.
48. Ruskamo S, Chukhlieb M, Vahokoski J, Bhargav SP, Liang F, Kursula I, et al. Juxtanodin is an intrinsically disordered F-actin-binding protein. *Sci Rep.* (2012) 2:899. doi: 10.1038/srep00899
49. Martins-de-Souza D, Cassoli JS, Nascimento JM, Hensley K, Guest PC, Pinzon-Velasco AM, et al. The protein interactome of collapsin response mediator protein-2 (CRMP2/DPYSL2) reveals novel partner proteins in brain tissue. *Proteomics Clin Appl.* (2015) 9:817–31. doi: 10.1002/prca.201500004/full
50. Vuaillat C, Varrin-Doyer M, Bernard A, Sagardoy I, Cavagna S, Chounlamountri I, et al. High CRMP2 expression in peripheral T lymphocytes is associated with recruitment to the brain during virus-induced neuroinflammation. *J Neuroimmunol.* (2008) 193:38–51. doi: 10.1016/j.jneuroim.2007.09.033
51. Myllykoski M, Baumann A, Hensley K, Kursula P. Collapsin response mediator protein 2: high-resolution crystal structure sheds light on small-molecule binding, post-translational modifications, and conformational flexibility. *Amino Acids.* (2017) 49:747–59. doi: 10.1007/s00726-016-2376-z

5

Connexin 30 Deficiency Attenuates Chronic but Not Acute Phases of Experimental Autoimmune Encephalomyelitis Through Induction of Neuroprotective Microglia

Mei Fang[1], *Ryo Yamasaki*[1], *Guangrui Li*[1], *Katsuhisa Masaki*[1], *Hiroo Yamaguchi*[1], *Atsushi Fujita*[1], *Noriko Isobe*[1,2] *and Jun-ichi Kira*[1*]

[1] *Department of Neurology, Neurological Institute, Graduate School of Medical Sciences, Kyushu University, Fukuoka, Japan,*
[2] *Department of Neurological Therapeutics, Neurological Institute, Graduate School of Medical Sciences, Kyushu University, Fukuoka, Japan*

***Correspondence:**
Jun-ichi Kira
kira@neuro.med.kyushu-u.ac.jp

Glial connexins (Cxs) form gap junction channels through which a pan-glial network plays key roles in maintaining homeostasis of the central nervous system (CNS). In multiple sclerosis (MS) and its animal model, experimental autoimmune encephalomyelitis (EAE), expression of astrocytic Cx43 is lost in acute lesions but upregulated in chronic plaques, while astrocytic Cx30 is very low in normal white matter and changes in its expression have not been convincingly shown. In Cx30 or Cx43 single knockout (KO) mice and even in Cx30/Cx43 double KO mice, acute EAE is unaltered. However, the effects of Cx30/Cx43 deficiency on chronic EAE remains to be elucidated. We aimed to clarify the roles of Cx30 in chronic neuroinflammation by studying EAE induced by myelin oligodendrocyte glycoprotein peptide 35–55 in Cx30 KO mice. We found that Cx30 deficiency improved the clinical symptoms and demyelination of chronic but not acute EAE without influencing $CD3^+$ T cell infiltration. Furthermore, increased ramified microglia in the naïve state and induced earlier and stronger microglial activation in the acute and chronic phases of EAE was observed. These activated microglia had an anti-inflammatory phenotype, as shown by the upregulation of arginase-1 and brain-derived neurotrophic factor and the downregulation of nitric oxide synthase 2. In the naïve state, Cx30 deficiency induced modest enlargement of astrocytic processes in the spinal cord gray matter and a partial reduction of Cx43 expression in the spinal cord white matter. These astrocytes in Cx30 KO mice showed earlier and stronger activation during the acute phase of EAE, with upregulated A2 astrocyte markers and a significant decrease in Cx43 in the chronic phases. Spinal cord neurons and axons were more preserved in Cx30 KO mice than in littermates in the chronic phase of EAE. These findings suggest that Cx30 deficiency increased ramified microglia in the CNS in the naïve state and improved chronic EAE through redirecting microglia toward an anti-inflammatory phenotype, suggesting a hitherto unknown critical role of astrocytic Cx30 in regulating microglial number and functional state.

Keywords: astrocyte, chronic neuroinflammation, connexin, experimental autoimmune encephalomyelitis, microglia, multiple sclerosis

INTRODUCTION

Multiple sclerosis (MS) is an inflammatory demyelinating disease of the central nervous system (CNS) (1). It initially presents as relapsing remitting MS (RRMS) but later evolves into secondary progressive MS (SPMS) in ~20% of patients, even after disease-modifying therapies (DMTs) are introduced (2, 3). Most DMTs, mainly targeting the peripheral immune system, can effectively reduce relapses in RRMS; however, they are of little benefit for chronic progression in SPMS (4–6). Thus, chronic progression in MS is currently a matter of concern for research and drug development. Recently, siponimod (7) and ozanimod (8), new functional antagonists of sphingosine-1-phosphate receptor 1 (S1P1), were reported to be effective for preventing disability progression in SPMS. These drugs may directly act on glial cells harboring S1P1 such as microglia and astroglia, in addition to their inhibitory effects on lymphocyte egress from the secondary lymphoid organs (9–11). In chronic MS lesions, persistent demyelination with varying degrees of remyelination and neuroaxonal degeneration are accompanied by the presence of activated microglia but few T cells (12, 13), suggesting a key role of microglia, which are not targeted by the peripherally acting DMTs, in chronic inflammation in SPMS.

Connexins (Cxs) form gap junction (GJ) channels, which allow the intercellular exchange of ions and secondary messengers (14). In the CNS, astrocytes express Cx43, Cx30, and Cx26, while oligodendrocytes express Cx47, Cx32, and Cx29 (15–17). These Cxs constitute a pan-glial network through GJ channels and play key roles in maintaining CNS homeostasis (18–20). We and others have reported dynamic changes of glial Cxs in MS and Baló's concentric sclerosis lesions (21–23). Oligodendrocytic Cx47 and Cx32 are persistently lost in acute and chronic MS plaques, while astrocytic Cx43 is lost in acute lesions and then upregulated in chronic astrogliotic plaques (22–24). Similar changes in Cx47, Cx32, and Cx43 were also observed in acute and chronic experimental autoimmune encephalomyelitis (EAE), an animal model of MS (25–28). These findings suggest the involvement of glial Cxs in inflammatory demyelination.

Consistent with this notion, oligodendrocytic Cx32 knockout (KO) mice developed aggravated acute and chronic EAE, with increased demyelination despite a similar degree of inflammation upon immunization with myelin oligodendrocyte glycoprotein (MOG), compared with wild type (WT) mice (25). By contrast, in astrocytic Cx30 or Cx43 single KO mice and even in Cx30/Cx43 double KO mice, acute EAE was unaltered (29). However, it remains to be elucidated whether a deficiency in Cx30 or Cx43 influences chronic EAE.

Because the expression level of astrocytic Cx30 is very low in normal white matter, changes of Cx30 in MS or EAE lesions have not been well demonstrated (22, 23, 30). Cx43 exists in both mature and immature astrocytes, while Cx30 is expressed only in mature astrocytes (31–33), thus gliotic scar astrocytes show an upregulation of Cx43 but no detectable changes of Cx30 (23). Similarly, cultured astrocytes express detectable levels of Cx43 but not Cx30, although they can express Cx30 after very long term culture (33, 34). These features of Cx30 make it difficult to study its dynamics and roles in inflammatory demyelination, and therefore there have been few studies of Cx30 in EAE. However, the non-channel functions of Cxs have recently gained increasing attention: Cx30 can change astrocyte morphology, thereby modulating astrocyte functions such as synaptic transmission (35). Cxs also inhibits DNA synthesis, which affects the gene expression network (36, 37).

In the present study, we aimed to clarify the roles of Cx30 in chronic neuroinflammation by studying chronic EAE in Cx30 KO mice. Here, we report Cx30 deficiency induces anti-inflammatory microglia and improves clinical symptoms and demyelination of chronic but not acute EAE.

MATERIALS AND METHODS

Ethics Statement

The experimental procedures were designed to minimize the number of animals used as well as animal suffering. All animal experiments were carried out according to the guidelines for proper conduct of animal experiments published by the Science Council of Japan and the ARRIVE (Animal Research: Reporting of *in vivo* Experiments) guidelines for animal research. Ethical approval for the study was granted by the Animal Care and Use Committee of Kyushu University (#A29-146-3).

Animals and Genotyping

Twelve-to-sixteen-week-old female Cx30 KO mice were used in this study. Cx30 KO mice (38) that had been backcrossed to C57BL/6J at the archiving center were purchased from the European Mouse Mutant Archive. C57BL/6 mice were purchased from KBT Oriental (Tosu, Japan). All mice were bred and maintained under specific pathogen free conditions in the Center of Biological Research, Graduate School of Medical Sciences, Kyushu University. The Cx30 KO mice were genotyped by PCR of DNA obtained from tail biopsies. Primer pairs for detecting Cx30 KO were Cx30 KO-1 (LACZ e Neo): 5′-GGT ACC TTC TAC TAA TTA GCTTGG-3′; Cx30 KO2 (LACZ e Neo): 5′-AGG TGG TAC CCA TTG TAG AGG AAG-3′; and Cx30 KO-3 (LACZ e Neo): 5′-AGC GAG TAA CAA CCC GTC GGA TTC-3′. The Cx30 KO and WT littermate DNA products were 460 and 544 bps in size, respectively. Cx30 KO mice and their littermates were principally used for the animal experiments, unless otherwise specified.

Induction and Clinical Evaluation of EAE

EAE was induced by immunization of mice with 200 μg of MOG_{35-55} peptide (TS-M704-P; MBL, Nagoya, Japan) in 50 μl phosphate buffered saline (PBS) emulsified in an equal volume of complete Freund's adjuvant (CFA) containing 1 mg/ml *Mycobacterium tuberculosis* H37RA (#231131; BD Difco, Lawrence, KS, USA), followed by intraperitoneal injections of 500 ng pertussis toxin (# 180-A1; List Biological Laboratories Inc., Campbell, CA, USA) on days 0 and 2. Mice were examined daily for signs of EAE and scored as follows: 0, no disease; 1, limp tail; 2, abnormal gait and hind limb weakness (shaking); 2.5, paralysis of one hind limb; 3, paralysis of two hind limbs; 3.5, ascending paralysis (able to move around); 4, tetraplegia; 5, moribund.

Tissue Preparation

Animals were deeply anesthetized by isoflurane (Pfizer Japan Inc., Tokyo, Japan), and perfused transcardially with PBS and then with 4% paraformaldehyde (PFA) in 0.1 M PBS. Spinal cords, brains and optic nerves were carefully dissected. The tissues were fixed overnight in cold 4% PFA at 4°C, then processed into paraffin sections (5 μm). For frozen sections (20 μm), spinal cords were harvested and fixed overnight in 4% PFA using the same protocol as above and sequentially displaced with 15 and 30% sucrose in PBS for 24 h each at 4°C. The resulting tissues were embedded in Tissue-Tek O.C.T. Compound (4583, Sakura Finetek, Torrance, CA, USA) and stored at −80°C.

Histopathological and Immunohistochemical Analyses

Paraffin-embedded sections of spinal cord were stained with hematoxylin and eosin (HE). Paraffin-embedded sections of optic nerves were subjected to immunohistochemistry using an indirect immunoperoxidase method. After deparaffinization, endogenous peroxidase was quenched with 0.3% hydrogen peroxide in absolute methanol for 30 min. The sections were permeabilized with 0.1% Triton in PBS (PBS-T) for 10 min, washed using Tris-HCl for 5 min, dipped in 10 mM citrate buffer, and then autoclaved (120°C, 10 min). All sections were cooled to room temperature and incubated with anti-brain-derived neurotrophic factor (BDNF) antibodies overnight at 4°C (**Supplementary Table 1**). The next day, after rinsing, sections were labeled with either a streptavidin-biotin complex or an enhanced indirect immunoperoxidase method using Envision (K4003, Dako, Glostrup, Denmark); 3,3-diaminobenzidine tetrahydrochloride (DAB; D5637, Sigma-Aldrich, Tokyo, Japan) was used for the DAB color reaction. Finally, sections were counterstained with hematoxylin.

Confocal Microscope Immunofluorescence Analysis

Paraffin sections of brain and optic nerves were deparaffinized in xylene and rehydrated through ethanol. After washing and autoclaving, sections were incubated with anti-arginasel, anti-nitric oxide synthase 2 (NOS2), anti-Iba-1, anti-glial fibrillary acidic protein (GFAP), anti-Cx43, anti-Cx30, anti-myelin basic protein (MBP), anti-NeuN, purified anti-neurofilament H (NF-H) (SMI-31), and anti-IL-34 antibodies (**Supplementary Table 1**) overnight at 4°C. The following day, the sections were washed, incubated with Alexa Fluor 488- or 546-conjugated secondary antibodies (1:1,000; Thermo Fisher, Rockford, IL, USA) and 4′,6-diamidino-2-phenylindole (DAPI; Sigma-Aldrich, Tokyo, Japan) overnight at 4°C, then dehydrated and sealed with Permafluor (#TA-030-FM; Thermo Scientific, Fremont, CA, USA). The frozen sections of spinal cords were cut at 20 μm with a cryostat microtome (Leica CM 1850, Leica Microsystems GmbH, Wetzlar, Germany) and floated in PBS-T. The sections were washed 3 times in PBS-T, blocked with 10% normal goat serum in PBS for 2 h, then incubated overnight at 4°C with anti-arginasel, anti-NOS2, anti-Cx30, anti-Cx43, anti-Iba-1, anti-GFAP, anti-CD45, anti-CD3, anti-C3, and anti-CD169 antibodies (**Supplementary Table 1**). The sections were also treated with anti-S100a10 antibody in the same way but without blocking by normal goat serum (**Supplementary Table 1**). After rinsing the next day, the sections were incubated with Alexa Fluor 488- or 546-conjugated secondary antibodies (1:1,000; Thermo Fisher) or FluoroMyelin Red Fluorescent Myelin Stain (1:1,000; #F34652; Thermo Fisher) and DAPI overnight at 4°C, then washed in PBS-T and sealed with Permafluor. Immunofluorescence was captured by a confocal laser microscope (Nikon A1; Nikon, Tokyo, Japan), equipped with 405, 488, and 561 nm laser lines, at the same magnification, laser intensity, gain, offset values, and pinhole settings. Quantification of immunofluorescence was performed using ImageJ version 1.6.0_24 (Windows version of NIH Image; downloaded from https://imagej.nih.gov/ij/download.html) on three-to-five lumbar spinal cord sections for each animal in each group.

Quantification of Myelin Density and Cell Infiltration in the Spinal Cord, Brain, and Optic Nerve

For the quantification of GFAP, Iba-I, Cx30, Cx43, CD3, CD169, CD45, S100A10, C3, BDNF, NOS2, and IL-34, fluorescent images from the anterior part of the lumbar spinal cord, cerebellum, cerebrum, and optic nerve were analyzed (ImageJ version 1.6.0_24) using the area fraction technique as previously described (39, 40). Briefly, identical microscope settings were applied to all photographs from each experiment and images from the same areas were acquired. Images were de-noised and set to the same threshold baseline across experimental groups for each antibody to measure the area of cellular staining, instead of cell density measurement or cell number counting, because most infiltrating cells were focally clustered. For the quantification of myelin and MBP immunostaining results, whole spinal cord images were captured under the microscope and separated into anterior or posterior parts for analysis. SMI-31 immunostaining images were captured under the microscope and spinal cord anterior white matter areas were used for analysis. Image analysis was performed using ImageJ software. Mean pixel intensity values were compared between genotypes (41). For the quantitative analyses of NeuN-positive cells, transverse sections of the spinal cord were divided into the left and right regions by a vertical line through the central canal. The size of each microscopic field was 1.6384 mm^2. The left or right positive cell region areas (0.33–0.44 mm^2) were calculated automatically by ImageJ. NeuN-positive cells were counted manually and used to calculate the cell density (neurons/mm^2) (42). The investigator performing the analysis was blinded to the genotypes. All assessments were made from three-to-five sections per mouse ($n = 3$ to 8 mice in each group). In the quantification graph, the mean value of three-to-five sections was used as scatter dots to represent each mouse.

Immunocolocalization Analysis

We delineated the same areas of focus in the spinal cord white matter, optic nerve, and arbor vitae of the cerebellum in all samples to be analyzed. Colocalization of arginase-1 and Iba-1 was expressed as a Pearson's correlation coefficient and the intensity correlation analysis plugin of ImageJ was used (43). Pearson's correlation values range from 1 to −1, with 1 representing complete positive correlation and −1 a negative correlation, with zero representing no correlation. All quantifications were obtained from a minimum of three sections from the spinal cord, optic nerve, cerebellum, and cerebrum per mouse.

Microglial Circularity Analysis

ImageJ was used to automatically calculate the circularity of microglial cells (circularity $= 4\pi S/L2$). Cells with circularity close to 1 were regarded as having a morphology close to round, indicating an activated state (44, 45).

Microglial Cell Isolation and Flow Cytometry

Brains and spinal cords were harvested and homogenized. Mononuclear cells were separated with a 30 and 70% Percoll (GE Healthcare, Tokyo, Japan) gradient as previously described (46). Cells were stained with anti-CD45-PerCP and anti-CD11b-PE/Cy7 antibodies, sorted and analyzed on a SH800 Cell Sorter (Sony Corporation, Tokyo, Japan).

Gene Expression Microarray

Total RNA was isolated from cells using an RNeasy Mini Kit (Qiagen) according to the manufacturer's instructions. RNA samples were quantified by an ND-1000 spectrophotometer (NanoDrop Technologies, Wilmington, DE, USA) and the quality was confirmed with a 2200 TapeStation (Agilent technologies, Santa Clara, CA, USA). Total RNA (2 ng) was amplified, labeled using a GeneChip® WT Pico Kit, and hybridized to an Affymetrix GeneChip® Mouse Transcriptome Array 1.0 according to the manufacturer's instructions (Affymetrix, Santa Clara, CA, USA). All hybridized microarrays were scanned by an Affymetrix scanner. Relative hybridization intensities and background hybridization values were calculated using the Affymetrix Expression Console®. These gene array assay results were uploaded to the gene expression omnibus repository (accession number is GSE68202) in the National Center for Biotechnology Information homepage (https://www.ncbi.nlm.nih.gov/geo/query/acc.cgi?acc=GSE112621).

Data Analysis and Filter Criteria

The raw signal intensities of all samples were normalized by a quantile algorithm with Affymetrix® Power Tool version 1.15.0 software. To identify upregulated or downregulated genes, we calculated Z-scores [Z] and ratios (non-log scaled fold-change) from the normalized signal intensities of each probe for comparison between control and experiment samples. Then, we established criteria for regulated genes: upregulated genes had a Z-score ≥ 2.0 and ratio ≥ 1.5-fold, and downregulated genes had a Z-score ≤ -2.0 and ratio ≤ 0.66. Gene set enrichment analysis (47, 48) (GSEA; www.broadinstitute.org/gsea) was performed to investigate deviations of particular gene sets (e.g., Anti-inflammatory set, Pro-inflammatory set; set S) according to a previous report (48, 49). Briefly, after we obtained expression data sets for each study group, we calculated an enrichment score (ES) that reflected the degree to which a set "S" was over-represented at the extremes (top or bottom) of the entire ranked list "L." The score was calculated by walking down the list L and increasing a running-sum statistic when we encountered a gene in S. The ES is the maximum deviation from zero encountered in the random walk. After the estimation of statistical significance of ES, we controlled the proportion of false positives by calculating the false discovery rate (FDR). When the normalized p-value was <0.05 and the FDR was <0.25, the ES was considered significant.

Statistical Analysis

Data are expressed as the mean ± standard error of mean (S.E.M.). The area under curve (AUC) of the overall disease severity was calculated for each mouse to compare the disease course of WT and KO mice using the non-parametric Mann-Whitney U-test (50) Here, acute (onset to day 24) and chronic phases (day 25 and thereafter) were separately analyzed. The postimmunization date when WT groups reached a peak score of 2 or higher was identified as the "peak" (51). The incidence, day of onset, and peak clinical score of EAE were compared using the unpaired t-test with Welch's correction. In EAE experiments, mice that died before the intended day of sacrifice were excluded from statistical analyses. Cell percentages and histological data were assessed by the unpaired t-test with Welch's correction, two-way ANOVA, or one-way ANOVA. A p-value < 0.05 was considered statistically significant. Analyses were performed using Graph Pad Prism 7.0 software (Graph Pad, La Jolla, CA, USA).

RESULTS

Cx30 Deficiency Induces Modest Morphological Changes and Cx43 Reduction in Spinal Cord Astrocytes but No Changes in Myelin Density

In WT littermate mice in the naïve state, Cx30 was expressed predominantly on astrocytes in the gray matter of the spinal cord, cerebellum and cerebrum, while Cx30 expression was very low in white matter astrocytes, including the optic nerve (**Figure 1A**; **Supplementary Figure 1**), which is consistent with our previous study in humans (22). By contrast, Cx30 was completely absent in Cx30 KO mice (**Figures 1A–C**; **Supplementary Figure 1**). GFAP immunostaining revealed neither morphological nor quantitative changes in $GFAP^+$ astrocytes in the white matter between WT and Cx30 KO mice, whereas $GFAP^+$ astrocytes in the gray matter had thicker processes and showed a tendency to be increased in Cx30 KO mice than in WT mice ($p = 0.0575$, **Figures 1A,D,E**).

Because astrocytic Cx30 and Cx43 have similar functions and partly overlapping permeation profiles (15), we examined whether Cx43 was upregulated to compensate for the lack of Cx30 in Cx30 KO mice. GFAP and Cx43 double immunostaining

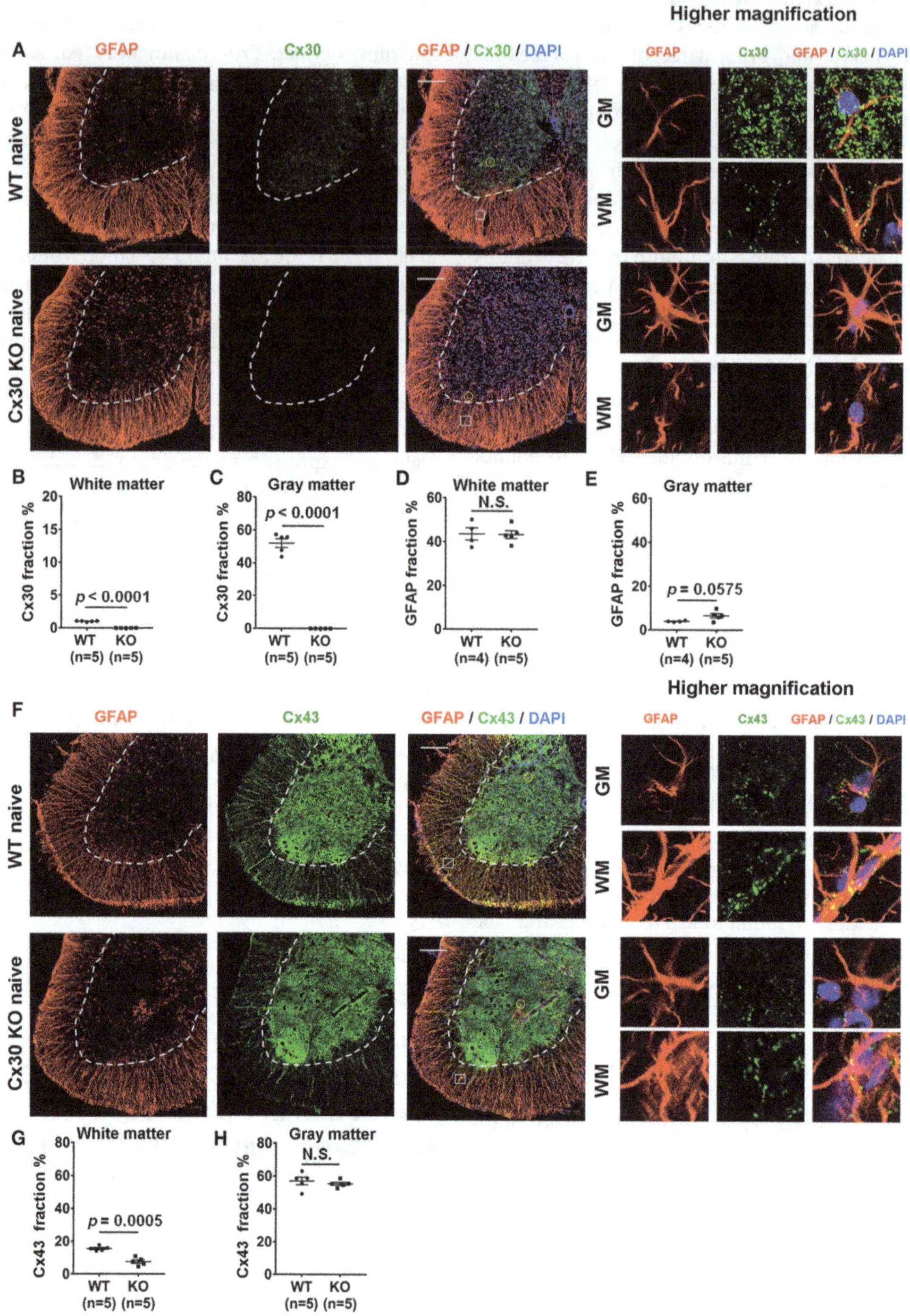

FIGURE 1 | Morphology and number of astrocytes, and expressions of Cx30 and Cx43 in WT and Cx30 KO mice. **(A)** Confocal images showing immunostaining for Cx30 and GFAP in the anterior part of spinal cord sections from naïve WT (littermate) and Cx30 KO mice. Higher magnification images show co-labeling of GFAP and Cx30 in single astrocytes, which are highlighted by a yellow circle in the gray matter or a white square in the white matter of each figure. Scale bars, 200 μm. **(B,C)** Quantification of Cx30$^+$ area percentages in the white **(B)** and gray **(C)** matter. **(D,E)** Quantification of GFAP$^+$ area percentages in the white **(D)** and gray **(E)** matter. **(F)** Confocal images showing immunostaining for GFAP and Cx43 in spinal cords from naïve WT (littermate) and Cx30 KO mice. Higher magnification images show co-labeling of GFAP and Cx43 in single astrocytes, which are highlighted by a yellow circle in the gray matter or a white square in the white matter of the figure. Scale bars, 200 μm. **(G,H)** Quantification of Cx43$^+$ area percentages in the white matter **(G)** and gray matter **(H)**. Means ± S.E.M. are shown. Statistical differences were determined by unpaired *t*-test with Welch's correction. N.S. = not significant, *n* indicates number of mice and each scatter dot represents individual mice in each group.

revealed that Cx43 was more abundant in the gray matter than in the white matter of the spinal cord in both WT and Cx30 KO mice (**Figures 1F–H**). There was no significant difference in Cx43 immunoreactivity in the spinal cord gray matter between WT and Cx30 KO mice, but Cx43 levels were significantly reduced in the spinal cord white matter of Cx30 KO mice compared with WT mice ($p = 0.0005$; **Figures 1F–H**). These findings are consistent with the observation that Cx30 but not Cx43 can compensate for other Cxs in CNS tissues (52). This suggests that Cx30 deficiency causes modest enlargement of astrocytic processes in the spinal gray matter and a partial reduction of Cx43 expression in spinal white matter astrocytes. However, myelin density did not differ significantly between Cx30 KO mice and WT littermates in the naive state by Fluoromyelin staining or MBP immunostaining (**Supplementary Figures 2A–D**).

Cx30 Deficiency Increases the Numbers of Ramified Microglia

Unexpectedly, Cx30 KO mice showed an apparent increase in the numbers of Iba-1^+ microglia in the spinal cord gray matter, optic nerve, cerebellum, and cerebrum compared with WT littermate mice ($p = 0.0055$, $p = 0.0274$, $p = 0.0015$, and $p = 0.0012$, respectively), but not in the spinal cord white matter (**Figures 2A–E**). Morphologically, microglia in Cx30 KO mice had thin soma and delicate radially-projecting processes (**Figure 2A** inset), indicating that these microglia were in a resting state (ramified phenotype). There were no significant differences in the microglia circularity index between Cx30 KO and WT mice in the spinal cord gray and white matter, optic nerve, cerebrum, and cerebellum (**Figures 2B–E**). Flow cytometric analyses demonstrated that numbers of $CD45^{dim}CD11b^+$ microglia in isolated viable cells from the brain were significantly increased in Cx30 KO mice compared with WT littermate mice ($p = 0.0025$; **Figures 2F,G**).

To further characterize the microglial phenotype in Cx30 KO mice, gene expression profiles were analyzed by RNA microarray using microglia isolated from the spinal cords and brains of naïve WT and Cx30 KO mice. Microglia from Cx30 KO mice showed similar expression levels of anti-inflammatory and pro-inflammatory genes to WT microglia in both the spinal cord and brain (**Table 1** and **Figure 3A**). GSEA analysis revealed similar gene enrichments in the spinal cord and brain between naive WT and KO mice (**Table 1** and **Figures 3B–E**). We also performed GSEA analysis to characterize the expression profiles of cytokines/chemokines, complement, alarmin, reactive oxygen species (ROS), MHC, and tumor genes. Among them, Cx30 KO microglia from the naïve spinal cord but not brain demonstrated significantly lower expression levels of cytokines/chemokines, alarmin, MHC, and tumor genes, indicating a less reactive state to inflammatory insults (**Table 1** and **Supplementary Figures 3A,C**). These findings indicate that the increase in microglia was widespread in the CNS of naïve Cx30 KO mice compared with WT mice; these microglial were not activated but rather in a resting state, with a ramified morphology and low cytokine/chemokine, alarmin, MHC, and tumor gene production.

Cx30 Deficiency Attenuates the Clinical Severity and Demyelination of Chronic but Not Acute EAE Without Influencing T Cell Infiltration

Cx30 KO mice did not show any significant differences in the incidence, onset day, and clinical severity (peak score and acute phase AUC from Day 9 to 24) of acute EAE compared with WT mice, in agreement with a previous study (29) (**Figure 4A**). By contrast, clinical severity in the chronic EAE phase (chronic phase AUC from Day 25 to 59) was significantly attenuated in Cx30 KO mice compared with WT mice. HE staining showed that the infiltration of inflammatory cells into the spinal cord was markedly reduced in Cx30 KO mice compared with WT mice in the chronic EAE phase (**Figure 4B**). Moreover, the extent of demyelination was significantly decreased in the chronic but not acute phase of EAE in Cx30 KO mice compared with WT mice, in both the anterior and posterior parts of the spinal cord ($p = 0.0031$ and $p = 0.002$, respectively, by Fluoromyelin staining; and $p = 0.0328$ and $p = 0.0167$, respectively, by MBP immunostaining; **Figures 4C–E, Supplementary Figures 2E,F**). $CD45^+$ immunocytes and $CD3^+$ T cells were not significantly different between Cx30 KO and WT mice in either acute or chronic phases, although $CD45^+$ cells tended to be increased in Cx30 KO mice compared with WT mice at acute phase ($p = 0.0622$; **Figures 4C,D,F**). We performed CD169 immunostaining to discriminate peripheral blood-borne macrophages from microglia and other immune cells, and found that $CD169^+$ macrophages were significantly lower in Cx30 KO mice compared with WT mice in the chronic phase ($p = 0.0336$), but not the acute phase (**Figures 5A–C**).

Microglia in Cx30 KO Mice Are Widespread and Highly Activated in the Chronic Phase of EAE

Intriguingly, Iba-1^+ microglial cell numbers were consistently greater in both the white and gray matter of the spinal cord in Cx30 KO mice compared with WT mice in the acute and chronic phases (white matter, $p = 0.0106$ on Day 13 and $p = 0.0274$ on Day 59; gray matter, $p = 0.0483$ on Day 13 and $p = 0.0111$ on Day 59; **Figures 5D,E,G**). The above-mentioned increased tendency of $CD45^+$ cells in the acute phase in Cx30 KO mice might be explained by the earlier and stronger increase of Iba-1^+ cells compared with WT mice. In the spinal cord white matter, microglial circularity was significantly greater in Cx30 KO mice than in WT mice in both the acute ($p = 0.045$) and chronic phases ($p = 0.0418$; **Figure 5H**). This increase in Iba-1^+ cells in the chronic phase of EAE was also observed in the optic nerve ($p = 0.0067$) and cerebellum ($p = 0.0312$) of Cx30 KO mice (**Supplementary Figures 4A,B,D,E**). In the cerebellum, microglial circularity was significantly greater ($p = 0.0121$) in Cx30 KO mice than in WT mice but there was no significant increase of microglial circularity in the optic nerve (**Supplementary Figures 4C,F**). These findings suggest that a widespread increase and activation of Iba-1^+ microglia in inflamed CNS tissues, especially the spinal cord white matter, is a characteristic feature of Cx30 KO mice.

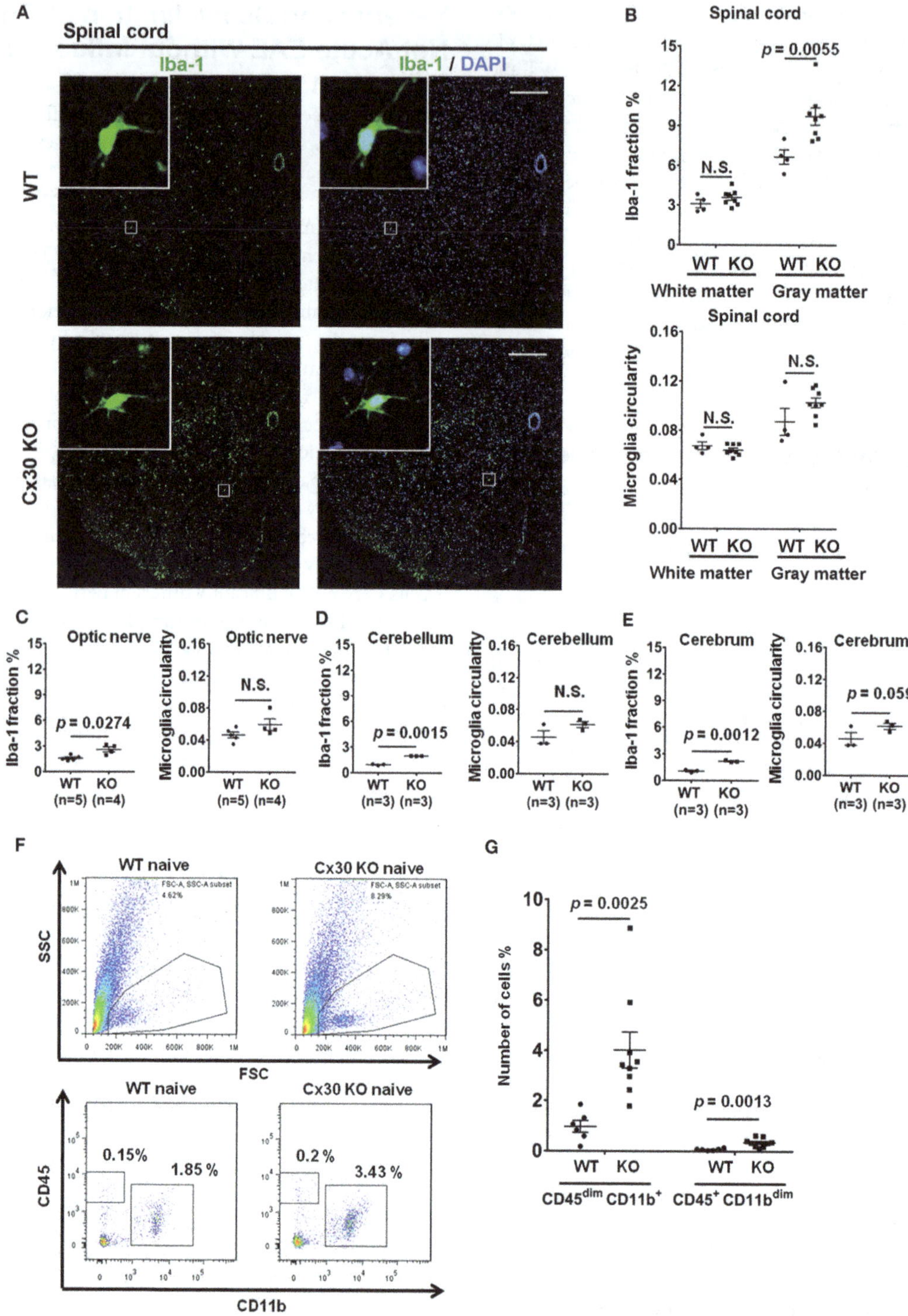

FIGURE 2 | Microglial morphology and numbers in CNS tissues of WT and Cx30 KO mice. **(A)** Representative images of Iba-1 immunostaining of naïve WT (littermate) and Cx30 KO mouse spinal cord. Scale bars, 200 μm. **(B–E)** Quantification of Iba-1^{+} cell area fractions and microglia circularity in the white and gray matter of the anterior spinal cord **(B)**, optic nerve **(C)**, cerebellum **(D)**, and cerebrum **(E)**. **(F)** Gating strategy used to determine viable mononuclear cells for further analysis. In the whole brain suspension, a gate was created on the non-debris population. Inside this population, the microglial cells were gated based on CD45/CD11b intensity. SSC, Side scatter; FSC, Forward scatter. Representative flow cytometric analysis of microglia (CD45^{dim} CD11b^{+} cells) isolated from WT (littermate) and Cx30 KO mouse brains. Numbers on plots are percentages of double-positive cells among the gated viable cells. **(G)** Percentages of CD45^{dim} CD11b^{+} microglia and CD45^{+} CD11b^{dim} cells in the total cell population (3×10^4) isolated from naïve WT (littermate) and Cx30 KO mouse brains. Data are from 6 WT mice and 9 Cx30 KO mice. Means ± S.E.M. are shown. Statistical differences were determined using the unpaired *t*-test with Welch's correction. N.S. = not significant. *n* indicates the number of mice and each scatter dot represents individual mice in each group.

TABLE 1 | Summary of GSEA results.

Gene category	Naive spinal cord	EAE spinal cord	Naive brain	EAE brain
	WT vs. Cx30 KO	WT vs. Cx30 KO	WT vs. Cx30 KO	WT vs. Cx30 KO
Pro-inflammatory	0.392 (WT)	0.007 (WT)	0.571 (Cx30 KO)	0.016 (WT)
Anti-inflammatory	0.083 (WT)	0.092 (WT)	0.234 (WT)	0.450 (WT)
Cytokines/Chemokines	<0.001 (WT)	<0.001 (WT)	0.773 (WT)	0.252 (Cx30 KO)
Complement	0.997 (Cx30 KO)	0.001 (WT)	0.576 (WT)	0.348 (Cx30 KO)
Alarmin	<0.001 (WT)	0.005 (WT)	0.898 (Cx30 KO)	0.061 (WT)
ROS	0.524 (WT)	0.005 (WT)	0.093 (Cx30 KO)	0.363 (Cx30 KO)
MHC	<0.001 (WT)	0.008 (WT)	0.173 (WT)	<0.001 (Cx30 KO)
Tumor	<0.001 (WT)	<0.001 (WT)	0.967 (Cx30 KO)	0.001 (Cx30 KO)

Normalized p-values by gene set enrichment analysis between WT (C57BL/6) and Cx30 KO mice are shown. Upregulated groups are indicated in parenthesis for each category.

Microglia in Cx30 KO EAE Mice Have an Anti-inflammatory Phenotype in the Chronic Phase of EAE by Gene Expression Microarrays

To further characterize the activated microglial phenotype in the chronic phase of EAE in Cx30 KO mice, we used MOG_{35-55}-induced EAE and isolated microglia from the spinal cords and brains of Cx30 KO and WT mice at Day 39 after immunization, when clinical scores and AUC in the chronic phase were significantly lower in Cx30 KO mice than in WT mice ($p = 0.0023$). Microglia isolated from Cx30 KO EAE spinal cords and brains had lower expression levels of pro-inflammatory genes, such as *IL-1b*, *Nos2*, *Tnf*, and *Ptgs2*, but no significant changes in anti-inflammatory gene levels, except for an increase in the *Mrc1*gene (**Figure 3F**). GSEA analysis revealed that microglia from Cx30 KO mouse spinal cord and brain had less pro-inflammatory gene expressions than those from WT mice in the chronic EAE phase (spinal cord, ES = 0.721, normalized $p = 0.007$, FDR = 0.018; brain, pro-inflammatory genes; ES = 0.643, normalized $p = 0.016$, FDR = 0.037; **Table 1** and **Figures 3G–J**). Furthermore, gene expressions of cytokines/chemokines, complements, alarmins, ROS, MHC, and tumor antigens in spinal cord but not brain microglia were significantly less in Cx30 KO than in WT mice in the chronic EAE phase (**Table 1** and **Supplementary Figures 3B,D**). These findings indicate that the increased numbers of activated microglia in Cx30 KO mice have a reduced pro-inflammatory phenotype, especially in the spinal cord, in the chronic EAE phase.

Cx30 KO Mice Upregulate Arginase-1 and BDNF but Downregulate NOS2 in the Chronic Phase of EAE

To confirm the anti-inflammatory nature of the activated microglia in the CNS tissues of Cx30 KO mice in the chronic EAE phase, we performed double-staining for Iba-1 and arginase-1, an anti-inflammatory gene. Colocalization of Iba-1 and arginase-1 was more frequently observed in the optic nerve and cerebellum of Cx30 KO mice compared with WT littermate mice ($p = 0.012$, and $p = 0.0041$, respectively; determined by higher mean Pearson's coefficient values; **Figures 6A–D**), although differences in colocalization levels between WT and Cx30 KO mice did not reach statistical significance in the spinal cord, possibly because of the infiltration of peripheral blood-borne macrophages (**Figures 6E,F**). Furthermore, in the optic nerve of Cx30 KO mice, BDNF immunoreactivity was significantly greater compared with WT mice ($p = 0.0019$; **Supplementary Figures 5A,B**). By contrast, NOS2 immunoreactivity in the optic nerve, cerebellum, and spinal cord white matter was significantly lower in Cx30 KO mice than in WT mice ($p = 0.0003$, $p = 0.0032$, and $p = 0.0047$, respectively; **Supplementary Figures 5C–H**). These findings indicate that microglia in Cx30 KO mice tended to have an anti-inflammatory phenotype, which is more evident in the CNS areas where peripheral blood-borne macrophages are rare during chronic EAE.

Cx30 Deficiency Induces the Earlier and Stronger Activation of A2 Astrocytes During EAE

Compared with naïve spinal cord, numbers of $GFAP^+$ astrocytes in the white and gray matter of the spinal cord increased significantly in the chronic EAE phase in both WT and Cx30 KO mice (white matter, $p = 0.0159$ and $p = 0.0003$, respectively; and gray matter, $p = 0.0008$ and $p = 0.0014$, respectively, at Day 59) but not in the acute phase, except for $GFAP^+$ astrocytes in the gray matter of Cx30 KO mice at Day 16 ($p = 0.0154$; **Figure 7A**; **Supplementary Figures 6A–D**). However, Cx30 KO mice had significantly more $GFAP^+$ astrocytes in the spinal cord white and gray matter (white matter; $p = 0.0341$ on Day 13 and gray matter; $p = 0.0006$ on Day 16) during the acute phase compared with WT mice, whereas this difference was not evident in the chronic phase in either the white or gray matter, suggesting the earlier and stronger activation of astrocytes in Cx30 KO mice (**Figures 7A–C**).

In WT mice, Cx30 immunoreactivity was unchanged throughout the clinical course of EAE in the spinal white matter, but compared with the naïve state it was increased significantly in the spinal cord gray matter in the chronic stage ($p = 0.0327$; **Figures 7A,D,E**; **Supplementary Figures 6E,F**). In Cx30 KO mice, Cx30 immunoreactivity was not detected at any stage

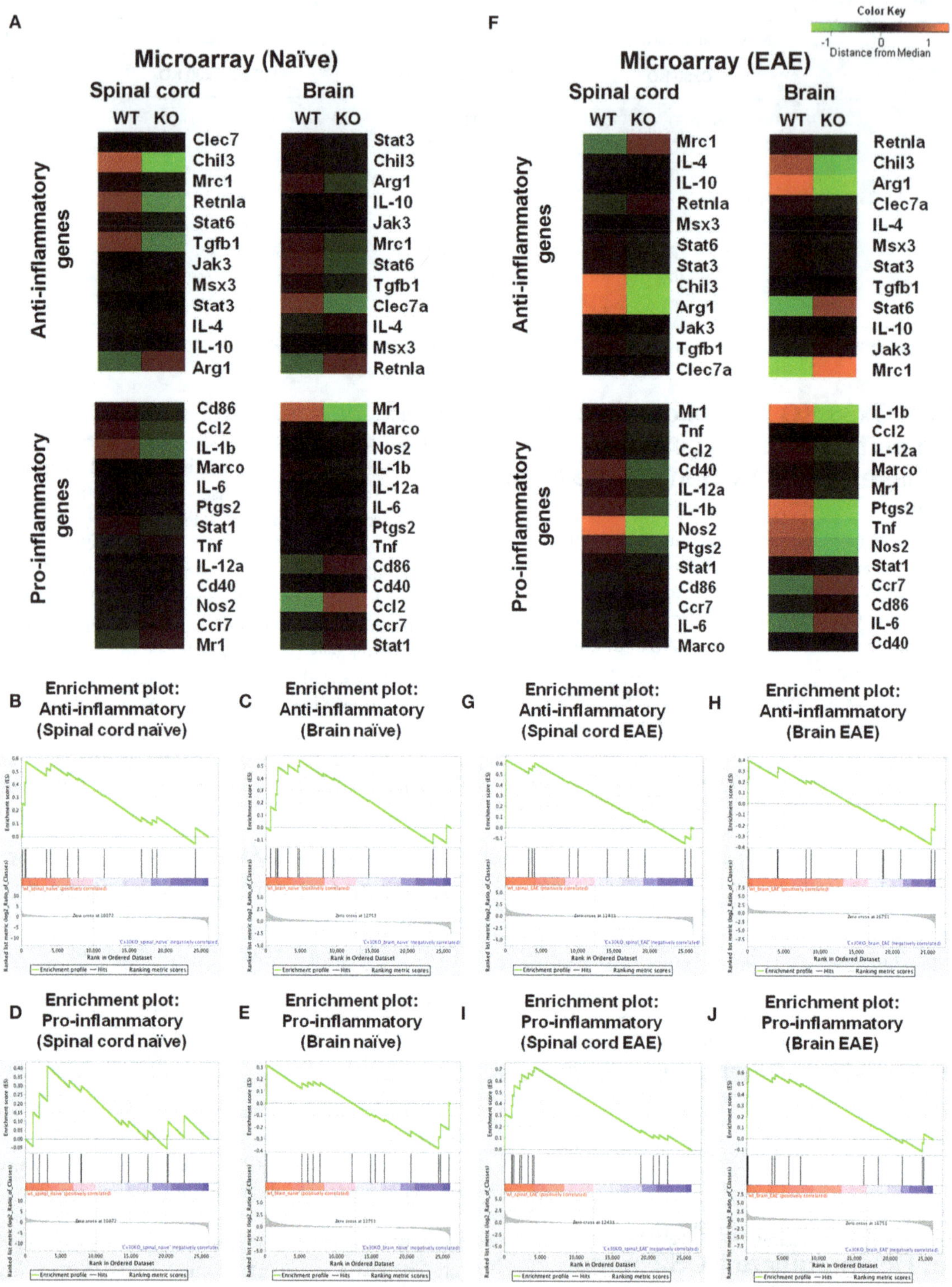

FIGURE 3 | Microarray analysis of microglia isolated from spinal cords and brains of WT (C57BL/6) and Cx30 KO mice. **(A)** Cluster analysis of gene expression arrays according to anti-inflammatory and pro-inflammatory genes of naïve brain and spinal cord from WT (C57BL/6) and Cx30 KO mice. Color keys on each column represent *Z* scores for each gene. **(B–E)** Enrichment plots for the anti-inflammatory **(B,C)** and pro-inflammatory **(D,E)** genes of naive spinal cords **(B,D)** and brains **(C,E)** from WT (C57BL/6) and Cx30 KO mice. **(F)** Cluster analysis of gene expression arrays according to anti-inflammatory and pro-inflammatory genes of chronic EAE brains and spinal cords from WT (C57BL/6) and Cx30 KO mice. Color keys on each column represent *Z* scores for each gene. **(G–J)** Enrichment plots for the anti-inflammatory **(G,H)** and pro-inflammatory **(I,J)** genes of chronic EAE spinal cords **(G,I)** and brains **(H,J)** from WT (C57BL/6) and Cx30 KO mice. The relative gene positions are indicated by the straight lines (line plot) under each graph. Lines clustered to the left represent higher ranked genes in the ranked list.

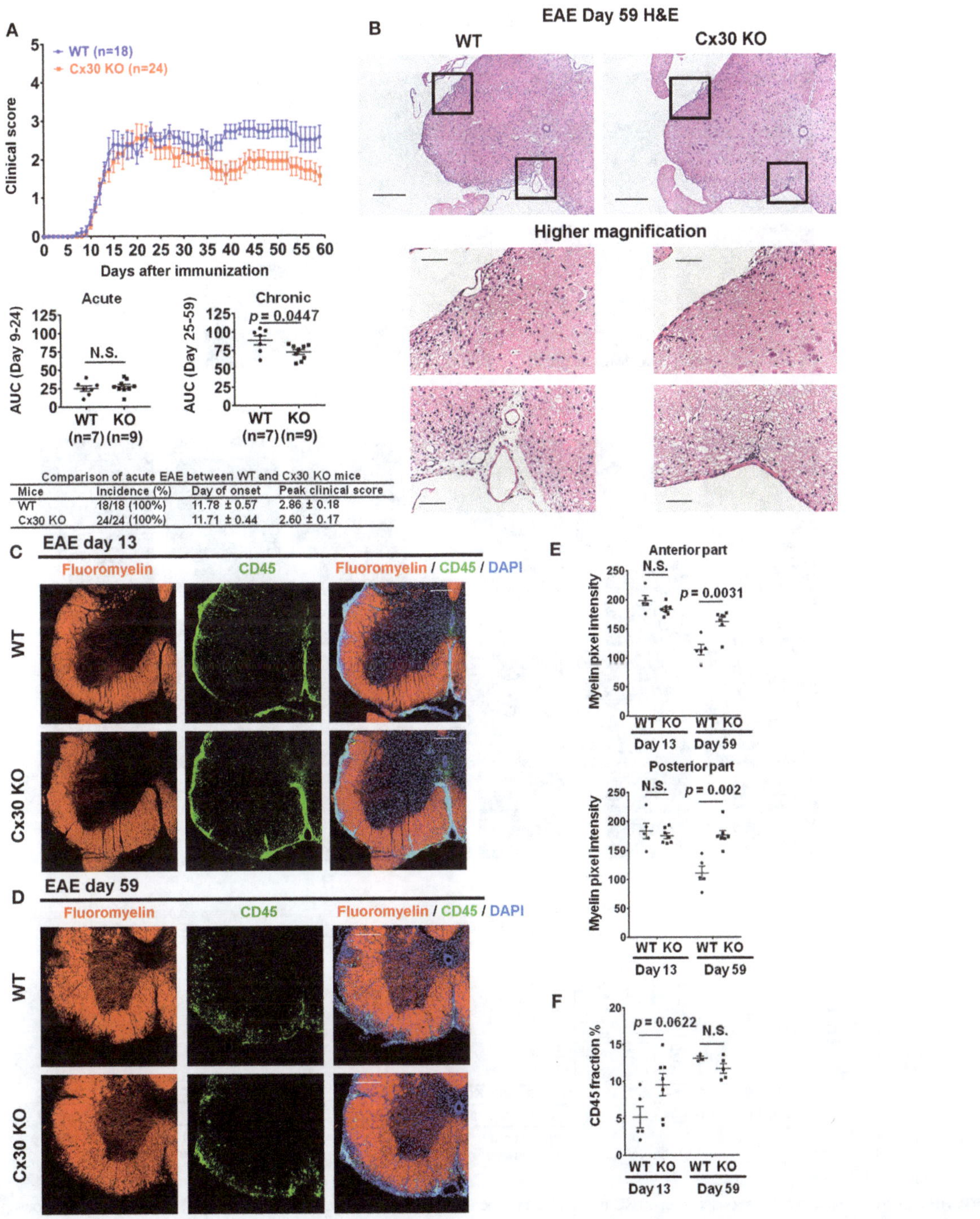

FIGURE 4 | Improvement of clinical severity and demyelination in the chronic but not acute phase of EAE in Cx30 KO mice. **(A)** EAE clinical score changes in WT (littermate) and Cx30 KO mice. The severity of disease was separately analyzed according to acute (Days 9–24) and chronic (Days 25–59) phases by evaluating the area under the curve (AUC). Data shown are from a single experiment representative of four independent experiments including a total of 42 mice; *p*-values of the AUC were determined by the Mann-Whitney *U*-test. There was no significant difference in incidence, day of onset, or peak clinical score between WT (littermate) and Cx30 KO mice in the acute EAE phase. Data for the following parameters are shown as the mean ± S.E.M.: day of EAE onset, and peak clinical score of mice that developed EAE. Statistical differences were determined using the unpaired *t*-test with Welch's correction. **(B)** HE staining of spinal cords in the chronic EAE phase (Day 59). Scale bars, 200 μm in the upper panels and 100 μm in the lower panels. **(C,D)** Confocal images showing immunostaining for Fluoromyelin and CD45 in spinal cord sections from WT (littermate) and Cx30 KO mice in the acute (Day 13) and chronic (Day 59) EAE phases. Scale bars, 200 μm. **(E)** Quantification of myelin density in the anterior and posterior parts of spinal cords from WT (littermate) and Cx30 KO mice in the acute (Day 13) and chronic (Day 59) EAE phases. **(F)** Quantification of the $CD45^+$ cell area fraction in the anterior spinal cords from WT (littermate) and Cx30 KO EAE mice in the acute (Day 13) and chronic EAE phases (Day 59). Statistical differences were determined using the unpaired *t*-test with Welch's correction. N.S. = not significant. *n* indicates the number of mice and each scatter dot represents individual mice in each group.

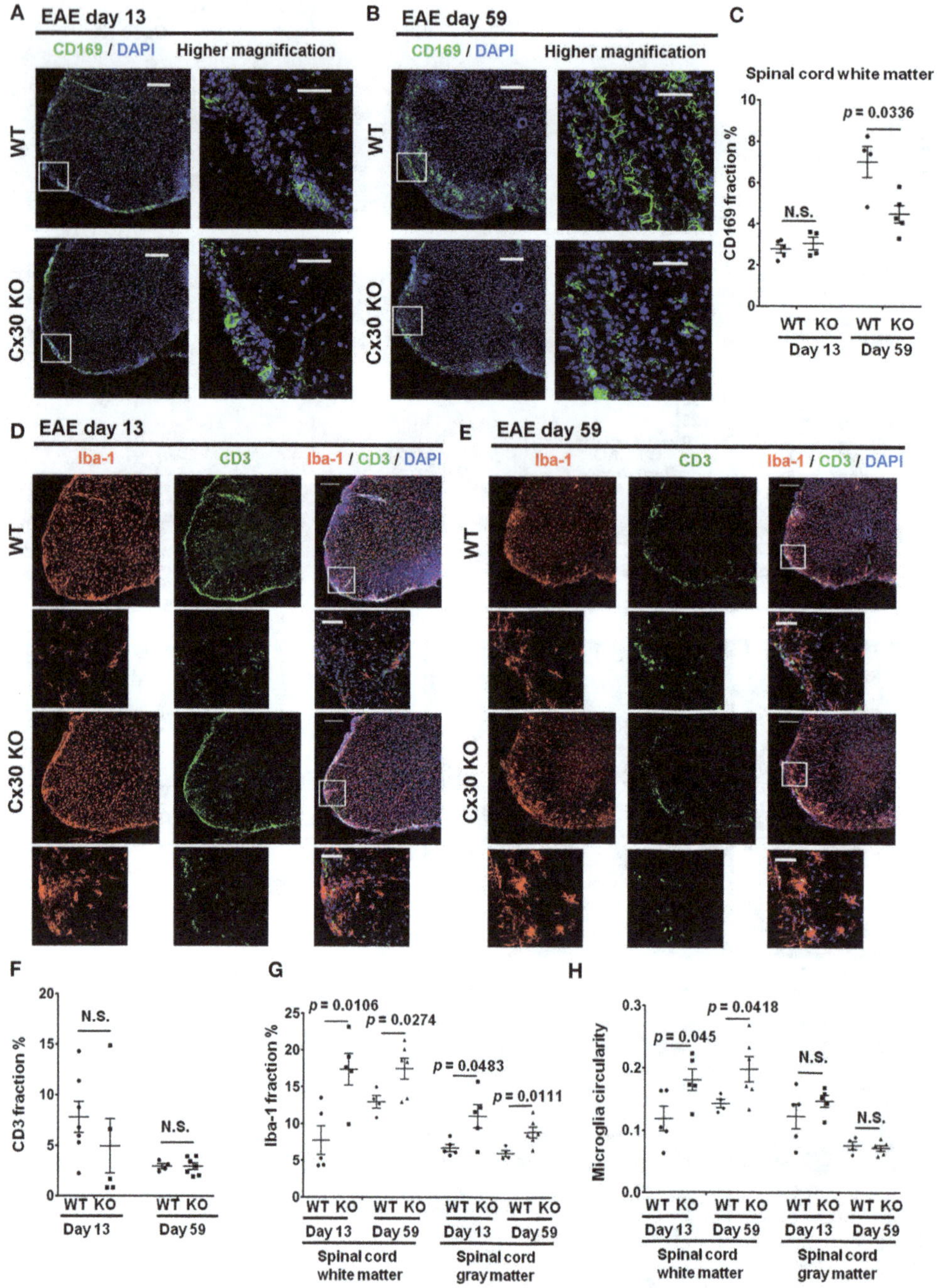

FIGURE 5 | Altered immune cell responses in Cx30 KO mice in the chronic EAE phase compared with WT mice. **(A,B)** Confocal images showing immunostaining of CD169 in spinal cord sections from WT (littermate) and Cx30 KO EAE mice in the acute (Day 13) and chronic (Day 59) EAE phase. Scale bars, 200 μm. Higher magnification images are CD169 in the spinal cord, which are highlighted by a white rectangular frame in the left panel of lower magnification images. **(C)** Quantification of the CD169$^+$ cell area fraction in the anterior spinal cord white matter from WT (littermate) and Cx30 KO EAE mice in the acute (Day 13) and chronic (Day 59) EAE phases. **(D,E)** Confocal images showing immunostaining for Iba-1 and CD3 in spinal cord sections from WT (littermate) and Cx30 KO EAE mice in the acute (Day 13) and chronic (Day 59) EAE phases. Scale bars, 200 μm. Higher magnification images show co-labeling of CD3 and Iba-1 in spinal cords, which are highlighted by a white rectangular frame in the lower magnification images above. **(F)** Quantification of the CD3$^+$ cell area fraction in the anterior spinal cords from WT (littermate) and Cx30 KO EAE mice in the acute (Day 13) and chronic (Day 59) EAE phases. **(G,H)** Quantification of the Iba-1$^+$ cell area fraction **(G)** and microglial circularity **(H)** in the spinal cord white and gray matter from WT (littermate) and Cx30 KO EAE mice in the acute (Day 13) and chronic (Day 59) EAE phase. Means $\pm$ S.E.M. are shown. Statistical differences were determined using the unpaired *t*-test with Welch's correction. N.S. = not significant. *n* indicates the number of mice and each scatter dot represents individual mice in each group.

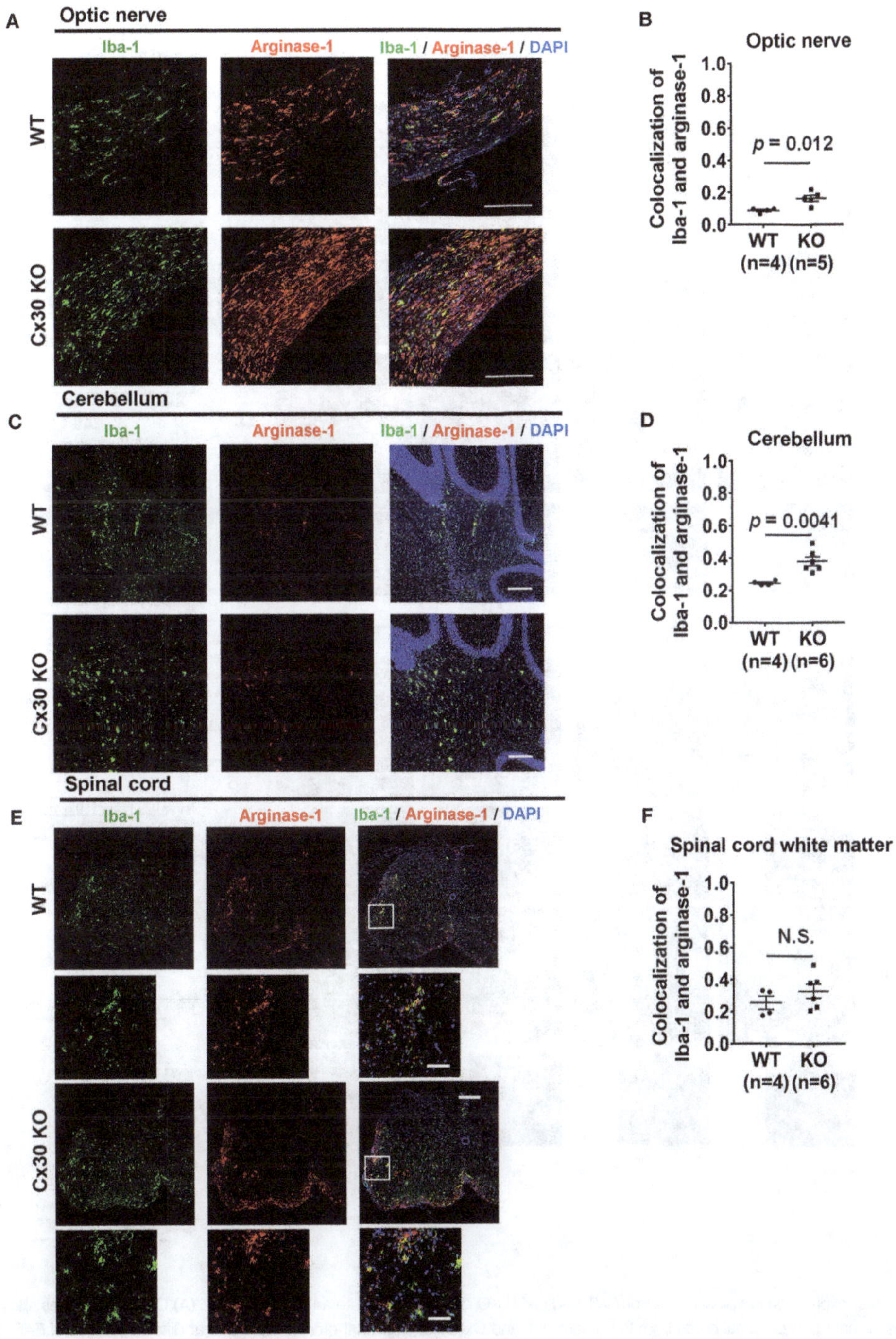

FIGURE 6 | Anti-inflammatory marker expression of microglia in WT and Cx30 KO mice with chronic EAE. **(A,C,E)** Confocal images showing immunostaining for Iba-1 and arginase-1 in optic nerves **(A)**, cerebellum **(C)**, and spinal cords **(E)** from WT (littermate) and Cx30 KO mice in the chronic EAE phase (Day 59). Scale bars, 200 μm. Each higher magnification image is from the white rectangular frame in the lower magnification image above. Scale bars in higher magnification images, 50 μm. **(B,D,F)** Colocalization analysis of arginase-1 and Iba-1 in optic nerves **(B)**, cerebellum **(D)**, and spinal cord white matter **(F)** from WT (littermate) and Cx30 KO mice in the chronic EAE phase, expressed as Pearson's correlation coefficients. Means ± S.E.M. are shown. Statistical differences were determined using the unpaired *t*-test with Welch's correction. N.S. = not significant. *n* indicates number of mice and each scatter dot represents individual mice in each group.

of EAE (**Figures 7A,D,E**). By contrast, Cx43 in the spinal cord white matter demonstrated a dynamic change during EAE in WT mice. Cx43 decreased significantly in the acute phase compared with the naïve state ($p = 0.0149$ on Day 13 and $p = 0.0067$ on Day 16) and then recovered to similar levels to the naïve state (significant increase compared with the peak day levels,

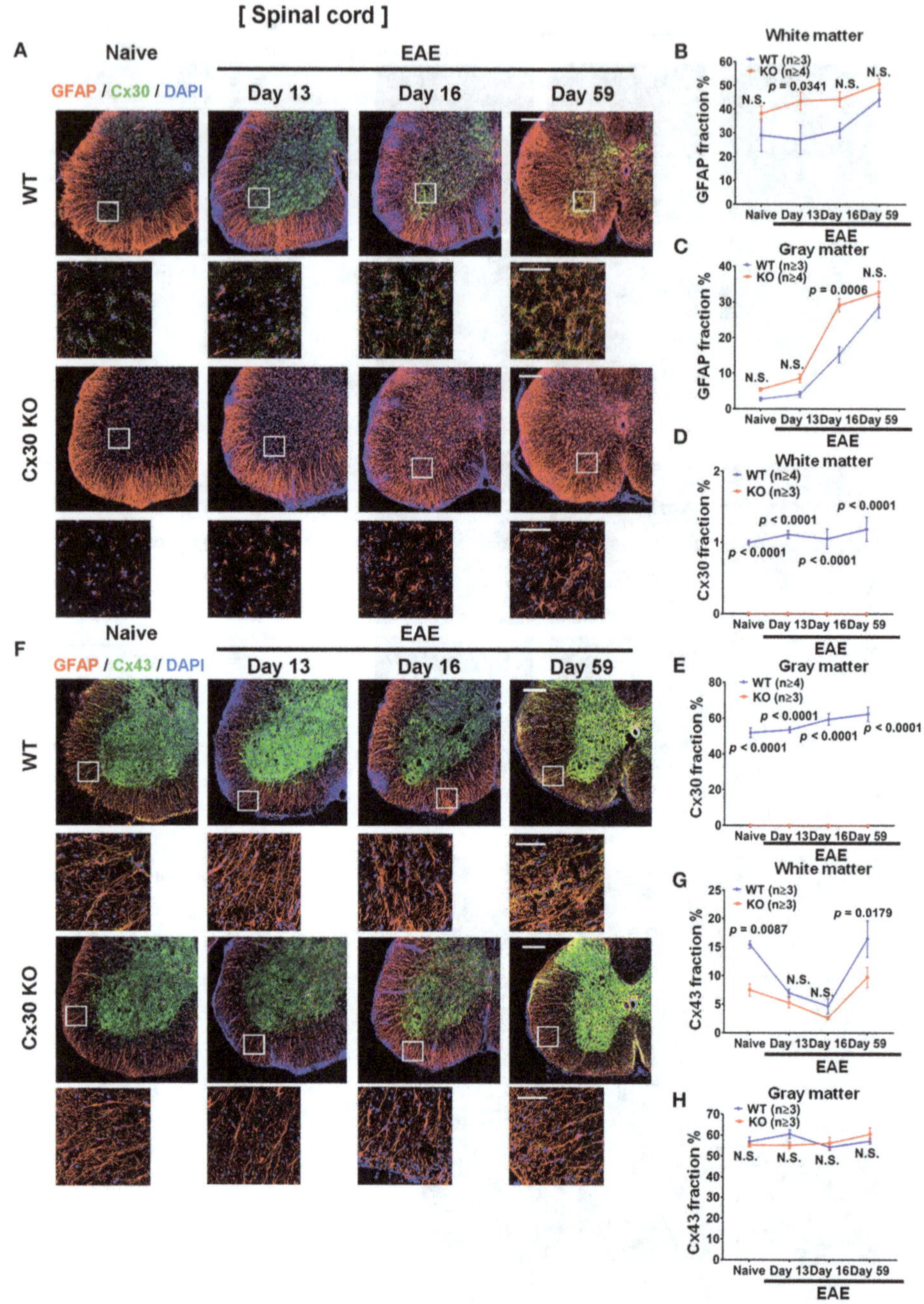

FIGURE 7 | Astrocytic marker expression in spinal cords from WT and Cx30 KO mice during acute and chronic EAE. **(A)** Confocal images showing immunostaining for Cx30 and GFAP in the anterior part of spinal cords from WT (littermate) and Cx30 KO mice in the naïve state and at different stages of EAE. Scale bars, 200 μm. Each higher magnification image is from the white rectangular frame in the lower magnification image above. Scale bars in higher magnification images, 50 μm. **(B,C)** Quantification of the GFAP$^+$ cell area fraction in the white **(B)** and gray **(C)** matter. **(D,E)** Quantification of the Cx30$^+$ cell area fraction in the white matter **(D)** and gray matter **(E)**. **(F)** Confocal images showing immunostaining for Cx43 and GFAP in the anterior part of spinal cords from WT (littermate) and Cx30 KO mice. Scale bars, 200 μm. Each higher magnification image is from the white rectangular frame in the lower magnification image above. Scale bars in higher magnification images, 50 μm. **(G,H)** Quantification of the Cx43$^+$ cell area fraction in the white **(G)** and gray **(H)** matter. Means ± S.E.M. are shown. Statistical differences were determined using two-way ANOVA. N.S. = not significant. *n* indicates number of mice in each group at different stages and each scatter dot represents the mean value for each group.

$p = 0.0147$; **Figures 7F,G; Supplementary Figure 6G**). A similar decrease of Cx43 in the acute phase and recovery of Cx43 in the chronic phase were also observed in Cx30 KO mice ($p = 0.0142$ at Day 16 and $p = 0.0026$ at Day 59 compared with Day 16; **Figures 7F,G; Supplementary Figure 6I**); however, Cx43 levels were significantly lower in Cx30 KO mice than in WT mice, in the naïve state and in the chronic EAE phase ($p = 0.0087$ and $p = 0.0179$, respectively) (**Figures 7F,G**). Cx43 expression in the gray matter did not show obvious changes in either WT or Cx30 KO mice (**Figures 7F,H; Supplementary Figures 6H,J**).

We examined A1 and A2 astrocyte markers based on a recent report (53). Immunostaining analyses for S100A10, a representative A2 astrocyte marker, revealed a successive increase in the spinal cord white matter during the course of EAE, which was highest in the chronic EAE stage, in both WT and Cx30 KO mice compared with the naïve state (not significant in either mouse strain on Day 13; not significant and $p = 0.0251$, respectively, on Day 16; $p = 0.0010$ and $p = 0.0002$, respectively, on Day 59; **Figures 8A,B; Supplementary Figures 6K,L**). Interestingly, this increase in S100A10 immunoreactivity was greater in Cx30 KO mice than in WT mice at all stages of EAE and the difference increased in the later stages of EAE ($p < 0.0001$ at Day 59; **Figures 8A,B**). By contrast, C3, an A1 astrocyte marker, sharply increased and peaked in the acute phase and then steadily decreased in the chronic phase compared with the naïve state in both WT and Cx30 KO mice ($p = 0.0174$ on Day 13, and $p = 0.0174$ on Day 16, respectively; **Figures 8C,D; Supplementary Figures 6M,N**). These findings suggest that the stronger activation of A2 astrocytes in Cx30 KO mice plays a role in inducing neuroprotective microglia, which attenuate EAE in the chronic phase.

Cx30 Deficiency Causes Less Neuronal Death in the Chronic Phase of EAE

Finally, because astrocytic Cx30 has close contact with neurons, we examined changes in neurons and axons in Cx30 KO mice during EAE. In the native state, the numbers of NeuN$^+$ cells and SMI-31$^+$ axonal density were not significantly different between Cx30 and WT littermate mice (**Figures 9A–D**). Although only SMI-31$^+$ axonal density decreased significantly in the chronic EAE phase compared with the naïve state in both WT and Cx30 KO mice ($p < 0.0001$, and $p = 0.0035$, respectively), Cx30 KO mice had significantly more NeuN$^+$ cells and SMI-31$^+$ remaining axons compared with WT mice in the chronic EAE phase ($p = 0.0376$, and $p = 0.0003$, respectively; **Figures 9E,F**). Because IL-34, expressed on CNS neurons, induces the differentiation of microglia to a neuroprotective phenotype (54), we examined its expression by immunostaining, and detected significantly more IL-34 in the spinal white matter of Cx30 KO mice than in WT mice in the chronic EAE phase (**Supplementary Figure 7**). These findings suggest less neuronal death and axonal loss in Cx30 KO mice compared with WT mice in the chronic phase of EAE, leading to more IL-34 production in Cx30 KO mice.

DISCUSSION

The main new findings in the present study are as follows: (1) Cx30 deficiency attenuated only chronic EAE clinically and pathologically without affecting T cell infiltration. (2) Cx30 deficiency increased the numbers of ramified microglia in the naïve state and induced earlier and more widespread activation of microglia in the acute and chronic phases of EAE. (3) These activated microglia in Cx30 KO mice were prone to differentiate toward an anti-inflammatory phenotype with less pro-inflammatory gene expression. (4) In the naïve state, Cx30 deficiency induced only a modest enlargement of astrocytic processes in the spinal gray matter and a partial reduction of Cx43 expression in the spinal white matter, whereas it caused earlier and stronger activation of astrocytes in the acute EAE phase, upregulated S100A10, a representative A2 astrocyte marker, and attenuated the recovery of Cx43 in the chronic phase. (5) Cx30 deficiency rescued more neurons and axons in the chronic EAE phase without influencing the quantity of neurons or axons in the naïve state.

According to the present study, Cx30 deficiency has no apparent influence on the clinical and histological severity of acute EAE, in accordance with a previous report describing that a single or double KO of Cx30 and/or Cx43 did not affect acute EAE (29). Collectively, this suggests that Cx30 does not modulate the peripheral immune system or alter the clinical course of acute EAE. Surprisingly, chronic EAE and demyelination were significantly attenuated by Cx30 deficiency. These differences in results between a previous study (29) and the current study might be attributable to a difference in the observation period. Thus, acute and chronic EAE are differentially regulated, at least in part, and Cx30 is mainly involved in the chronic phase, when microglia and astrocytes are postulated to be key players (55, 56).

We demonstrated the attenuation of chronic EAE by Cx30 deficiency without influencing T cell infiltration, which further underlines the importance of microglia and astrocytes in the chronic phase of EAE. In naïve Cx30 KO mice, increased microglia were observed throughout the CNS; however, these microglia retained a ramified morphology without a significant increase in circularity. Consistent with this morphology, they had similar expression levels of pro-inflammatory genes to WT microglia by RNA microarray. During the chronic EAE phase in Cx30 KO mice, there were increased numbers and more activated microglia in the spinal cord and the brain, which had reduced pro-inflammatory gene expression compared with WT mice. Indeed, microglia in Cx30 KO mice had lower expressions of *IL-1b*, *Nos2*, *Tnf*, and *Ptgs2* and a higher expression of *Mrc1*. IL-1β, tumor necrosis factor-α, NOS2, and prostaglandin-endoperoxide synthase-2, also known as cyclooxygenase-2, are well-known pro-inflammatory molecules involved in neuroinflammation (57–61). Mannose receptor C-type 1 (Mrcl), downregulated by IFN-γ (62), and upregulated by IL-4 (63), is expressed at high levels during the resolution of inflammation where it has a critical role in the removal of inflammatory glycoproteins (64). We also immunohistochemically observed the increased expression of arginase-1 and BDNF and the decreased expression of NOS2 in the optic nerve, cerebrum, and cerebellum. Although such changes were not clear in inflamed spinal cord lesions, the increased infiltration of peripheral blood-borne pro-inflammatory macrophages, reported to be abundant in chronic EAE (65) and shown as a significant increase of CD169$^+$ cells in the chronic EAE phase in the present study, might have obscured

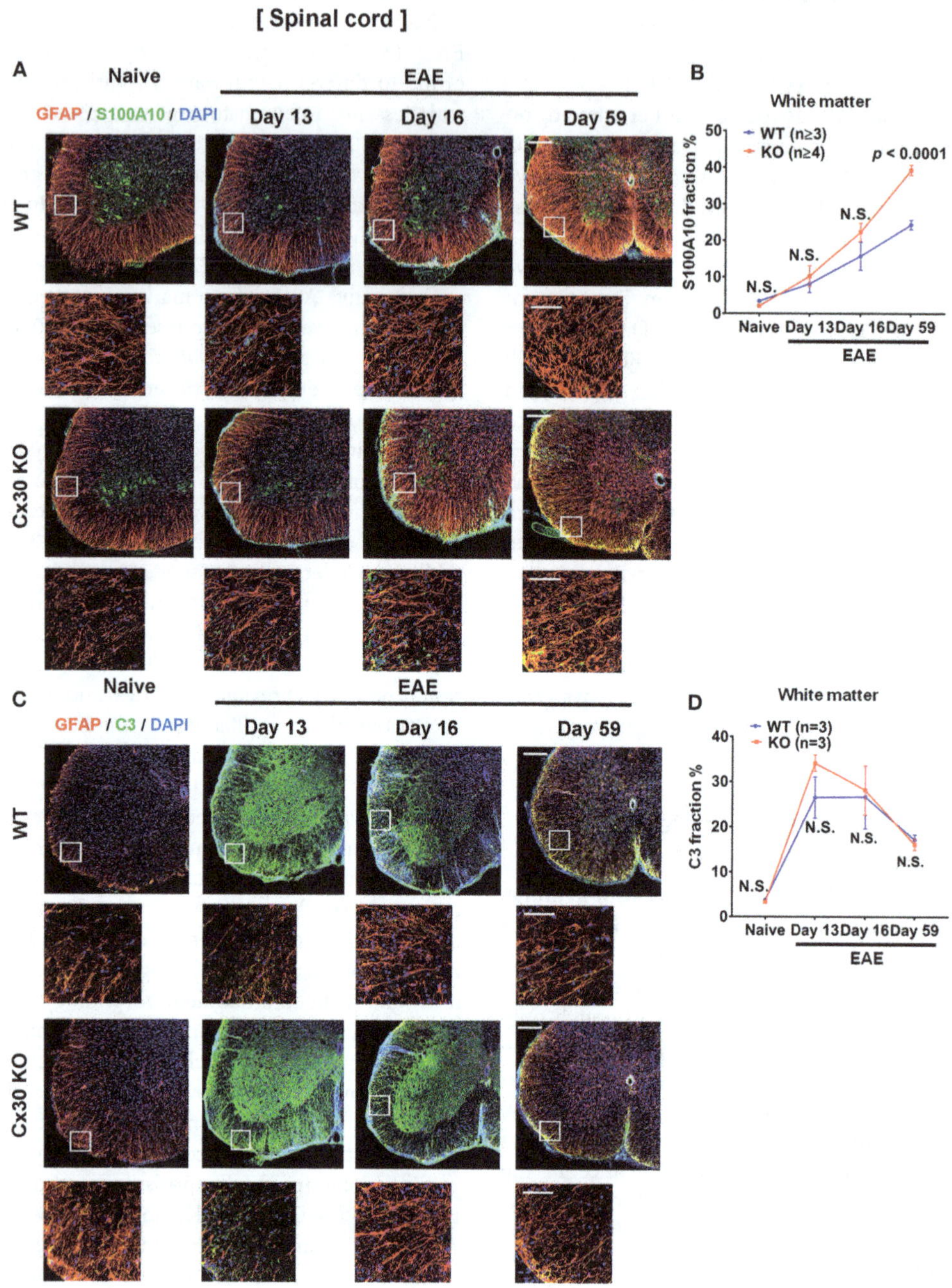

FIGURE 8 | A1 and A2 astrocyte marker expression in spinal cords from WT and Cx30 KO mice during acute and chronic EAE. **(A)** Confocal images showing immunostaining for S100A10 and GFAP in spinal cords from WT (littermate) and Cx30 KO mice. Scale bars, 200 μm. Each higher magnification image is from the white rectangular frame in the lower magnification image above. Scale bars in higher magnification images, 50 μm. **(B)** Quantification of the S100A10$^+$ cell fraction in the spinal cord white matter. **(C)** Confocal images showing immunostaining for GFAP and C3 in spinal cords from WT (littermate) and Cx30 KO mice. Scale bars, 200 μm. **(D)** Quantification of the C3$^+$ cell fraction in the spinal cord white matter. Each higher magnification image is from the white rectangular frame in the lower magnification image above. Scale bars in higher magnification images, 50 μm. Means ± S.E.M. are shown. Statistical differences were determined using two-way ANOVA. N.S. = not significant. *n* indicates number of mice in each group at different stages and each scatter dot represents the mean value for each group.

the reduced pro-inflammatory nature of Cx30 KO mouse spinal cord microglia.

Notably, spinal cord but not brain microglia had significantly lower expressions of cytokines/chemokines, alarmins, and MHC genes in Cx30 KO than in WT mice, suggesting spinal cord microglia are less reactive to inflammatory insults than brain microglia in the naïve state in Cx30 KO mice. In the chronic EAE phase, cytokines/chemokines, complements, alarmins, ROS, and MHC gene expressions in microglia were significantly lower in Cx30 KO than in WT mice in the spinal cord but not in the brain,

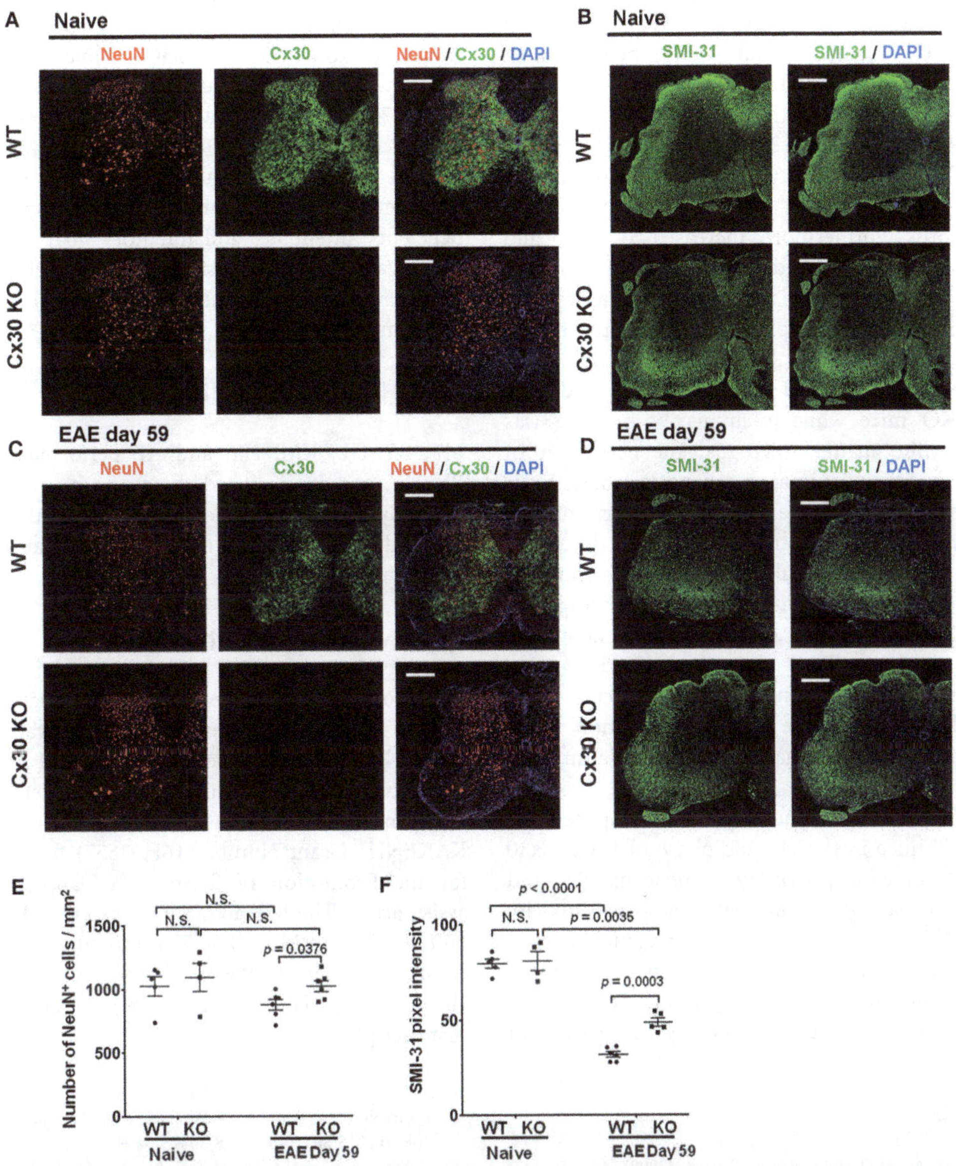

FIGURE 9 | NeuN and SMI-31 immunostaining of spinal cords from WT and Cx30 KO mice with or without EAE. **(A,C)** Confocal images showing immunostaining for Cx30 and NeuN in spinal cords from WT (littermate) and Cx30 KO mice in the naive state **(A)** and chronic EAE phase (Day 59) **(C)**. Scale bars, 200 μm. **(B,D)** Confocal images showing immunostaining for SMI-31 in spinal cord sections from WT (littermate) and Cx30 KO EAE mice in the naive state **(B)** and chronic EAE phase (Day 59) **(D)**. Scale bars, 200 μm. **(E)** Quantification of NeuN$^+$ cell numbers/mm^2 of spinal cord in the naive state or chronic EAE phase. **(F)** Quantification of SMI-31 density in anterior white matter regions of the spinal cord from WT (littermate) and Cx30 KO EAE mice in the naive state and chronic EAE phase (Day 59). Means ± S.E.M. are shown. Statistical differences were determined using the unpaired *t*-test with Welch's correction. N.S. = not significant. *n* indicates the number of mice and each scatter dot represents individual mice in each group.

indicating that spinal cord microglia have a tendency to have a reduced pro-inflammatory and increased anti-inflammatory phenotype compared with brain microglia in Cx30 KO mice.

Earlier and stronger activation of astrocytes in EAE was another characteristic feature of Cx30 KO mice. S100A10, a neuroprotective A2 astrocyte-related gene product (53), was increasingly expressed in the spinal cord white matter as EAE proceeded from the acute to chronic phase. Although the precise functions of astrocytic S100A10 remain to be elucidated, it was reported to be required for membrane repair (66), cell proliferation (67), and inhibition of cell apoptosis by interaction with Bcl-xL/Bcl-2-associated death promoter (68). Thus, S100A10 expressed in astrocytes might be beneficial for tissue repair. These findings collectively suggest that Cx30-deficient astrocytes may be prone to differentiate toward an A2 astrocyte phenotype upon activation. In addition, these Cx30-deficient astrocytes showed less Cx43 immunoreactivity in the astrogliotic scar in the chronic

EAE phase as well as in the naïve state. The overexpression of Cx43 might propagate inflammatory mediators through homotypic Cx43 GJ channels and Cx43 hemichannels (69–72). Thus, the downregulation of Cx43 on Cx30-deficient astrocytes may also function in suppressing chronic neuroinflammation.

Increased numbers of GFAP^{+} astrocytes were present in the white matter compared with the gray matter of Cx30 KO mice spinal cords. Furthermore, increased S100A10 and decreased Cx43 levels were observed in the spinal white matter, suggesting white matter astrocytes may exhibit earlier and stronger activation toward an A2 phenotype than gray matter astrocytes in the Cx30 KO spinal cord. Because increased microglia numbers were observed in spinal white and gray matter in Cx30 KO mice while a circularity increase was detected only in white matter microglia, the activation of microglia toward an anti-inflammatory phenotype may occur more strongly in the spinal white matter than in the gray matter. Collectively, earlier and stronger astroglial activation toward an A2 phenotype occurred in the spinal white matter, which might partly explain the induction of anti-inflammatory microglia in Cx30 KO mice spinal white matter. Such microglial activation occurred even in the acute EAE phase in Cx30 KO mice; however, this effect might not be sufficient in the acute phase when CD3^{+} T cells mainly induce acute inflammation, while becoming evident in the chronic phase when glial inflammation predominates.

Interestingly, Cx30 KO mice had more remaining neurons and axons than WT mice in the chronic phase of EAE. Cx30 on astrocytes exists in close proximity to neurons (32) and Cx30 hemichannels release glutamate that exerts excitotoxicity on neurons (54, 73). Thus, Cx30 deficiency may confer survival of neurons and axons. Neuronal IL-34 is a potent activator for microglia toward a neuroprotective phenotype (74). Accordingly, we hypothesized that the earlier and stronger activation of astroglia toward an A2 phenotype in Cx30 KO mice in the spinal white matter induced anti-inflammatory microglia (75, 76). Increased axonal IL-34 in Cx30 KO mice may also contribute to the induction of anti-inflammatory microglia in the chronic EAE phase (74), which might dampen chronic neuroinflammation.

In conclusion, Cx30 on astrocytes plays a significant role in perpetuating neuroinflammation in chronic EAE by augmenting pro-inflammatory glial responses. How Cx30 deficiency attenuates inflammatory glial responses should be investigated in future studies, and might provide valuable information for new therapeutic strategies for chronic glial inflammation in MS.

AUTHOR CONTRIBUTIONS

MF, RY, GL, KM, HY, and AF performed experiments. MF, RY, HY, and JK designed the research. MF, RY, KM, NI, and JK analyzed the data and provided scientific suggestions. MF, RY, and JK drafted the manuscript. All authors reviewed the manuscript.

ACKNOWLEDGMENTS

This work was supported in part by Glial Assembly Grants-in-Aid for Scientific Research on Innovative Areas (MEXT KAKENHI Grant Numbers 25117001 and 25117012) from the Ministry of Education, Culture, Sports, Science and Technology of Japan, and a Grant-in-Aid for Scientific Research (A) (JSPS KAKENHI Grant Number 16H02657) from the Japan Society for the Promotion of Science. We appreciate the technical assistance of The Research Support Center, Research Center for Human Disease Modeling, Kyushu University Graduate School of Medical Sciences. We thank Ann Turnley, PhD, from Edanz Group (www.edanzediting.com/ac) for editing a draft of this manuscript.

REFERENCES

1. Compston A, Coles A. Multiple sclerosis. *Lancet* (2008) 372:1502–17. doi: 10.1016/s0140-6736(08)61620-7
2. Tremlett H, Zhao Y, Devonshire V. Natural history of secondary-progressive multiple sclerosis. *Multiple Sclerosis J.* (2008) 14:314–24. doi: 10.1177/1352458507084264
3. Scalfari A, Neuhaus A, Daumer M, Muraro PA, Ebers GC. Onset of secondary progressive phase and long-term evolution of multiple sclerosis. *J Neurol Neurosurg Psychiatr.* (2013) 85:67–75. doi: 10.1136/jnnp-2012-304333
4. Kappos L, Kuhle J, Multanen J, Kremenchutzky M, di Cantogno E, Cornelisse V. et al. Factors influencing long-term outcomes in relapsing–remitting multiple sclerosis: PRISMS-15. *J Neurol Neurosurg Psychiatr.* (2015) 86:1202–7. doi: 10.1136/jnnp-2014-310024
5. Lorscheider J, Jokubaitis VG, Spelman T, Izquierdo G, Lugaresi A, Havrdova E, et al. Anti-inflammatory disease-modifying treatment and short-term disability progression in SPMS. *Neurology* (2017) 89:1050–9. doi: 10.1212/WNL.0000000000004330
6. Ontaneda D, Fox RJ, Chataway J. Clinical trials in progressive multiple sclerosis: lessons learned and future perspectives. *Lancet Neurol.* (2015) 14:208–223. doi: 10.1016/S1474-4422(14)70264-9
7. Kappos L, Bar-Or A, Cree BA, Fox RJ, Giovannoni G, Gold R, et al. Siponimod versus placebo in secondary progressive multiple sclerosis (EXPAND): a double-blind, randomised, phase 3 study. *Lancet* (2018) 391:1263–73. doi: 10.1016/S0140-6736(18)30475-6
8. Cohen JA, Arnold DL, Comi G, Bar-Or A, Gujrathi S, Hartung JP, et al. Safety and efficacy of the selective sphingosine 1-phosphate receptor modulator ozanimod in relapsing multiple sclerosis (RADIANCE): a randomised, placebo-controlled, phase 2 trial. *Lancet Neurol.* (2016) 15:373–81. doi: 10.1016/S1474-4422(16)00018-1
9. O'sullivan SA, O'sullivan C, Healy LM, Dev KK, Sheridan GK. Sphingosine 1-phosphate receptors regulate TLR 4-induced CXCL 5 release from astrocytes and microglia. *J Neurochem.* (2018) 144:736–47. doi: 10.1111/jnc.14313
10. Healy LM, Sheridan GK, Pritchard AJ, Rutkowska A, Mullershausen F, Dev KK. Pathway specific modulation of S1P1 receptor signalling in rat and human astrocytes. *Br J Pharmacol.* (2013) 169:1114–29. doi: 10.1111/bph.12207
11. Choi JW, Gardell SE, Herr DR, Rivera R, Lee C-W, Noguchi K, et al. FTY720 (fingolimod) efficacy in an animal model of multiple sclerosis requires astrocyte sphingosine 1-phosphate receptor 1 (S1P1) modulation. *Proc Natl Acad Sci.* (2011) 108:751–6. doi: 10.1073/pnas.1014154108
12. Mahad DH, Trapp BD, Lassmann H. Pathological mechanisms in progressive multiple sclerosis. *Lancet Neurol.* (2015) 14:183–93. doi: 10.1016/S1474-4422(14)70256-X
13. Prineas JW, Kwon EE, Cho ES, Sharer LR, Barnett MH, Oleszak EL, et al. Immunopathology of secondary-progressive multiple sclerosis. *Ann Neurol.* (2001) 50:646–57. doi: 10.1002/ana.1255

14. J.-Hervé C, Derangeon M. Gap-junction-mediated cell-to-cell communication. *Cell Tissue Res.* (2013) 352:21–31. doi: 10.1007/s00441-012-1485-6
15. Nagy J, Patel D, Ochalski P, Stelmack G. Connexin30 in rodent, cat and human brain: selective expression in gray matter astrocytes, co-localization with connexin43 at gap junctions and late developmental appearance. *Neuroscience* (1999) 88:447–68. doi: 10.1016/S0306-4522(98)00191-2
16. Rash J, Yasumura T, Davidson K, Furman C, Dudek FE, Nagy J. Identification of cells expressing Cx43, Cx30, Cx26, Cx32 and Cx36 in gap junctions of rat brain and spinal cord. *Cell Commun Adhesion* (2001) 8:315–20. doi: 10.3109/15419060109080745
17. Rouach N, Avignone E, Meme W, Koulakoff A, Venance L, Blomstrand F, et al. Gap junctions and connexin expression in the normal and pathological central nervous system. *Biol Cell* (2002) 94:457–75. doi: 10.1016/S0248-4900(02)00016-3
18. Cotrina ML, Lin JH-C, Alves-Rodrigues A, Liu S, Li J, Azmi-Ghadimi H, et al. Connexins regulate calcium signaling by controlling ATP release. *Proc Natl Acad Sci.* (1998) 95:15735–40. doi: 10.1073/pnas.95.26.15735
19. Spray D, Harris A, Bennett M. Gap junctional conductance is a simple and sensitive function of intracellular p*Science* (1981) 211:712–5. doi: 10.1126/science.6779379
20. Stout CE, Costantin JL, Naus CC, Charles AC. Intercellular calcium signaling in astrocytes via ATP release through connexin hemichannels. *J Biol Chem.* (2002) 277:10482–8. doi: 10.1074/jbc.M109902200
21. Markoullis K, Sargiannidou I, Schiza N, Hadjisavvas A, Roncaroli F, Reynolds R, et al. Gap junction pathology in multiple sclerosis lesions and normal-appearing white matter. *Acta Neuropathol.* (2012) 123:873–86. doi: 10.1007/s00401-012-0978-4
22. Masaki K, Suzuki SO, Matsushita T, Matsuoka T, Imamura S, Yamasaki R, et al. Connexin 43 astrocytopathy linked to rapidly progressive multiple sclerosis and neuromyelitis optica. *PLoS ONE* (2013) 8:e72919. doi: 10.1371/journal.pone.0072919
23. Masaki K, Suzuki SO, Matsushita T, Yonekawa T, Matsuoka T, Isobe N, et al. Extensive loss of connexins in Baló's disease: evidence for an auto-antibody-independent astrocytopathy via impaired astrocyte–oligodendrocyte/myelin interaction. *Acta Neuropathol.* (2012) 123:887–900. doi: 10.1007/s00401-012-0972-x
24. Brand-Schieber E, Werner P, Iacobas DA, Iacobas S, Beelitz M, Lowery SL, et al. Connexin43, the major gap junction protein of astrocytes, is down-regulated in inflamed white matter in an animal model of multiple sclerosis. *J Neurosci Res.* (2005) 80:798–808. doi: 10.1002/jnr.20474
25. Markoullis K, Sargiannidou I, Gardner C, Hadjisavvas A, Reynolds R, Kleopa KA. Disruption of oligodendrocyte gap junctions in experimental autoimmune encephalomyelitis. *Glia* (2012) 60:1053–66. doi: 10.1002/glia.22334
26. Roscoe W, Kidder G, Karlik S. Experimental allergic encephalomyelitis in connexin 43–heterozygous mice. *Cell Commun Adhesion* (2007) 14:57–73. doi: 10.1080/15419060701459569
27. Roscoe W, Messersmith E, Meyer-Franke A, Wipke B, Karlik S. Connexin 43 gap junction proteins are up-regulated in remyelinating spinal cord. *J Neurosci Res.* (2007) 85:945–953. doi: 10.1002/jnr.21194
28. Theotokis P, Kleopa KA, Touloumi O, Lagoudaki R, Lourbopoulos A, Nousiopoulou E, et al. Connexin43 and connexin47 alterations after neural precursor cells transplantation in experimental autoimmune encephalomyelitis. *Glia* (2015) 63:1772–83. doi: 10.1002/glia.22843
29. Lutz SE, Raine CS, Brosnan CF. Loss of astrocyte connexins 43 and 30 does not significantly alter susceptibility or severity of acute experimental autoimmune encephalomyelitis in mice. *J Neuroimmunol.* (2012) 245:8–14. doi: 10.1016/j.jneuroim.2012.01.007
30. Dahl E, Manthey D, Chen Y, Schwarz H-J, Chang YS, Lalley PA, et al. Molecular cloning and functional expression of mouse connexin-30, a gap junction gene highly expressed in adult brain and skin. *J Biol Chem.* (1996) 271:17903–10. doi: 10.1074/jbc.271.30.17903
31. Dermietzel R, Traub O, Hwang T, Beyer E, Bennett M, Spray D, et al. Differential expression of three gap junction proteins in developing and mature brain tissues. *Proc Natl Acad Sci.* (1989) 86:10148–52. doi: 10.1073/pnas.86.24.10148
32. Koulakoff A, Ezan P, Giaume C. Neurons control the expression of connexin 30 and connexin 43 in mouse cortical astrocytes. *Glia* (2008) 56:1299–311. doi: 10.1002/glia.20698
33. Kunzelmann P, Schröder W, Traub O, Steinhäuser C, Dermietzel R, Willecke K. Late onset and increasing expression of the gap junction protein connexin30 in adult murine brain and long-term cultured astrocytes. *Glia* (1999) 25:111–9.
34. Watanabe M, Masaki K, Yamasaki R, Kawanokuchi J, Takeuchi H, Matsushita T, et al. Th1 cells downregulate connexin 43 gap junctions in astrocytes via microglial activation. *Sci Rep.* (2016) 6:38387. doi: 10.1038/srep38387
35. Pannasch U, Freche D, Dallérac G, Ghézali G, Escartin C, Ezan P, et al. Connexin 30 sets synaptic strength by controlling astroglial synapse invasion. *Nat Neurosci.* (2014) 17:549–58. doi: 10.1038/nn.3662
36. Kardami E, Dang X, Iacobas DA, Nickel BE, Jeyaraman M, Srisakuldee W, et al. The role of connexins in controlling cell growth and gene expression. *Prog Biophys Mol Biol.* (2007) 94:245–64. doi: 10.1016/j.pbiomolbio.2007.03.009
37. Zhou JZ, Jiang JX. Gap junction and hemichannel-independent actions of connexins on cell and tissue functions–an update. *FEBS Lett.* (2014) 588:1186–92. doi: 10.1016/j.febslet.2014.01.001
38. Teubner B, Michel V, Pesch J, Lautermann J, Cohen-Salmon M, Söhl G, et al. Connexin30 (Gjb6)-deficiency causes severe hearing impairment and lack of endocochlear potential. *Hum Mol Genet.* (2003) 12:13–21. doi: 10.1093/hmg/ddg001
39. Evonuk KS, Baker BJ, Doyle RE, Moseley CE, Sestero CM, Johnston BP, et al. Inhibition of system xc– transporter attenuates autoimmune inflammatory demyelination. *J Immunol.* (2015) 195:450–63. doi: 10.4049/jimmunol.1401108
40. Li G, Yamasaki R, Fang M, Masaki K, Ochi H, Matsushita T, et al. Novel disease-modifying anti-rheumatic drug iguratimod suppresses chronic experimental autoimmune encephalomyelitis by down-regulating activation of macrophages/microglia through an NF-κB pathway. *Sci Rep.* (2018) 8:1933. doi: 10.1038/s41598-018-20390-5
41. Grishchuk Y, Peña KA, Coblentz J, King VE, Humphrey DM, Wang SL, et al. Impaired myelination and reduced brain ferric iron in the mouse model of mucolipidosis IV. *Dis Models Mech.* (2015) 8:1591–601. doi: 10.1242/dmm.021154
42. Doeppner TR, Kaltwasser B, Bähr M, Hermann DM. Effects of neural progenitor cells on post-stroke neurological impairment—a detailed and comprehensive analysis of behavioral tests. *Front Cell Neurosci.* (2014) 8:338. doi: 10.3389/fncel.2014.00338
43. Ramírez-Franco JJ, Munoz-Cuevas FJ, Luján R, Jurado S. Excitatory and inhibitory neurons in the hippocampus exhibit molecularly distinct large dense core vesicles. *Front Cell Neurosci.* (2016) 10:202. doi: 10.3389/fncel.2016.00202
44. Fernández-Arjona M, Grondona JM, Granados-Durán P, Fernández-Llebrez P, López-Ávalos MD. Microglia morphological categorization in a rat model of neuroinflammation by hierarchical cluster and principal components analysis. *Front Cell Neurosci.* (2017) 11:235. doi: 10.3389/fncel.2017.00235
45. Yamasaki R, Fujii T, Wang B, Masaki K, Kido MA, Yoshida M, et al. Allergic inflammation leads to neuropathic pain via glial cell activation. *J Neurosci.* (2016) 36:11929–45. doi: 10.1523/JNEUROSCI.1981-16.2016
46. Cardona AE, Huang D, Sasse ME, Ransohoff RM. Isolation of murine microglial cells for RNA analysis or flow cytometry. *Nat Protocols* (2006) 1:1947–51. doi: 10.1038/nprot.2006.327
47. Katayama Y, Nishiyama M, Shoji H, Ohkawa Y, Kawamura A, Sato T, et al. CHD8 haploinsufficiency results in autistic-like phenotypes in mice. *Nature* (2016) 537:675. doi: 10.1038/nature19357
48. Subramanian A, Tamayo P, Mootha VK, Mukherjee S, Ebert BL, Gillette MA, et al. Gene set enrichment analysis: a knowledge-based approach for interpreting genome-wide expression profiles. *Proc Natl Acad Sci.* (2005) 102:15545–50. doi: 10.1073/pnas.0506580102
49. Zabala A, Vazquez-Villoldo N, Rissiek B, Gejo J, Martin A, Palomino A, et al. P2X4 receptor controls microglia activation and favors remyelination

in autoimmune encephalitis. *EMBO Mol Med.* (2018) 2018:e8743. doi: 10.15252/emmm.201708743

50. Tietz SM, Zwahlen M, Haghayegh Jahromi N, Baden P, Lazarevic I, Enzmann G, et al. Refined clinical scoring in comparative EAE studies does not enhance the chance to observe statistically significant differences. *Eur J Immunol.* (2016) 46:2481–3. doi: 10.1002/eji.201546272
51. Ji N, Kovalovsky A, Fingerle-Rowson G, Guentzel MN, Forsthuber TG. Macrophage migration inhibitory factor promotes resistance to glucocorticoid treatment in EAE. *Neurol Neuroinflamm.* (2015) 2:e139. doi: 10.1212/NXI.0000000000000139
52. Theis M, Giaume C. Connexin-based intercellular communication and astrocyte heterogeneity. *Brain Res.* (2012) 1487:88–98. doi: 10.1016/j.brainres.2012.06.045
53. Liddelow SA, Guttenplan KA, Clarke LE, Bennett FC, Bohlen CJ, Schirmer L, et al. Neurotoxic reactive astrocytes are induced by activated microglia. *Nature* (2017) 541:481–7. doi: 10.1038/nature21029
54. Mizuno T, Doi Y, Mizoguchi H, Jin S, Noda M, Sonobe Y, et al. Interleukin-34 selectively enhances the neuroprotective effects of microglia to attenuate oligomeric amyloid-β neurotoxicity. *Am J Pathol.* (2011) 179:2016–27. doi: 10.1016/j.ajpath.2011.06.011
55. Mayo L, Trauger SA, Blain M, Nadeau M, Patel B, Alvarez JI, et al. Regulation of astrocyte activation by glycolipids drives chronic CNS inflammation. *Nat Med.* (2014) 20:1147–56. doi: 10.1038/nm.3681
56. Rasmussen S, Wang Y, Kivisäkk P, Bronson RT, Meyer M, Imitola J, et al. Persistent activation of microglia is associated with neuronal dysfunction of callosal projecting pathways and multiple sclerosis-like lesions in relapsing–remitting experimental autoimmune encephalomyelitis. *Brain* (2007) 130:2816–29. doi: 10.1093/brain/awm219
57. Rothwell NJ, Luheshi GN. Interleukin 1 in the brain: biology, pathology and therapeutic target. *Trends Neurosci.* (2000) 23:618–25. doi: 10.1016/S0166-2236(00)01661-1
58. Liu JS-H, Zhao M-L, Brosnan CF, Lee SC. Expression of inducible nitric oxide synthase and nitrotyrosine in multiple sclerosis lesions. *Am J Pathol.* (2001) 158:2057–66. doi: 10.1016/S0002-9440(10)64677-9
59. Sharief M, Noori M, Ciardi M, Cirelli A, Thompson E. Increased levels of circulating ICAM-1 in serum and cerebrospinal fluid of patients with active multiple sclerosis. correlation with TNF-α and blood-brain barrier damage. *J Neuroimmunol.* (1993) 43:15–21. doi: 10.1016/0165-5728(93)90070-F
60. Rieckmann P, Albrecht M, Kitze B, Weber T, Tumani H, Broocks A, et al. Tumor necrosis factor-α messenger RNA expression in patients with relapsing-remitting multiple sclerosis is associated with disease activity. *Annal Neurol.* (1995) 37:82–8. doi: 10.1002/ana.410370115
61. Kurumbail RG, Kiefer JR, Marnett LJ. Cyclooxygenase enzymes: catalysis and inhibition. *Curr Opin Struct Biol.* (2001) 11:752–60. doi: 10.1016/S0959-440X(01)00277-9
62. Mokoena T, Gordon S. Human macrophage activation. Modulation of mannosyl, fucosyl receptor activity *in vitro* by lymphokines, gamma and alpha interferons, and dexamethasone. *J Clin Invest.* (1985) 75:624–31. doi: 10.1172/JCI111740
63. Stein M, Keshav S, Harris N, Gordon S. Interleukin 4 potently enhances murine macrophage mannose receptor activity: a marker of alternative immunologic macrophage activation. *J Exp Med.* (1992) 176:287–92. doi: 10.1084/jem.176.1.287
64. Andreou KE, Soto MS, Allen D, Economopoulos V, de Bernardi A, Larkin JR, et al. Anti-inflammatory microglia/macrophages as a potential therapeutic target in brain metastasis. *Front Oncol.* (2017) 7:251. doi: 10.3389/fonc.2017.00251
65. Berard JL, Kerr BJ, Johnson HM, David S. Differential expression of SOCS1 in macrophages in relapsing-remitting and chronic EAE and its role in disease severity. *Glia* (2010) 58:1816–26. doi: 10.1002/glia.21051
66. Rezvanpour A, Santamaria-Kisiel L, Shaw GS. The S100A10-annexin A2 complex provides a novel asymmetric platform for membrane repair. *J Biol Chem.* (2011) 286:40174–83. doi: 10.1074/jbc.M111.244038
67. Li J, Riau AK, Setiawan M, Mehta JS, Ti S-E, Tong L, Tan DT, et al. S100A expression in normal corneal-limbal epithelial cells and ocular surface squamous cell carcinoma tissue. *Mol Vis.* (2011) 17:2263.
68. Hsu SY, Kaipia A, Zhu L, Hsueh AJ. Interference of BAD (Bcl-xL/Bcl-2-associated death promoter)-induced apoptosis in mammalian cells by 14-3-3 isoforms and P11. *Mol Endocrinol.* (1997) 11:1858–67.
69. Chen MJ, Kress B, Han X, Moll K, Peng W, Ji RR, et al. Astrocytic CX43 hemichannels and gap junctions play a crucial role in development of chronic neuropathic pain following spinal cord injury. *Glia* (2012) 60:1660–70. doi: 10.1002/glia.22384
70. Cronin M, Anderson PN, Cook JE, Green CR, Becker DL. Blocking connexin43 expression reduces inflammation and improves functional recovery after spinal cord injury. *Mol Cell Neurosci.* (2008) 39:152–60. doi: 10.1016/j.mcn.2008.06.005
71. Huang C, Han X, Li X, Lam E, Peng W, Lou N, et al. Critical role of connexin 43 in secondary expansion of traumatic spinal cord injury. *J Neurosci.* (2012) 32:3333–8. doi: 10.1523/JNEUROSCI.1216-11.2012
72. Takeuchi H, Jin S, Wang J, Zhang G, Kawanokuchi J, Kuno R, et al. Tumor necrosis factor-α induces neurotoxicity via glutamate release from hemichannels of activated microglia in an autocrine manner. *J Biol Chem.* (2006) 281:21362–68. doi: 10.1074/jbc.M600504200
73. Hansen DB, Braunstein TH, Nielsen MS, MacAulay N. Distinct permeation profiles of the connexin 30 and 43 hemichannels. *FEBS Lett.* (2014) 588:1446–57. doi: 10.1016/j.febslet.2014.01.036
74. Wang Y, Szretter KJ, Vermi W, Gilfillan S, Rossini C, Cella M, et al. IL-34 is a tissue-restricted ligand of CSF1R required for the development of Langerhans cells and microglia. *Nat Immunol.* (2012) 13:753. doi: 10.1038/ni.2360
75. Cekanaviciute E, Dietrich HK, Axtell RC, Williams AM, Egusquiza R, Wai KM, et al. Astrocytic TGF-β signaling limits inflammation and reduces neuronal damage during central nervous system Toxoplasma infection. *J Immunol.* (2014) 2014:1303284. doi: 10.4049/jimmunol.1303284
76. Cekanaviciute E, Fathali N, Doyle KP, Williams AM, Han J, Buckwalter MS. Astrocytic transforming growth factor-beta signaling reduces subacute neuroinflammation after stroke in mice. *Glia* (2014) 62:1227–40. doi: 10.1002/glia.22675

6

Myelin Oligodendrocyte Glycoprotein Antibody-Associated Disorders: Toward a New Spectrum of Inflammatory Demyelinating CNS Disorders?

Franziska Di Pauli and Thomas Berger*

Clinical Department of Neurology, Medical University of Innsbruck, Innsbruck, Austria

***Correspondence:**
Thomas Berger
thomas.berger@meduniwien.ac.at

Inflammatory demyelinating CNS syndromes include, besides their most common entity multiple sclerosis (MS), several different diseases of either monophasic or recurrent character—including neuromyelitis optica spectrum disorders (NMOSDs) and acute disseminated encephalomyelitis (ADEM). Early diagnostic differentiation is crucial for devising individual treatment strategies. However, due to overlapping clinical and paraclinical features diagnosis at the first demyelinating event is not always possible. A multiplicity of potential biological markers that could discriminate the different diseases was studied. As the use of autoantibodies in patient management of other autoimmune diseases, is well-established and evidence for the critical involvement of B cells/antibodies in disease pathogenesis in inflammatory demyelinating CNS syndromes increases, antibodies seem to be valuable diagnostic tools. Since the detection of antibodies against aquaporin-4 (AQP-4), the understanding of immunopathogenesis and diagnostic management of NMOSDs has dramatically changed. However, for most inflammatory demyelinating CNS syndromes, a potential antigen target is still not known. A further extensively studied possible target structure is myelin oligodendrocyte glycoprotein (MOG), found at the outermost surface of myelin sheaths and oligodendrocyte membranes. With detection methods using cell-based assays with full-length, conformationally correct MOG, antibodies have been described in early studies with a subgroup of patients with ADEM. Recently, a humoral immune reaction against MOG has been found not only in monophasic diseases, but also in recurrent non-MS diseases, particularly in pediatric patients. This review presents the findings regarding MOG antibodies as potential biological markers in discriminating between these different demyelinating CNS diseases, and discusses recent developments, clinical implementations, and data on immunopathogenesis of MOG antibody-associated disorders.

Keywords: multiple sclerosis, myelin oligodendrocyte glycoprotein antibody-associated disorders, neuromyelitis optica spectrum disease, inflammatory demyelinating CNS syndromes, clinically isolated syndrome

INTRODUCTION

Inflammatory demyelinating CNS diseases are a heterogeneous group, covering monophasic and multiphasic diseases, prognoses ranging from benign to fulminant, and a variety of different treatment responses. Although the sensitivity and specificity of diagnostic criteria, particularly for multiple sclerosis (MS), the most common demyelinating CNS disease, have significantly improved (1), misdiagnosis is not infrequent and occurs in up to 10% of cases (2). Differential diagnoses are beside other neurological non-inflammatory diseases, in particular neuromyelitis optica spectrum disorder (NMOSD), acute disseminated encephalomyelitis (ADEM), multiphasic disseminated encephalomyelitis (MDEM), and atypical demyelinating CNS syndromes (3, 4). Diagnosis is based on a combination of anamnesis, clinical presentation, and radiological findings (1, 5, 6) and allows, for the most part, correct stratification.

Given the recommendation for early treatment initiation in MS, and the availability of highly effective treatments (7), in the last few years efforts have been made to establish the diagnosis as early as possible. However, this in turn increases the risk of beginning a possibly harmful treatment regimen in patients without MS. The first detection of a laboratory biomarker in MS concerned the description of oligoclonal bands (OCBs) more than 60 years ago (8). However, so far analysis of the target antigen of an intrathecal immunoreaction has not been successful, and no specific antibodies have been found to be associated with MS (9).

In 2004, a change in the diagnosis and research of inflammatory demyelinating CNS diseases was evoked with the description of specific autoantibodies in patients with NMOSD (10). These antibodies are directed against aquaporin-4 (AQP-4), an abundant water channel in the CNS on astrocytic endfeets (11). However, a subgroup of clinically defined NMOSD patients are seronegative, and no marker is so far established for other differential diagnoses (12).

In animal models of MS (experimental autoimmune encephalomyelitis, EAE) a well-known target structure is myelin oligodendrocyte glycoprotein (MOG) (13), a protein comprising 245 amino acids that is exclusively expressed on the outermost surface of the myelin sheath and oligodendrocyte plasma membrane in the CNS, and which is easily accessible by a humoral immune reaction (14, 15). After passive immunization with tissue homogenates of CNS, the predominant antigen target in EAE is MOG, and inflammatory and demyelinating changes are enhanced by MOG antibodies (16–19). Furthermore, in combination with complement, demyelination, and diseases relapses have been induced and MOG antibodies seem to be involved in macrophage mediated myelin destruction/phagocytosis (12).

Given these promising results, a multiplicity of studies have attempted to identify MOG antibodies in demyelinating CNS diseases. Numerous techniques and heterogeneous study populations have been included in these, leading to conflicting and inconsistent data on the prognostic and diagnostic value in MS (20–24). However, the establishment of methods similar to that used for the analysis of AQP-4 directed antibodies has enabled the reliable detection of antibodies against native correctly folded and glycosylated MOG (12, 25). With these cell-based assays, a humoral immune response against MOG has been consistently identified—initially in ADEM and subsequently in a subgroup of particular pediatric patients with inflammatory demyelinating CNS diseases (20, 22, 24, 26).

In the last few years, the MOG antibody-associated disorder spectrum has been rapidly broadening, making more data regarding clinical, radiological, and laboratory findings available, as well as elucidating immunopathogenesis. The current paper discusses the developing clinical spectrum, histopathological data, and immunopathogenesis, alongside the implications of the same for daily clinical practice.

CLINICAL PRESENTATION AND PROGNOSIS OF MOG ANTIBODY-ASSOCIATED DISORDERS

The first evidence for the potential use of antibodies against native MOG as a biological marker for ADEM was published by O'Connor et al. (26). Self-assembling radiolabelled MOG tetramers were established and a humoral immunoreactivity against MOG reliably identified in a subgroup of children with ADEM. Initially, these antibodies seemed to be associated with monophasic disease courses, predominantly present in children with an ADEM-like onset (27–29). Subsequent studies, however, revealed that the spectrum of MOG antibody-associated disorders is much broader. MOG antibodies have been found to be present in a subset of patients with ADEM, NMOSD, monophasic, and recurrent optic neuritis (ON), and transverse myelitis (TM), demyelinating syndromes overlapping with anti-NMDA receptor encephalitis or glycine receptor alpha 1 subunit antibody positive ON, **Figure 1** (26, 27, 29–48). It is now well-accepted that MOG antibodies are in particular associated with ON and TM (49). In MS, a humoral immune response against MOG is only rarely seen (12). In atypical MS with a distinct clinical phenotype of e.g., severe brainstem and spinal cord involvement, immunoreactivity against MOG has been described in up to 5% of cases (50). In this subgroup, frequent relapses and insufficient responses to disease-modifying treatment seem to be a common feature. As co-incidence of MOG and AQP-4 immunoreactivity is an exception, disease mechanisms have been suggested to be at least partly different in these two entities (24).

However, clinical MOG antibody-positive patients can present with an NMOSD phenotype. Mader et al. were the first to describe the presence of MOG antibodies in this patient group

---

Abbreviations: ADEM, acute disseminated encephalomyelitis; ADEMON, acute disseminated encephalomyelitis followed by optic neuritis; AQP-4, aquaporin-4; CSF, cerebrospinal fluid; CRION, chronic relapsing inflammatory optic neuropathy; EAE, experimental autoimmune encephalomyelitis; LETM, longitudinally extensive transverse myelitis; MDEM, multiphasic disseminated encephalomyelitis; MS, multiple sclerosis; MOG, myelin oligodendrocyte glycoprotein; NMOSD, neuromyelitis optica spectrum disorder; OCBs, oligoclonal bands; ON, optic neuritis; RON, recurrent optic neuritis; TM, transverse myelitis.

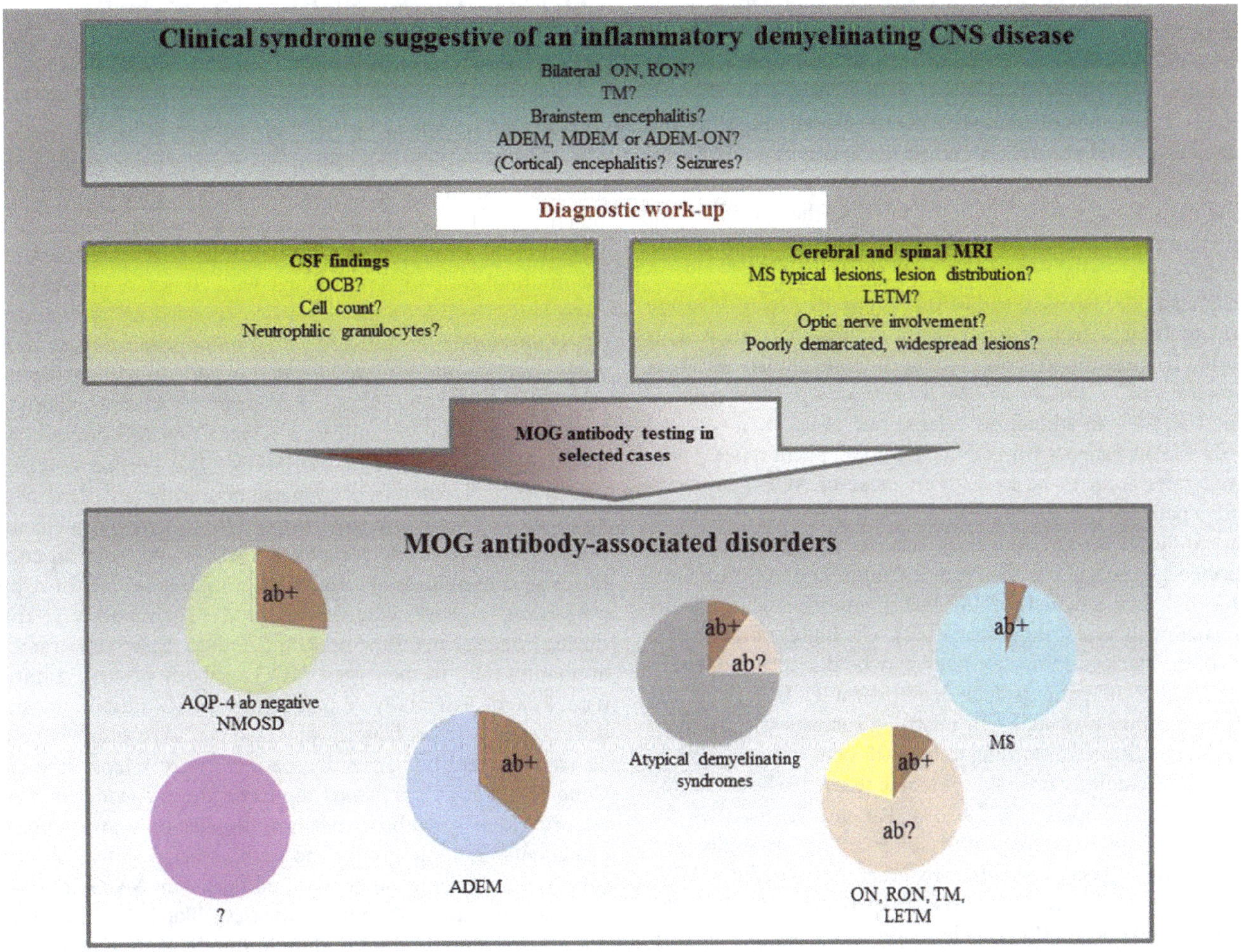

FIGURE 1 | Spectrum of MOG antibody-associated disorders.

(51). Subsequent studies supported the results: overall, in AQP-4 negative patients, MOG antibodies have a prevalence of 25% (12). In contrast to AQP-4 antibody-associated disorders with the well-defined clinical phenotype of NMOSD, in MOG antibody-associated disorders, the clinical presentation is less well-defined. Still, particularly in children, the sensitivity in ADEM is highest, at an average of 36% in different studies (12).

The two largest cohorts looking at the clinical features of MOG antibody-associated disorders were recently published (49, 52). Clinical presentation based on a trimodal distribution with age clusters of <20 years, 20–45 years, and >45 years, ADEM was most common in the age group <20 years; whereas ON (20–45 years) and bilateral ON (>45 years) were more frequent in adult patients with MOG antibody positive disorders (52). A short TM occurred in 14% of patients >45 years, but was rarely described in younger patients. The age-dependent clinical presentation was confirmed in a further study, with a predominance of ON found in adult onset MOG antibody-associated disorders, compared to a predominance of ADEM-like patterns in children as well as better recovery from neurological symptoms in children (53). The second largest study to include MOG antibody positive patients supported ON/TM as the main manifestations, given they represented clinical onset in over 90% of adult patients (49). However, NMOSD criteria (54) were fulfilled in only 19% of patients. Interestingly, in this study population, an encephalogenic phenotype was described with clinical signs of meningeal symptoms, retrograde amnesia, and seizures—uncommon symptoms in classical MS. Furthermore, seizures and encephalitis-like presentations are more common in MOG antibody-associated disorders compared to AQP-4 antibody positive diseases (55). Three recent case reports also found MOG antibodies to be associated with clinical presentation of cortical encephalitis and steroid responsiveness (56–58), indicating a new phenotype of MOG antibody-associated disorders.

Initial studies assumed MOG antibody-associated disorders to be monophasic, but it is now well-known that monophasic and recurrent diseases are both associated with MOG antibodies (59). In children, MOG antibodies are predictive not only of non-MS disease with a specificity of 100% but also of a recurrent non-MS disease course with a specificity of 75% including

NMOSD, recurrent ON (RON), MDEM, and ADEM followed by optic neuritis (ADEMON) (48). Overall, 39% of MOG antibody positive children have been found to have a recurrent disease course, but only 5% a typical MS. It is important to note that as low levels of MOG antibodies were also measured in healthy and other neurological controls, a cut-off for positivity was in most studies defined as ≥1:160 (12). However, this study introduced a new cut-off for seropositivity, to increase the specificity for prediction of non-MS diseases with only a moderate decrease of sensitivity, at a titer of ≥1:1,280 (48).

Higher age, female sex, and MRI findings atypical of MS were found to be risk factors for a recurrent disease course. This reported risk was found to vary across different studies. Relapses were observed in 36% of 252 MOG antibody positive patients in the UK, with an annualized relapse rate of 0.2 (52), with the highest risk in patients with ON or NMOSD phenotypes. These relapse rates seem to be lower than those of AQP-4 antibody positive patients (37, 39, 49, 60). However, disease reoccurrence of up to 80% with an annualized relapse rate of 0.9 has been described as associated with a humoral immune reaction against MOG (61); in particular, a NMOSD phenotype seemed to be correlated with a relapsing disease (62). The highly variable data on further attacks and relapse rates may be due to the different characteristics of patients included for study, as well as the higher detection probability in relapsing diseases compared to monophasic diseases according to study design.

In several studies, a favorable outcome seemed to be associated with MOG antibodies (34, 39, 63). Patients seropositive for MOG antibodies less frequently suffer motor disability and have a better EDSS score after recovery compared to AQP-4 antibody positive patients (37). In patients with TM, the presence of MOG antibodies has also been associated with a better recovery from acute attack, indeed similar frequency of severe attacks at onset and similar relapse rates to AQP-4 antibody-associated disorders (64). Although, MOG antibody-associated ON is mainly a recurrent disease, accompanied by severe visual loss in the acute phase, visual recovery was found to be good (65); the outcome was better in MOG- compared to AQP-4 antibody positive patients correlating with a better preserved retinal fiber layer thickness (65, 66). However, in another study, severe functional loss was described in nearly half of MOG antibody positive patients and retinal axonal damage was similar in both conditions (61, 67). In a recent study, visual function outcomes and ambulation were significantly better in MOG antibody-associated disorders than in AQP-4 antibody-associated disorders; indeed, permanent disability was described in nearly half of the patients after a median disease duration of 16 months, and permanent bladder and erectile dysfunction in ~1 quarter of the MOG antibody positive patients (52). In a subgroup of adult MOG antibody positive patients, severe disease courses and lack of response to DMT were also noted (50). Though more data are necessary to confidently evaluate the prognostic value of MOG antibodies regarding disability, data indicates a favorable outcome at least in the majority of patients; however, severe disease courses with pronounced functional loss are possible, and may warrant early immunotherapy.

LONGITUDINAL ANALYSIS OF MOG ANTIBODIES: IMPLICATIONS FOR CLINICAL PRACTICE

Prognostic assessment in MOG antibody positive patients who have had their first demyelinating event, with a possibility of an ensuing multiphasic disease course, is a challenge in clinical practice, and has important implications regarding further initiation of disease-modifying treatment. An association of longitudinal antibody level change with clinical course has been suggested (28, 29). Studies have also revealed an association of MOG antibody titer decrease with a monophasic disease course compared to stable or increasing titer in patients with multiphasic diseases (36, 45, 49, 50, 68). Persistent MOG antibodies have been predominantly found in recurrent non-MS diseases such as MDEM, NMOSD, and ADEMON (48). Furthermore, in a cohort of ON patients, 98% presented with persistent MOG antibodies, and of these 80% relapsed (65). A recent publication on adult and pediatric seropositive ADEM patients supported the clinical usefulness of serial MOG antibody testing for relapse prediction, as 88% with persistent MOG antibodies relapsed during long-term follow-up compared to 12% with transient antibodies (69). In the largest MOG antibody positive cohort to date, 72% of patients were persistently MOG antibody positive during the disease course; of these, 60% relapsed, whereas all transient antibody positive patients were relapse-free (52). Cobo-Calvo et al. confirmed the trend toward association of a relapsing disease with persistent antibodies only in a subgroup of patients; in some groups, no such association was observed (49). Similarly, Duignan et al. found persistent MOG antibodies in relapsing and monophasic diseases alike (70). In addition, one study showed that in adult MS patients, a subgroup had an immunoreactivity against MOG as well as associated severe brainstem and spinal cord involvement, frequent relapses, and a less favorable treatment response, with fluctuating and non-persistent antibody levels (50).

Promising results for the use of MOG antibodies as treatment biomarkers were published in 2017 in a study showing conversion to seronegativity during immune-directed therapies. The conversion was found to be a predictive marker for disease-free activity during the subsequent disease course (71). Although there is evidence for the potential use of serial testing as a long-term disease marker and potential treatment marker, more prospective data are necessary for the final evaluation of the predictive value of serial MOG antibody testing, as the results are in part inconsistent, and severe, relapsing disease courses have been described in patients with decreasing/disappearing antibody levels.

PARACLINICAL FINDINGS AND MOG ANTIBODIES

In ADEM, an intrathecal IgG synthesis as measured by IgG index or OCBs, is rare (72)—in contrast with MS, in which OCBs are present in over 90% of cases. OCBs are included in recent diagnostic MS criteria, and count for dissemination in time (1). Similar findings have been confirmed for MOG antibody-associated disorders: OCBs are uncommon, occurring in ~10% of cases, and cerebrospinal fluid (CSF) reactivity to MOG has only been shown in cases of high serum levels (27, 28, 46, 73). These findings indicate a peripheral production of MOG antibodies and secondary diffusion in the CNS similar to that in NMOSD (74). Possible explanations include: a direct CNS infection with leakage of CNS antigens in the periphery, and a secondary peripheral immune reaction against MOG (20); or a peripheral infection that stimulates MOG antibody production via molecular mimicry (20, 22).

Other routine CSF analyses were also comparable between MOG antibody-associated disorders and NMOSD. CSF pleocytosis was detected in 55–70% of cases, with neutrophilic granulocytes in more than half of patients and cell counts higher than in typical MS (37, 61, 75). In addition, similarities were found between CSF cytokine profiles in MOG antibody-associated disorders and AQP-4 antibody-associated NMOSD, with a predominant up-regulation of T helper 17 related cytokines in the latter, whereas in MS, T helper 1 related cytokines were found (75, 76), suggesting shared immunological pathomechanisms in the two diseases.

Besides clear differences in clinical and laboratory findings, MRI also provides a useful means of discriminating MOG antibody-associated disorders from other CNS demyelinating diseases, in particular MS. Brain MRI abnormalities at onset range from 40 to 77% (41, 49, 61, 77, 78) and supratentorial lesions have been found in nearly half of patients during the disease course and brainstem, respectively, cerebellar lesions in one third of the patients. Brain MRI abnormalities are associated with pathological CSF findings (49). According to the typical clinical manifestations of TM, the most common imaging finding is a longitudinally extensive transverse myelitis (LETM) or a short TM (61). In MOG antibody-associated ON, typical imaging characteristics are a contrast enhancement of the optic nerve, a perineural enhancement in a proportion of the patients, and in 80%, more than half of the pre-chiasmic optic nerve length being affected (65, 79). Lesion distribution in children seems to be age-dependent, with poorly demarcated, widespread lesions in younger children, in contrast with a normal brain MRI in older children (80). It has been possible to distinguish MOG antibody-associated NMOSD from MS with a specificity of 95% and a sensitivity of 91% by employing predefined MRI criteria for lesion distribution, including Dawson's fingers, subcortical *U* fiber lesions, and lesions adjacent to the lateral ventricles, as typical for MS (81). A subsequent study confirmed these results, and was able to accurately discriminate MS from MOG antibody-associated disorders by the presence of ovoid lesions adjacent to the body of the lateral ventricles, Dawson's fingers, and T1 hypointense lesions, whereas fluffy lesions and three lesions or less were typical for MOG antibody-associated disorders (82). However, there was an overlap between MRI characteristics for AQP-4 and MOG antibody-associated disorders. Moreover, a further study could not identify typical radiological features to discriminate between the diseases; indeed, thalamus, and pons lesions were more common in MOG antibody-associated disorders, and in 16% of patients, a cortical involvement, and in 6% a leptomeningeal enhancement, was described (49).

Although MRI is variable in MOG antibody-associated disorders, depending on the clinical presentation and age of the patient, it is an important diagnostic tool. In the absence of an unique imaging finding, typical features of MOG antibody positive patients are characterized as a normal brain MRI or large, confluent, poorly marginated MRI lesions (if clinically presenting with ADEM), LETM, perineural enhancement of the optic nerve, brainstem and hypothalamic lesions, and a leukodystrophy-like MRI pattern (25, 83).

DIAGNOSTIC RECOMMENDATIONS FOR MOG ANTIBODY-ASSOCIATED DISORDERS

The International Panel on Diagnosis of Multiple Sclerosis published in 2017 its most recent diagnostic criteria for MS. The revised diagnostic criteria were based on further knowledge of a combination of clinical, MRI, and CSF findings, and emphasized the important role of OCBs in the diagnosis of MS and in reducing the risk of misdiagnosis (1). Although MOG antibody testing was not included in the revised criteria, due to a lack of full validation of antibody testing, special clinical situations were described for which antibody testing was recommended.

NMOSD and MS are often precisely discriminated by clinical and paraclinical features (84), of which the important therapeutic consequences regarding DMT requires special attention. NMOSD, therefore, should be considered in every suspected case of MS (1). The presence of antibodies against MOG and AQP-4 should be tested for in patients with clinical symptoms suggestive of NMOSD, such as bilateral ON, severe brainstem involvement, or LETM, in special patient groups with a high risk of NMOSD, if there is evidence of large cerebral lesions, if MS criteria of dissemination in space are not fulfilled, or if brain MRI is normal (1). As lack of OCBs is a very rare finding in typical MS; MOG antibody testing should be considered in OCB negative MS patients. In pediatric onset MS, antibody testing can support the diagnosis of AQP-4 negative NMOSD, ADEM followed by RON or with including chronic relapsing inflammatory optic neuropathy (CRION). In 2017, Hacohen et al. more precisely described the routine diagnostic use of MOG antibody testing for pediatric patients in clinical practice, and proposed a diagnostic algorithm for any episode of CNS demyelination (83). According to the revised McDonald criteria, first of all the diagnosis of MS should be evaluated by spinal and brain MRI and CSF findings. Given the 2010 McDonald diagnostic criteria (85), in this cohort diagnosis MS is also reliable in children independent of age and no further diagnostic steps are required. However, if there are features of NMOSD or ADEM in cases where the patient is AQP-4 antibody negative, MOG antibody analysis is strongly recommended. In contrast, preceding criteria advised to apply the McDonald criteria with caution for children under 12 years, as the validation of the predictive value is lacking (86). In addition, MOG antibodies are much more frequent in children; therefore, less stringent indications for antibody testing should be implemented in the clinical practice.

Other red flags indicating the usefulness of MOG antibody testing identified in the study of Hacohen et al. included poorly marginated lesions located in the cerebellar peduncle and a leukodystrophy-like MRI pattern. As MOG antibody positive patients have distinct clinical features (being young, less frequent area postrema syndrome, typically presenting ADEM initially, lower disability during follow-up, a longer time interval till the first relapse), the authors regard MOG antibody-associated disorder as a new phenotype, discriminating it in terms of its diagnostic algorithm from MS, AQP-4 antibody positive NMOSD, and antibody-negative recurrent demyelinating syndrome (83).

Due to the rising relevance, in 2018 an international recommendation based on expert consensus was proposed for indication of antibody testing for patients with a demyelinating CNS disease of suspected autoimmune etiology and either a monophasic or relapsing disease course (25). Jarius et al. proposed the urgent necessity of stringent indications for MOG antibody testing, as screening for a rare biomarker in large, unselected patient cohorts significantly decreases the predictive power of a test (25). This limitation applies particularly to adult patients, as in children MOG antibodies are more common. Based on a combination of clinical, imaging, and laboratory findings, MOG antibody testing should be performed in patients with high risk of a MOG antibody-associated disorder and/or in the case of findings that are atypical for MS. Concrete antibody testing indications are: "Monophasic or relapsing acute ON, myelitis, brainstem encephalitis, encephalitis, or any combination thereof, AND radiological or, only in patients with a history of ON, electrophysiological (VEP) findings compatible with CNS demyelination" (25). In addition, at least one further finding is necessary, of clearly defined MRI, Fundoscopy, CSF, or clinical features, or typical treatment response. Among others, a progressive disease course, progressive lesion load shown by MRI during clinically inactive time periods, AQP-4 AND MOG antibody positivity, and MOG IgM antibodies are regarded as red flags for a false positive result.

As discussed above, no exact clinically unique phenotype has been identified in patients with MOG antibodies. However, MOG antibody-associated disorders share similar features and a common treatment response, making their inclusion in diagnostic criteria for all patient age ranges of important clinical relevance. Therefore, two research groups independently suggested diagnostic criteria for MOG antibody-associated disorders, the newly introduced entity was termed as "MOG encephalomyelitis" (25), respectively, "MOG IgG associated disorders" (69). Jarius et al. propose the possible diagnostic criteria for "MOG encephalomyelitis" in adult patients, as including MOG antibody seropositive patients with either a monophasic or relapsing ON, TM, brainstem encephalitis, or encephalitis (or a combination of these syndromes), if MRI or electrophysiological findings are compatible with CNS demyelination (25). In the second proposal for diagnostic criteria of Lopez-Chiriboga et al., similar findings are required: MOG-IgG seropositivity measured by a cell-based assay with clinical findings of ADEM, ON, CRION, TM, brain or brainstem syndrome compatible with demyelination, or any combination of the described syndromes, after exclusion of other differential diagnoses (69).

These suggested criteria are preliminary: validation experiments are essential for confirming final use in clinical practice. Furthermore, depending on future data and antibody testing methods, which may offer improvements in sensitivity and specificity, adaptions will be necessary. In particular in large, experienced MS centers, screening for MOG antibody positivity in typical MS cohorts, and critical consideration of results, could yield enhanced knowledge of the whole spectrum of MOG antibody positive disorders.

HOW TO TEST FOR MOG ANTIBODIES

Several detection methods have been applied in identifying MOG antibodies in inflammatory demyelinating CNS diseases. Given the inconsistent results generated by ELISA and immunoblot in MS patients, these techniques are now regarded as obsolete (21). However, reliable results have been recorded with cell-based assays expressed in human cells using immunofluorescence or fluorescence-activated cell sorting. With this method, the expression of natural conformation full length native MOG at the cell surface is possible, and subsequently, so is the detection of antibodies targeting human MOG. Different expression vectors, cell lines, and read-out systems have been reliably used. Immunohistochemistry is not recommended, due to reduced sensitivity depending on the tissue donor, and limited data regarding specificity (12, 87). As mentioned above, a cut-off is important, as in healthy individuals as well as other neurological controls, low-titer antibodies are detectable, leading to a lack of disease specificity for low-titer MOG antibodies. Most studies have used a cut-off of $\geq$1:160 (88). A higher prognostic specificity has been described using a higher cut-off titer for positivity, but further prospective studies are required for the evaluation of optimal cut-off.

Waters et al. were able to improve the test using an IgGI-specific secondary antibody, in response to the problem of cross-reactivity of the anti-human IgG secondary antibody with IgM and IgA antibodies. This optimization increased the specificity of the MOG antibody assay in cases of non-MS disease, and the method provided class II evidence for the discrimination of non-MS CNS demyelinating disorders from MS (89). As an alternative, IgG Fc antibodies can be used (25). As data suggests peripheral production of MOG antibodies, analysis of serum samples results in higher specificity than CSF samples (28, 46), and CSF analysis is only recommended in rare cases (46).

Although the value of longitudinal testing warrants further evaluation, the current authors recommend serial analysis of positive patients at 6–12 months. As there is no evidence for seroconversion from negative to positive (48), there is no expectation of additional information by retesting negative patients during the disease course. However, as there is no gold standard for MOG antibody analysis, in particular cases with clinical and paraclinical findings suggestive for a MOG antibody associated disorder retesting is reasonable.

LESSONS FROM NEUROPATHOLOGY

Only limited data, mainly by single case reports, are available regarding MOG antibody positive patients and underlying histopathology. However, the existent neuropathological findings are consistent and show in most cases MS pattern II pathology (12). To the current authors' knowledge, to date only nine cases with available neuropathology are described in the literature, **Table 1** (47, 56, 58, 90–94). Most cases revealed MS pattern II lesions with demyelination, relatively preserved axons, pre-oligodendrocytes, an absence of myelin, and myelin-laden macrophages. The inflammatory hallmark is an infiltrate consisting of T cells as well as a complement and antibodies (12)—indicative of humoral pathogenesis in these cases. The clinical presentation of MOG antibody positive patients with MS pattern II pathology varies, and includes cases with CIS, MS, NMOSD, recurrent LETM followed by tumefactive lesions, and atypical inflammatory demyelinating CNS syndromes (47, 58, 90–94). Tough the clinical presentation corresponded to NMOSD, the typical pathological hallmarks of NMOSD with AQP-4 and astrocyte loss, necrosis, complement activation, focal perivascular or confluent extensive demyelination, eosinophilic, and neutrophilic cell infiltration (95), and thickened hyalinized vessel walls (96) were missing.

Similar results have been obtained for ADEM. No clinical ADEM MOG antibody positive case to date, according to the diagnostic criteria, has the ADEM typical neuropathological findings with perivenous demyelination (compared to confluent demyelination in MS) (97) and cortical microglial activation (35). In accordance with this, it has previously been shown that 9% of patients with ADEM according to clinical criteria were misdiagnosed, since the pathology was MS typical and the patients developed MS during long-term follow-up (97). Complications in ADEM diagnosis are still possible with biopsy, as an overlap of confluent and perivenous demyelination has been described. However, two recently published MOG antibody positive cases presented with a distinct pathology and clinical presentation (56, 58). In the first case, a bilateral cortical frontal steroid-responsive encephalitis with ADEM-like lesions and ON was associated with MOG antibodies and mild inflammatory changes with intact myelin sheaths (56). Comparably, in the second case, of cerebral cortical encephalomyelitis, epilepsy, and steroid responsiveness, biopsy revealed slight inflammation without distinct demyelination, and in contrast to the first case, mild loss of MOG (58). Whether these two cases extended the spectrum of MOG antibody-associated disorders to a subgroup of cortical inflammatory encephalitis without pronounced demyelination needs to be further elucidated.

To summarize the available rare data, MOG antibody-associated disorders seem to be mainly associated with MS pattern II pathology, independent of clinical features, pointing to a distinct humoral-mediated disease group of demyelinating CNS diseases.

EVIDENCE FOR THE PATHOGENIC ROLE OF MOG ANTIBODIES

In animal models, it is well-established that MOG antibodies have a pathogenic effect (12); however, in humans, the role of MOG antibodies in disease pathogenesis is less clear and still under debate, including the subjects of direct, antibody-mediated cell induced tissue destruction or their presence of a bystander phenomenon.

Initial studies showing evidence for a pathogenic effect of humoral immune response against MOG involved purified human MOG antibodies; these antibodies were able to induce cell death of MOG-expressing cells, as well as natural killer-cell mediated cell death, with the extent of cell damage dependent on antibody levels (27, 30). In addition, MOG antibodies belong mainly to the complement binding IgG1 subtype, and have been found to be able to activate the complement cascade, finally leading to complement-dependent destruction of MOG expressing cells (31, 51). A disruption of the oligodendrocyte cytoskeleton, with the effect of a functional modification, has been described (73); however, results from *in vivo* studies of the ability of MOG antibodies to damage tissue are inconclusive. Patient purified antibodies injected in EAE increased demyelination (30), and reversibly damaged axons, though no inflammatory reaction or complement deposition was induced (98). One possible explanation is that human and rodent MOG differs, and human MOG antibodies do not recognize rodent MOG (99).

However, in CNS antigen-presenting cells (APCs), accumulation of MOG antibodies has been described, with a subsequent activation of autoreactive T cells, as well as a MOG antibody induced Fc-mediated APC recognition of MOG, followed by induction of peripheral autoreactive T cells (100, 101). A recent study confirmed the pathogenic effect on rodents of affinity-purified MOG antibodies transferred from patients. These purified MOG antibodies were not only able to mediate MS pattern II pathology with typical immunoglobulin-mediated tissue destruction, but also induce, in combination with MOG reactive T-cells, a clinical disease with enhanced T-cell recruitment and reaction (102). Importantly, results revealed that MOG antibodies alone did not induce inflammation and tissue destruction—their interdependence with T-cells was required to evolve their pathogenic potential.

Evidence is arising that MOG antibodies have a pathogenic potential, but the exact pathomechanism and the synergy with T cells requires further elucidation. However, if MOG antibodies are mainly bystanders and only slightly contribute to disease development and pathogenesis, their important role as disease biomarkers is obvious.

TREATMENT

As there have been no controlled treatment trials in MOG antibody positive diseases, therapy regimes are based on the suspected individual prognosis and clinical experiences.

TABLE 1 | Histopathological findings in MOG antibody-associated disorders. Modified after (12, 24).

Sex	Age	Clinical diagnosis	Neuropathological classification	Inflammatory infiltrates and confluent demyelination[a]	Perivascular complement deposition and/or AQP-4 loss[b]	Eosinophilic cell infiltration[b]	Comment	References
M	71	Fulminant encephalomyelitis	MS pattern II, in addition lesions with complement activation and AQP4 loss	+	+ in a single lesion of optic chiasm	nr	Late seroconversion to low-titer AQP-4 antibody positivity during disease course	(91)
M	46	Encephalitis, ADEM-like lesions and unilateral optic neuritis	Mild inflammatory changes	na	na	na	No demyelinating lesions	(56)
F	29	Cerebral cortical encephalitis with epilepsy and bilateral optic neuritis	Inflammatory infiltrates in the cortex and subcortex	na	na	na	No demyelinating lesions	(58)
F	63	CIS	MS pattern II	+	–	–	–	(93)
W	49	RRMS	MS pattern II	+	–	–	–	(90)
M	49	ADEM	MS pattern II with an overlap of MS pattern III	+	–	–	Oligodendrocyte apoptosis and loss	(94)
M	34	ADEM	MS pattern II	+	–	–	–	
F	66	Recurrent myelitis and brainstem involvement followed by tumefactive bilateral lesions	MS pattern II	+	–	–	–	(92)
F	67	NMOSD, recurrent myelitis followed by cerebral tumefactive lesions	No pattern classification, inflammatory demyelination without astrocyte loss	+	nr	nr	–	(47)

[a] *Typical neuropathological findings of MS and NMOSD.*
[b] *Typical neuropathological findings of NMOSD, nr, not reported; na, not applicable.*

In an acute attack, similar approaches are used as in other inflammatory demyelinating CNS diseases such as MS (intravenous methylprednisolone and plasma exchange). A favorable recovery has been demonstrated in 70–90% of patients given intravenous methylprednisolone (39, 103). Long-term treatment with corticosteroids reduces the risk of relapse and cessation has been associated with breakthrough disease (103). Jarius et al. describe similar results, with a full recovery in 50% of cases, partial recovery in 44%, and no recovery in 6% (61). Of particular importance is that tapering or finishing of corticosteroids was followed by a flare-up of the disease and early relapses (25, 52, 103). Thus, some authors have favored long-term steroid treatment over 6 months, given alongside other immunomodulatory or immunosuppressive drugs. When there is suggestion of an antibody-mediated immune reaction, plasma exchange, which is normally initiated if corticosteroid therapy is insufficient, is promising for managing the acute attack. Use of plasma exchange seems to be associated in several reports with a better outcome and improved neurological deficits after the failure of corticosteroids (50, 80). However, though plasma exchange seems mainly to be followed by a good functional outcome, in a substantial proportion of patients, only partial recovery was achieved (61). On balance, plasma exchange seems to be a reasonable therapy after the treatment failure of corticosteroids, or in selected patients as an early treatment option.

A challenge in MOG antibody-associated disorders is the choice of long-term immunotherapy, since clinical courses and prognoses substantially vary between individuals. When considering the underlying pathogenesis as involving B cells and antibodies, therapies directing the humoral immune response may prove most promising.

Although the data shows that recurrent disabling disease courses are common with MOG antibody-associated disorders, they are treated less often than AQP-4 associated diseases (104). Only 40% received a long-term maintenance therapy (52). As mentioned above, a combination of corticosteroids and other immune-mediated therapies seems favorable. Ramanathan et al. found a reduction of relapse rates with different immunotherapies such as azathioprine, rituximab, and mycophenolate, maintenance corticosteroids and rituximab being most effective in preventing disease activity (103). In addition, further studies confirmed the positive effect of immunosuppression/immunomodulation, including azathioprine, methotrexate, and rituximab, on the risk of relapse and the annualized relapse rate (23, 49, 52), in particular if treatment is maintained for more than 3 months (52). Recently, a study including children with relapsing MOG antibody associated disorders demonstrated a benefit of intravenous immunoglobulins on the annualized relapse rate (78). Classical MS drugs such as natalizumab, interferon, and glatirameracetat showed no treatment efficacy (61). To the knowledge of the current authors, so far only one case has been published detailing treatment with alemtuzumab, a highly effective treatment in MS. Similar to reports of alemtuzumab use in AQP-4 antibody NMOSD (105), treatment failed and disease activity resumed (106). The failure of a treatment effective in MS is well-known in NMOSD, suggesting a distinct pathomechanism in antibody-associated disorders. In conclusion, promising treatment regimes include maintenance corticosteroids and rituximab, although for a more definitive statement, prospective controlled trials are required.

CONCLUSION

Inflammatory demyelinating CNS diseases include a broad spectrum of different diseases, among which single diseases might show distinct clinical phenotypes and prognoses. For disease stratification, prognostic evaluation, treatment decisions, and patient counseling an early diagnosis is important. Diagnostic procedures now include a combination of clinical, imaging, and laboratory findings. However, correct diagnosis at disease onset is still a challenge and an exact prognostic estimation regarding occurrence of relapses and disability is remains out of reach. Biomarker research has therefore been a focus of interest for several decades, given that in MS, in particular, new treatment allows for early therapy initiation. However, since newly available treatments are not only more effective but also more aggressive, carrying more side effects and risks, overtreatment should be avoided.

Over the past few years our knowledge of clinical, imaging, and laboratory data regarding MOG antibody-associated disorders has evolved. Clear differences in this spectrum have not only been found with MS, but also, to a lesser degree, with AQP-4 associated disorders. Although there is no unique clinical phenotype, clinical presentation, prognosis, and treatment response is distinct in this demyelinating CNS disease subgroup. In particular, in MOG antibody-associated NMOSD a different immunopathogenesis, with an oligodendrogliopathy rather than a classical astrocytopathy, is suggested. These differences are mirrored in the histopathological findings of MOG antibody-associated disorders, where there is a preponderance of MS pattern II findings. This finding is clearly different from AQP-4 associated disorders, and suggests that other therapeutic strategies might be promising. An integration of the two diseases would be short-sighted, as there are not only important implications for further research but also for patient counseling and treatment considerations.

Various research groups have published diagnostic recommendations for MOG antibody-associated disorders and introduced them as a new spectrum disorder. International cooperation for the development of diagnostic consensus criteria, either as stand-alone or for inclusion in the MS or NMOSD criteria, would constitute further important progress. In addition, serial testing is now upcoming in the generation of prognostic, and perhaps also therapeutic, biomarkers; its routine use in clinical practice warrants further prospective trials, in particular for patients undergoing long-term treatment. Overall, MOG antibody-associated disorders should, it is suggested, be classified as distinct spectrum disorders, though research is still in its early stages in understanding the exact underlying pathomechanism and its prognostic implications.

AUTHOR CONTRIBUTIONS

All authors listed have made a substantial, direct and intellectual contribution to the work, and approved it for publication.

REFERENCES

1. Thompson AJ, Banwell BL, Barkhof F, Carroll WM, Coetzee T, Comi G, et al. Diagnosis of multiple sclerosis: 2017 revisions of the McDonald criteria. *Lancet Neurol.* (2018) 17:162–73. doi: 10.1016/S1474-4422(17)30470-2
2. Solomon AJ, Weinshenker BG. Misdiagnosis of multiple sclerosis: frequency, causes, effects, and prevention. *Curr Neurol Neurosci Rep.* (2013) 13:403. doi: 10.1007/s11910-013-0403-y
3. Brownlee WJ, Hardy TA, Fazekas F, Miller DH. Diagnosis of multiple sclerosis: progress and challenges. *Lancet* (2017) 389:1336–46. doi: 10.1016/S0140-6736(16)30959-X
4. Hoftberger R, Lassmann H. Inflammatory demyelinating diseases of the central nervous system. *Handb Clin Neurol.* (2017) 145:263–83. doi: 10.1016/B978-0-12-802395-2.00019-5
5. Karussis D. The diagnosis of multiple sclerosis and the various related demyelinating syndromes: a critical review. *J Autoimmun.* (2014) 48–9:134–42. doi: 10.1016/j.jaut.2014.01.022
6. Beesley R, Anderson V, Harding KE, Joseph F, Tomassini V, Pickersgill TP, et al. Impact of the 2017 revisions to McDonald criteria on the diagnosis of multiple sclerosis. *Mult Scler.* (2018) 24:1786–7. doi: 10.1177/1352458518778007
7. Thompson AJ, Baranzini SE, Geurts J, Hemmer B, Ciccarelli O. Multiple sclerosis. *Lancet* (2018) 391:1622–36. doi: 10.1016/S0140-6736(18)30481-1
8. Yahr MD, Goldensohn SS, Kabat EA. Further studies on the gamma globulin content of cerebrospinal fluid in multiple sclerosis and other neurological diseases. *Ann N Y Acad Sci.* (1954) 58:613–24. doi: 10.1111/j.1749-6632.1954.tb54099.x
9. Weissert R. Adaptive immunity is the key to the understanding of autoimmune and paraneoplastic inflammatory central nervous system disorders. *Front Immunol.* (2017) 8:336. doi: 10.3389/fimmu.2017.00336
10. Lennon VA, Wingerchuk DM, Kryzer TJ, Pittock SJ, Lucchinetti CF, Fujihara K, et al. A serum autoantibody marker of neuromyelitis optica: distinction from multiple sclerosis. *Lancet* (2004) 364:2106–12. doi: 10.1016/S0140-6736(04)17551-X
11. Lennon VA, Kryzer TJ, Pittock SJ, Verkman AS, Hinson SR. IgG marker of optic-spinal multiple sclerosis binds to the aquaporin-4 water channel. *J Exp Med.* (2005) 202:473–7. doi: 10.1084/jem.20050304
12. Peschl P, Bradl M, Hoftberger R, Berger T, Reindl M. Myelin oligodendrocyte glycoprotein: deciphering a target in inflammatory demyelinating diseases. *Front Immunol.* (2017) 8:529. doi: 10.3389/fimmu.2017.00529
13. Lebar R, Boutry JM, Vincent C, Robineaux R, Voisin GA. Studies on autoimmune encephalomyelitis in the guinea pig. II An *in vitro* investigation on the nature, properties, and specificity of the serum-demyelinating factor. *J Immunol.* (1976) 116:1439–46.
14. Gardinier MV, Amiguet P, Linington C, Matthieu JM. Myelin/oligodendrocyte glycoprotein is a unique member of the

immunoglobulin superfamily. *J Neurosci Res.* (1992) 33:177–87. doi: 10.1002/jnr.490330123
15. Kroepfl JF, Viise LR, Charron AJ, Linington C, Gardinier MV. Investigation of myelin/oligodendrocyte glycoprotein membrane topology. *J Neurochem.* (1996) 67:2219–22.
16. Lebar R, Lubetzki C, Vincent C, Lombrail P, Boutry JM. The M2 autoantigen of central nervous system myelin, a glycoprotein present in oligodendrocyte membrane. *Clin Exp Immunol.* (1986) 66:423–34.
17. Linington C, Lassmann H. Antibody responses in chronic relapsing experimental allergic encephalomyelitis: correlation of serum demyelinating activity with antibody titre to the myelin/oligodendrocyte glycoprotein (MOG). *J Neuroimmunol.* (1987) 17:61–9.
18. Linington C, Bradl M, Lassmann H, Brunner C, Vass K. Augmentation of demyelination in rat acute allergic encephalomyelitis by circulating mouse monoclonal antibodies directed against a myelin/oligodendrocyte glycoprotein. *Am J Pathol.* (1988) 130:443–54.
19. Lebar R, Baudrimont M, Vincent C. Chronic experimental autoimmune encephalomyelitis in the guinea pig. Presence of anti-M2 antibodies in central nervous system tissue and the possible role of M2 autoantigen in the induction of the disease. *J Autoimmun.* (1989) 2:115–32.
20. Reindl M, Di Pauli F, Rostasy K, Berger T. The spectrum of MOG autoantibody-associated demyelinating diseases. *Nat Rev Neurol.* (2013) 9:455–61. doi: 10.1038/nrneurol.2013.118
21. Berger T, Reindl M. Antibody biomarkers in CNS demyelinating diseases - a long and winding road. *Eur J Neurol.* (2015) 22:1162–8. doi: 10.1111/ene.12759
22. Ramanathan S, Dale RC, Brilot F. Anti-MOG antibody: the history, clinical phenotype, and pathogenicity of a serum biomarker for demyelination. *Autoimmun Rev.* (2016) 15:307–24. doi: 10.1016/j.autrev.2015.12.004
23. Dos Passos GR, Oliveira LM, da Costa BK, Apostolos-Pereira SL, Callegaro D, Fujihara K, et al. MOG-IgG-associated optic neuritis, encephalitis, and myelitis: lessons learned from neuromyelitis optica spectrum disorder. *Front Neurol.* (2018) 9:217. doi: 10.3389/fneur.2018.00217
24. Weber MS, Derfuss T, Metz I, Bruck W. Defining distinct features of anti-MOG antibody associated central nervous system demyelination. *Ther Adv Neurol Disord.* (2018) 11. doi: 10.1177/1756286418762083
25. Jarius S, Paul F, Aktas O, Asgari N, Dale RC, de Seze J, et al. MOG encephalomyelitis: international recommendations on diagnosis and antibody testing. *J Neuroinflamm.* (2018) 15:134. doi: 10.1186/s12974-018-1144-2
26. O'Connor KC, McLaughlin KA, De Jager PL, Chitnis T, Bettelli E, Xu C, et al. Self-antigen tetramers discriminate between myelin autoantibodies to native or denatured protein. *Nat Med.* (2007) 13:211–7. doi: 10.1038/nm1488
27. Brilot F, Dale RC, Selter RC, Grummel V, Kalluri SR, Aslam M, et al. Antibodies to native myelin oligodendrocyte glycoprotein in children with inflammatory demyelinating central nervous system disease. *Ann Neurol.* (2009) 66:833–42. doi: 10.1002/ana.21916
28. Di Pauli F, Mader S, Rostasy K, Schanda K, Bajer-Kornek B, Ehling R, et al. Temporal dynamics of anti-MOG antibodies in CNS demyelinating diseases. *Clin Immunol.* (2011) 138:247–54. doi: 10.1016/j.clim.2010.11.013
29. Probstel AK, Dornmair K, Bittner R, Sperl P, Jenne D, Magalhaes S, et al. Antibodies to MOG are transient in childhood acute disseminated encephalomyelitis. *Neurology* (2011) 77:580–8. doi: 10.1212/WNL.0b013e318228c0b1
30. Zhou D, Srivastava R, Nessler S, Grummel V, Sommer N, Bruck W, et al. Identification of a pathogenic antibody response to native myelin oligodendrocyte glycoprotein in multiple sclerosis. *Proc Natl Acad Sci USA.* (2006) 103:19057–62. doi: 10.1073/pnas.0607242103
31. McLaughlin KA, Chitnis T, Newcombe J, Franz B, Kennedy J, McArdel S, et al. Age-dependent B cell autoimmunity to a myelin surface antigen in pediatric multiple sclerosis. *J Immunol.* (2009) 183:4067–76. doi: 10.4049/jimmunol.0801888
32. Selter RC, Brilot F, Grummel V, Kraus V, Cepok S, Dale RC, et al. Antibody responses to EBV and native MOG in pediatric inflammatory demyelinating CNS diseases. *Neurology* (2010) 74:1711–5. doi: 10.1212/WNL.0b013e3181e04096
33. Lalive PH, Hausler MG, Maurey H, Mikaeloff Y, Tardieu M, Wiendl H, et al. Highly reactive anti-myelin oligodendrocyte glycoprotein antibodies differentiate demyelinating diseases from viral encephalitis in children. *Mult Scler.* (2011) 17:297–302. doi: 10.1177/1352458510389220
34. Kitley J, Woodhall M, Waters P, Leite MI, Devenney E, Craig J, et al. Myelin-oligodendrocyte glycoprotein antibodies in adults with a neuromyelitis optica phenotype. *Neurology* (2012) 79:1273–7. doi: 10.1212/WNL.0b013e31826aac4e
35. Rostasy K, Mader S, Schanda K, Huppke P, Gartner J, Kraus V, et al. Anti-myelin oligodendrocyte glycoprotein antibodies in pediatric patients with optic neuritis. *Arch Neurol* (2012) 69:752–6. doi: 10.1001/archneurol.2011.2956
36. Rostasy K, Mader S, Hennes EM, Schanda K, Gredler V, Guenther A, et al. Persisting myelin oligodendrocyte glycoprotein antibodies in aquaporin-4 antibody negative pediatric neuromyelitis optica. *Mult Scler.* (2013) 19:1052–9. doi: 10.1177/1352458512470310
37. Kitley J, Waters P, Woodhall M, Leite MI, Murchison A, George J, et al. Neuromyelitis optica spectrum disorders with aquaporin-4 and myelin-oligodendrocyte glycoprotein antibodies: a comparative study. *JAMA Neurol.* (2014) 71:276–83. doi: 10.1001/jamaneurol.2013.5857
38. Ramanathan S, Reddel SW, Henderson A, Parratt JD, Barnett M, Gatt PN, et al. Antibodies to myelin oligodendrocyte glycoprotein in bilateral and recurrent optic neuritis. *Neurol Neuroimmunol Neuroinflamm.* (2014) 1:e40. doi: 10.1212/NXI.0000000000000040
39. Sato DK, Callegaro D, Lana-Peixoto MA, Waters PJ, de Haidar Jorge FM, Takahashi T, et al. Distinction between MOG antibody-positive and AQP4 antibody-positive NMO spectrum disorders. *Neurology* (2014) 82:474–81. doi: 10.1212/WNL.0000000000000101
40. Titulaer MJ, Hoftberger R, Iizuka T, Leypoldt F, McCracken L, Cellucci T, et al. Overlapping demyelinating syndromes and anti-N-methyl-D-aspartate receptor encephalitis. *Ann Neurol.* (2014) 75:411–28. doi: 10.1002/ana.24117
41. Hacohen Y, Absoud M, Deiva K, Hemingway C, Nytrova P, Woodhall M, et al. Myelin oligodendrocyte glycoprotein antibodies are associated with a non-MS course in children. *Neurol Neuroimmunol Neuroinflamm.* (2015) 2:e81. doi: 10.1212/NXI.0000000000000081
42. Ketelslegers IA, Van Pelt DE, Bryde S, Neuteboom RF, Catsman-Berrevoets CE, Hamann D, et al. Anti-MOG antibodies plead against MS diagnosis in an Acquired Demyelinating Syndromes cohort. *Mult Scler.* (2015) 21:1513–20. doi: 10.1177/1352458514566666
43. Martinez-Hernandez E, Sepulveda M, Rostasy K, Hoftberger R, Graus F, Harvey RJ, et al. Antibodies to aquaporin 4, myelin-oligodendrocyte glycoprotein, and the glycine receptor alpha1 subunit in patients with isolated optic neuritis. *JAMA Neurol.* (2015) 72:187–93. doi: 10.1001/jamaneurol.2014.3602
44. Probstel AK, Rudolf G, Dornmair K, Collongues N, Chanson JB, Sanderson NS, et al. Anti-MOG antibodies are present in a subgroup of patients with a neuromyelitis optica phenotype. *J Neuroinflamm.* (2015) 12:46. doi: 10.1186/s12974-015-0256-1
45. Baumann M, Hennes EM, Schanda K, Karenfort M, Kornek B, Seidl R, et al. Children with multiphasic disseminated encephalomyelitis and antibodies to the myelin oligodendrocyte glycoprotein (MOG): Extending the spectrum of MOG antibody positive diseases. *Mult Scler.* (2016) 22:1821–9. doi: 10.1177/1352458516631038
46. Jarius S, Ruprecht K, Kleiter I, Borisow N, Asgari N, Pitarokoili K, et al. MOG-IgG in NMO and related disorders: a multicenter study of 50 patients. Part 1: Frequency, syndrome specificity, influence of disease activity, long-term course, association with AQP4-IgG, and origin. *J Neuroinflamm.* (2016) 13:279. doi: 10.1186/s12974-016-0717-1
47. Wang JJ, Jaunmuktane Z, Mummery C, Brandner S, Leary S, Trip SA. Inflammatory demyelination without astrocyte loss in MOG antibody-positive NMOSD. *Neurology* (2016) 87:229–31. doi: 10.1212/WNL.0000000000002844
48. Hennes EM, Baumann M, Schanda K, Anlar B, Bajer-Kornek B, Blaschek A, et al. Prognostic relevance of MOG antibodies in children with an acquired demyelinating syndrome. *Neurology* (2017) 89:900–8. doi: 10.1212/WNL.0000000000004312
49. Cobo-Calvo A, Ruiz A, Maillart E, Audoin B, Zephir H, Bourre B, et al. Clinical spectrum and prognostic value of CNS MOG autoimmunity in adults: the MOGADOR study. *Neurology* (2018) 90:e1858–e1869. doi: 10.1212/WNL.0000000000005560

50. Spadaro M, Gerdes LA, Krumbholz M, Ertl-Wagner B, Thaler FS, Schuh E, et al. Autoantibodies to MOG in a distinct subgroup of adult multiple sclerosis. *Neurol Neuroimmunol Neuroinflamm.* (2016) 3:e257. doi: 10.1212/NXI.0000000000000257
51. Mader S, Gredler V, Schanda K, Rostasy K, Dujmovic I, Pfaller K, et al. Complement activating antibodies to myelin oligodendrocyte glycoprotein in neuromyelitis optica and related disorders. *J Neuroinflamm.* (2011) 8:184. doi: 10.1186/1742-2094-8-184
52. Jurynczyk M, Messina S, Woodhall MR, Raza N, Everett R, Roca-Fernandez A, et al. Clinical presentation and prognosis in MOG-antibody disease: a UK study. *Brain* (2017) 140:3128–38. doi: 10.1093/brain/awx276
53. Chen L, Chen C, Zhong X, Sun X, Zhu H, Li X, et al. Different features between pediatric-onset and adult-onset patients who are seropositive for MOG-IgG: a multicenter study in South China. *J Neuroimmunol.* (2018) 321:83–91. doi: 10.1016/j.jneuroim.2018.05.014
54. Wingerchuk DM, Banwell B, Bennett JL, Cabre P, Carroll W, Chitnis T, et al. International consensus diagnostic criteria for neuromyelitis optica spectrum disorders. *Neurology* (2015) 85:177–89. doi: 10.1212/WNL.0000000000001729
55. Hamid SHM, Whittam D, Saviour M, Alorainy A, Mutch K, Linaker S, et al. Seizures and encephalitis in myelin oligodendrocyte Glycoprotein IgG disease vs Aquaporin 4 IgG disease. *JAMA Neurol.* (2018) 75:65–71. doi: 10.1001/jamaneurol.2017.3196
56. Fujimori J, Takai Y, Nakashima I, Sato DK, Takahashi T, Kaneko K, et al. Bilateral frontal cortex encephalitis and paraparesis in a patient with anti-MOG antibodies. *J Neurol Neurosurg Psychiatry* (2017) 88:534–6. doi: 10.1136/jnnp-2016-315094
57. Ogawa R, Nakashima I, Takahashi T, Kaneko K, Akaishi T, Takai Y, et al. MOG antibody-positive, benign, unilateral, cerebral cortical encephalitis with epilepsy. *Neurol Neuroimmunol Neuroinflamm.* (2017) 4:e322. doi: 10.1212/NXI.0000000000000322
58. Ikeda T, Yamada K, Ogawa R, Takai Y, Kaneko K, Misu T, et al. The pathological features of MOG antibody-positive cerebral cortical encephalitis as a new spectrum associated with MOG antibodies: a case report. *J Neurol Sci.* (2018) 392:113–5. doi: 10.1016/j.jns.2018.06.028
59. Narayan R, Simpson A, Fritsche K, Salama S, Pardo S, Mealy M, et al. MOG antibody disease: a review of MOG antibody seropositive neuromyelitis optica spectrum disorder. *Mult Scler Relat Disord.* (2018) 25:66–72. doi: 10.1016/j.msard.2018.07.025
60. van Pelt ED, Wong YY, Ketelslegers IA, Hamann D, Hintzen RQ. Neuromyelitis optica spectrum disorders: comparison of clinical and magnetic resonance imaging characteristics of AQP4-IgG versus MOG-IgG seropositive cases in the Netherlands. *Eur J Neurol.* (2016) 23:580–7. doi: 10.1111/ene.12898
61. Jarius S, Ruprecht K, Kleiter I, Borisow N, Asgari N, Pitarokoili K, et al. MOG-IgG in NMO and related disorders: a multicenter study of 50 patients. Part 2: Epidemiology, clinical presentation, radiological and laboratory features, treatment responses, and long-term outcome. *J Neuroinflamm.* (2016) 13:280. doi: 10.1186/s12974-016-0718-0
62. Hamid SHM, Whittam D, Mutch K, Linaker S, Solomon T, Das K, et al. What proportion of AQP4-IgG-negative NMO spectrum disorder patients are MOG-IgG positive? A cross sectional study of 132 patients. *J Neurol.* (2017) 264:2088–94. doi: 10.1007/s00415-017-8596-7
63. Sepulveda M, Armangue T, Martinez-Hernandez E, Arrambide G, Sola-Valls N, Sabater L, et al. Clinical spectrum associated with MOG autoimmunity in adults: significance of sharing rodent MOG epitopes. *J Neurol.* (2016) 263:1349–60. doi: 10.1007/s00415-016-8147-7
64. Cobo-Calvo A, Sepulveda M, Bernard-Valnet R, Ruiz A, Brassat D, Martinez-Yelamos S, et al. Antibodies to myelin oligodendrocyte glycoprotein in aquaporin 4 antibody seronegative longitudinally extensive transverse myelitis: clinical and prognostic implications. *Mult Scler.* (2016) 22:312–9. doi: 10.1177/1352458515591071
65. Chen JJ, Flanagan EP, Jitprapaikulsan J, Lopez-Chiriboga ASS, Fryer JP, Leavitt JA, et al. Myelin Oligodendrocyte Glycoprotein Antibody (MOG-IgG)-positive optic neuritis: clinical characteristics, radiologic clues and outcome. *Am J Ophthalmol.* (2018) 195:8–15. doi: 10.1016/j.ajo.2018.07.020
66. Stiebel-Kalish H, Lotan I, Brody J, Chodick G, Bialer O, Marignier R, et al. Retinal nerve fiber layer may be better preserved in MOG-IgG versus AQP4-IgG optic neuritis: a cohort study. *PLoS ONE* (2017) 12:e0170847. doi: 10.1371/journal.pone.0170847
67. Pache F, Zimmermann H, Mikolajczak J, Schumacher S, Lacheta A, Oertel FC, et al. MOG-IgG in NMO and related disorders: a multicenter study of 50 patients. Part 4: Afferent visual system damage after optic neuritis in MOG-IgG-seropositive versus AQP4-IgG-seropositive patients. *J Neuroinflamm.* (2016) 13:282. doi: 10.1186/s12974-016-0720-6
68. Lechner C, Baumann M, Hennes EM, Schanda K, Marquard K, Karenfort M, et al. Antibodies to MOG and AQP4 in children with neuromyelitis optica and limited forms of the disease. *J Neurol Neurosurg Psychiatry* (2016) 87:897–905. doi: 10.1136/jnnp-2015-311743
69. Lopez-Chiriboga AS, Majed M, Fryer J, Dubey D, McKeon A, Flanagan EP, et al. Association of MOG-IgG serostatus with relapse after acute disseminated encephalomyelitis and proposed diagnostic criteria for MOG-IgG-associated disorders. *JAMA Neurol.* (2018) 75:1355–63. doi: 10.1001/jamaneurol.2018.1814
70. Duignan S, Wright S, Rossor T, Cazabon J, Gilmour K, Ciccarelli O, et al. Myelin oligodendrocyte glycoprotein and aquaporin-4 antibodies are highly specific in children with acquired demyelinating syndromes. *Dev Med Child Neurol.* (2018) 60:958–62. doi: 10.1111/dmcn.13703
71. Hyun JW, Woodhall MR, Kim SH, Jeong IH, Kong B, Kim G, et al. Longitudinal analysis of myelin oligodendrocyte glycoprotein antibodies in CNS inflammatory diseases. *J Neurol Neurosurg Psychiatry* (2017) 88:811–7. doi: 10.1136/jnnp-2017-315998
72. Dale RC, Brilot F, Banwell B. Pediatric central nervous system inflammatory demyelination: acute disseminated encephalomyelitis, clinically isolated syndromes, neuromyelitis optica, and multiple sclerosis. *Curr Opin Neurol.* (2009) 22:233–40. doi: 10.1097/WCO.0b013e32832b4c47
73. Dale RC, Tantsis EM, Merheb V, Kumaran RY, Sinmaz N, Pathmanandavel K, et al. Antibodies to MOG have a demyelination phenotype and affect oligodendrocyte cytoskeleton. *Neurol Neuroimmunol Neuroinflamm.* (2014) 1:e12. doi: 10.1212/NXI.0000000000000012
74. Jarius S, Franciotta D, Paul F, Ruprecht K, Bergamaschi R, Rommer PS, et al. Cerebrospinal fluid antibodies to aquaporin-4 in neuromyelitis optica and related disorders: frequency, origin, and diagnostic relevance. *J Neuroinflamm.* (2010) 7:52. doi: 10.1186/1742-2094-7-52
75. Kaneko K, Sato DK, Nakashima I, Ogawa R, Akaishi T, Takai Y, et al. CSF cytokine profile in MOG-IgG+ neurological disease is similar to AQP4-IgG+ NMOSD but distinct from MS: a cross-sectional study and potential therapeutic implications. *J Neurol Neurosurg Psychiatry* (2018) 89:927–36. doi: 10.1136/jnnp-2018-317969
76. Kothur K, Wienholt L, Tantsis EM, Earl J, Bandodkar S, Prelog K, et al. B Cell, Th17, and neutrophil related cerebrospinal fluid cytokine/chemokines are elevated in MOG antibody associated demyelination. *PLoS ONE* (2016) 11:e0149411. doi: 10.1371/journal.pone.0149411
77. Mariotto S, Ferrari S, Monaco S, Benedetti MD, Schanda K, Alberti D, et al. Clinical spectrum and IgG subclass analysis of anti-myelin oligodendrocyte glycoprotein antibody-associated syndromes: a multicenter study. *J Neurol.* (2017) 264:2420–30. doi: 10.1007/s00415-017-8635-4
78. Hacohen Y, Wong YY, Lechner C, Jurynczyk M, Wright S, Konuskan B, et al. Disease course and treatment responses in children with relapsing myelin oligodendrocyte glycoprotein antibody-associated disease. *JAMA Neurol.* (2018) 75:478–87. doi: 10.1001/jamaneurol.2017.4601
79. Biotti D, Bonneville F, Tournaire E, Ayrignac X, Dalliere CC, Mahieu L, et al. Optic neuritis in patients with anti-MOG antibodies spectrum disorder: MRI and clinical features from a large multicentric cohort in France. *J Neurol.* (2017) 264:2173–5. doi: 10.1007/s00415-017-8615-8
80. Baumann M, Grams A, Djurdjevic T, Wendel EM, Lechner C, Behring B, et al. MRI of the first event in pediatric acquired demyelinating syndromes with antibodies to myelin oligodendrocyte glycoprotein. *J Neurol.* (2018) 265:845–55. doi: 10.1007/s00415-018-8781-3
81. Jurynczyk M, Tackley G, Kong Y, Geraldes R, Matthews L, Woodhall M, et al. Brain lesion distribution criteria distinguish MS from AQP4-antibody NMOSD and MOG-antibody disease. *J Neurol Neurosurg Psychiatry* (2017) 88:132–6. doi: 10.1136/jnnp-2016-314005
82. Jurynczyk M, Geraldes R, Probert F, Woodhall MR, Waters P, Tackley G, et al. Distinct brain imaging characteristics of autoantibody-mediated

CNS conditions and multiple sclerosis. *Brain* (2017) 140:617–27. doi: 10.1093/brain/aww350
83. Hacohen Y, Mankad K, Chong WK, Barkhof F, Vincent A, Lim M, et al. Diagnostic algorithm for relapsing acquired demyelinating syndromes in children. *Neurology* (2017) 89:269–78. doi: 10.1212/WNL.0000000000004117
84. Tan CT, Mao Z, Qiu W, Hu X, Wingerchuk DM, Weinshenker BG. International consensus diagnostic criteria for neuromyelitis optica spectrum disorders. *Neurology* (2016) 86:491–2. doi: 10.1212/WNL.0000000000002366
85. Polman CH, Reingold SC, Banwell B, Clanet M, Cohen JA, Filippi M, et al. Diagnostic criteria for multiple sclerosis: 2010 revisions to the McDonald criteria. *Ann Neurol.* (2011) 69:292–302. doi: 10.1002/ana.22366
86. Krupp LB, Tardieu M, Amato MP, Banwell B, Chitnis T, Dale RC, et al. International Pediatric Multiple Sclerosis Study Group criteria for pediatric multiple sclerosis and immune-mediated central nervous system demyelinating disorders: revisions to the 2007 definitions. *Mult Scler.* (2013) 19:1261–7. doi: 10.1177/1352458513484547
87. Reindl M, Jarius S, Rostasy K, Berger T. Myelin oligodendrocyte glycoprotein antibodies: how clinically useful are they? *Curr Opin Neurol.* (2017) 30:295–301. doi: 10.1097/WCO.0000000000000446
88. Di Pauli F, Reindl M, Berger T. New clinical implications of anti-myelin oligodendrocyte glycoprotein antibodies in children with CNS demyelinating diseases. *Mult Scler Relat Disord.* (2018) 22:35–7. doi: 10.1016/j.msard.2018.02.023
89. Waters P, Woodhall M, O'Connor KC, Reindl M, Lang B, Sato DK, et al. MOG cell-based assay detects non-MS patients with inflammatory neurologic disease. *Neurol Neuroimmunol Neuroinflamm.* (2015) 2:e89. doi: 10.1212/NXI.0000000000000089
90. Konig FB, Wildemann B, Nessler S, Zhou D, Hemmer B, Metz I, et al. Persistence of immunopathological and radiological traits in multiple sclerosis. *Arch Neurol.* (2008) 65:1527–32. doi: 10.1001/archneur.65.11.1527
91. Di Pauli F, Hoftberger R, Reindl M, Beer R, Rhomberg P, Schanda K, et al. Fulminant demyelinating encephalomyelitis: insights from antibody studies and neuropathology. *Neurol Neuroimmunol Neuroinflamm.* (2015) 2:e175. doi: 10.1212/NXI.0000000000000175
92. Spadaro M, Gerdes LA, Mayer MC, Ertl-Wagner B, Laurent S, Krumbholz M, et al. Histopathology and clinical course of MOG-antibody-associated encephalomyelitis. *Ann Clin Transl Neurol.* (2015) 2:295–301. doi: 10.1002/acn3.164
93. Jarius S, Metz I, Konig FB, Ruprecht K, Reindl M, Paul F, et al. Screening for MOG-IgG and 27 other anti-glial and anti-neuronal autoantibodies in 'pattern II multiple sclerosis' and brain biopsy findings in a MOG-IgG-positive case. *Mult Scler.* (2016) 22:1541–9. doi: 10.1177/1352458515622986
94. Kortvelyessy P, Breu M, Pawlitzki M, Metz I, Heinze HJ, Matzke M, et al. ADEM-like presentation, anti-MOG antibodies, and MS pathology: TWO case reports. *Neurol Neuroimmunol Neuroinflamm.* (2017) 4:e335. doi: 10.1212/NXI.0000000000000335
95. Lucchinetti CF, Guo Y, Popescu BF, Fujihara K, Itoyama Y, Misu T. The pathology of an autoimmune astrocytopathy: lessons learned from neuromyelitis optica. *Brain Pathol.* (2014) 24:83–97. doi: 10.1111/bpa.12099
96. Mandler RN, Davis LE, Jeffery DR, Kornfeld M. Devic's neuromyelitis optica: a clinicopathological study of 8 patients. *Ann Neurol.* (1993) 34:162–8. doi: 10.1002/ana.410340211
97. Young NP, Weinshenker BG, Parisi JE, Scheithauer B, Giannini C, Roemer SF, et al. Perivenous demyelination: association with clinically defined acute disseminated encephalomyelitis and comparison with pathologically confirmed multiple sclerosis. *Brain* (2010) 133(Pt 2):333–48. doi: 10.1093/brain/awp321
98. Saadoun S, Waters P, Owens GP, Bennett JL, Vincent A, Papadopoulos MC. Neuromyelitis optica MOG-IgG causes reversible lesions in mouse brain. *Acta Neuropathol Commun.* (2014) 2:35. doi: 10.1186/2051-5960-2-35
99. Mayer MC, Breithaupt C, Reindl M, Schanda K, Rostasy K, Berger T, et al. Distinction and temporal stability of conformational epitopes on myelin oligodendrocyte glycoprotein recognized by patients with different inflammatory central nervous system diseases. *J Immunol.* (2013) 191:3594–604. doi: 10.4049/jimmunol.1301296
100. Flach AC, Litke T, Strauss J, Haberl M, Gomez CC, Reindl M, et al. Autoantibody-boosted T-cell reactivation in the target organ triggers manifestation of autoimmune CNS disease. *Proc Natl Acad Sci USA.* (2016) 113:3323–8. doi: 10.1073/pnas.1519608113
101. Kinzel S, Lehmann-Horn K, Torke S, Hausler D, Winkler A, Stadelmann C, et al. Myelin-reactive antibodies initiate T cell-mediated CNS autoimmune disease by opsonization of endogenous antigen. *Acta Neuropathol.* (2016) 132:43–58. doi: 10.1007/s00401-016-1559-8
102. Spadaro M, Winklmeier S, Beltran E, Macrini C, Hoftberger R, Schuh E, et al. Pathogenicity of human antibodies against myelin oligodendrocyte glycoprotein. *Ann Neurol.* (2018) 84:315–28. doi: 10.1002/ana.25291
103. Ramanathan S, Mohammad S, Tantsis E, Nguyen TK, Merheb V, Fung VSC, et al. Clinical course, therapeutic responses and outcomes in relapsing MOG antibody-associated demyelination. *J Neurol Neurosurg Psychiatry* (2017) 89:127–37. doi: 10.1136/jnnp-2017-316880
104. Hoftberger R, Sepulveda M, Armangue T, Blanco Y, Rostasy K, Calvo AC, et al. Antibodies to MOG and AQP4 in adults with neuromyelitis optica and suspected limited forms of the disease. *Mult Scler.* (2015) 21:866–74. doi: 10.1177/1352458514555785
105. Kowarik MC, Hoshi M, Hemmer B, Berthele A. Failure of alemtuzumab as a rescue in a NMOSD patient treated with rituximab. *Neurol Neuroimmunol Neuroinflamm.* (2016) 3:e208. doi: 10.1212/NXI.0000000000000208
106. Wildemann B, Jarius S, Schwarz A, Diem R, Viehover A, Hahnel S, et al. Failure of alemtuzumab therapy to control MOG encephalomyelitis. *Neurology* (2017) 89:207–9. doi: 10.1212/WNL.0000000000004087

7

Bioinformatics Analyses Determined the Distinct CNS and Peripheral Surrogate Biomarker Candidates Between Two Mouse Models for Progressive Multiple Sclerosis

Seiichi Omura [1,2]***, Fumitaka Sato*** [1,2]***, Nicholas E. Martinez*** [2]***, Ah-Mee Park*** [1]***, Mitsugu Fujita*** [1]***, Nikki J. Kennett*** [3]***, Urška Cvek*** [4]***, Alireza Minagar*** [5]***, J. Steven Alexander*** [5,6] ***and Ikuo Tsunoda*** [1,2,5*]

[1] Department of Microbiology, Kindai University Faculty of Medicine, Osakasayama, Japan, [2] Department of Microbiology and Immunology, Louisiana State University Health Sciences Center-Shreveport, Shreveport, LA, United States, [3] Department of Pathology, University of Utah, Salt Lake City, UT, United States, [4] Department of Computer Science, Louisiana State University Shreveport, Shreveport, LA, United States, [5] Department of Neurology, Louisiana State University Health Sciences Center-Shreveport, Shreveport, LA, United States, [6] Department of Molecular and Cellular Physiology, Louisiana State University Health Sciences Center-Shreveport, Shreveport, LA, United States

****Correspondence:***
Ikuo Tsunoda
itsunoda@med.kindai.ac.jp

Previously, we have established two distinct progressive multiple sclerosis (MS) models by induction of experimental autoimmune encephalomyelitis (EAE) with myelin oligodendrocyte glycoprotein (MOG) in two mouse strains. A.SW mice develop ataxia with antibody deposition, but no T cell infiltration, in the central nervous system (CNS), while SJL/J mice develop paralysis with CNS T cell infiltration. In this study, we determined biomarkers contributing to the homogeneity and heterogeneity of two models. Using the CNS and spleen microarray transcriptome and cytokine data, we conducted computational analyses. We identified up-regulation of immune-related genes, including immunoglobulins, in the CNS of both models. Pro-inflammatory cytokines, interferon (IFN)-γ and interleukin (IL)-17, were associated with the disease progression in SJL/J mice, while the expression of both cytokines was detected only at the EAE onset in A.SW mice. Principal component analysis (PCA) of CNS transcriptome data demonstrated that down-regulation of prolactin may reflect disease progression. Pattern matching analysis of spleen transcriptome with CNS PCA identified 333 splenic surrogate markers, including *Stfa2l1*, which reflected the changes in the CNS. Among them, we found that two genes (*PER1/MIR6883* and *FKBP5*) and one gene (*SLC16A1/MCT1*) were also significantly up-regulated and down-regulated, respectively, in human MS peripheral blood, using data mining.

Keywords: multi-variate analysis, primary progressive EAE, principal component analysis (PCA), pattern matching, data mining

INTRODUCTION

Multiple sclerosis (MS) is an inflammatory demyelinating disease of the central nervous system (CNS) (1). World-wide, MS affects about 2.5 million people (2). Although the precise etiology of MS remains unclear, MS has been proposed to be a disease caused by interactions between autoimmunity, microbial infections, and/or genetic factors (3). The clinical courses of MS are classified into four types: (1) clinically isolated syndrome (CIS), (2) relapsing-remitting (RR), (3) primary progressive (PP), (4) secondary progressive (SP) (4). CIS is a first clinical episode with CNS inflammation and demyelination (5). RR-MS is defined by "relapses" (disease attacks) with periods of "remission" (recovery) and is the most frequent occurring. SP-MS is defined by an initial RR disease course followed by continuous disease progression. Approximately 95% of RR-MS patients develop SP-MS (6). PP-MS progresses continuously from the onset without recovery. There is no biomarker that can be used to classify or predict clinical courses of the four subtypes of MS (7).

Neuroimaging studies suggest that MS lesions shifted from inflammatory demyelination to neurodegeneration during the disease progression (8, 9). In contrast, neuropathology studies suggest that the pathogenesis of MS remained the same throughout the course (10, 11). There was neither a definite mechanistic explanation of how the pathogenesis shifts from inflammatory demyelination to neurodegeneration in all MS cases, nor an explanation of whether the two conflicting views based on neuroimaging or neuropathology observations can be reconciled. The different views on disease pathogenesis in MS could be attributed to the fact that each view is based on one aspect of the disease: neuroimaging or histological changes. Alternatively, MS pathogenesis might differ among individual patients (12). The neuropathological view might be based on MS patients whose effector mechanism remains the same during the disease course, while the neuroimaging view could be based on the patient subgroup whose effector mechanism changes during the disease course. We hypothesized that inconsistencies of effectiveness of treatment, neuroimaging and neuropathology among progressive MS patients could be heterogeneities of the pathogenesis of MS.

Clinical courses of animal models for MS are also variable. Experimental autoimmune encephalomyelitis (EAE) can be induced by sensitization with CNS antigens, including myelin basic protein (MBP), myelin proteolipid protein (PLP), and myelin oligodendrocyte glycoprotein (MOG) (3, 13). The clinical course of EAE can be RR, PP, and SP, which are similar to the various forms of MS: RR-MS, PP-MS, and SP-MS, respectively. Several EAE models with different clinical courses have been established: RR-course in SJL/J mice with $PLP_{139-151}$, $PLP_{178-191}$, or MOG_{92-106}, PP-, and SP-course in A.SW mice with MOG_{92-106} and SJL/J mice with MOG_{92-106} and additional treatment (ultraviolet irradiation, injection of *Bordetella Pertussis*, apoptotic cell, or curdlan) (14–17). Monophasic EAE can also be induced in PL/J mice with MBP_{1-11} and C57BL/6 mice with MOG_{35-55} (18, 19). In this study, we used two PP-EAE models, A.SW mice sensitized with MOG_{92-106} and SJL/J mice sensitized with MOG_{92-106} and curdlan. Previously, we reported that A.SW mice sensitized with MOG_{92-106} developed PP-EAE with large areas of demyelination, immunoglobulin deposition, neutrophil infiltration, and spleen atrophy (14, 16).

Systemic and multivariate analyses of data from animal models for MS are powerful methods to characterize each model. In MS, microarray analyses have been performed mainly using peripheral blood lymphocytes. Several reports showed that various genes related to the immune response, apoptosis, and cell cycle progression were up- or down-regulated in disease (20, 21), while microarray analyses using human CNS tissues have been limited by its nature (22). In most microarray analyses in EAE, genes related to the immune response, such as cytokines, chemokines, and complement components, are known to be up-regulated in the CNS (23–26).

We aimed to determine CNS biomarkers and peripheral surrogate markers that could characterize the two PP-EAE models induced in A.SW and SJL/J mice. We have conducted microarray and bioinformatics analyses, using the brains and spleens which reflect the changes in the CNS and peripheral lymphoid organs, respectively. There were differences in numbers of genes that were up- and down-regulated in the brains and spleens between A.SW and SJL/J mice with PP-EAE, while immune response-related genes were highly up-regulated in the brains and erythrocyte-related genes highly down-regulated in the spleens from both mouse strains. Pathway analysis showed that Fc receptor and complement-related genes were up-regulated in both mouse strains' brains, but pro-inflammatory cytokine-related genes were up-regulated only in SJL/J mouse brains. Genes irrelevant to immune responses were down-regulated in the spleens of PP-EAE mice, and the expression of T helper (Th)1/Th2-related genes differed between A.SW and SJL/J mouse brains. Principal component analysis (PCA) of transcriptome data of brains and spleens separated between control and EAE groups. Pattern matching analysis between brain PCA data and spleen transcriptome data identified the spleen surrogate marker candidates that reflect the gene expression patterns in the brain. Translational application of our bioinformatics approach would be useful to identify the brain biomarkers and peripheral surrogate markers for MS.

MATERIALS AND METHODS

Animal Experiments

To induce PP-EAE, 5-week-old female nine SJL/J mice and 13 A.SW mice (The Jackson Laboratory, Bar Harbor, ME) were sensitized in the base of the tail with 100 nmol of MOG_{92-106} peptide (DEGGYTCFFRDHSYQ, Core Facility, University of Utah Huntsman Cancer Institute, Salt Lake City, UT) in complete Freund's adjuvant (CFA) (14–16). On day −1 prior to MOG injection, 5 mg curdlan (a Th17 inducer produced by *Alcaligenes faecalis var. myxogenes*, Wako Pure Chemical Industries, Osaka, Japan) in PBS was injected for SJL/J mice intraperitoneally (27). To induce RR-EAE, six SJL/J mice were sensitized $PLP_{139-151}$ (HSLGKWLGHPDKF) in CFA (28). Mice were given standard laboratory rodent chow and water *ad libitum*. All experimental procedures were reviewed and approved by the Institutional

Animal Care and Use Committee of Louisiana State University Health Sciences Center (LSUHSC)-Shreveport, and performed according to the criteria outlined by the National Institutes of Health (NIH) (29).

Clinical signs of EAE and body weights were monitored daily (14, 30). Mice were euthanized at disease peak and remission of RR-EAE and at latent period, onset and peak of PP-EAE (**Figure 1**). At each time point, brains and spleens were harvested from three to six mice per group and frozen immediately in liquid nitrogen.

RNA Preparation

Brains and spleens from three to six mice per group were homogenized individually in TRI-Reagent® (Molecular Research Center, Cincinnati, OH), using the Kinematica Polytron™ homogenizer (Kinematica, Bohemia, NY). Total RNA was extracted with an RNeasy Mini Kit (Qiagen, Germantown, MD) according to the manufacturer's instructions from brain and spleen homogenate. DNase treatment was performed during RNA isolation with an RNase-Free DNase Set (Qiagen). All samples were purified to an absorbance ratio (A260/A280) between 1.9 and 2.1 (31).

Real-Time PCR

We reverse-transcribed 1 μg of total RNA into cDNA, using ImProm-II™ Reverse Transcription System (Promega Corporation, Madison, WI) ($n = 3$–7). We mixed 50 ng of cDNA with RT^2 Fast SYBER® Green qPCR Master Mixes (Qiagen) and primer set. The mixture was amplified and monitored using iCycler iQ System (Bio-Rad Laboratories, Hercules, CA). The following primer sets were purchased from Real Time Primers (Elkins Park, PA): interferon (IFN)-γ, interleukin (IL)-17A, chemokine (C-X-C motif) ligand 13 (CXCL13), lipocalin 2 (LCN2), CD3 antigen γ subunit (CD3G), Kell blood group (KEL), and stefin A2 like 1 (STFA2L1). The results were normalized using housekeeping genes, glyceraldehyde-3-phosphate dehydrogenase (*Gapd*) or phosphoglycerate kinase 1(*Pgk1*) (32, 33).

Microarray Analysis

We used total RNA samples of brains and spleens from three mice with PP-EAE at the disease peak and three age-matched control mice for each mouse strain. We conducted microarray analyses, using Affymetrix GeneChip® Mouse Gene 1.0 ST Array (Affymetrix, Santa Clara, CA), according to the manufacturer's instruction. The data were visualized and quantified by Affymetrix GeneChip Command Console (AGCC), and normalized by Robust Multi-array Average (RMA) using Expression Console. Data were analyzed using the Ingenuity Pathway Analysis® (Qiagen), NetAffx database (Affymetrix; http://www.affymetrix.com/index.affx), and Mouse Genome Informatics (The Jackson Laboratory, Bar Harbor, ME; http://www.informatics.jax.org/). The datasets generated and/or analyzed during the current study are available in the Gene Expression Omnibus (GEO; http://www.ncbi.nlm.nih.gov/geo/) repository in National Center for Biotechnology Information (NCBI) (Accession number: GSE99300).

Bioinformatics and Statistics Analyses

Volcano Plot

We drew a volcano plot, using the OriginPro 8.1 (OriginLab Corporation, Northampton, MA), to visualize significance and fold changes of transcriptome data (34–36). In the volcano plot, log ratios (logarithms of fold changes to base 2) of gene expression in the brains and spleens from EAE mice compared with age-matched control mice were used as an x-axis and the logarithms of P values to base 10 were used as a y-axis.

Heat Map

We drew heat maps to determine the expression patterns of top 20 up- or down-regulated genes of brain and spleen samples from EAE mice, and compared the expression levels between EAE vs. control groups, using R version 3.2.2 and the programs "gplots" and "genefilter" (37). A list of abbreviations of genes is shown in **Supplemental Table 1**.

K-means Clustering

To find the differences of gene expression patterns between organs or mouse strains, we conducted k-means clustering using an R package "cclust" (37). We used Davies-Bouldin index (38) to determine the optimum number of clusters and obtained the lowest score (0.78), when microarray data were separated into 35 clusters (**Supplemental Figure 2**). Graphs were drawn using 240 genes (top 80, middle 80, and bottom 80 genes) in each cluster. A radar chart was drawn using the expression patterns of cluster center genes.

Ingenuity Pathway Analysis (IPA)

To classify the genes functionally, we used IPA (Qiagen) where we entered the genes whose genes were over- or under-transcribed more than 2-fold compared with control samples (P values <0.05). IPA shows possible networks involved in microarray profiles by the IPA Network Generation Algorithm (39). The algorithm clustered and classified the entered genes, which generated the networks, each of which was composed of three canonical pathways. The networks were ranked by the network score. The network score was calculated based on the right-tailed Fisher's Exact Test that uses several parameters, including the numbers of network eligible molecules in the network, the given dataset, and the IPA database. We focused the networks whose network score was higher than 35, since the only networks with high network scores have interpretable connections.

Principal Component Analysis (PCA)

Using PCA, we reduced the dimensionality of a microarray data set consisting of 28,853 mRNA expression signals into two components, principal component (PC) 1 and PC2 (37, 40, 41). PCA was conducted as an "unsupervised" analysis to clarify the variance among microarray data from brain and spleen samples using an R program "prcomp," as we described previously (37, 42). The proportion of variance was also calculated to determine the percentage of variance explained by each PC, while factor loading for PC1 or PC2 was used to rank a set of genes contributing to PC1 or PC2 values.

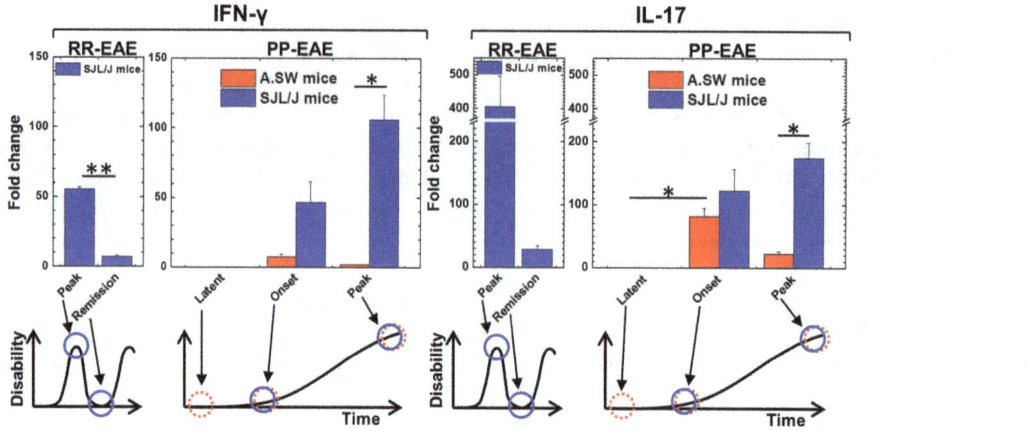

FIGURE 1 | Kinetics of interferon (IFN)-γ and interleukin (IL)-17 expression of relapsing-remitting (RR)-experimental autoimmune encephalomyelitis (EAE) and primary progressive (PP)-EAE in SJL/J mice (blue column) and A.SW mice (red column). Expression of IFN-γ and IL-17 in brains were determined by real-time PCR. Expression levels were shown as fold changes compared with three control mice of each strain. In SJL/J mice with RR-EAE, both IFN-γ and IL-17 levels were high at the disease peak and low during remission ($n = 3$, at each time point). On the other hand, in PP-EAE, expression levels of both IFN-γ and IL-17 were associated with disease activity in SJL/J mice with EAE ($n = 3$, at each time point), while they increased at the onset (no increase at latent period) but decreased at the disease peak in A.SW mice with EAE ($n = 3$–6, at each time point). Data are presented as means ± standard error of the mean (SEM). $^*P < 0.05$, $^{**}P < 0.001$, ANOVA.

Pattern Matching Analysis

To find the splenic genes whose expression patterns correlated with PC1 values in PCA of the brains, we conducted a pattern matching analysis based on correlation (43), using the R. We focused the genes whose expression levels, compared with control samples, were up- or down-regulated more than 2-fold, and whose correlation coefficients (r) were more than 0.8 or < -0.8.

Data Mining on Human MS Transcriptome Database

We obtained the gene expression profile datasets relevant to MS patients from GEO profile database (https://www.ncbi.nlm.nih.gov/geoprofiles/), using search keywords with the gene symbols identified in the current study as follows:

"multiple sclerosis"[All Fields] AND "Homo sapiens"[Organism] AND "peripheral blood"[All Fields] AND "disease state"[Flag Information] AND (gene symbols connected by OR). The data were processed according to the instructions of GEO profile database (44), and the differentially expressed genes ($P < 0.05$) between MS patients and controls were extracted.

Statistics

The data were shown as mean ± standard error of the mean (SEM). Statistical comparisons were conducted using the Student t test or analysis of variance (ANOVA), using the OriginPro 8.1. $P < 0.05$ was considered as significant difference.

RESULTS

Levels of IFN-γ and IL-17 Were Associated With Disease Activity of PP-EAE in SJL/J Mice, but Not in A.SW Mice

The precise effector mechanism of PP-MS is currently unknown. Since the pro-inflammatory cytokines, IFN-γ, and IL-17 have been shown to be key effector molecules in many, but not all EAE models (15, 16, 45–48), we first examined the kinetics of IFN-γ and IL-17 in animal models for PP-MS, using two mouse strains. We induced PP-EAE with MOG_{92-106} in A.SW mice as we described previously (14–16). We also induced PP-EAE in SJL/J mice with MOG_{92-106} sensitization, 1 day after injection of curdlan. In SJL/J mice, disease continuously progressed until mice became moribund without remission within 20 days after initial clinical signs (**Supplemental Figure 1**). A.SW mice developed ataxic EAE and weight loss 1 month post induction (p.i.) of EAE (14, 16), while SJL/J mice developed classical EAE with tail and limb paralysis and weight loss in both PP- and RR-EAE.

Using real-time PCR, we conducted a time course analysis of IFN-γ and IL-17 mRNA levels in the brains of A.SW and SJL/J mice with PP-EAE (**Figure 1**). For comparison, we also used brain samples from SJL/J mice with RR-EAE. In both RR-EAE and PP-EAE in SJL/J mice, clinical signs were associated with increased levels of both IFN-γ and IL-17 in the brain. However, in PP-EAE in A.SW mice, the levels of IFN-γ and IL-17 increased at the disease onset, but declined during the disease progression. These results suggested that the effector mechanisms in disease progression of SJL/J mice and A.SW mice differed at the disease peak. Thus, we decided to analyze potentially distinct pathomechanisms of disease progression between A.SW and SJL/J mice with PP-EAE.

Volcano Plots of Brain and Spleen Transcriptome Data Showed Overall Greater Changes in SJL/J Mice, While A.SW Mice Had More Down-Regulated Spleen Genes

To compare the potentially distinct effector mechanisms during the disease progression between A.SW and SJL/J mice, we conducted conventional "supervised" two-way comparison analyses of the brain and spleen transcriptome data at the disease peak from the two mouse strains with PP-EAE. First, using volcano plots, we visualized the numbers of genes whose expression levels were significantly ($P < 0.05$) up- or down-regulated more than 2-fold compared with control samples (**Figures 2A,B**). In the brain, higher numbers of genes were up- or down-regulated in SJL/J mice than in A.SW mice, suggesting that molecular changes in SJL/J mice could be more complex than in A.SW mice (**Figure 2A**). On the other hand, in the spleen, the numbers of down-regulated genes were higher in A.SW mice, while those of up-regulated genes were higher in SJL/J mice (**Figure 2B**). An increased number of down-regulated genes in A.SW mouse spleen seemed to be associated with spleen weight changes at disease peak in PP-EAE, where the spleen of A.SW mice, but not SJL/J mice, showed significant atrophy (16).

Heat Maps Revealed the Up-Regulation of Immune Response-Related Genes in the Brains and Down-Regulation of Erythrocyte-Related Genes in the Spleens From Both Mouse Strains

Next, to visualize the differences in most highly up- or down-regulated genes in the brains and spleens, we drew heat maps, using microarray data at the disease peak (**Figures 2C–F**). Overall, heat maps of each organ (brain or spleen) were similar among samples from A.SW and SJL/J mice. Most of the highly up- or down-regulated genes in each organ in A.SW mice were also up- or down-regulated in SJL/J mice. On the other hand, heat maps between brains and spleens were different regardless of the mouse strains. Only serine (or cysteine) peptidase inhibitor, clade A, member 3N (*Serpina3n*) was highly up-regulated in both brains and spleens in both mouse strains. In the heat maps based on brain gene expression levels from A.SW (**Figure 2C**) and SJL/J mice (**Figure 2D**), commonly up-regulated genes included: lipocalin 2 (*Lcn2*); chemokines, such as chemokine (C-X-C motif) ligand 13 (*Cxcl13*); and chemokine (C-C motif) ligand 3 (*Ccl3*); complement-related genes, *C3* and complement component 3a receptor (*C3ar1*); immunoglobulin (*Igkv1-110*); MHC class II-related genes, *H2-Aa* and *Cd74* (CLIP). Serine (or cysteine) peptidase inhibitor, clade B, member 1a (*Serpinb1a*), and UDP galactosyltransferase 8A (*Ugt8a*) were down-regulated in common.

In the spleen heat maps based on gene expression levels from A.SW (**Figure 2E**) and SJL/J mice (**Figure 2F**), several genes, including pyruvate dehydrogenase kinase, isoenzyme 4 (*Pdk4*), testis specific gene A13 (*Tsga13*), and *Serpina3n*, were up-regulated in common, while erythrocyte-related genes, such as glycophorin A (*Gypa*), Kell blood group (*Kel*), Rh blood group, D antigen (*Rhd*), and claudin 13 (*Cldn13*) (49), were down-regulated significantly. On the other hand, lactotransferrin (*Ltf*) and lymphocyte antigen 6 complex, locus G (*Ly6g/Gr1*, a granulocyte marker) (50) showed different expression patterns between the spleens of two mouse strains with PP-EAE, down-regulation in A.SW mice and up-regulation in SJL/J mice. In addition, tryptase α/β 1 (*Tpsab1*) and γ-aminobutyric acid (GABA) A receptor, subunit θ (*Gabrq*) were up-regulated only in the spleen of A.SW mice, while immune response-related genes, such as chitinase-like 3 (*Chil3*), interferon induced transmembrane protein 6 (*Ifitm6*), and haptoglobin (*Hp*), were up-regulated only in the spleen of SJL/J mice.

K-means Clustering Revealed the Different Expression Patterns of Genes Between the Brains and Spleens of A.SW and SJL/J Mice With PP-EAE

To further identify the genes that had distinct expression patterns among the transcriptome data from brains and spleens of A.SW and SJL/J mice with PP-EAE at the disease peak, we divided all genes into 35 clusters, using *k*-means clustering, based on Davies-Bouldin Index (**Supplemental Figures 2, 3**). The centroid genes of the 14 of 35 clusters showed substantial changes (>2- or <1/2-fold compared with controls), at least, in one organ or in one mouse strain (**Supplemental Figures 3, 4**, lists of genes in each cluster were shown in **Supplemental Tables 2–15**). A radar chart for centroid genes of each cluster showed that, in most clusters, gene expression levels in one organ between the two mouse strains were similar, while those between brains vs. spleens were different (a radar chart using the 14 clusters in **Figure 3A**; radar chart using all the 35 clusters in **Supplemental Figure 4**). The radar chart showed that, in most clusters, the gene expression patterns in one organ between the two mouse strains were similar, while those between brain and spleen were different.

The genes in the spleen were up-regulated in cluster 3 and down-regulated in cluster 22 in both mouse strains, while there were no substantial changes (log ratios ≈0, compared with controls) in cluster 3 or 22 in the two mouse brain samples (**Figure 3B**). Cluster 3 included stefins (*Stfa1* and *Stfa2l1*) (**Supplemental Table 4**), while cluster 22 included erythrocyte-related genes, such as *Kel*, *Rhd*, and *Gypa* (**Supplemental Table 10**). On the other hand, the genes in clusters 8 and 25 were up-regulated only in the brains, but not in the spleens, in both mouse strains. Immune response-related genes were included in clusters 8 and 25: *Cxcl9*, *Cxcl10*, and *Cd3g* in cluster 8; *Lcn2*, *Cd74*, and *H2-Aa* in cluster 25 (**Supplemental Tables 6, 12**). Some genes in cluster 8 were up-regulated only in the brains of SJL/J mice (e.g., *Cd3g*: 1.3-fold in A.SW mice, 4.9-fold in SJL/J mice), while several genes in cluster 25 were only down-regulated in A.SW mouse spleens (e.g., *Lcn2*: 0.3-fold). Up-regulation of *Cd3g* in SJL/J mouse brain, but not A.SW mouse brain, was consistent with our previous histological finding that CNS $CD3^+$ T cell infiltration was seen only in SJL/J mice (14, 16). Thus, *k*-means clustering clearly showed that groups of immune response-related genes were induced in each organ commonly in two mouse strains, but differentially between brains vs. spleens at the peak of disease progression. However, *k*-means clustering alone was insufficient to identify individual genes that were expressed differentially between the two strains, requiring further analyses.

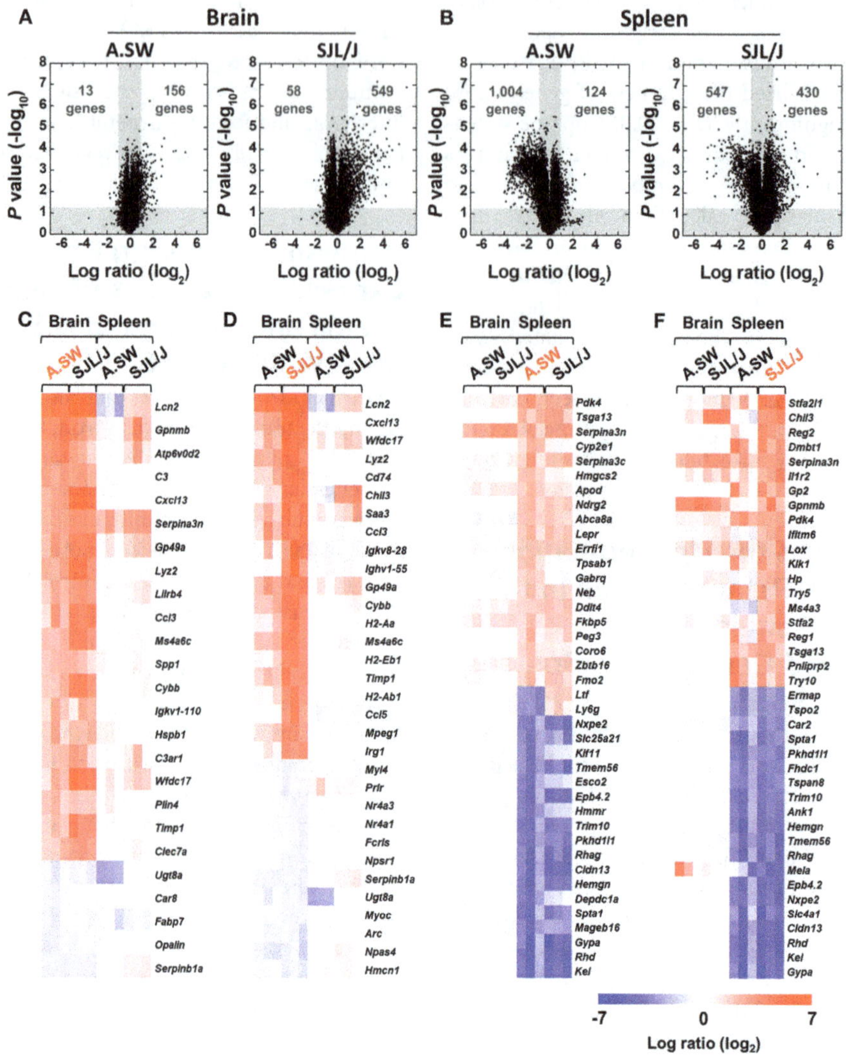

FIGURE 2 | (A,B) Volcano plots of up- or down-regulated genes in the brains **(A)** and spleens **(B)** of PP-EAE mice. Gene expression profiles in the brains and spleens of three mice with PP-EAE at the disease peak and three age-matched control mice for each mouse strain were determined by microarray. Fold changes were calculated by division of signal values of EAE samples by those of controls. *P* values were calculated using the Student *t* test. Dots in the white areas were genes whose expressions were up- or down-regulated more than 2-fold ($\log_2$ ratio = 1, compared with controls), significantly ($P < 0.05$). In the brain, SJL/J mice had substantially higher numbers of both up- and down-regulated genes, compared with A.SW mice. On the other hand, in the spleen, SJL/J mice had a higher number of up-regulated genes, but a lower number of down-regulated genes, compared with A.SW mice. **(C–F)** Heat maps of identified genes among most highly up- or down-regulated 20 genes in the brains and spleens at disease peak of PP-EAE. Red, blue, and white indicate up-regulation, down-regulation, and no change, respectively. **(C)** In the brains of A.SW mice with PP-EAE, significantly up-regulated genes included: lipocalin 2 (*Lcn2*), complement-related genes, and chemokines. **(D)** In the brains of SJL/J mice with PP-EAE, *Lcn2*, chemokine-, MHC molecule-, and immunoglobulin-related genes were highly up-regulated. **(E,F)** In the spleens of both A.SW **(E)** and SJL/J **(F)** mice with PP-EAE, erythrocyte-related genes were down-regulated significantly. Overall, heat maps between A.SW and SJL/J mice were similar in the brains or spleens. A list of abbreviations of genes is shown in **Supplemental Table 1**.

Brain Pathway Analysis Revealed That Fc Receptor and Complement-Related Genes Were Up-Regulated in Both Mouse Strains Brains, but Pro-inflammatory Cytokine-Related Genes Were Up-Regulated Only in SJL/J Mice

Using the IPA, we clustered and categorized the genes up- or down-regulated in the brains and spleens of mouse models for PP-EAE (**Figures 3C–F**). The IPA identified one network in A.SW mice and five networks in SJL/J mice with a high network score (>35). The network identified in the brains of A.SW mice was categorized as "Cell-To-Cell Signaling and Interaction," "Hematological System Development and Function" and "Immune Cell Trafficking" (**Figure 3C**). This network contained up-regulation of immune response-related genes: particularly MHC molecules [*H2-Aa* (MHC class II), *H2-Q2* (MHC class I), and *Cd74* (invariant polypeptide of MHC class II molecule)]; immunoglobulin-related genes, including immunoglobulin J chain (*Igj*) (51) and Fc receptors (*Fcgr2a*,

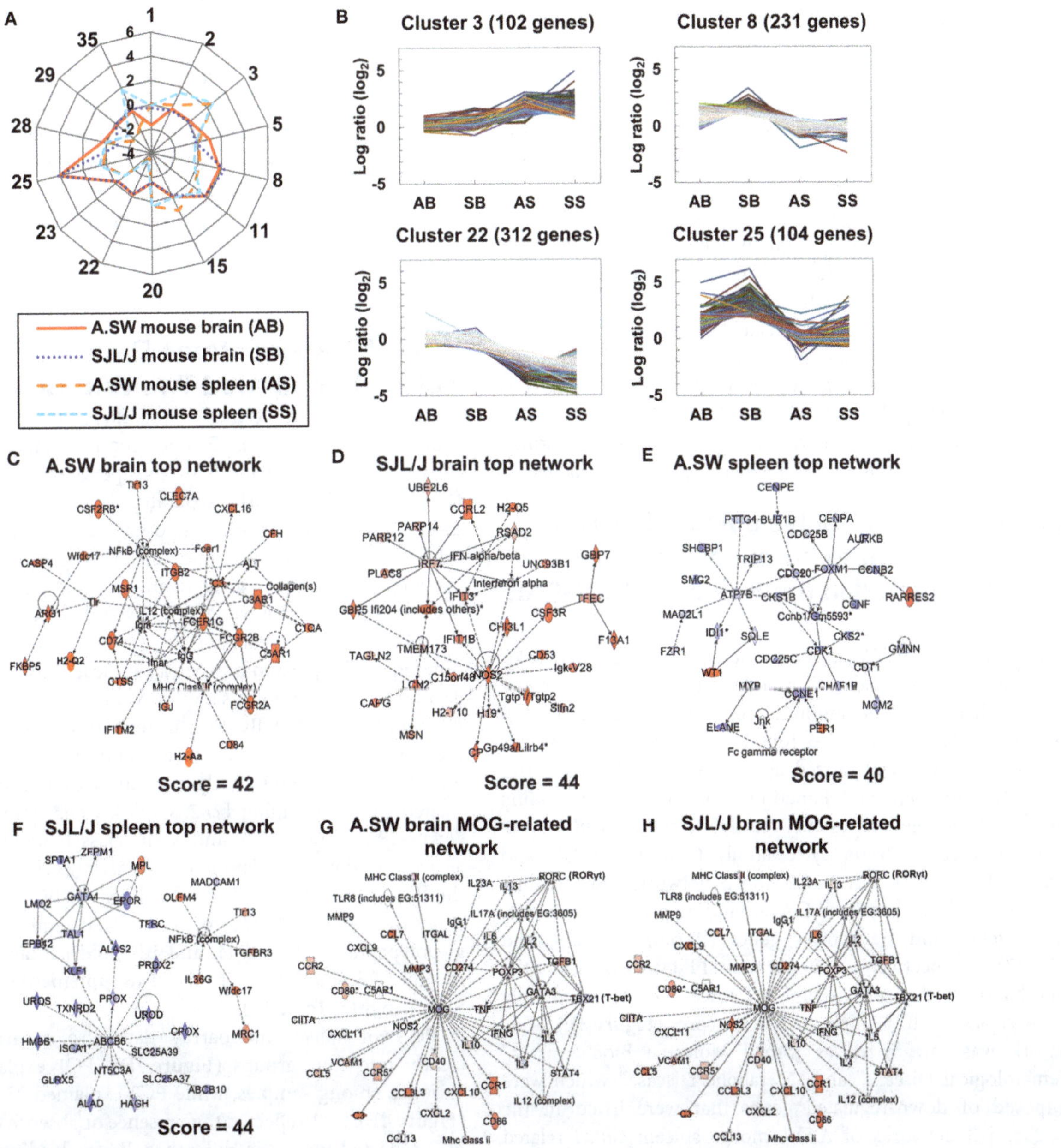

FIGURE 3 | (A,B) *K*-means clustering for brain and spleen microarray data from two models. **(A)** A radar chart of 14 cluster center genes whose log ratios were higher than 1 or lower than −1, at least in one organ or in one mouse strain, compared with controls, among the total 35 clusters. **(B)** Dynamic expression patterns of four clusters. AB, SB, AS, and SS indicate A.SW mouse brain, SJL/J mouse brain, A.SW mouse spleen, and SJL/J mouse spleen, respectively. We used microarray data from three PP-EAE and three naïve mice of each strain (the total number of mice = 12). Genes in cluster 3 were up-regulated in the spleens of both models. Genes in cluster 8 were up-regulated in the brains of SJL/J mice. Genes in cluster 22 were down-regulated in the spleens of both models. Genes in cluster 25 were up-regulated in the brains of both models. **(C–H)** Gene networks up-regulated in the brains or down-regulated in the spleens from two models. Transcriptome data at disease peak were clustered and categorized by the Ingenuity Pathway Analysis (IPA) Network Generation. **(C)** The top network in the brains of A.SW mice was categorized as "Cell-To-Cell Signaling and Interaction," "Hematological System Development and Function," and "Immune Cell Trafficking," which were composed of Fc receptor and complement-related genes. **(D)** The top network in SJL/J mouse brain was categorized as "Immunological Disease," "Endocrine System Disorders," and "Gastrointestinal Disease," which were composed of IFN-α/β-induced genes and nitric oxide synthase 2 (*Nos2*). **(E)** The top network in A.SW mouse spleen was categorized as "Cell Cycle," "Reproductive System Development and Function," and "Cancer" which were composed of cell cycle-related genes. **(F)** The top network in SJL/J mouse spleen was categorized as "Small Molecule Biochemistry," "Hematological Disease," and "Metabolic Disease" which were composed of GATA1- and transporter-related genes. **(G,H)** Up- or down-regulated genes associated with MOG in the brains of A.SW mice **(G)** and SJL/J mice **(H)**. Pro-inflammatory genes were down-regulated in A.SW mice and up-regulated in SJL/J mice, while Th2-associated genes were up-regulated in A.SW mice and down-regulated in SJL/J mice. Red and blue nodes indicate up- and down-regulated genes, respectively. Solid and dashed lines indicated direct and indirect connections, respectively. Score = network score.

Fcgr2b, *Fcer1a*, and *Fcer1g*); and complement-related genes, including complement component 3 (*C3*), C3a receptor 1 (*C3ar1*), C5a receptor 1 (*C5ar1*), complement component factor h (*Cfh*), and C1q α chain (*C1qa*) (52, 53).

In the brains of SJL/J mice, all five networks with a high network score were associated with immune responses (**Figure 3D** and **Supplemental Figure 5**). The top 1 network was categorized as "Immunological Disease," "Endocrine System Disorders," and "Gastrointestinal Disease" (**Figure 3D**). The network was composed of up-regulated genes related to IFN-α/β and nitric oxide synthase 2 (*Nos2*). The top 2 network contained similar genes to the top 1 network of A.SW mouse brain, such as Fc receptor and complement-related genes, while substantial up-regulation of the genes related to IL-6-related genes and costimulatory molecules *Cd80*/*Cd86* (B7-1/B7-2) was seen only in SJL/J mice (**Supplemental Figure 5**). All the top 3, 4, and 5 networks were associated with pro-inflammatory cytokines, IL-1β, tumor necrosis factor (TNF)-α, and IFN-γ, respectively.

Spleen Pathway Analysis Revealed That Genes Irrelevant to Immune Responses Down-Regulated in the Spleens of PP-EAE Mice

In the spleen of A.SW mice, we identified three networks, which were composed of mainly down-regulated genes that are irrelevant to immune responses (**Figure 3E** and **Supplemental Figure 6**). The top 1 network in the spleens of A.SW mice was categorized as "Cell Cycle," "Reproductive System Development and Function," and "Cancer," including down-regulated genes: cyclin family (*Ccne1*, *Ccnb1*, and *Ccnb2*) and cell division cycle family (*Cdc20*, *Cdc25b*, and *Cdc25c*) (**Figure 3E**). The top 2 and 3 networks were mainly composed of down-regulated GATA binding protein 1 (*Gata1*)-related genes and transporter genes (*Abcb6*, *Slc25a39*, and *Slc25a37*), respectively (**Supplemental Figure 6**). On the other hand, in the spleens of SJL/J mice, we identified only one network with a high network score (**Figure 3F**). The network was categorized as "Small Molecule Biochemistry," "Hematological Disease," and "Metabolic Disease," which were composed of down-regulated genes that were listed in the top 2 and 3 networks of A.SW mouse spleen: *Gata1*-related genes and transporter genes (*Abcb6*, *Slc25a39*, and *Slc25a37*). *Gata1*-related genes are essential for normal hematopoiesis, particularly erythropoiesis (54), while transporter genes are cell membrane proteins that control the uptake and efflux of various compounds (55, 56). The network also included up-regulated genes, such as Toll-like receptor 13 (*Tlr13*) and transforming growth factor (TGF) β receptor III (*Tgfbr3*).

MOG-related Pathway Analysis Revealed That Expression of Th1/Th2-Related Genes Differed Between Two Mouse Brains

In both mouse strains, we also determined the gene expression changes in a MOG-related network in the brains, using IPA (**Figures 3G,H**). *Mog* itself was down-regulated in both mouse strains (A.SW, 0.81-fold, $P < 0.05$; SJL/J, 0.85-fold, $P < 0.05$). The gene expression of several cytokines and chemokines was up-regulated similarly in both mouse strains, including *Cxcl10*, *Ccr1*, and *Il6*. However, some pro-inflammatory genes, such as *Ifng*, *Cxcl11*, *Mmp9*, and *Nos2*, were down-regulated in A.SW mice (**Figure 3G**), while they were up-regulated in SJL/J mice (**Figure 3H**). On the other hand, Th2-related genes (*Gata3* and *Il5*, but not *Il4*) were up-regulated in A.SW mice, while they were down-regulated in SJL/J mice.

PCA of Transcriptome Data of Brains and Spleens Separated Two EAE Groups

To identify the molecules (biomarkers) that distinguish the samples between PP-EAE and control mice, we analyzed microarray data, using an unsupervised approach, PCA (**Figure 4**). PCA clearly separated brain samples into four groups, each of which was composed of samples from A.SW and SJL/J mice with PP-EAE, and their control mice (**Figure 4A**), showing that distinct gene expression patterns were present between the four groups. PCA showed that PC1 likely reflected the presence or absence of EAE, while PC2 reflected strain differences. Proportion of variance indicated that PC1 explained 33% of variance among samples, while PC2 explained 20% of variance (**Figure 4B**). By using factor loading for PC1, we ranked the genes that contributed to the PC1 values (**Figure 4C** and **Supplemental Table 16**). Up-regulation of immune response-related genes, including *Lcn2*, *Cxcl13*, *Chil3*, immunoglobulins (*Igkv8-28* and *Ighv1-55*), and MHC class II molecule (*H2-Aa*), as well as down-regulation of prolactin (*Prl*), contributed to the PC1 values. Among factor loadings for PC2, although most genes were unidentified, cytochrome P450, family two, subfamily g, polypeptide 1 (*Cyp2g1*), and BPI fold containing family B, member 9B (*Bpifb9b*) were listed (**Supplemental Figure 7** and **Supplemental Table 17**).

PCA of spleen microarray data also separated samples clearly into four groups (**Figure 4D**). PC1 explained 40% of variance among samples, while PC2 explained 23% of variance (**Figure 4E**). PC1 reflected the presence or absence of EAE, while PC2 reflected the strain difference. Factor loading showed that stefin A2 like 1 (*Stfa2l1*), deleted in malignant brain tumors 1 (*Dmbt1*), and trypsin genes (*Try5* and *Try10*) contributed to the PC1 values positively, while erythrocyte-related genes (*Gypa*, *Kel*, *Rhd*, and *Cldn13*) contributed to the PC1 value negatively (**Figure 4F** and **Supplemental Tables 18, 19**). Among top or bottom 100 genes that were listed in factor loading for PC1 values, only three genes, *Chil3*, *Serpina3n*, and leucine-rich α-2-glycoprotein 1 (*Lrg1*), were in common in the brains and spleens: *Chil3*, which is also known as *Ym1*, is rodent-specific chitinase-like protein and associated with Th2 inflammation (57), *Serpina3n* is an inhibitor of granzyme b (58), and *Lrg1* is related to TGF-β signaling pathway (59). Thus, most CNS gene expression changes seemed to occur independently from those in the peripheral lymphoid organs, during the disease progression of EAE.

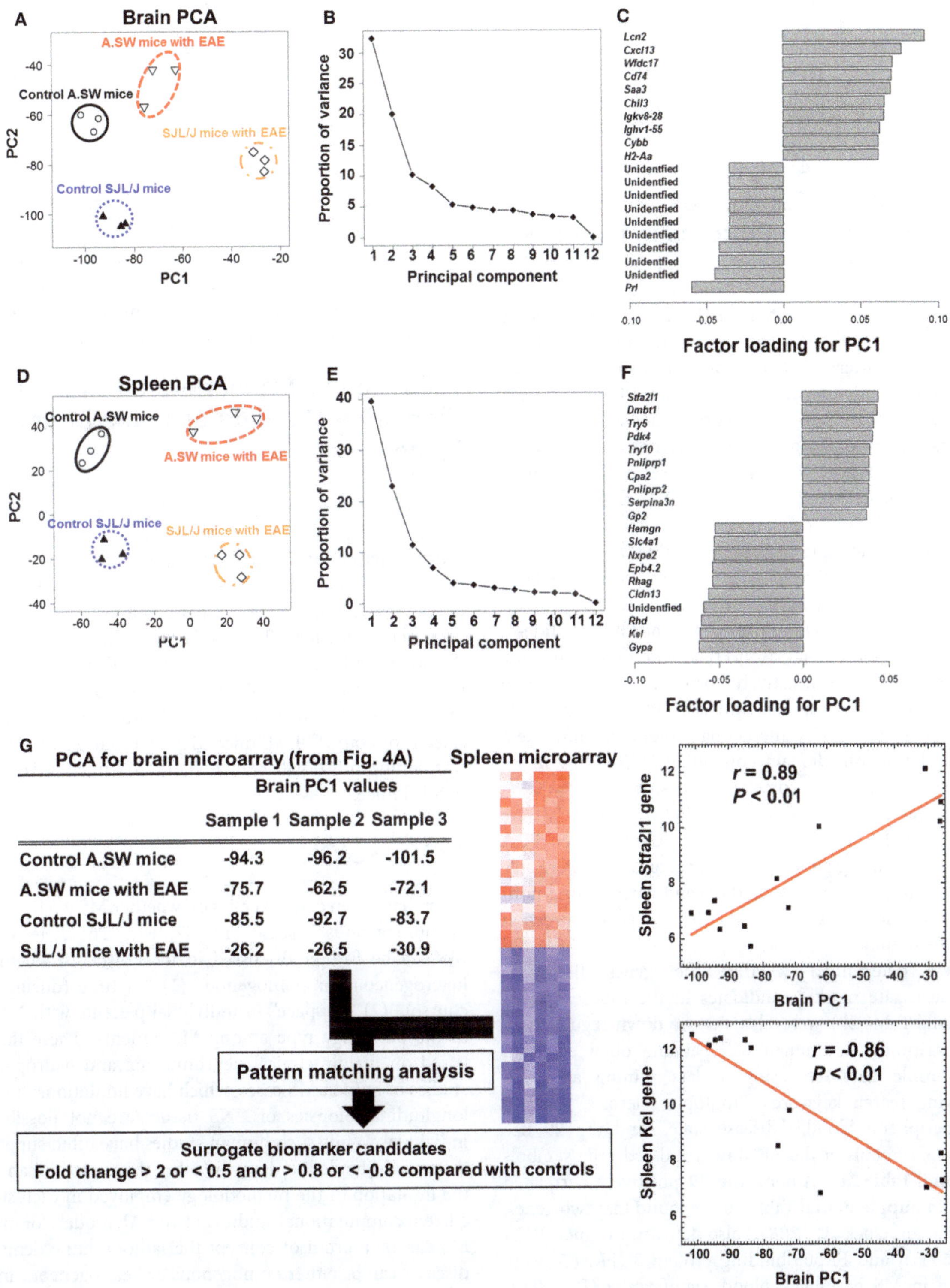

FIGURE 4 | (A–F) Principal component analysis (PCA) of transcriptome data of brains and spleens from A.SW and SJL/J mice with PP-EAE and control mice. PCA separated the samples into four groups in both brains **(A)** and spleens **(D)**, where principal component (PC) 1 reflected the presence of EAE, while PC2 reflected strain difference. The proportion of variance showed that PC1 explained variance among samples 33% in the brains **(B)** and 40% in the spleens **(E)**. In the brain **(C)**, factor loading for PC1 showed that up-regulation of immune response-related genes, including lipocalin 2 (*Lcn2*), CXCL13, and immunoglobulins, and down-regulation of prolactin (*Prl*) contributed to PC1 values. In the factor loading for PC1 of spleen PCA **(F)**, stefin A2 like 1 (*Stfa2l1*) and erythrocyte-related genes (*Gypa*, *Kel*, and *Rhd*) contributed to PC1 distribution positively and negatively, respectively. Transcriptome data from three PP-EAE and three naïve mice of each strain were used. **(G)** A flow

(Continued)

FIGURE 4 | chart of pattern matching analysis using brain PC1 values and spleen microarray data from A.SW and SJL/J mice. To find peripheral surrogate biomarkers that reflect the changes in the brain, we conducted pattern matching analysis. Genes whose fold changes were >2 or <0.5 with correlation coefficients of >0.8 or <-0.8 were identified as surrogate marker candidates (**Supplemental Table 15**). *Stfa2l1* and *Kel* genes, which were up- and down-regulated significantly in the spleens of PP-EAE mice, respectively, were strongly correlated with brain PC1 values (*Stfa2l1*: $r = 0.89$, $P < 0.01$; *Kel*: $r = -0.86$, $P < 0.01$). We used microarray data of brains and spleens of three mice with PP-EAE and three age-matched control mice for each mouse strain (the total number of mice = 12).

Pattern Matching Analysis Showed Spleen Surrogate Marker Candidates That Reflect the Gene Expression Patterns in the Brain

In the above PCA, we attempted to find peripheral surrogate markers that reflect the changes in the brain. However, we were not able to identify the common genes using factor loading for PC1 among the brain and spleen transcriptome data. Thus, we conducted a pattern matching analysis using brain PC1 values and spleen microarray data from two PP-EAE models and controls; pattern matching analysis allowed us to find splenic genes whose expression patterns matched the PC1 values of brain samples (**Figure 4G**). When the results were sorted by correlation coefficients (r >0.8 or <-0.8) and expression ratios (>2- or <1/2-fold, compared with controls), 333 genes showed strong correlation (**Supplemental Table 20**). Among the 333 genes, we found 29 splenic genes positively correlated with the brain PC1 values, including adhesion G protein-coupled receptor G2 (*Adgrg2*), *Lrg1*, and phosphoinositide-3-kinase interacting protein 1 (*Pik3ip1*). On the other hand, we found 304 splenic genes negatively correlated with the brain PC1 values, including progestin and adipoQ receptor family member IX (*Paqr9*), RAB3A interacting protein (rabin3)-like 1 (*Rab3il1*), and Josephin domain containing 2 (*Josd2*). Among the positively and negatively correlated genes, *Stfa2l1* ($r = 0.89$) and erythrocyte-related genes, including *Kel* ($r = -0.86$), were listed in the top 10 of factor loading for PC1 in spleen PCA (**Figure 4F**). Thus, using pattern matching analysis, we were able to find the peripheral surrogate marker candidates among non-immune-related molecules that could reflect the gene expression changes in the brain.

Next, we determined whether the genes listed as peripheral surrogate marker candidates in the mouse spleens (**Supplemental Table 20**) were also up- or down-regulated in blood transcriptome of human MS patients obtained from the GEO profile database, using a data mining approach with following search keywords: "multiple sclerosis," "Homo sapiens," "peripheral blood," "disease state," and the 29 up-regulated gene symbols or the 304 downregulated gene symbols (**Supplemental Table 21**). Among the 29 positively correlated genes listed in **Supplemental Table 20**, we found that two genes, period circadian clock 1 [*PER1*, also known as microRNA 6883 (*MIR6883*)] and FK506 binding protein 5 (*FKBP5*) were up-regulated in MS peripheral blood, significantly ($P < 0.01$, **Supplemental Table 21**). Among the 304 negatively correlated genes, we found that only one gene, solute carrier family 16 member 1 [*SLC16A1*, also known as monocarboxylate transporter (MCT) 1] was down-regulated in MS peripheral blood, significantly ($P < 0.05$, **Supplemental Table 21**). Up-regulation of *Per1* and down-regulation *SLC16A1* were found in the data set (60) from 12 MS patients compared with 15 unaffected controls, whose other clinical data were not available. Upregulation of *FKBP5* was found in the data set of peripheral blood cells from three MS patients with high serum levels of transmembrane-type semaphorin (Sema4A) (but not from MS patients with low Sema4A levels), compared with four healthy controls with low serum levels of Sema4A (61).

Validation of Transcriptome Data of Biomarker Candidates in the Brains and Spleens

To validate transcriptome data of brain and spleen samples, we conducted real-time PCR for the representative genes listed in the clustering, PCA factor loading and pattern matching data (**Supplemental Figure 8**). The expression patterns of *Cxcl13*, *Lcn2*, and *Cd3g* in the brain samples and those of *Kel* and *Stfa2l1* in the spleen samples between microarray and real-time PCR data were consistent. The levels of *Cxcl13*, *Lcn2*, and *Cd3g* in the brains with PP-EAE were higher in SJL/J mice than in A.SW mice. Similarly, in the spleen, the expression of *Stfa2l1* was also up-regulated. On the other hand, *Kel* was down-regulated in the spleens of both PP-EAE mice. Expression of *Lcn2* in the spleens was significantly down-regulated in A.SW mice and up-regulated in SJL/J mice.

DISCUSSION

There have been controversies on whether MS is a heterogeneous or homogenous disease (12, 47, 62). The heterogeneity of MS can be further discussed in three aspects; whether MS is heterogeneous or homogenous (1) "in time (during the time course)," (2) "in space" in individual patients with MS, and (3) in the pathology type among MS patients. These theories are based on mainly clinical neuroimaging and neuropathological studies of human MS cases, which have limitations; for example, longitudinal biopsies of CNS tissues are not possible in one individual. While such human studies have often supported one theory, and tended to deny the other theories, this can be due to the limitation of the methodology employed in each study. Our current computational studies of two EAE models for progressive MS can be a proof of concept that autoimmune demyelinating diseases can be either homogenous or heterogeneous in all three aspects, to some extent.

First, "Is MS a heterogeneous in time?" in other word, "Is MS a 1-stage or 2-stage disease (47)?" The "1-stage" disease theory is that the pathophysiology (effector mechanism) of MS is the same during the entire course of MS in individual patients. The "2-stage" disease theory is that CNS tissue damage is caused by inflammation in Stage 1, while neurodegeneration in Stage 2 is independent of inflammation, leading to disease progression. While some neuropathology studies in MS supported the 1-stage disease theory, neuroimaging and clinical studies, such as drug responses and epidemiological data, supported the 2-stage disease theory (63, 64).

In our current study, when we assessed kinetics of IFN-γ and IL-17 levels, these pro-inflammatory cytokines were associated with disease activities in RR-EAE and PP-EAE in SJL/J mice (common effector mechanism in initiation, acute attack, and disease progression), while IFN-γ and IL-17 levels in PP-EAE in A.SW mice were up-regulated only in disease initiation, but declined at disease peak. Since these results suggested that another effector mechanism independent of the pro-inflammatory responses could contribute to disease progression in A.SW mice, we further conducted transcriptome analyses of the CNS at disease peak of PP-EAE in both mouse strains. Volcano plots of transcriptome data showed the different number of up- or down-regulated genes between brains and spleens or between A.SW and SJL/J mice. While many genes were up-regulated in the brains and down-regulated in the spleens, down-regulation of genes in the spleen may be associated with splenic atrophy (16). Heat maps showed highly up-regulated genes in each brain and spleen of two mouse strains as a result of "supervised" two-way comparison. In the brains of both models, several genes were up-regulated in common. Among the genes, *Lcn2* was the most highly up-regulated gene, which has been reported as an immune mediator of EAE and MS (65, 66). Glycoprotein nonmetastatic melanoma B (*Gpnmb*) is a type I transmembrane protein which works in various biological processes, such as inflammation (67, 68). Activation of complement components, including *C3*, plays a pivotal role by recruiting inflammatory cells, increasing myelin phagocytosis by macrophages, and exerting direct cytotoxic effects on oligodendrocytes (69). *Cxcl13* attracts B lymphocytes and Th cells via chemokine receptor CXCR5 (70) and can be used as a biomarker of inflammation in MS (71). Since *Cybb/Nox2* was also up-regulated, oxidative stress may be related to damage in the brain (72).

In the spleens of both models, we found significant down-regulation of *Kel*, *Rhd*, *Gypa*, and *Cldn13*, which have been reported as erythrocyte-related genes (**Figures 2E,F**) (49). This is consistent with splenic pathway analysis data (**Figure 3F** and **Supplemental Figure 6A**), in which we found down-regulation of *Gata1*-related genes that are essential for erythropoiesis (54). *Stfa2l1*, which acts as a cathepsin inhibitor, was up-regulated in common and could regulate antigen presentation processes involved in immune response and autoimmune diseases (73). Interestingly, two neutrophil-associated proteins, *Ltf*, and *Ly6g* were down-regulated in A.SW spleens, but up-regulated in SJL/J spleens. *Ltf* is a protein contained in secondary granules of neutrophils and can ameliorate the signs of EAE (74), while *Ly6g* is expressed in neutrophils and can regulate leukocyte activation and adhesion (75). Distinct expression of these genes suggested the different role of neutrophils in two PP-EAE models.

Interestingly, our bioinformatics analyses, including pathway analyses and PCA, demonstrated that antibody-mediated pathophysiology (composed of immunoglobulin-, complement-, and FcR-related molecules) seemed to be active in both mouse strains. We confirmed the presence of immunoglobulin deposition and complement receptor positive cells by immunohistochemistry (data not shown). In PP-EAE in SJL/J mice, bioinformatics analyses also showed that the top network present in the CNS was associated with pro-inflammatory responses composed of most major inflammatory pathways, including those of IFN-α/β, IFN-γ, IL-17, IL-6, TNF-α, and IL-1β. Thus, in SJL/J mice, the pro-inflammatory effector mechanism could play a pathogenic role during the entire course (here, the disease might look a homogeneous disease, if one focuses only on these pro-inflammatory responses), while the antibody-mediated effector mechanism also seemed to be active at disease peak in both mouse strains (**Figure 5**). On the other hand, downregulation of prolactin also contributed to the separation between EAE and control groups in PCA. Prolactin is secreted not only by the anterior pituitary but also extra-pituitary tissues including immune cells, while prolactin receptor is found on lymphocytes and other immune cells (76). Prolactin has several roles including immunomodulation and remyelination. Although our current PCA demonstrated downregulation of prolactin could be associated with EAE progression, prolactin has been suggested to exacerbate other EAE models (77). Similarly, in human MS, an association between prolactin levels and disease activities remains controversial (76). Ysrraelit and Correale proposed that prolactin may exert dual and opposing effects in MS and that caution must be taken when prolactin levels are manipulated in MS.

However, these results do not deny the possibility of disease progression based on the 1-stage disease theory, since uncontrolled pro-inflammatory cellular responses alone can lead to disease progression regardless of the presence of involvement of antibody and complement, in theory. Indeed, many experimentally proven encephalitogenic antigens, including MBP, PLP, and neurofilament light chain (NF-L), can induce only pathogenic T cell responses that cause neurological deficits (antibodies to MBP, PLP, and NF-L do not cause tissue or cell injury because their epitopes are not expressed on cell surface) (78).

Our bioinformatics transcriptome analyses also addressed the second question, "Is MS pathology homogeneous or heterogeneous in space, in one patient, and at one time point?" or "Is there only one pathology (one effector mechanism) present in the CNS or are multiple different pathologies simultaneously present in the CNS in one patient?" At the disease peak of A.SW mice with PP-EAE, we identified only one major effector mechanism (= antibody and complement-mediated tissue damage), while two effector mechanisms may be involved in SJL/J mice: (1) antibody and complement-mediated tissue damage and (2) pro-inflammatory $CD3^+$ T cell-mediated tissue damage. Histologically, in SJL/J mice, we found that some areas showed antibody deposition without T cell infiltration and other areas contained T cell infiltration with or without antibody deposition (data not shown). These results suggested that CNS demyelinating pathology can be homogenous (contain one pathology type) or can be heterogeneous (contain more than two pathologies) in a single individual. In most CNS peptide-induced

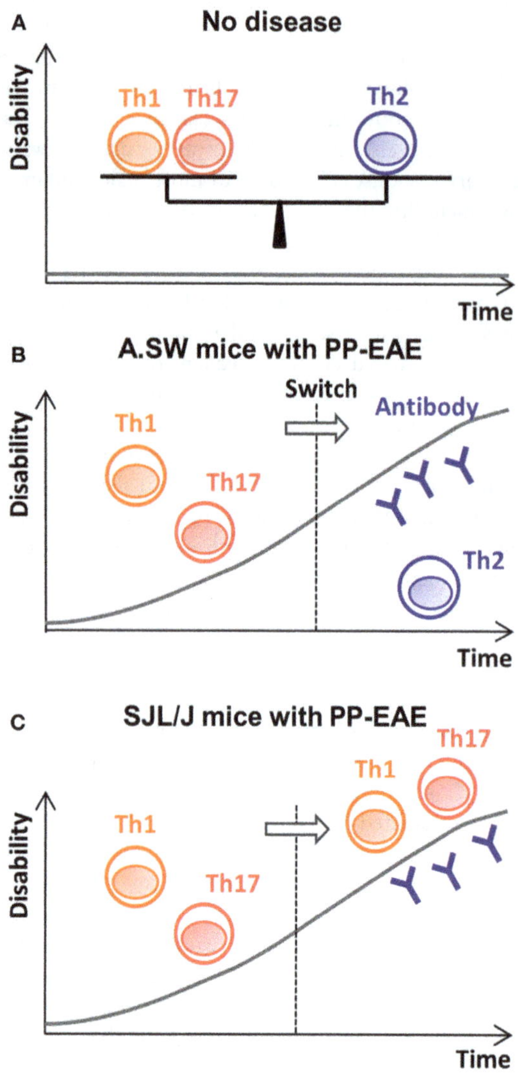

FIGURE 5 | The disease theories in A.SW and SJL/J mice with PP-EAE. **(A)** When Th1/Th17 cells vs. Th2 cells is well-balanced, no disease is induced. **(B)** In A.SW mice, increased Th1/Th17 immune responses initiate disease. Later, the Th1/Th17 responses decline, and increased Th2 immune responses help auto-antibody production. Here, effector mechanism switches from proinflammatory Th1/Th17 responses (first stage) to antibody-mediated pathology (second stage). **(C)** In SJL/J mice, while Th1/Th17 cells play an effector role during the entire disease course, anti-myelin antibody also contributes to disease progression at the "second" stage.

EAE models, pathology has been shown to be homogeneous since most peptides are either major T cell epitopes or B cell epitopes, but not both. In contrast, multiple effector mechanisms as well as heterogeneous neuropathology can be present in one single EAE model, when EAE is induced with encephalitogens that have both T-cell and B-cell epitopes [for example, MOG_{92-106} (current experiment) and brain homogenates].

Our results also addressed the third question, "Is MS pathophysiology homogeneous (common) in all MS patients, or are there heterogeneities in pathophysiology among MS patients?" Our current experiments showed that a single encephalitogen (MOG_{92-106}) can cause two different pathophysiologies (pro-inflammatory and antibody-mediated). This supports a concept and clinical pathology findings that MS neuropathology is heterogeneous. However, this does not deny the presence of possible common (homogeneous) pathologic component of demyelinating diseases. For example, in our current studies, the antibody-mediated tissue damage seemed to be a common effector mechanism in two PP-EAE models; we also found that some genes, such as *Lcn2* and *Chil3*, were commonly up-regulated in two models. In addition, common neuropathology and effector components have been demonstrated among several different EAE models that were induced with different encephalitogenic antigens. For example, EAE can be induced in SJL/J mice or C57BL/6 mice, using different encephalitogens, such as $PLP_{139-151}$, $PLP_{178-192}$, MOG_{92-106}, and MOG_{35-55} (13, 79). Here, neuropathology and pro-inflammatory immune responses in EAE induced with these different peptides were overall indistinguishable (14, 28, 80). In this context, it should also be noted that virus-induced demyelinating models share a common pathology and effector mechanism (3). Therefore, in theory, the cause of MS (several different autoantigens or even viruses) can be homogeneous or heterogeneous. Here, one autoantigen can cause different (heterogeneous) pathology depending on the genetic background or the presence of adjuvant (which mimics polymicrobial infection). On the other hand, several different autoantigens (different causes) can induce the same (homogeneous) pathology in the CNS of MS patients.

In this study, we have also conducted splenic transcriptome analyses to find peripheral surrogate markers that reflect the change in the CNS. In clinical studies in MS, while some reports showed that immune profiles in the blood reflected disease activity, others showed that peripheral profiles did not reflect the change in the CNS (81, 82). Using heat map and network/pathway analyses, we found that highly up-regulated and down-regulated genes and pathways were different between the spleens and brains in both mouse strains. Interestingly, in splenic pathway analysis, both mouse strains had down-regulation of GATA1-related genes and transporter genes (**Figure 3F** and **Supplemental Figures 6A,B**), while only A.SW mice had down-regulation of a network related to the cell cycle (**Figure 3E**). Cell cycle arrest could occur in the atrophic spleen with apoptosis in A.SW mice with progressive EAE, as we reported previously (16). Thus, A.SW mice had an additional major change in the network, comparing with SJL/J mice; this is in contrast to the CNS network profiles where SJL/J mice had an additional effector mechanism, comparing with A.SW mice.

We also conducted PCA using splenic transcriptome data from A.SW and SJL/J mice. Although PC1 values reflected the presence or absence of EAE in both the CNS and spleens, we did not find commonly up- or down-regulated genes contributing to PC1 between the brain and spleen factor loading for PC1. Thus, both supervised two-way comparison and unsupervised PCA showed that there were only three genes in common between the brains and spleens: *Chil3*, *Serpina3n*, and *Lrg1*. This could be consistent with a hypothesis that immune responses in progressive MS are sequestered from the systemic immune responses; the pathophysiology in the CNS at this stage may occur within the intact blood-brain barrier, and be independent of systemic immune responses (83).

On the other hand, our pattern matching analyses between the brain PC1 (that may reflect brain disease) and spleen transcriptome data showed that the pattern changes in a set of peripheral genes were significantly correlated with the brain PC1 values. Interestingly, the splenic genes showed the significant correlation with brain PC1 values were not immune-mediated genes. Although the causal relationship between the brain pathophysiology and splenic transcriptome changes is unclear, these set of splenic genes could be used as surrogate markers, or may be the contributing factor and/or outcomes of the pathology in the CNS. Among the genes listed as peripheral surrogate marker candidates (**Supplemental Table 20**), three genes, *PER1*, *FKBP5*, and *SLC16A1* were up- or down-regulated significantly in the peripheral blood data sets from MS patients, although these data sets were from small numbers of patients with unknown clinical histories (**Supplemental Table 21**). *PER1* encodes microRNA6883, which is associated with circadian rhythm (84). *FKBP5* is a member of immunophilin protein family which works in immunoregulation and interacts with the progesterone receptor and GATA-2 (85). *SLC16A1* encodes the MCT1, whose inhibition has been found to modulate T cell responses (86, 87). This is the first report showing the association between these three genes and MS. Peripheral surrogate marker candidates identified in this study might be worth monitoring in MS blood samples.

AUTHOR CONTRIBUTIONS

AM, JA, and IT conceived and supervised the project. SO and NK designed the experiments. SO, FS, and NM conducted the experiments. SO, A-MP, MF, and UC conducted bioinformatics analyses. SO and IT wrote the manuscript. All authors read and approved the final manuscript.

FUNDING

This work was supported by an Institutional Development Award (IDeA) from the National Institute of General Medical Science of the NIH (5P30GM110703, IT), the fellowships from the Malcolm Feist Cardiovascular Research Endowment, LSUHSC-Shreveport (SO and FS), Science Research Promotion Fund from the Promotion and Mutual Aid Corporation for Private Schools of Japan (FS), Faculty Assistance and Development Research Grant from the Kindai University Research Enhancement Grant (SO and FS), and KAKENHI from the Japan Society for the Promotion of Science [JSPS, Grant-in-Aid for Scientific Research (B)-MEXT KAKENHI Grant #15K08975 (A-MP), Grant-in-Aid for Young Scientists (B) KAKENHI, JP17K15628 (FS), and Grants-in-Aid for Scientific Research-KAKENHI, 16H07356 (IT)].

ACKNOWLEDGMENTS

We thank Elaine Cliburn Stewart, Sadie Faith Pearson, Lesya Ekshyyan, and Paula Polk for excellent technical assistance. We also thank Drs. Tsutomu Mori and Takashi Kawamura, Department of Human Life Sciences, Fukushima Medical University School of Nursing, for helpful comments.

REFERENCES

1. Willenborg DO, Staykova MA. Cytokines in the pathogenesis and therapy of autoimmune encephalomyelitis and multiple sclerosis. *Adv Exp Med Biol.* (2003) 520:96–119. doi: 10.1007/978-1-4615-0171-8_7
2. Browne P, Chandraratna D, Angood C, Tremlett H, Baker C, Taylor BV, et al. Atlas of multiple sclerosis 2013: a growing global problem with widespread inequity. *Neurology.* (2014) 83:1022–4. doi: 10.1212/WNL.0000000000000768
3. Sato F, Omura S, Martinez NE, Tsunoda I. Animal models of multiple sclerosis. In: Minagar A, editor. *Neuroinflammation*. 2nd ed. Burlington, MA: Academic Press (2018). p. 37–72.
4. Katz Sand I. Classification, diagnosis, and differential diagnosis of multiple sclerosis. *Curr Opin Neurol.* (2015) 28:193–205. doi: 10.1097/WCO.0000000000000206
5. Miller DH, Chard DT, Ciccarelli O. Clinically isolated syndromes. *Lancet Neurol.* (2012) 11:157–69. doi: 10.1016/S1474-4422(11)70274-5
6. Ebers GC. Prognostic factors for multiple sclerosis: the importance of natural history studies. *J Neurol.* (2005) 252 (Suppl. 3) iii15-iii20. doi: 10.1007/s00415-005-2012-4
7. Rudick RA. The elusive biomarker for personalized medicine in multiple sclerosis: the search continues. *Neurology.* (2012) 79:498–9. doi: 10.1212/WNL.0b013e318259e13a
8. Kalinski P, Moser M. Consensual immunity: success-driven development of T-helper-1 and T-helper-2 responses. *Nat Rev Immunol.* (2005) 5:251–60. doi: 10.1038/nri1569
9. Yanagawa K, Kawachi I, Toyoshima Y, Yokoseki A, Arakawa M, Hasegawa A, et al. Pathologic and immunologic profiles of a limited form of neuromyelitis optica with myelitis. *Neurology.* (2009) 73:1628–37. doi: 10.1212/WNL.0b013e3181c1deb9
10. Lucchinetti C, Brück W, Parisi J, Scheithauer B, Rodriguez M, Lassmann H. Heterogeneity of multiple sclerosis lesions: implications for the pathogenesis of demyelination. *Ann Neurol.* (2000) 47:707–17. doi: 10.1002/1531-8249(200006)47:6%3C707::AID-ANA3%3E3.0.CO;2-Q
11. Breij ECW, Brink BP, Veerhuis R, van den Berg C, Vloet R, Yan R, et al. Homogeneity of active demyelinating lesions in established multiple sclerosis. *Ann Neurol.* (2008) 63:16–25. doi: 10.1002/ana.21311
12. Sato F, Martinez NE, Omura S, Tsunoda I. Heterogeneity versus homogeneity of multiple sclerosis. *Expert Rev Clin Immunol.* (2011) 7:165–7. doi: 10.1586/eci.11.3
13. Didonna A. Preclinical models of multiple sclerosis: advantages and limitations towards better therapies. *Curr Med Chem.* (2016) 23:1442–59. doi: 10.2174/0929867323666160406121218
14. Tsunoda I, Kuang L-Q, Theil DJ, Fujinami RS. Antibody association with a novel model for primary progressive multiple sclerosis: induction of relapsing-remitting and progressive forms of EAE in $H2^s$ mouse strains. *Brain Pathol.* (2000) 10:402–18. doi: 10.1111/j.1750-3639.2000.tb00272.x
15. Tsunoda I, Kuang L-Q, Igenge IZ, Fujinami RS. Converting relapsing remitting to secondary progressive experimental allergic encephalomyelitis (EAE) by ultraviolet B irradiation. *J Neuroimmunol.* (2005) 160:122–34. doi: 10.1016/j.jneuroim.2004.11.007
16. Tsunoda I, Libbey JE, Kuang L-Q, Terry EJ, Fujinami RS. Massive apoptosis in lymphoid organs in animal models for primary and

secondary progressive multiple sclerosis. *Am J Pathol.* (2005) 167:1631–46. doi: 10.1016/S0002-9440(10)61247-3

17. Libbey JE, Cusick MF, Tsunoda I, Fujinami RS. Antiviral CD8$^+$ T cells cause an experimental autoimmune encephalomyelitis-like disease in naive mice. *J Neurovirol.* (2012) 18:45–54. doi: 10.1007/s13365-012-0077-2
18. Mendel I, Kerlero de Rosbo N, Ben-Nun A. A myelin oligodendrocyte glycoprotein peptide induces typical chronic experimental autoimmune encephalomyelitis in H-2^b mice: fine specificity and T cell receptor Vβ expression of encephalitogenic T cells. *Eur J Immunol.* (1995) 25:1951–9. doi: 10.1002/eji.1830250723
19. Deng C, Minguela A, Hussain RZ, Lovett-Racke AE, Radu C, Ward ES, et al. Expression of the tyrosine phosphatase Src homology 2 domain-containing protein tyrosine phosphatase 1 determines T cell activation threshold and severity of experimental autoimmune encephalomyelitis. *J Immunol.* (2002) 168:4511–8. doi: 10.4049/jimmunol.168.9.4511
20. Satoh J, Nakanishi M, Koike F, Miyake S, Yamamoto T, Kawai M, et al. Microarray analysis identifies an aberrant expression of apoptosis and DNA damage-regulatory genes in multiple sclerosis. *Neurobiol Dis.* (2005) 18:537–50. doi: 10.1016/j.nbd.2004.10.007
21. Singh MK, Scott TF, LaFramboise WA, Hu FZ, Post JC, Ehrlich GD. Gene expression changes in peripheral blood mononuclear cells from multiple sclerosis patients undergoing beta-interferon therapy. *J Neurol Sci.* (2007) 258:52–9. doi: 10.1016/j.jns.2007.02.034
22. Kinter J, Zeis T, Schaeren-Wiemers N. RNA profiling of MS brain tissues. *Int MS J.* (2008) 15:51–8.
23. Baranzini SE, Bernard CCA, Oksenberg JR. Modular transcriptional activity characterizes the initiation and progression of autoimmune encephalomyelitis. *J Immunol.* (2005) 174:7412–22. doi: 10.4049/jimmunol.174.11.7412
24. Brand-Schieber E, Werner P, Iacobas DA, Iacobas S, Beelitz M, Lowery SL, et al. Connexin43, the major gap junction protein of astrocytes, is down-regulated in inflamed white matter in an animal model of multiple sclerosis. *J Neurosci Res.* (2005) 80:798–808. doi: 10.1002/jnr.20474
25. Gilgun-Sherki Y, Barhum Y, Atlas D, Melamed E, Offen D. Analysis of gene expression in MOG-induced experimental autoimmune encephalomyelitis after treatment with a novel brain-penetrating antioxidant. *J Mol Neurosci.* (2005) 27:125–35. doi: 10.1385/JMN:27:1:125
26. Roscoe WA, Welsh ME, Carter DE, Karlik SJ. VEGF and angiogenesis in acute and chronic $MOG_{(35-55)}$ peptide induced EAE. *J Neuroimmunol.* (2009) 209:6–15. doi: 10.1016/j.jneuroim.2009.01.009
27. Libbey JE, Tsunoda I, Fujinami RS. Studies in the modulation of experimental autoimmune encephalomyelitis. *J Neuroimmune Pharmacol.* (2010) 5:168–75. doi: 10.1007/s11481-010-9215-x
28. Tsunoda I, Kuang L-Q, Tolley ND, Whitton JL, Fujinami RS. Enhancement of experimental allergic encephalomyelitis (EAE) by DNA immunization with myelin proteolipid protein (PLP) plasmid DNA. *J Neuropathol Exp Neurol.* (1998) 57:758–67. doi: 10.1097/00005072-199808000-00005
29. Sato F, Kawai E, Martinez NE, Omura S, Park AM, Takahashi S, et al. T-bet, but not Gata3, overexpression is detrimental in a neurotropic viral infection. *Sci Rep.* (2017) 7:10496. doi: 10.1038/s41598-017-10980-0
30. McRae BL, Vanderlugt CL, Dal Canto MC, Miller SD. Functional evidence for epitope spreading in the relapsing pathology of experimental autoimmune encephalomyelitis. *J Exp Med.* (1995) 182:75–85. doi: 10.1084/jem.182.1.75
31. Martinez NE, Sato F, Kawai E, Omura S, Takahashi S, Yoh K, et al. Th17-biased RORγt transgenic mice become susceptible to a viral model for multiple sclerosis. *Brain Behav Immun.* (2014) 43:86–97. doi: 10.1016/j.bbi.2014.07.008
32. Boda E, Pini A, Hoxha E, Parolisi R, Tempia F. Selection of reference genes for quantitative real-time RT-PCR studies in mouse brain. *J Mol Neurosci.* (2009) 37:238–53. doi: 10.1007/s12031-008-9128-9
33. Martinez NE, Karlsson F, Sato F, Kawai E, Omura S, Minagar A, et al. Protective and detrimental roles for regulatory T cells in a viral model for multiple sclerosis. *Brain Pathol.* (2014) 24:436–51. doi: 10.1111/bpa.12119
34. Chen JJ, Wang S-J, Tsai C-A, Lin C-J. Selection of differentially expressed genes in microarray data analysis. *Pharmacogenomics J.* (2007) 7:212–20. doi: 10.1038/sj.tpj.6500412
35. Oberg AL, Mahoney DW, Eckel-Passow JE, Malone CJ, Wolfinger RD, Hill EG, et al. Statistical analysis of relative labeled mass spectrometry data from complex samples using ANOVA. *J Proteome Res.* (2008) 7:225–33. doi: 10.1021/pr700734f
36. Li W. Volcano plots in analyzing differential expressions with mRNA microarrays. *J Bioinform Comput Biol.* (2012) 10:1231003. doi: 10.1142/S0219720012310038
37. Omura S, Kawai E, Sato F, Martinez NE, Chaitanya GV, Rollyson PA, et al. Bioinformatics multivariate analysis determined a set of phase-specific biomarker candidates in a novel mouse model for viral myocarditis. *Circ Cardiovasc Genet.* (2014) 7:444–54. doi: 10.1161/CIRCGENETICS.114.000505
38. Davies DL, Bouldin DW. A cluster separation measure. *IEEE Trans Pattern Anal Mach Intell.* (1979) 1:224–7. doi: 10.1109/TPAMI.1979.4766909
39. Savli H, Szendröi A, Romics I, Nagy B. Gene network and canonical pathway analysis in prostate cancer: a microarray study. *Exp Mol Med.* (2008) 40:176–85. doi: 10.3858/emm.2008.40.2.176
40. Ringnér M. What is principal component analysis? *Nat Biotechnol.* (2008) 26:303–4. doi: 10.1038/nbt0308-303
41. Loke P, Favre D, Hunt PW, Leung JM, Kanwar B, Martin JN, et al. Correlating cellular and molecular signatures of mucosal immunity that distinguish HIV controllers from noncontrollers. *Blood.* (2010) 115:e20–32. doi: 10.1182/blood-2009-12-257451
42. Chaitanya GV, Omura S, Sato F, Martinez NE, Minagar A, Ramanathan M, et al. Inflammation induces neuro-lymphatic protein expression in multiple sclerosis brain neurovasculature. *J Neuroinflamm.* (2013) 10:125. doi: 10.1186/1742-2094-10-125
43. Pavlidis P, Noble WS. Analysis of strain and regional variation in gene expression in mouse brain. *Genome Biol.* (2001) 2:research0042. doi: 10.1186/gb-2001-2-10-research0042
44. Barrett T, Edgar R. Mining microarray data at NCBI's gene expression omnibus (GEO)*. *Methods Mol Biol.* (2006) 338:175–90. doi: 10.1385/1-59745-097-9:175
45. Lafaille JJ, Van de Keere F, Hsu AL, Baron JL, Haas W, Raine CS, et al. Myelin basic protein-specific T helper 2 (Th2) cells cause experimental autoimmune encephalomyelitis in immunodeficient hosts rather than protect them from the disease. *J Exp Med.* (1997) 186:307–12. doi: 10.1084/jem.186.2.307
46. Komiyama Y, Nakae S, Matsuki T, Nambu A, Ishigame H, Kakuta S, et al. IL-17 plays an important role in the development of experimental autoimmune encephalomyelitis. *J Immunol.* (2006) 177:566–73. doi: 10.4049/jimmunol.177.1.566
47. Martinez NE, Sato F, Omura S, Minagar A, Alexander JS, Tsunoda I. Immunopathological patterns from EAE and Theiler's virus infection: is multiple sclerosis a homogenous 1-stage or heterogenous 2-stage disease? *Pathophysiology.* (2013) 20:71–84. doi: 10.1016/j.pathophys.2012.03.003
48. Martinez NE, Sato F, Omura S, Kawai E, Takahashi S, Yoh K, et al. RORγ, but not T-bet, overexpression exacerbates an autoimmune model for multiple sclerosis. *J Neuroimmunol.* (2014) 276:142–9. doi: 10.1016/j.jneuroim.2014.09.006
49. Thompson PD, Tipney H, Brass A, Noyes H, Kemp S, Naessens J, et al. Claudin 13, a member of the claudin family regulated in mouse stress induced erythropoiesis. *PLoS ONE.* (2010) 5:e12667. doi: 10.1371/journal.pone.0012667
50. Bamezai A. Mouse Ly-6 proteins and their extended family: markers of cell differentiation and regulators of cell signaling. *Arch Immunol Ther Exp.* (2004) 52:255–66.
51. Koshland ME. Structure and function of the J chain. *Adv Immunol.* (1975) 20:41–69. doi: 10.1016/S0065-2776(08)60206-0
52. Ingram G, Loveless S, Howell OW, Hakobyan S, Dancey B, Harris CL, et al. Complement activation in multiple sclerosis plaques: an immunohistochemical analysis. *Acta Neuropathol Commun.* (2014) 2:53. doi: 10.1186/2051-5960-2-53
53. Kouser L, Madhukaran SP, Shastri A, Saraon A, Ferluga J, Al-Mozaini M, et al. Emerging and novel functions of complement protein C1q. *Front Immunol.* (2015) 6:317. doi: 10.3389/fimmu.2015.00317
54. Crispino JD, Horwitz MS. GATA factor mutations in hematologic disease. *Blood.* (2017) 129:2103–10. doi: 10.1182/blood-2016-09-687889
55. Löscher W, Potschka H. Blood-brain barrier active efflux transporters: ATP-binding cassette gene family. *NeuroRx.* (2005) 2:86–98. doi: 10.1602/neurorx.2.1.86

56. Schlessinger A, Matsson P, Shima JE, Pieper U, Yee SW, Kelly L, et al. Comparison of human solute carriers. *Protein Sci.* (2010) 19:412–28. doi: 10.1002/pro.320
57. Lee CG, Da Silva CA, Dela Cruz CS, Ahangari F, Ma B, Kang M-J, et al. Role of chitin and chitinase/chitinase-like proteins in inflammation, tissue remodeling, and injury. *Annu Rev Physiol.* (2011) 73:479–501. doi: 10.1146/annurev-physiol-012110-142250
58. Ang LS, Boivin WA, Williams SJ, Zhao H, Abraham T, Carmine-Simmen K, et al. Serpina3n attenuates granzyme B-mediated decorin cleavage and rupture in a murine model of aortic aneurysm. *Cell Death Dis.* (2011) 2:e209. doi: 10.1038/cddis.2011.88
59. Zhong D, He G, Zhao S, Li J, Lang Y, Ye W, et al. LRG1 modulates invasion and migration of glioma cell lines through TGF-β signaling pathway. *Acta Histochem.* (2015). doi: 10.1016/j.acthis.2015.05.001
60. Kamppinen AK, Saarela J. *Expression Data From Peripheral Blood Mononuclear Cells in Multiple Sclerosis Patients and Controls. Gene Expression Omnibus.* (2011). Available online at: https://www.ncbi.nlm.nih.gov/geo/query/acc.cgi?acc=GSE21942
61. Nakatsuji Y, Okuno T, Moriya M, Sugimoto T, Kinoshita M, Takamatsu H, et al. *Sema4A, a Novel Serum Marker of Multiple Sclerosis, Implicates Th17 Pathology and Efficacy of Interferon-β.* Gene Expression Omnibus (2011). Available online at: https://www.ncbi.nlm.nih.gov/geo/query/acc.cgi?acc=GSE26484
62. Weiner HL. The challenge of multiple sclerosis: how do we cure a chronic heterogeneous disease? *Ann Neurol.* (2009) 65:239–48. doi: 10.1002/ana.21640
63. Leray E, Yaouanq J, Le Page E, Coustans M, Laplaud D, Oger J, et al. Evidence for a two-stage disability progression in multiple sclerosis. *Brain.* (2010) 133:1900–13. doi: 10.1093/brain/awq076
64. Edan G, Leray E. A new treatment era in multiple sclerosis: clinical applications of new concepts. *J Neurol Sci.* (2011) 306:170–2. doi: 10.1016/j.jns.2010.09.018
65. Berard JL, Zarruk JG, Arbour N, Prat A, Yong VW, Jacques FH, et al. Lipocalin 2 is a novel immune mediator of experimental autoimmune encephalomyelitis pathogenesis and is modulated in multiple sclerosis. *Glia.* (2012) 60:1145–59. doi: 10.1002/glia.22342
66. Marques F, Mesquita SD, Sousa JC, Coppola G, Gao F, Geschwind DH, et al. Lipocalin 2 is present in the EAE brain and is modulated by natalizumab. *Front Cell Neurosci.* (2012) 6:33. doi: 10.3389/fncel.2012.00033
67. Huang J-J, Ma W-J, Yokoyama S. Expression and immunolocalization of Gpnmb, a glioma-associated glycoprotein, in normal and inflamed central nervous systems of adult rats. *Brain Behav.* (2012) 2:85–96. doi: 10.1002/brb3.39
68. Järve A, Mühlstedt S, Qadri F, Nickl B, Schulz H, Hübner N, et al. Adverse left ventricular remodeling by glycoprotein nonmetastatic melanoma protein B in myocardial infarction. *FASEB J.* (2017) 31:556–68. doi: 10.1096/fj.201600613R
69. Chen Y, Li R, Wu AM, Shu YQ, Lu ZQ, Hu XQ. The complement and immunoglobulin levels in NMO patients. *Neurol Sci.* (2014) 35:215–20. doi: 10.1007/s10072-013-1481-y
70. Lalor SJ, Segal BM. Lymphoid chemokines in the CNS. *J Neuroimmunol.* (2010) 224:56–61. doi: 10.1016/j.jneuroim.2010.05.017
71. Alvarez E, Piccio L, Mikesell RJ, Klawiter EC, Parks BJ, Naismith RT, et al. CXCL13 is a biomarker of inflammation in multiple sclerosis, neuromyelitis optica, and other neurological conditions. *Mult Scler.* (2013) 19:1204–8. doi: 10.1177/1352458512473362
72. Fischer MT, Sharma R, Lim JL, Haider L, Frischer JM, Drexhage J, et al. NADPH oxidase expression in active multiple sclerosis lesions in relation to oxidative tissue damage and mitochondrial injury. *Brain.* (2012) 135:886–899. doi: 10.1093/brain/aws012
73. Bilodeau M, MacRae T, Gaboury L, Laverdure J-P, Hardy M-P, Mayotte N, et al. Analysis of blood stem cell activity and cystatin gene expression in a mouse model presenting a chromosomal deletion encompassing *Csta* and *Stfa2l1*. *PLoS ONE.* (2009) 4:e7500. doi: 10.1371/journal.pone.0007500
74. Zimecki M, Kocięba M, Chodaczek G, Houszka M, Kruzel ML. Lactoferrin ameliorates symptoms of experimental encephalomyelitis in Lewis rats. *J Neuroimmunol.* (2007) 182:160–6. doi: 10.1016/j.jneuroim.2006.10.008
75. Abbitt KB, Cotter MJ, Ridger VC, Crossman DC, Hellewell PG, Norman KE. Antibody ligation of murine Ly-6G induces neutropenia, blood flow cessation, and death via complement-dependent and independent mechanisms. *J Leukoc Biol.* (2009) 85:55–63. doi: 10.1189/jlb.0507305
76. Ysrraelit MC, Correale J. Impact of sex hormones on immune function and multiple sclerosis development. *Immunology.* (2019) 156:9–22. doi: 10.1111/imm.13004
77. Oki S. Novel mechanism and biomarker of chronic progressive multiple sclerosis. *Clin Exp Neuroimmunol.* (2018) 9:25–34. doi: 10.1111/cen3.12449
78. Puentes F, van der Star BJ, Victor M, Kipp M, Beyer C, Peferoen-Baert R, et al. Characterization of immune response to neurofilament light in experimental autoimmune encephalomyelitis. *J Neuroinflamm.* (2013) 10:118. doi: 10.1186/1742-2094-10-118
79. Tsunoda I, Fujinami RS. Two models for multiple sclerosis: experimental allergic encephalomyelitis and Theiler's murine encephalomyelitis virus. *J Neuropathol Exp Neurol.* (1996) 55:673–86. doi: 10.1097/00005072-199606000-00001
80. Tsunoda I, Tanaka T, Terry EJ, Fujinami RS. Contrasting roles for axonal degeneration in an autoimmune versus viral model of multiple sclerosis: when can axonal injury be beneficial? *Am J Pathol.* (2007) 170:214–26. doi: 10.2353/ajpath.2007.060683
81. Frisullo G, Plantone D, Marti A, Iorio R, Damato V, Nociti V, et al. Type 1 immune response in progressive multiple sclerosis. *J Neuroimmunol.* (2012) 249:112–6. doi: 10.1016/j.jneuroim.2012.04.019
82. Gurevich M, Achiron A. The switch between relapse and remission in multiple sclerosis: Continuous inflammatory response balanced by Th1 suppression and neurotrophic factors. *J Neuroimmunol.* (2012) 252:83–8. doi: 10.1016/j.jneuroim.2012.07.014
83. Lassmann H, van Horssen J, Mahad D. Progressive multiple sclerosis: pathology and pathogenesis. *Nat Rev Neurol.* (2012) 8:647–56. doi: 10.1038/nrneurol.2012.168
84. Burioka N, Fukuoka Y, Takata M, Endo M, Miyata M, Chikumi H, et al. Circadian rhythms in the CNS and peripheral clock disorders: function of clock genes: influence of medication for bronchial asthma on circadian gene. *J Pharmacol Sci.* (2007) 103:144–9. doi: 10.1254/jphs.FMJ06003X4
85. Magklara A, Smith CL. A composite intronic element directs dynamic binding of the progesterone receptor and GATA-2. *Mol Endocrinol.* (2009) 23:61–73. doi: 10.1210/me.2008-0028
86. Murray CM, Hutchinson R, Bantick JR, Belfield GP, Benjamin AD, Brazma D, et al. Monocarboxylate transporter MCT1 is a target for immunosuppression. *Nat Chem Biol.* (2005) 1:371–6. doi: 10.1038/nchembio744
87. Gray AL, Coleman DT, Shi R, Cardelli JA. Monocarboxylate transporter 1 contributes to growth factor-induced tumor cell migration independent of transporter activity. *Oncotarget.* (2016) 7:32695–706. doi: 10.18632/oncotarget.9016

8

The Selective HDAC6 Inhibitor ACY-738 Impacts Memory and Disease Regulation in an Animal Model of Multiple Sclerosis

*Patrizia LoPresti**

Department of Psychology, University of Illinois at Chicago, Chicago, IL, United States

Correspondence:
Patrizia LoPresti
lopresti@uic.edu

Multiple sclerosis (MS) is a complex disease characterized by autoimmune demyelination and progressive neurodegeneration. Pathogenetic mechanisms of the disease remain largely unknown. Changes in synaptic functions have been reported; however, the significance of such alterations in the disease course remains unclear. Furthermore, the therapeutic potential of targeting synapses is not well-established. Synapses have key signaling elements that regulate intracellular transport and overall neuronal health. Histone deacetylase (HDAC)6 is a microtubule-associated deacetylase. The interaction between HDAC6 and microtubules is augmented by HDAC6 inhibitors. In this study, experimental autoimmune encephalomyelitis (EAE) mice, an animal model of MS, were treated with the HDAC6 inhibitor drug ACY-738 (20 mg/kg) on day 9 and day 10 post-immunization. Mice were assessed for working memory using the cross-maze test at 10 days post-immunization (d.p.i.), whereas disease scores were recorded over approximately 4 weeks post-immunization. We observed that ACY-738 delayed disease onset and reduced disease severity. Most importantly, ACY-738 increased short-term memory in a manner sensitive to disease severity. We induced EAE disease with various amounts of myelin oligodendrocyte glycoprotein (MOG35-55). EAE mice receiving 100 μg of MOG35-55 and treated with ACY-738 had a statistically significant increase in short term-memory compared to naive mice. Additionally, EAE mice receiving 50 μg MOG35-55 and treated with ACY-738 had a statistically significant increase in short term-memory when compared to EAE mice without drug treatment. In contrast, ACY-738 did not change short-term memory in EAE mice immunized with 200 μg of MOG35-55. Because ACY-738 increases short-term memory only with lower amounts of EAE-inducing reagents, we hypothesize that the inflammatory-demyelinating environment induced by higher amount of EAE-inducing reagents overpowers (at day 10 post-immunization) the synaptic molecules targeted by ACY-738. These studies pave the way for developing ACY-738-like compounds for MS patients and for using ACY-738 as a probe to elucidate disease-sensitive changes at the synapses occurring early in the disease course.

Keywords: multiple sclerosis, drug therapy, memory, neurodegeneration, disability, CNS repair

INTRODUCTION

Multiple sclerosis (MS) is a central nervous system (CNS) neurodegenerative disease. The causes of this devastating disease are largely unknown, although autoimmune demyelination and brain inflammation are considered pivotal in the CNS damage that occurs throughout the disease course. In both MS and experimental autoimmune encephalomyelitis (EAE) (an animal model of MS), there are changes in synaptic transmission and function (1, 2) linked to the neurodegeneration, which eventually emerges during the disease with devastating clinical outcomes. Ziehn et al. (3) described deficits in memory function at 40 days post-immunization (d.p.i.) in EAE mice during the chronic form of the disease. Acharjee et al. (4) described emotional and cognitive deficits in chronic EAE during the presymptomatic stage, between 6 and 8 d.p.i. Further, LoPresti (5) identified subclinical, progressive memory decline in the relapsing-remitting (RR) EAE. Indeed, in this model, memory function was not significantly different among groups; however, memory decline occurred over time, with an initial apparent improvement in memory function as early as 10 d.p.i. Although memory function progressively declined, mobility impairment recovered, suggesting that the disease has both progressive and remitting components. Overall, such studies have elucidated that changes in synaptic transmission occur at a relatively early stage during the disease, often subclinically, such early changes may eventually be responsible for late neurodegeneration (6).

The cytoskeleton at the synapse has received attention for its role in synaptic plasticity regulation and various neuropsychiatric diseases (7). At the synapse, key functional interactions involve tubulin, end-binding proteins (EBs), Ankyrin, and actin (8). Such protein-protein interactions at the synapse regulate synaptic function and plasticity. Histone deacetylase (HDAC)6 is a microtubule-associated deacetylase (9), and such protein-protein interaction increases with administration of HDAC6 inhibitors. HDAC6 inhibitors also promote the interaction of HDAC6 with EBs (10).

HDACs are a class of enzymes targeting both histone and non-histone substrates. Non-histone substrates include transcription factors, cytoskeletal proteins, metabolic enzymes, and chaperones (11). HDAC classes consist of 18 types. HDAC6 is localized predominantly in the cytoplasm and does not deacetylate histones *in vivo* (11). The main substrate for HDAC6 is α-tubulin, although additional substrates have been identified. Such substrates include Hsp90 (heat shock protein 90) (12), cortactin (cortical actin binding protein) (13), and beta-catenin (14). Beta-catenin regulates cell–cell adhesion and gene transcription.

In vivo treatment with HDAC6 inhibitors increases brain α-tubulin acetylation, with no changes in acetylation levels of histones (15). Although the loss of HDAC6 does not cause toxicity, apoptosis, or major neurodevelopmental defects in rodents, it causes an antidepressant-like phenotype and memory deficits (16–19).

In this study, we analyzed EAE mice after treatment for only 2 days with the HDAC6 inhibitor ACY-738 and observed that ACY-738 delayed disease onset and attenuated disease severity. In addition, we observed that short-term memory in the cross-maze test was improved in EAE mice treated with the drug at 9 and 10 d.p.i. and tested at 10 d.p.i. Such effect was sensitive to the amount of reagent used to induce the disease.

MATERIALS AND METHODS

EAE Induction

To induce EAE, we used an emulsion obtained from Hooke Lab (EK-0111, Hooke Kit™) and Pertussis toxin (#10033-540, Enzo Life Sciences; VWR). The emulsion from Hooke lab (see **Supplementary Table 1A**) contained ~1 mg/mL of myelin oligodendrocyte glycoprotein (MOG35-55) and ~5 mg/mL of killed *Mycobacterium tuberculosis* H37/Ra (MT). We injected the emulsion at volumes of 200, 100, and 50 µL. Thus, 200 µL contained 200 µg of MOG35-55 and 1 mg of MT, 100 µL contained 100 µg of MOG35-55 and 0.5 mg of MT, and 50 µL contained 50 µg MOG35-55 and 0.250 mg MT. Pertussis toxin (200 ng/100 µL/mouse) remained constant for all experiments and was injected intraperitoneally (ip) on the day of immunization and 2 days later. With higher amounts of reagents, we observed a more severe form of the disease, with a persistent severe disease score above two at 3 weeks post-immunization. With lower amounts of reagents, most of the mice recovered from a severe disease score above two. The mice were examined for ~4 weeks post-immunization. The amounts used in this study to induce chronic (CH) vs. relapsing-remitting (RR)-EAE are included in **Supplementary Table 1A**, together with a summary of previous work showing various concentrations of the reagents used to induce either CH- or RR-EAE (**Supplementary Table 1B**).

C57BL/6 female mice between 7 and 8 weeks of age were ordered from Jackson Laboratory and housed for 1 week before EAE induction. Mice were immunized subcutaneously (sc) (200 µL/mouse) with 200 µg/mouse of MOG35–55 peptide emulsion in complete Freund's adjuvant (CFA) (EK-0111, Hooke Kit™). Experiments were also performed with volumes of 100 µL/mouse and 50 µL/mouse (from kit EK-0111, Hooke Kit™). Pertussis toxin (200 ng/100 µL/mouse) remained constant for all experiments and was injected ip on the day of immunization and 2 days later. EAE mice were graded on a scale of 0–5: 0, no disease; 1, limp tail; 2, hind limb weakness; 3, one or two hind limb paralysis; 4, hind and fore limb paralysis; and 5, moribund and death (5). Disease scores were the averages obtained at each time point from five mice/group/experiment. Mean disease scores (±SEM) were calculated from these disease scores. We collected 44 disease scores per group from seven experiments.

Drug Treatment

ACY-738 powder (Celgene Corporation, Acetylon Pharmaceuticals) was dissolved in dimethyl sulfoxide (DMSO) and diluted in phosphate-buffered saline (PBS) for ip injection of 200 µL (20 mg/kg) on days 9 and 10 post-immunization. The drug was injected on day 9 (~1:00 p.m.) and day 10 (~12:00 p.m.) post-immunization; mice were tested in the cross-maze test on day 10 post-immunization. The EAE mice treated with the drug (EAE+ D) were tested starting 1 hour and 30 min after the last drug injection.

Cross-Maze Exploration Test

The Cross-maze exploration test was performed to evaluate spatial working memory using a protocol described previously (5). Briefly, each mouse was placed in the center of a four-arm cross-maze apparatus and was permitted to enter each arm freely (each arm was marked A, B, C, or D). Each mouse was evaluated for up to 31 entries. An entry occurred when all four paws entered the arm. An alternation occurred when an entry occurred into each of the four distinct arms (e.g., A, D, C, B, or C, D, A, B; but not D, A, C, A). Percentage of alternation was used as an indicator of memory strength, when successive entries took place into the four arms in overlapping quadruple sets. Data are indicated as percent alternation, an indicator of short-term memory. Percent alternation value is equal to the ratio of actual/possible alternations ×100 (5). Data are presented as mean ± SEM in the **Table 2**, and are presented as mean ± SE in the corresponding histogram.

Statistical Analysis

Each experiment comprised five mice/group. Disease scores were the averages calculated from five mice per group at distinct times. Forty-four disease scores were collected per group and from seven independent experiments. Mean disease scores (±SEM) were calculated from the disease scores. Mean disease scores (±SEM) were compared with independent samples t-test. We measured mean disease scores between 11 and 14, 15 and 18, and 19 and 32 d.p.i. In **Table 1**, "n" represents the number of disease scores obtained over time and from distinct experiments. In addition to independent samples t-test, statistical analysis was performed using mixed effects linear regression model. Clustering of observations within experiments (ICC = 0.46, $z = 2.01$, $p = 0.0224$) was accounted for with a random intercept term.

For the cross-maze test, we applied independent samples t-test and one-way ANOVA. At each dosage level, one-way ANOVA with **two** degrees of freedom was used to test the null hypothesis of equal means across all the three groups (naïve, EAE, and EAE + D). Pairwise comparisons were made using independent samples t-test and the more conservative Tukey's test. One-way ANOVA was used to compare the overall mean response across the three dosage levels. For the independent samples t-test, we used GraphPad QuickCalcs online program. For one-way ANOVA and mixed effects linear regression model, we used the PROC ANOVA in SAS version 9.4.

For disease scores, $p < 0.05$ was considered statistically significant using the independent samples t-test. For behavioral test, $p < 0.05$ was considered statistically significant using the independent samples t-test and one-way ANOVA (** $p < 0.05$). One asterisk (*$p < 0.05$, independent samples t-test) denotes $p < 0.1$ with one-way ANOVA.

RESULTS

The Selective HDAC6 Inhibitor ACY-738 Regulates Experimental Autoimmune Encephalomyelitis Disease

Drug administration on days 9 and 10 post-immunization (20 mg/kg) reduced disease severity in both RR and CH EAE. Representative examples are provided in **Figure 1A** for RR-EAE and in **Figure 1B** for CH-EAE. Disease score was the average calculated from five mice/group, indicated in blue for EAE mice and in red for EAE + D mice (**Figures 1A,B**).

Disease scores collected at distinct times over ~4 weeks post-immunization were obtained from seven independent experiments. Disease score was the average calculated from five mice/group at a specific time and from distinct experiments. The experiments included both RR- and CH-EAE disease. **Table 1A** shows that of the 44 disease scores, twenty-five disease scores were higher than 1.5 in EAE mice; whereas only seven disease scores were higher than 1.5 in EAE + D mice. In addition, we calculated mean disease scores (±SEM) from disease scores taken at various times during the disease and from independent experiments. Early in the disease (11–14 d.p.i.), mean disease score was 1.160 ± 0.248 in EAE mice vs. 0.360 ± 0.160 in EAE + D mice, with a statistically significant difference of $p = 0.0267$ ($n = 5$, where n indicates the number of disease scores). During the mid phase of the disease (15–18 d.p.i.), mean disease score was 1.989 ± 0.205 in EAE mice vs. 0.989 ± 0.114 in EAE + D mice, with a statistically significant difference of $p = 0.0001$ ($n = 18$). At the end of disease course (19–32 d.p.i.), mean disease score was 1.657 ± 0.220 in EAE mice vs. 0.857 ± 0.175 in EAE + D mice, with a statistically significant difference of $p = 0.0069$ ($n = 21$). Thus, the difference between untreated and treated groups reached statistical significance (independent samples t-test) over the entire course of the disease. In addition, by combining all the disease scores collected from the various experiments at various times, the cumulative disease score was 76.4 in EAE mice vs. 37.6 in EAE + D mice, which showed an overall reduction in disease severity of about 50%.

In addition, mixed effects linear regression model revealed that the effects of treated vs. untreated was −0.67 ($p = 0.0188$), indicating that the disease score was 0.67 less in the treated animals than in the untreated animals at any time point. Estimated means from the linear regression model and results of the independent samples t-test of the main effects indicate a statistically significant reduction in disease score with treatment ($p = 0.0188$). The estimates from the model accounted for the clustering of repeated measures, whereas the independent samples t-test assumed each of the two compared groups were a set of independent observations. In contrast, the estimated slope in EAE mice was −0.003 ($p = 0.8471$), whereas in EAE + D mice, it was 0.00 ($p = 1.000$). The two parallel lines across time for EAE and EAE + D mice had a common slope of −0.0015 ($p = 0.8907$), indicating a slight decrease that was not statistically significant. Thus, the slope was the same in both groups, suggesting that the disease, although diminished in its severity secondary to drug treatment, was not altered in its dynamics; i.e., the disease displayed similar trends in EAE vs. EAE + D mice, although EAE + D had significantly lower disease scores (**Figure 1C**, **Table 1B**).

Notably, drug treatment delayed disease onset. Disease onset occurred between 11 and 14 d.p.i. **Figure 1A** shows that in RR-EAE +D mice, the disease had not yet started at 14 d.p.i., whereas EAE mice with no drug treatment already

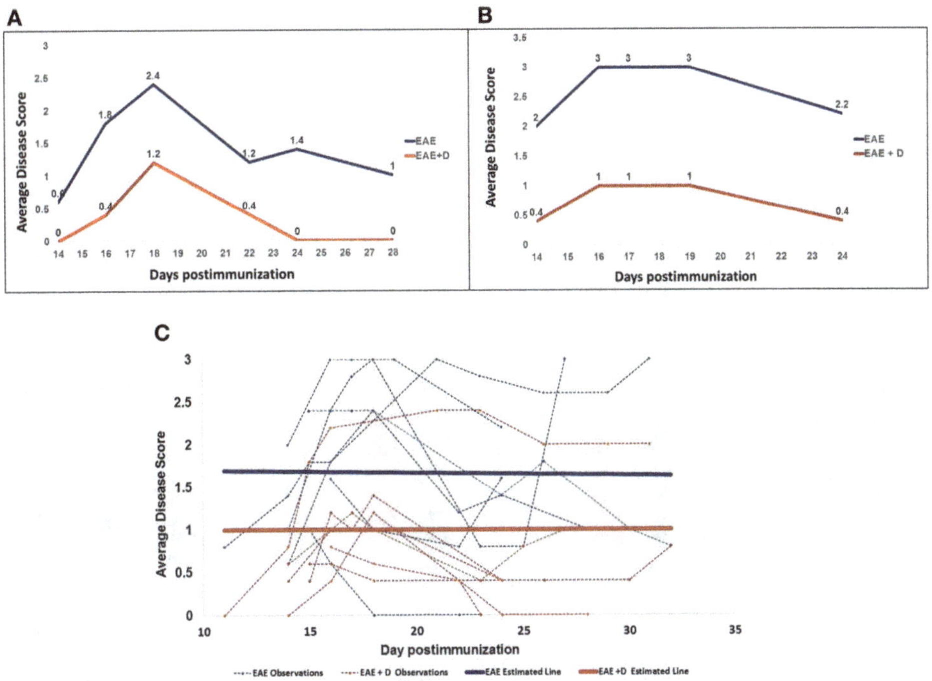

FIGURE 1 | The selective HDAC6 inhibitor ACY-738 regulates experimental autoimmune encephalomyelitis in both Relapsing-Remitting **(A)** and Chronic **(B)** EAE mice. **(C)** Shows all disease scores and an estimated line for the disease scores.

TABLE 1 | (A) Disease score analysis with *t*-test and **(B)** Disease score analysis with mixed effects linear regression model.

(A)

Treatment	Disease score ≥ 1.5	Mean disease score ± SEM at 11–14 d.p.i.	Mean disease score ± SEM at 15–18 d.p.i.	Mean disease score ± SEM at 19–32 d.p.i.	Cumulative disease score
EAE	25/44	1.160 ± 0.248	1.989 ± 0.205	1.657 ± 0.220	76.4
EAE + D	7/44	0.36 ± 0.160	0.989 ± 0.114	0.857 ± 0.175	37.6
		$n = 5$; $p = 0.0267$**	$n = 18$; $p = 0.0001$**	$n = 21$; $p = 0.0069$**	$n = 44$

(B)

	Disease score				*t*-test for EAE vs. EAE + D
	Mean	**SE**	**95% C.I.**		$t = 2.40$, do = 74, $p = 0.0188$
EAE	1.670	0.197	1.241	2.100	
EAE + D	1.000	0.197	0.570	1.430	

The drug administered on days 9 and 10 post-immunization (20 mg/kg) reduced disease severity in both Relapsing-Remitting (RR) ***(A)*** *and Chronic (CH)* ***(B)*** *EAE mice.* ***Figures 1A,B*** *have the disease scores. Each disease score is the average obtained from five mice/group, in blue for EAE mice and in red for EAE + D mice.* ***Figure 1C*** *shows all disease scores collected from seven experiments at distinct times, together with an estimated line for the disease scores of EAE (blue) and EAE + D (red) mice.*

In ***(A)****, n represents the number of disease scores. Among the 44 disease scores per group, EAE mice had twenty-five over 1.5, whereas EAE + D mice had only seven over 1.5.* ***(A)*** *has mean disease scores (± SEM) during early (11–14 d.p.i.), mid phase (15–18 d.p.i.), and at the end of disease course (19–32 d.p.i.) with statistically significant differences in EAE vs. EAE + D mice over the course of the entire disease. The cumulative disease score (from all the disease scores) shows also an overall decrease in disease severity of about 50% in EAE+D mice.* ***(B)*** *displays the statistical analysis with a linear regression model and statistically significant differences between EAE and EAE + D mice (Mean = 1,670 and 1,000, respectively; p = 0.0188). n indicates the number of disease scores. Disease score is the average obtained from five mice/group. **p < 0.05.*

exhibited mobility defects revealed by disease scores above zero. Such delay in disease onset was striking when a high dose (50 mg/kg) of a single drug injection was administered at 10 d.p.i. (**Supplementary Material**). In this experiment conducted with five mice per group, differences were evident at 11 d.p.i. (24 hours post-treatment), suggesting that the drug abruptly halted the disease.

The Selective HDAC6 Inhibitor ACY-738 Regulates Short-Term Memory in a Manner Sensitive to Disease Severity

We measured short-term memory with the cross-maze test at day 10 post-immunization. We combined the data from three independent experiments performed with mice receiving 200

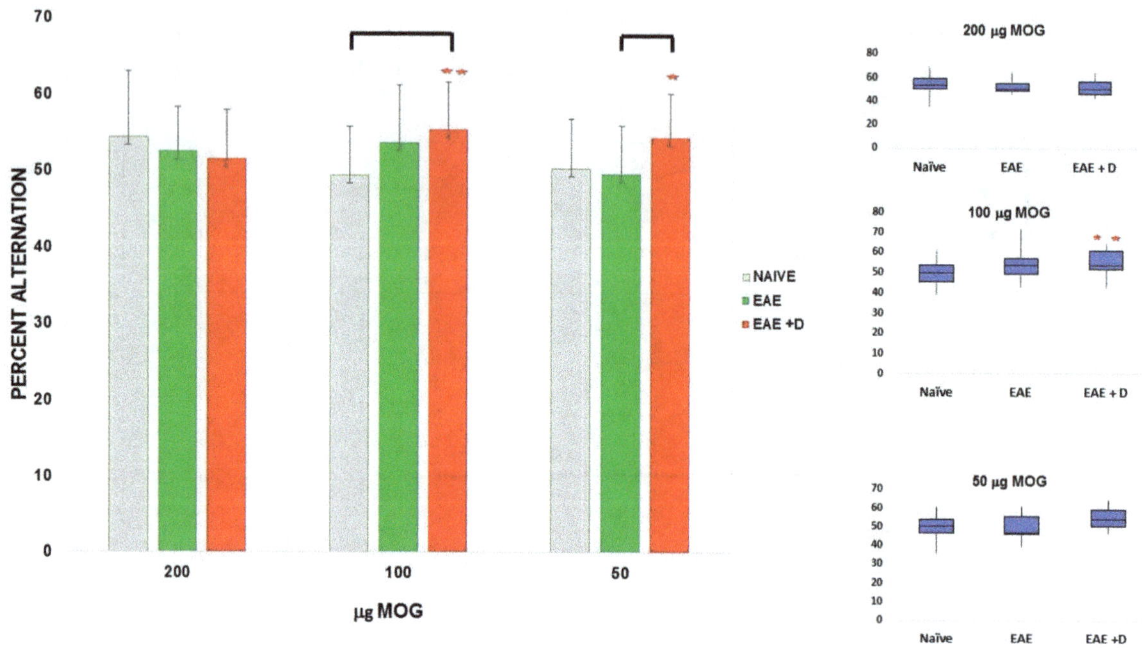

FIGURE 2 | The selective HDAC6 inhibitor ACY-738 regulates short-term memory in a manner sensitive to disease severity. $^{**}p < 0.05$ independent samples t-test and one-way ANOVA. $^{*}p < 0.05$ independent samples t-test.

TABLE 2 | The selective HDAC6 inhibitor ACY-738 regulates short-term memory in a manner sensitive to disease severity.

MOG35-55	NAÏVE (N)		EAE (E)		EAE + D (ED)		*p*-values			
µg	*n*	*t* test mean ± SEM	*n*	*t* test mean ± SEM	*n*	*t* test mean ± SEM	N vs. E	N vs. ED	E vs. ED	One-way ANOVA
200	15	54.3 ± 2.2	15	52.4 ± 1.5	15	51.4 ± 1.8	0.4854	0.3335	0.6950	0.5569
100	20	49.3 ± 1.4	20	53.6 ± 1.7	19	55.3 ± 1.5	0.0613	0.0058**	0.4562	0.0234**
50	15	50.2 ± 1.7	15	49.5 ± 1.6	15	54.3 ± 1.5	0.7633	0.0828	0.0396*	0.0890

*Naïve mice were not administered any drug. EAE was induced with various amounts of EAE-inducing reagents (200, 100, and 50 µg MOG35-55). Data are presented as mean ± SEM in the Table, and as mean ± SE in the corresponding histogram. Comparison with independent samples t-test revealed that in EAE mice administered 100 µg MOG35-55, the difference between Naïve and EAE + D mice was statistically significant (p = 0.0058). This difference was also statistically significant at α = 0.05 using Tukey's studentized range test. Comparison with independent samples t-test revealed that in mice receiving 50 µg MOG35-55, the difference between EAE and EAE + D mice was also statistically significant (p = 0.0396). One-way ANOVA revealed a statistically significant difference in the group administered 100 µg MOG35-55 (F = 4.02, p = 0.0234) and in the group administered 50 µg MOG35-55 (F = 2.56, p = 0.0890). One-way ANOVA data are displayed as boxplots. In boxplots, the central black line represents the median, the bottom and top boundaries represent quartiles. n indicates the number of mice. **p < 0.05 independent samples t-test and one-way ANOVA. *p < 0.05 independent samples t-test.*

µg MOG35-55. No significant differences among the groups were observed. We combined the data from four independent experiments performed with 100 µg MOG35-55. A statistically significant difference between Naïve and EAE + D groups was observed. We combined the data from three independent experiments performed with 50 µg MOG35-55. A statistically significant difference between EAE and EAE + D groups was noted (**Figure 2** and **Table 2**).

Experiments With 200 µg MOG35-55

Fifteen mice ($n = 5$ each for Naïve, EAE, and EAE + D) were used for each experiment. Each experiment was repeated three times, and the data obtained with the cross-maze test on day 10 post-immunization were combined. We observed that the difference between Naïve and EAE mice was not statistically significant (mean ± SEM, 54.3 ± 2.2 vs. 52.4 ± 1.5, respectively; $p = 0.4854$). The difference between Naïve and EAE + D mice was not statistically significant (mean ± SEM, 54.3 ± 2.2 vs. 51.4 ± 1.8, respectively; $p = 0.3335$). In addition, the difference between EAE and EAE + D mice was not statistically significant (mean ± SEM, 52.4 ± 1.5 vs. 51.4 ± 1.8, respectively; $p = 0.6950$). There were also no statistically significant differences across the means of the three groups as determined by one-way ANOVA ($F = 0.59$, $p = 0.5569$).

Experiments With 100 µg MOG35-55

Fifteen mice ($n = 5$ each for Naïve, EAE, and EAE + D) were used for each experiment. Each experiment was repeated four times, and the data were combined. In one of the experiments, only fourteen mice were analyzed ($n = 5$ each for Naïve and EAE, and $n = 4$ for EAE + D). We observed that the difference between Naïve and EAE mice was not statistically significant (mean ± SEM, 49.3 ± 1.4 vs. 53.6 ± 1.7, respectively; $p = 0.0613$); whereas the difference between Naïve and EAE + D mice was statistically significant (mean ± SEM, 49.3 ± 1.4 vs. 55.3 ± 1.5, respectively; $p = 0.0058$). Such difference was significant at $\alpha = 0.05$ using Tukey's studentized range test. In contrast, the difference between EAE and EAE + D mice was not statistically significant (mean ± SEM, 53.6 ± 1.7 vs. 55.3 ± 1.5, respectively; $p = 0.4562$). One-way ANOVA, revealed a statistically significant difference between the three group means (F = 4.02, df = 2, $p = 0.0234$).

Experiments With 50 μg MOG35-55

Fifteen mice ($n = 5$ each for Naïve, EAE, and EAE + D) were used for each experiment. Each experiment was repeated three times, and the data were combined. We found that the difference between Naïve and EAE mice was not statistically significant (mean ± SEM, 50.2 ± 1.7 vs. 49.5 ± 1.6, respectively; $p = 0.7633$). The difference between Naïve and EAE + D mice was not statistically significant (mean ± SEM, 50.2 ± 1.7 vs. 54.3 ± 1.5, respectively; $p = 0.0828$). In contrast, the difference between EAE and EAE + D mice was statistically significant (mean ± SEM, 49.5 ± 1.6 vs. 54.3 ± 1.5, respectively; $p = 0.0396$). There was a statistically significant difference between group means as determined by one-way ANOVA (F = 2.56, df = 2, $p = 0.0890$). The contrast between EAE vs. EAE+ D was significant using a independent samples t-test but not under the more conservative Tukey's test. Comparison of all the data in the group with 200, 100, and 50 μg MOG35-55 revealed no statistically significant differences across the group means as determined by one-way ANOVA (F = 0.57, df = 2, $p = 0.5665$) (data not shown).

DISCUSSION

The positive effects of ACY-738 on disease course occurred after one or two injections, and protection occurred within 24 hours post-treatment. Work by Ren et al. (20) showed that ACY-738 decreased innate and adaptive immune responses in a model of systemic lupus erythematosus; ACY-738 reduced disease pathogenesis by altering differentiation of T and B cells (21). However, these positive effects were observed after long-term treatment lasting several weeks. We did not assess the mechanisms by which ACY-738 protects from EAE disease; however, the beneficial outcomes within 24 hours post-treatment may be related to an effect of ACY-738 on the neuronal cytoskeleton and/or secondary to a lethal, acute, effect of ACY-738 against cells attacking myelin. Indeed, it was previously shown that ACY-738 induces cell death *in vitro* when used at high concentrations (22). In addition, Guo et al. (23) reported that HDAC6 inhibition reverses axonal transport defects in motor neurons derived from FUS-ALS patients. Mutations in FUS (fused in sarcoma) cause amyotrophic lateral sclerosis (ALS). It is known that early in EAE, axonal transport deficits are present, and reduced levels of KIF5A (kinesin heavy chain isoform 5A) were reported in MS patients (6, 24, 25). Thus, part of the beneficial effects observed for the disease course could be secondary to positive regulation of axonal transport exerted by ACY-738. Indeed, the inhibition of HDAC6 may regulate both anterograde and retrograde transport due to the regulation of kinesin and dynein motors (26).

Acetylation of α-tubulin occurs at lysine 40 at the inner surface. Additional sites of acetylation have been identified in both α- and β- tubulin (27). Further studies are required to determine the functional consequences of HDAC6 inhibitors on post-translational modification of these various sites of tubulin. This information could facilitate effective pharmacological targeting of cytoskeleton dynamics at the synapse, with beneficial impacts on axonal transport regulation.

Drugs such as TSA (Trichostatin A) or SAHA (suberoyl + anilide + hydroxamic acid) inhibit both HDAC6 and class I isoforms, whereas drugs such as tubacin and tubastatin A selectively inhibit HDAC6 (11, 28, 29). Interestingly, ACY-738 is a selective inhibitor of HDAC6 and has the unique property of rapid distribution in the brain, with a short plasma half-life of 12 min (11).

Pathways that regulate synaptic plasticity are critical for brain health and prevention of neuropsychiatric and degenerative diseases (7). In this study, we developed an experimental model that can establish pharmacological targets at the synaptic cytoskeleton upon which ACY-738 acts. Further, ACY-738 will allow us to investigate how short-term memory is regulated. While the role of HDAC6 in synaptic plasticity and memory is established (30), the dynamics of cytoskeletal interactions at the synapse require additional investigation. Our model may reveal dynamic regulation at synapses that requires pharmacologic rescue to treat selective memory deficits during various diseases of the CNS.

Jochems et al. (11) reported that upon acute treatment, ACY-738 improved ambulation levels and decreased anxiety. Majid et al. (31) showed that ACY-738 improved Alzheimer's disease phenotype in amyloid precursor protein/presenilin 1 mice. In particular, this study indicated that drug administration increased cognition; however, the drug was administered for 21 and 90 days. In addition, Selenica et al. (32) showed that tubastatin A, a selective HDAC6 inhibitor, improved memory and reduced total tau levels in a mouse model of tau deposition. However, the mice were treated for 2 months. Zhang et al. (33) used tubastatin A and ACY-1215 to rescue cognitive deficits in a mouse model of Alzheimer's disease and found that both tubastatin A and ACY-1215 reduced behavioral deficits, amyloid-β load, and tau hyperphosphorylation. However, the mice were treated for 20 consecutive days; ACY-1215 is a selective HDAC6 inhibitor. In contrast, in this study, we analyzed mice after treatment with ACY-738 for only two days and observed an increase of short-term memory.

The cross-maze test relies on working memory, which depends on selected CNS areas including the hippocampus, septum, basal forebrain, and prefrontal cortex. The cytoskeleton at the synapse has a role in synaptic plasticity regulation and various neuropsychiatric diseases (7). Protein-protein interactions at the synapse regulate synaptic function and plasticity. At the synapse, key functional interactions involve tubulin, EBs, ankyrins, and actin (8). HDAC6 inhibitors increase the interaction of HDAC6 with microtubules and EBs (10).

HDAC6 also regulates growth factor-induced actin remodeling and endocytosis (34); thus, HDAC6 inhibitors may also alter functional regulation of actin. Anxiety- and depression-like behaviors were described in EAE mice before any motor defect became apparent (2, 4), so our experimental conditions may have brought the antidepressive properties of ACY-738 to light (11). Finally, the positive effects on memory may be partly explained by enhancement of stress resilience through HDAC6-mediated regulation of glucocorticoid receptor chaperone dynamics (11). In this respect, additional studies are necessary to elucidate the mechanisms by which ACY-738 acts on memory regulation. Nicotine, previously shown to inhibit HDAC6 and chaperone-dependent activation of glucocorticoid receptors in cultured cells, had a neuroprotective effect in an experimental model of MS (35, 36). In summary, with the aim of developing the most effective treatments for MS patients, future studies should aim to understand similarities and differences among various inhibitors directed at HDAC6, so selective drugs of such class with the highest safety and efficacy could provide breakthrough therapy for the neurodegeneration in patients affected by MS.

AUTHOR CONTRIBUTIONS

The author confirms being the sole contributor of this work and has approved it for publication.

FUNDING

This work was supported by Celgene Corporation/ Acetylon Pharmaceuticals. The funders had no role in study design, data collection and analysis, decision to publish, or preparation of the manuscript.

ACKNOWLEDGMENTS

PL thanks Professor Sally Freels (Division of Epidemiology and Biostatistics, School of Public Health, University of Illinois at Chicago) for assistance in preparing sections related to the Statistical Analysis.

REFERENCES

1. Centonze D, Muzio L, Rossi S, Furlan R, Bernardi G, Martino G. The link between inflammation, synaptic transmission and neurodegeneration in multiple sclerosis. *Cell Death Differ.* (2010) 17:1083–91. doi: 10.1038/cdd.2009.179
2. Haji N, Mandolesi G, Gentile A, Sacchetti L, Fresegna D, Rossi S, et al. TNF-α-mediated anxiety in a mouse model of multiple sclerosis. *Exp Neurol.* (2012) 237:296–303. doi: 10.1016/j.expneurol.2012.07.010
3. Ziehn MO, Avedisian AA, Tiwari-Woodruff S, Voskuhl RR. Hippocampal CA1 atrophy and synaptic loss during experimental autoimmune encephalomyelitis, EAE. *Lab Invest.* (2010) 90:774–86. doi: 10.1038/labinvest.2010.6
4. Acharjee S, Nayani N, Tsutsui M, Hill MN, Ousman SS, Pittman QJ. Altered cognitive-emotional behavior in early experimental autoimmune encephalitis–cytokine and hormonal correlates. *Brain Behav Immun.* (2013) 33:164–72. doi: 10.1016/j.bbi.2013.07.003
5. LoPresti P. Glatiramer acetate guards against rapid memory decline during relapsing-remitting experimental autoimmune encephalomyelitis. *Neurochem Res.* (2015) 40:473–9. doi: 10.1007/s11064-014-1491-z
6. LoPresti P. Silent free fall at disease onset, a perspective on therapeutics for progressive multiple sclerosis. *Front Neurol.* (2018) 9:973. doi: 10.3389/fneur.2018.00973
7. Forrest MP, Parnell E, Penzes P. Dendritic structural plasticity and neuropsychiatric disease. *Nat Rev Neurosci.* (2018) 19:215–34. doi: 10.1038/nrn.2018.16
8. Smith KR, Penzes P. Ankyrins: roles in synaptic biology and pathology. *Mol Cell Neurosci.* (2018) 91:131–9. doi: 10.1016/j.mcn.2018.04.010
9. Hubbert C, Guardiola A, Shao R, Kawaguchi Y, Ito A, Nixon A, et al. HDAC6 is a microtubule-associated deacetylase. *Nature.* (2002) 417:455–8. doi: 10.1038/417455a
10. Zilberman Y, Ballestrem C, Carramusa L, Mazitschek R, Khochbin S, Bershadsky A. Regulation of microtubule dynamics by inhibition of the tubulin deacetylase HDAC6. *J Cell Sci.* (2009) 122:3531–41. doi: 10.1242/jcs.046813
11. Jochems J, Boulden J, Lee BG, Blendy JA, Jarpe M, Mazitschek R, et al. Antidepressant-like properties of novel HDAC6-selective inhibitors with improved brain bioavailability. *Neuropsychopharmacology.* (2014) 239:389–400. doi: 10.1038/npp.2013.207
12. Kovacs JJ, Murphy PJ, Gaillard S, Zhao X, Wu JT, Nicchitta CV, et al. HDAC6 regulates Hsp90 acetylation and chaperone-dependent activation of glucocorticoid receptor. *Mol Cell.* (2005) 18:601–7. doi: 10.1016/j.molcel.2005.04.021
13. Zhang X, Yuan Z, Zhang Y, Yong S, Salas-Burgos A, Koomen J, et al. HDAC6 modulates cell motility by altering the acetylation level of cortactin. *Mol Cell.* (2007) 27:197–213. doi: 10.1016/j.molcel.2007.05.033
14. Li Y, Zhang X, Polakiewicz RD, Yao TP, Comb MJ. HDAC6 is required for epidermal growth factor-induced beta-catenin nuclear localization. *J Biol Chem.* (2008) 283:12686–90. doi: 10.1074/jbc.C700185200
15. Rivieccio MA, Brochier C, Willis DE, Walker BA, D'Annibale MA, McLaughlin K, et al. HDAC6 is a target for protection and regeneration following injury in the nervous system. *Proc Natl Acad Sci USA.* (2009) 106:19599–604. doi: 10.1073/pnas.0907935106
16. Haberland M, Montgomery RL, Olson EN. The many roles of histone deacetylases in development and physiology: implications for disease and therapy. *Nat Rev Genet.* (2009) 10:32–42. doi: 10.1038/nrg2485
17. Du G, Liu X, Chen X, Song M, Yan Y, Jiao R, et al. Drosophila histone deacetylase 6 protects dopaminergic neurons against -synuclein toxicity by promoting inclusion formation. *Mol Biol Cell.* (2010) 21:2128–37. doi: 10.1091/mbc.e10-03-0200
18. Govindarajan N, Rao P, Burkhardt S, Sananbenesi F, Schlüter OM, Bradke F, et al. Reducing HDAC6 ameliorates cognitive deficits in a mouse model for Alzheimer's disease. *EMBO Mol Med.* (2012) 5:52–63. doi: 10.1002/emmm.201201923
19. Zhang Y, Kwon S, Yamaguchi T, Cubizolles F, Rousseaux S, Kneissel M, et al. Mice lacking histone deacetylase 6 have hyperacetylated tubulin but are viable and develop normally. *Mol Cell Biol.* (2008) 28:1688–701. doi: 10.1128/MCB.01154-06
20. Ren J, Liao X, Vieson MD, Chen M, Scott R, Kazmierczak J, et al. Selective HDAC6 inhibition decreases early stage of lupus nephritis by down-regulating both innate and adaptive immune responses. *Clin Exp Immunol.* (2018) 191:19–31. doi: 10.1111/cei.13046
21. Regna NL, Vieson MD, Luo XM, Chafin CB, Puthiyaveetil AG, Hammond SE, et al. Specific HDAC6 inhibition by ACY-738 reduces SLE pathogenesis in NZB/W mice. *Clin Immunol.* (2016) 162:58–73. doi: 10.1016/j.clim.2015.11.007
22. Mithraprabhu S, Khong T, Jones SS, Spencer A. Histone deacetylase (HDAC) inhibitors as single agents induce multiple myeloma cell death principally through the inhibition of class I HDAC. *Br J Haematol.* (2013) 162:559–62. doi: 10.1111/bjh.12388
23. Guo W, Naujock M, Fumagalli L, Vandoorne T, Baatsen P, Boon R, et al. HDAC6 inhibition reverses axonal transport defects in motor neurons derived from FUS-ALS patients. *Nat Commun.* (2017) 8:861. doi: 10.1038/s41467-017-00911-y
24. Errea OBM, Gonzalez-Franquesa A, Garcia-Roves P, Villoslada P. The disruption of mitochondrial axonal transport is an early

event in neuroinflammation. *J Neuroinflamm.* (2015) 12:152–67. doi: 10.1186/s12974-015-0375-8
25. Sorbara CD, Wagner NE, Ladwig A, Nikić I, Merkler D, Kleele T, et al. Pervasive axonal transport deficits in multiple sclerosis models. *Neuron.* (2014) 84:1183–90. doi: 10.1016/j.neuron.2014.11.006
26. Chen S, Owens GC, Makarenkova H, Edelman DB. HDAC6 regulates mitochondrial transport in hippocampal neurons. *PLoS ONE.* (2010) 5:e10848. doi: 10.1371/journal.pone.0010848
27. Sadoul K, Khochbin S. The growing landscape of tubulin acetylation: lysine 40 and many more. *Biochem J.* (2016) 473:1859–68. doi: 10.1042/BCJ20160172
28. Bertrand P. Inside HDAC with HDAC inhibitors. *Eur J Med Chem.* (2010) 45:2095–116. doi: 10.1016/j.ejmech.2010.02.030
29. Butler KV, Kalin J, Brochier C, Vistoli G, Langley B, Kozikowski AP. Rational design and simple chemistry yield a superior, neuroprotective HDAC6 inhibitor, tubastatin A. *J Am Chem Soc.* (2010) 132:10842–6. doi: 10.1021/ja102758v
30. Perry S, Kiragasi B, Dickman D, Ray A. The role of histone deacetylase 6 in synaptic plasticity and memory. *Cell Rep.* (2017) 8:1337–45. doi: 10.1016/j.celrep.2017.01.028
31. Majid T, Griffin D, Criss ZII, Jarpe M, Pautler RG. Pharmocologic treatment with histone deacetylase 6 inhibitor (ACY-738) recovers Alzheimer's disease phenotype in amyloid precursor protein/presenilin 1 (APP/PS1) mice. *Alzheimers Dement.* (2015) 1:170–81. doi: 10.1016/j.trci.2015.08.001
32. Selenica ML, Benner L, Housley SB, Manchec B, Lee DC, Nash KR, et al. Histone deacetylase 6 inhibition improves memory and reduces total tau levels in a mouse model of tau deposition. *Alzheimers Res Ther.* (2014) 6:12. doi: 10.1186/alzrt241
33. Zhang L, Liu C, Wu J, Tao JJ, Sui XL, Yao ZG, et al. Tubastatin A/ACY-1215 improves cognition in Alzheimer's disease transgenic mice. *J Alzheimers Dis.* (2014) 41:1193–205. doi: 10.3233/JAD-140066
34. Gao YS, Hubbert CC, Lu J, Lee YS, Lee JY, Yao TP. Histone deacetylase 6 regulates growth factor-induced actin remodeling and endocytosis. *Mol Cell Biol.* (2007) 27:8637–47. doi: 10.1128/MCB.00393-07
35. Sun LC, Lin JT, Li W, Zhang L, Zhou TL, Zhang XY. Nicotine inhibits histone deacetylase 6 activity and chaperone-dependent activation of the glucocorticoid receptor in A549 cells. *Chin Med J.* (2012) 125:662–6. doi: 10.3760/cma.j.issn.0366-6999.2012.04.019
36. Naddafi F, Reza Haidari M, Azizi G, Sedaghat R, Mirshafiey A. Novel therapeutic approach by nicotine in experimental model of multiple sclerosis. *Innov Clin Neurosci.* (2013) 10:20–5. doi: 10.1007/s13760-014-0392-x

9

Pathogenic Mechanisms Associated With Different Clinical Courses of Multiple Sclerosis

*Hans Lassmann**

Center for Brain Research, Medical University of Vienna, Vienna, Austria

Correspondence:
Hans Lassmann
hans.lassmann@meduniwien.ac.at

In the majority of patients multiple sclerosis starts with a relapsing remitting course (RRMS), which may at later times transform into secondary progressive disease (SPMS). In a minority of patients the relapsing remitting disease is skipped and the patients show progression from the onset (primary progressive MS, PPMS). Evidence obtained so far indicate major differences between RRMS and progressive MS, but no essential differences between SPMS and PPMS, with the exception of a lower incidence in the global load of focal white matter lesions and in particular in the presence of classical active plaques in PPMS. We suggest that in MS patients two types of inflammation occur, which develop in parallel but partially independent from each other. The first is the focal bulk invasion of T- and B-lymphocytes with profound blood brain barrier leakage, which predominately affects the white matter, and which gives rise to classical active demyelinated plaques. The other type of inflammation is a slow accumulation of T-cells and B-cells in the absence of major blood brain barrier damage in the connective tissue spaces of the brain, such as the meninges and the large perivascular Virchow Robin spaces, where they may form aggregates or in most severe cases structures in part resembling tertiary lymph follicles. This type of inflammation is associated with the formation of subpial demyelinated lesions in the cerebral and cerebellar cortex, with slow expansion of pre-existing lesions in the white matter and with diffuse neurodegeneration in the normal appearing white or gray matter. The first type of inflammation dominates in acute and relapsing MS. The second type of inflammation is already present in early stages of MS, but gradually increases with disease duration and patient age. It is suggested that $CD8^+$ T-lymphocytes remain in the brain and spinal cord as tissue resident cells, which may focally propagate neuroinflammation, when they re-encounter their cognate antigen. B-lymphocytes may propagate demyelination and neurodegeneration, most likely by producing soluble neurotoxic factors. Whether lymphocytes within the brain tissue of MS lesions have also regulatory functions is presently unknown. Key open questions in MS research are the identification of the target antigen recognized by tissue resident $CD8^+$ T-cells and B-cells and the molecular nature of the soluble inflammatory mediators, which may trigger tissue damage.

Keywords: relapsing remitting MS, secondary progressive MS, primary progressive MS, inflammation, demyelination, neurodegeneration

INTRODUCTION

Multiple sclerosis is a chronic inflammatory disease of the central nervous system which leads to the formation of focal confluent lesions of primary demyelination in the white and gray matter and to diffuse damage and neurodegeneration in the entire brain (1). In general the disease starts in patients in the third decade of life with a relapsing and remitting clinical course. On average after 10–15 years the disease in the majority of patients converts into a course of slow progression (secondary progressive MS). In a subset of patients, in particular in those with higher age at onset, the disease starts with a progressive course [primary progressive MS; (2)]. It is currently an open debate, whether primary progressive MS is a distinct disease entity or whether it just represents part of the variable clinical disease spectrum (3–5). This question has major pathogenic implications. Most researchers regard MS as a primary inflammatory disease, in which demyelination and tissue injury is driven by immune mediated mechanisms throughout all different stages and in all different courses (6, 7). In this case PPMS would be just a clinical variant of a common disease process. The other view suggests that MS is a primary neurodegenerative disease, which is modified and amplified by the inflammatory process. In this situation PPMS could reflect the primary disease process of MS and the other courses (RRMS and SPMS) are those, modified by an inflammatory reaction (3).

There is no doubt that major differences exist between the relapsing and progressive stages of MS and this is also reflected by the different response to currently available immunosuppressive or immunomodulatory treatments (8, 9). However, there is an overlap in pathological features, pathogenic mechanisms and therapeutic responses between relapsing and progressive MS (10, 11). In particular, evidence for subclinical disease activity, defined by the presence of new focal contrast enhancing lesions, can be present in patients with SPMS as well as PPMS. For this reason, it has been suggested to classify MS patients, who have entered the progressive disease stage into those with or without evidence of disease activity and with or without disease progression (2). The consequence of such a clinical disease classification could be to skip the distinction between primary and secondary progressive MS. Whether this may be justified or not and what are the pathogenic implications will be discussed in this review article.

CLINICAL COURSE, EPIDEMIOLOGY, AND GENETICS

Clinical and MRI Features

The term primary progressive MS clinically defines a disease, which develops with increase of neurological deficits in the absence of prior or intermittent exacerbations and remissions. This differs from the relapsing-remitting course of the disease, characterized by new bouts of the disease followed by stages of clinical remission. Relapsing/remitting MS may after several years of disease duration, and when patients have reached a moderate level of clinical disability (EDSS scape 3–4), transform into a secondary progressive disease course (12, 13). While disease relapses are associated with new and contrast enhancing lesions in MRI, the brain and spinal cord changes during progressive disease were thought to be reflected by a steady increase of brain and spinal cord atrophy. However, using more sophisticated tools for clinical monitoring of the patients, as for instance applied in controlled therapeutic trials, it turned out that a significant proportion of patients with PPMS and SPMS show signs of clinical or MRI-based "disease activity" (2) as defined above. Overall, no qualitative differences regarding disease activity between PPMS and SPMS were found, although, as reflected by the original disease definitions, relapses associated with new focal white matter lesions are less frequent in PPMS. Similarly, no essential differences between SPMS and PPMS were seen by MRI (14).

The average disease onset in patients with RRMS is within the third decade of life. In contrast disease onset in patients with PPMS peaks in the 5th decade of life, which is similar to the age, when patients with RRMS tend to convert into SPMS (15, 16). Clinical disease severity and the speed of disease progression is highly variable between patients, but on average the speed of progression is similar between patients with PPMS and SPMS, and is independent from the severity of previous relapses of the disease (12, 13).

GENETICS

The male to female ratio in patients with RRMS and SPMS is 1:3, while patients with PPMS show a lower female predominance (10, 17). Interestingly, disease risk is also transferred from unaffected females to their MS affected offspring than from males, raising the possibilities of the involvement of mitochondrial genes, epigenetic effects or a pathogenic role of intrauterine exposure to exogenous risk factors (18). Genome wide association studies have now identified numerous gene regions, associated with increased disease susceptibility, each of the individual genes providing only a very minor effect (19, 20). Interestingly nearly all of the gene regions identified so far contain genes involved in immune mechanisms, which is in line with clinical, immunological, and neuropathological data defining MS as an immune mediated disease. Importantly, within the familial risk in multiplex families there is no clear discrimination between the different MS courses. Thus, within the same family different patients may develop relapsing, secondary or primary progressive MS, although the concordance rate of clinical courses is moderately increased in siblings of the PPMS cohort (21, 22). In line with these observations, so far no clear differences in genetic associations became evident between PPMS and other disease forms in genome wide association studies (23). However, recent studies suggest that different genes may be associated with relapse risk vs. the speed of EDSS increase (24) and genetic variants, described to be pathogenic in some neurodegenerative diseases, have been identified in a (small) subset of patients with PPMS, but not in patients with other disease courses (23). One of these examples is a variant of a gene involved in transcriptional regulation (NR1H3), which was only found to be associated with PPMS, but not with other disease forms (25). This observation, however, also highlights a caveat regarding the interpretation of such data, since it has not been confirmed in a detailed analysis of the much larger dataset (26). Overall, however, these data indicate that there is a basic polygenic pattern determining the global MS risk and this is the same for all disease courses and involves immune mediated mechanisms (27), while the development of progressive disease may be additionally fostered by genetic variants associated with lipid metabolism or neurodegeneration. However, this may not apply for all, but only for a small subset of patients with PPMS.

IMMUNOLOGY AND BIOMARKERS

Many immunological studies have been performed with the aim to identify MS specific biomarkers and disease mechanisms and to find markers able to predict clinical disease course and outcome. These data are summarized in comprehensive recent review articles (28, 29). Besides MRI and markers related to therapy (induction of blocking antibodies) or JC virus infection, they include markers for neurodegeneration, such as neurofilaments, markers for astrocytic activation (e.g., chitinase or GFAP). Neurofilament protein detected in the serum or cerebrospinal fluid appears to be a good marker for the extent of active neurodegeneration, but this is not MS specific. Chitinase may be a good marker for active disease in relapsing remitting disease, reflecting the degree of astrocyte activation, or damage in active lesions.

So far the highest clinical relevance is reported for the presence of intrathecal immunoglobulin synthesis, reflected by an increased IgG index and oligoclonal bands. It is associated with MS with high sensitivity, but found also in other (chronic) inflammatory diseases of the central nervous system (30). Regarding PPMS its presence is an important paraclinical marker for diagnosis and, thus, detection of intrathecal IgG synthesis has been re-introduced into the new diagnostic criteria (31). Cytokines, chemokines, and adhesion molecules have been analyzed and a comprehensive immunophenotyping of inflammatory cells in the cerebrospinal fluid has been performed as well. Overall these studies showed increased levels in MS serum and CSF, being most significantly altered in patients with (active) RRMS followed by patients with SPMS and PPMS (32–34). These markers have some clinical value for diagnosis and monitoring of disease activity, but none of them have turned out to specific for MS. In addition, so far no specific serum or CSF marker profile has been identified, which allows the distinction between SPMS and PPMS.

To overcome this problem, the question regarding potential biomarkers for MS diagnosis and clinical subtypes has recently been approached with an innovative technology. By using an unbiased simultaneous screening for the concentration of 1.128 proteins together with new machine learning and bioinformatics technology, CSF protein profiles were established in a large sample of patients with RRMS, SPMS, and PPMS and the findings were compared with those seen in patients with other inflammatory and non-inflammatory CNS diseases (35). Using these new tools profiles were detected, which allowed to differentiate between MS and other inflammatory or non-inflammatory CNS diseases and to clearly separate RRMS from progressive forms of the disease. However, no significant differences appeared in the comparison between SPMS and PPMS. Deciphering the biomarker profile defined important pathogenic pathways. The protein profiles, which allowed the best differentiation between MS and other inflammatory CNS diseases, were those related to B-cell and Plasma cell function. This may represent an independent confirmation of the long standing observation that intrathecal immunoglobulin synthesis occurs in MS patients (30, 36). However, it also is in line with observations from pathology, that the contribution of B-cells differentiates MS lesions from non-MS inflammatory brain diseases better than it is the case for T-cell subsets or the activation of macrophages and microglia (37, 38). However, this profound B-cell component in the inflammatory response may not be specific for MS, since it is apparently also seen in certain other chronic human inflammatory diseases of the central nervous system, such as neurotuberculosis, borreliosis, lues, and others (39–41).

The CSF protein profiles most significantly associated with progressive MS were related to the formation of tertiary lymph follicles, and these markers were also associated with the extent of subpial cortical demyelinating pathology (42). Other markers being prominent in patients with progressive disease were related to innate immunity activation and oxidative injury as well as markers, which reflect neuronal and axonal injury, such as for instance neurofilament protein (42–44).

In another approach an un-biased metabolomic plasma profiling has been performed in PP vs. RRMS patients and the data were further compared to those obtained from patients with Parkinson's disease and healthy controls (45). The most dramatic metabolic changes were seen in PPMS patients and were mainly related to decreased profiles of glycerophospholipids and linoleic acid metabolism. These changes were not only present in the global MS population in comparison to controls, but even allowed to discriminate PPMS from RRMS. SPMS patients were not included in this study. It remains unresolved, whether these lipid changes just reflect the higher degree of global demyelination and neurodegeneration in progressive MS vs. RRMS. In addition, information on these lipid changes in proper disease controls with brain inflammation, demyelination or neurodegeneration is very limited.

Overall the immunological and metabolic data suggest that there are quantitative differences in immunological and neurobiological marker profiles between relapsing and progressive MS, which indicate that inflammation (systemic and intrathecal) is more pronounced in patients with relapsing disease and neurodegenerative events are more severe in the progressive stage of the disease. However, such differences vanish, when SPMS and PPMS patients are directly compared.

NEUROPATHOLOGY AND IMMUNOPATHOLOGY

There are several pathological hallmarks, which distinguish MS from other diseases of the central nervous system (1). The

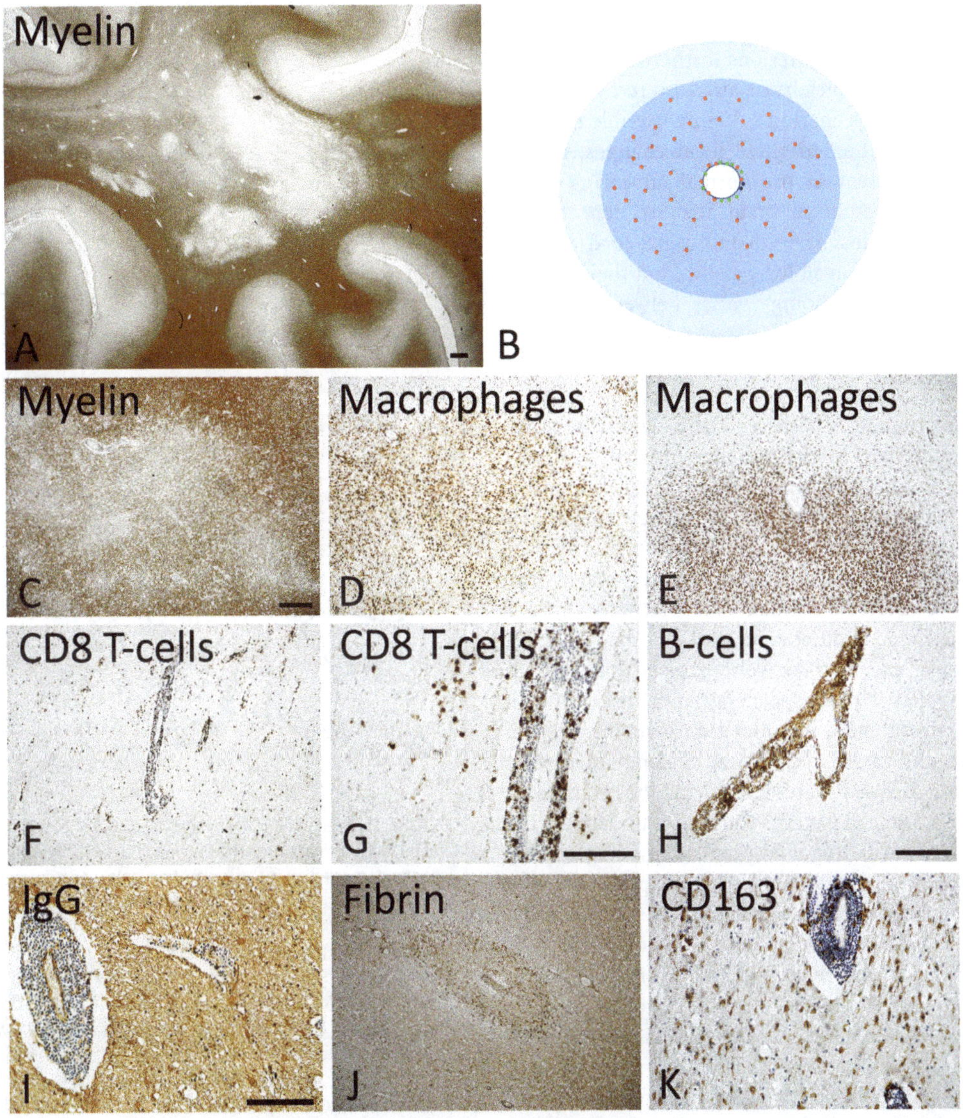

FIGURE 1 | Active Lesions in early MS (acute and RRMS). **(A)** The dominant pathology in early MS is the presence of focal confluent demyelinated lesions in the white matter, many of them being in the stage of activity; section of a patient with acute multiple sclerosis, stained for myelin by immunohistochemistry for proteolipid protein. Magnification bar: 1 mm. **(B)** The classical active lesions in early MS develop around a central vein with inflammatory infiltrates, composed of $CD8^+$ T-cells (red), CD20 positive B-cells (green), and few plasma cells (blue). While B-cells and plasma cells mainly remain in the perivascular space, the $CD8^+$ T-cells also diffusely infiltrate the lesion parenchyme. The lesion (blue) is massively infiltrated by macrophages. Many of the lymphocytes are in the process of passing the vessel wall and this is associated with profound blood brain barrier leakage. This results in profound edema, which expands beyond the area of active demyelination (light blue). **(C–E)** Myelin staining (immunocytochemistry for proteolipid protein) shows patchy areas of active demyelination, which is associated with dense infiltration of the tissue by macrophages **(D,E)**. **(F, G)** Immunohistochemistry for the T-cell marker CD8 shows perivascular accumulation of T-cells, and their diffuse infiltration of the lesion parenchyme. **(H)** The perivascular inflammatory infiltrates contain numerous $CD20^+$ B-lymphocytes. **(I,J)** Staining for IgG reveals massive leakage of the blood brain barrier and only a small number of IgG containing plasma cells in the perivascular space **(I)**; the profound blood brain barrier leakage is also reflected by extensive leakage of fibrinogen through the inflamed vessels **(J)**. **(K)** A subset of macrophages expresses the activation marker CD163, a feature which is typically found in active MS lesions. The magnification bars in the figures **(C,G,I)** represent 100 μm. Similar histological images as shown in this figure have been previously published. Structure of the lesions: Frischer et al. (46); Inflammatory reaction: Frischer et al. (47); Machado Santos et al. (37); Microglia and macrophages: Zrzavy et al. (38); Fibrin and blood brain barrier injury: Hochmeister et al. (48).

most specific pathological changes are focal lesions with primary demyelination and astrocytic scaring, which develop on the background of a chronic inflammatory process (**Figure 1**). These lesions are not restricted to the white matter, but are also abundant in the gray matter of the cortex, the deep brain stem nuclei and the spinal cord (49–51). Primary demyelination means that myelin sheaths and their supporting cells, the oligodendrocytes, are destroyed, while axons are at least in part preserved. However, axonal and neuronal injury in gray and white matter lesions is pronounced. When it passes the threshold of functional compensation its extent is currently the best pathological predictor for permanent neurological deficit in the patients (52). Focal demyelinated lesions in the white and gray matter can be partly or completely repaired by remyelination, although the degree of remyelination is highly variable between patients (53, 54). In addition to these focal changes, diffuse neurodegeneration is present in the normal appearing white and gray matter, which results in brain atrophy, reflected by profound focal and diffuse loss of brain and spinal cord volume. All these changes are present in all MS patients, but their relative contribution to the global pathology varies between different patients and different forms, courses, or stages of the disease.

Inflammation

MS is a chronic inflammatory disease of the central nervous. Inflammation, characterized by the presence of perivascular T- and B-lymphocytes and their dispersion into the parenchyma, is most pronounced in patients, who have died in early stages after disease onset and declines with age of the patients and disease duration [(47); **Figure 1**]. However, even in the progressive stage of the disease pronounced inflammation is present, which is quantitatively in the range of other acute and chronic infectious or inflammatory diseases and massively exceeds that seen in patients with metabolic or neurodegenerative diseases (37). In progressive disease pronounced inflammation is mainly seen in those patients with clinical or radiological evidence of disease activity or of ongoing disease progression during the last months or year (**Figures 2, 3**), while in patients with stable disease during the last year prior to death and/or at very late disease stages tissue infiltration by leukocytes may decrease to levels present in age matched controls (47). In these patients ongoing active axonal injury, detected by focal accumulation of amyloid precursor protein as a marker for disturbance of fast axonal transport, has also declined to the levels seen in age matched controls (47). This adaptive inflammatory process is associated with microglia activation and infiltration of the tissue by macrophages, which is most extensive at sites of active demyelination and neurodegeneration, but, in particular in patients with progressive disease, diffusely affects also the normal appearing white and gray matter.

Similarly as in other chronic inflammatory diseases of the human CNS, inflammatory cells from the adaptive immune system mainly consist of MHC Class I restricted $CD8^+$ T-cells, while MHC class II restricted $CD4^+$ T-cells are rare or even absent [(55, 56); **Figure 1**]. These T-cells display the phenotype of resident memory cells and show focally restricted activation within active lesions (37, 57). It has been suggested from experience obtained in models of autoimmune encephalomyelitis that $CD4^+$ T-cells are the major drivers of the inflammatory process, a concept that is also supported by the genetic association of MS with MHC class II haplotypes and of molecules involved in the regulation of MHC Class II restricted T-cell mediated inflammation (27). However, at the time, when new lesions and neurodegeneration appear in the nervous system, only sparse or even no $CD4^+$ T-cells are present in the tissue (37, 57). Thus, $CD4^+$ T-cells may be involved in the initiation of the immune response in MS patients, but less in the effector stage

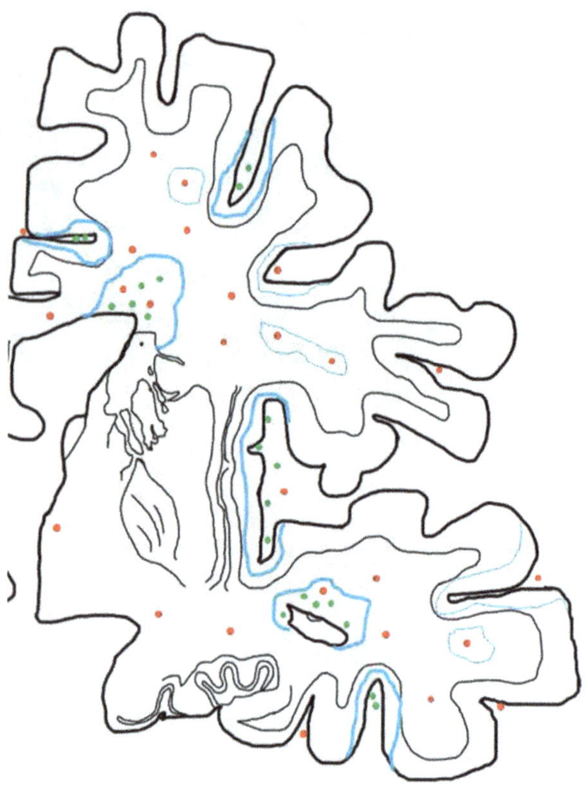

FIGURE 2 | Inflammatory reaction in the brain of patients with progressive MS and its relation to active demyelination and neurodegeneration. The inflammatory reaction in the brain of patients with progressive MS is mainly seen in the large connective tissue spaces of the meninges and the periventricular Virchow Robin spaces. These inflammatory sites mainly contain $CD8^+$ T-cells, a major component of $CD20^+$ B-cells and a variable number of plasma cells and may in their most severe manifestations become organized in structures with features of tertiary lymph follicles (green dots). In addition there are perivascular cuffs mainly composed of $CD8^+$ T-cells, which are more broadly dispersed within the white matter of the brain (red dots). Inflammation with T-cells, B-cells and Plasma cells (green dots) is associated with slow expansion of demyelinated lesions, defined by a rim of activated microglia cells, which in part contain early myelin degradation products in the cortex and the white matter (thick blue lines). Active demyelination and diffuse tissue injury occurs at a distance from the lymphocytic infiltrates and may, thus, be propagated by a soluble demyelinating or neurotoxic factor. Inactive plaques (thin green lines) can still be centered by a vein with a dominant infiltrate by $CD8^+$ T-cells (red dots).

of brain inflammation, immune mediated demyelination and neurodegeneration. In contrast to many other acute of chronic inflammatory brain diseases, cells from the B-cell lineage are a major component of the adaptive immune inflammation in the brain and spinal cord of MS patients (37). They consist in the early stage and in early lesions mainly of $CD20^+$ B-cells, while during lesion maturation and in the progressive stage of the disease plasma-blasts and plasma cells dominate (37, 47). Their possible role in the propagation of demyelination and neurodegeneration is indicated by the highly effective therapeutic response of MS patients in clinical trials targeting B-cells by antibodies against CD20 (58, 59). B-cells in MS lesions may

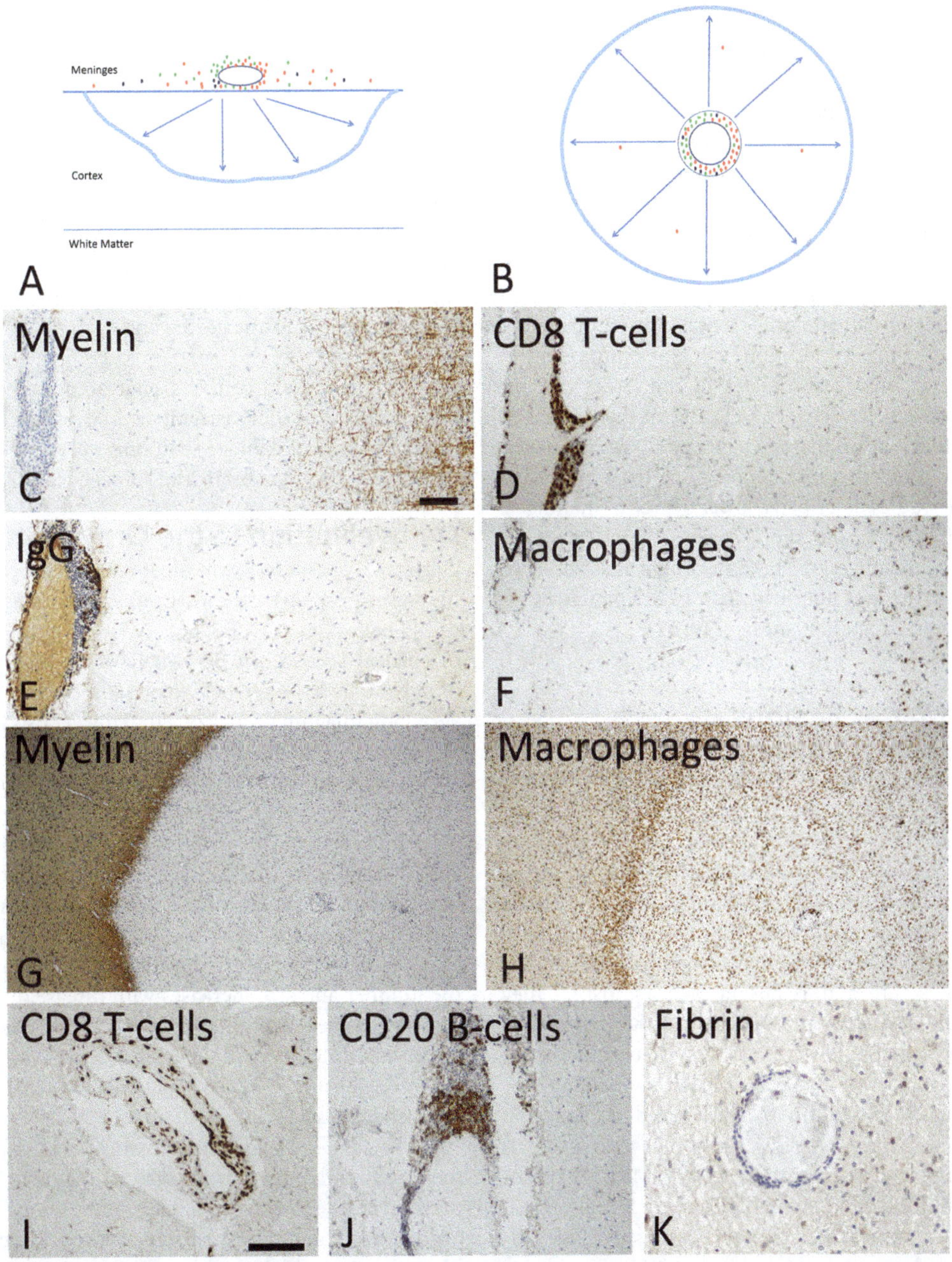

FIGURE 3 | Slowly expanding lesions in the progressive stage of MS in the cortex and the white matter. **(A)** Active cortical lesions are associated with inflammatory infiltrates in the meninges, which are composed of CD8$^+$ T-cells (red), CD20$^+$ B-cells (green) and plasma cells (blue). Active demyelination occurs at a distance of the inflammatory infiltrates and is associated with activated microglia (blue lesion rim). The lesions gradually expand from the pial surface of the cortex toward the depth of the gray matter. Lymphocyte infiltrates are rare or completely absent in the cortical tissue and in particular at the zone of active demyelination. It is suggested that the inflammatory infiltrates in the meninges produce a soluble factor, which induces demyelination and neurodegeneration either directly or indirectly through microglia activation (arrows). **(B)** In slowly expanding lesions in the white matter T-cell, B-cell and plasma cell infiltrates are present in the large perivascular Virchow Robin spaces. Active demyelination and neurodegeneration occurs at a distance and is associated with microglia activation. Also in these lesions it is suggested that demyelination and neurodegeneration is driven by a soluble factor, produced by the perivascular lymphocytes or plasma cells (arrows). **(C–F)** Active cortical lesion in a patient with progressive MS. Subpial myelin is completely lost in an area with meningeal inflammation **(C)**; CD8$^+$ T-cells are present in the meningeal infiltrates, but do not enter the cortical parenchyme **(D)**; The meningeal infiltrates also contain IgG positive plasma cells **(E)**, there is however no indication of IgG leakage from the vessels into the tissue, suggesting an intact blood brain barrier. Activated microglia and macrophages are seen at the site of active demyelination in the depth of the gray matter **(F)**. **(G,H)** Slowly expanding lesion in the white matter of a patient with progressive MS. The inactive plaque center contains vessels with perivascular cuffs of lymphocytes but the active demyelination at the lesion edge is associated with a rim of activated microglia **(G,H)**. Lymphocytes, such as for instance CD8$^+$ T-cells and B-cells are present in the large perivascular space of the vessels, but there is little or no infiltration into the lesion parenchyme **(I,J)**. No fibrinogen leakage is observed around inflamed vessels, indicating intact blood brain barrier function **(K)**. Magnification bar representative for all images: 100 μm. Similar histological images as shown in this figure have been previously published. Structure of the lesions: Frischer et al. (46); Inflammatory reaction: Frischer et al. (47); Machado Santos et al. (37); Microglia and macrophages: Zrzavy et al. (38); Fibrin and blood brain barrier injury: Hochmeister et al. (48).

augment T-cell mediated inflammation for instance through effective auto-antigen presentation, but may also have direct effects in disease pathogenesis. In this line some data suggest that B-cells within the central nervous system of MS patients produce factors that can trigger demyelination and neurodegeneration *in vitro* (60, 61). In addition, however, plasma cells in MS lesions express interleukin 10, suggesting a potential regulatory role (37).

It has been suggested that lymphocyte infiltration is less pronounced in patients with primary progressive compared to secondary progressive MS (62), but this observation was restricted to the analysis of focal white matter lesions and based on a limited number of patients only. It was not confirmed in a more recent study (47). In addition, a major component of the inflammatory response accumulates in the large Virchow Robin spaces of periventricular veins (63) and in the meninges, where they may form inflammatory aggregates, which in the most severe variants reveal the structure of tertiary lymphatic follicles (64). Some studies described a lower degree of meningeal inflammation and in particular the absence of tertiary follicle like structures in the meninges of PPMS in comparison to SPMS patients (65, 66), but this was not the case in PPMS patients with rapid disease progression in other studies (49, 67).

Focal White Matter Lesions

The inflammatory process in MS is associated with the formation of different focal lesion types in the white matter of the brain and spinal cord. They include classical active lesions with pronounced blood brain barrier injury, chronic active or slowly expanding lesions with a low degree of demyelinating activity at the lesion edge and no major blood brain barrier damage, inactive lesions and remyelinated shadow plaques (46, 68, 69). While classical active focal white matter lesions are most numerous in patients with early disease (acute and relapsing MS; **Figure 1**), they become rare in the patients who have entered the progressive stage. In the latter patients slowly expanding or chronic active lesions contribute on average 30% of all focal demyelinated or remyelinated plaques [(46); **Figure 3**]. Their speed of expansion is very low and longitudinal follow up for several years is necessary to document their enlargement at 7T MRI (70). MRI studies indicate that focal white matter lesions are less abundant in patients with primary vs. secondary progressive MS (71, 72). However, very large neuropathological studies on more than 300 patient autopsies did not reveal significant differences between PPMS and SPMS patients in the global extent of white matter plaques or the relative incidence of different focal white matter lesions, such as active, chronic active (slowly expanding), or inactive plaques (46, 69). This discrepancy between MRI and pathology data may in part be due to a sampling bias in pathology, where the selection of tissue areas for detailed analysis is focused on brain areas with macroscopically visible lesions. In this line, a study focusing on the analysis of very large hemispheric and double hemispheric MS brain section showed a lower incidence of active white matter lesions and more remyelinated plaques in the brain of patients with PPMS compared to SPMS, but this study was based on a rather small sample of patients (73).

The issue is further complicated by the observation of a subset of MS patients, who present with a cortico/spinal variant of multiple sclerosis. In these patients focal demyelinated white matter lesions are present only in the spinal cord and are associated with extensive cortical demyelination and neurodegeneration (74). They were present in cohorts of SPMS as well as of PPMS. Such patients show diffuse mainly periventricular white matter abnormalities in the brain in MRI. The nature of these diffuse white matter abnormalities is currently unresolved, but may be due to a combination of diffuse white matter inflammation, secondary degeneration due to neuronal loss in the cortex and age related comorbidity, such as small vessel disease [leukoarayosis; (74), see Figure 1 in (67)]. An extreme variant of this scenario appears to be a condition, designated as cortical variant of MS, which appears to be due to severe cortical damage with only very sparse and small white matter lesions in the brain and spinal cord (67, 75).

Demyelination in the Gray Matter

Cortical lesions, present in the forebrain, the cerebellum, and the hippocampus, have recently been identified as a major substrate of MS pathology [(49, 65, 66, 76–78); **Figure 3**]. More than 90% of cortical lesions can be visualized by post mortem scanning of the brain by high field magnetic resonance imaging using very long imaging times (79, 80). However so far, their detection in the living patients *in vivo* is very incomplete, depicting only an estimate of 10–15% of cortical demyelination, even when ultra-high field MRI is applied (81). Most lesions depicted in MRI are cortico/subcortical or intra-cortical, while the most abundant subpial lesions largely remain unrecognized. Cortical lesions, including the subpial lesions, may already arise in the early stages of MS, being present in brain biopsies or autopsies of patients with a disease duration of weeks to months (82), but the number and size increases with disease duration, thus being most extensive in patients with progressive disease (49). So far no significant differences in the incidence and size of cortical lesions have been observed between patients with primary or secondary progressive disease.

As discussed above, subpial cortical lesions are associated with meningeal inflammation (**Figure 3**). Meningeal inflammation is present in the form of diffuse infiltrates or of inflammatory aggregates containing densely packed T-cells, B-cells, and Plasma cells, which in most severe forms resemble tertiary lymphatic follicles (64). The severity of meningeal inflammation correlates with the extent of subpial cortical demyelination and neurodegeneration (83). Neuropathology, based on a limited number of cases, indicated that tertiary lymph follicles in the meninges are a feature of patients with secondary progressive disease (65), being absent in patients with primary progressive MS (66). However, this does not appear to be the case in PPMS patients with rapid disease progression (49). Furthermore, the presence of tertiary lymph follicles is not mandatory for active cortical demyelination, since active cortical lesions are also present in cases with lower degree and more diffuse meningeal inflammation.

While lymphocytes and plasma cells are restricted to the meninges, active cortical demyelination occurs in an outside/in gradient and is associated with microglia activation at the site of active myelin destruction (49, 84). These observations indicate that active demyelination and neurodegeneration in the cortex may be driven by a soluble factor, produced in the meningeal inflammatory infiltrates, either directly or indirectly through microglia activation (42, 84, 85). The existence of such a soluble demyelinating or neurotoxic factor has been described in the serum and cerebrospinal fluid of MS patients decades ago (86) and it seems to be produced by B-lymphocytes (60, 61). Although the nature of the demyelinating or neurotoxic factor has so far not been identified, several potential candidates have been suggested, including ceramide (87) or semaphorin 4A (88).

Cortical demyelination is accompanied by profound axonal and neuronal degeneration (50, 89). It results in profound neuronal loss following a gradient from the meningeal surface toward the depth of the cortical ribbon (84). Although neuronal loss in the cortex is highest in demyelinated lesions, it is also present in the normal appearing cortex (74).

Other gray matter areas, affected in the disease process of MS are the deep gray matter nuclei, including the thalamus, hypothalamus and basal ganglia as well as the gray matter of the spinal cord (50, 90, 91). As in the cerebral cortex these structures contain focal demyelinated plaques, but active lesions at these sites are not associated with meningeal, but perivascular inflammation. As in cortical lesions, active demyelination expands at a distance from the lymphocytic perivascular infiltrates and is associated with microglia activation. In contrast to cortical lesions, demyelinated plaques in deep gray matter nuclei are already present at early stages of MS and their number and size only moderately increases with disease duration (50). In addition to the presence of focal demyelinated lesions there is also a profound diffuse neuronal loss within the deep gray matter nuclei, associated with inflammation and oxidative injury, which may reflect augmentation of oxidative injury by the high iron content in the deep gray matter nuclei (50).

Diffuse Injury in the Normal Appearing White and Gray Matter

Diffuse injury in the normal appearing white matter is prominent in the MS brain and spinal cord, in particular in patients in the progressive stage of the disease. It consists of small perivascular inflammatory infiltrates, some diffuse infiltration of the tissue, predominantly by CD8$^+$ T-lymphocytes, diffuse axonal injury with secondary demyelination, reactive astrocytic scaring and global microglia activation. The average axonal loss in focal white matter lesions is in the range of 60% (52, 92, 93). The extent of cortical demyelination in the brain of patients with progressive MS is extensive (49) and can affect in extreme cases up to 90% of the cortical ribbon. Within the cortical lesions, but also in the surrounding normal appearing cortex, neuronal loss is seen, which may reach up to 60% of cortical nerve cells (84). Thus, a major part of the axonal neurodegeneration in the white matter appears to be due to secondary Wallerian degeneration as a consequence of axonal trans-section in plaques and neuronal loss in the gray matter (94). Wallerian tract degeneration in the human brain is a very slow process, reflected by the presence of degenerating axons even months after the focal trans-section in a lesion. Thus, ongoing axonal demise in the normal appearing white matter in the absence of lesions with active demyelination may to a major part reflect secondary anterograde or retrograde degeneration as a consequence of axonal or neuronal damage, that has occurred even months before.

Alternatively, diffuse neurodegeneration in the normal appearing gray and white matter may occur independently of focal lesions. Diffuse axonal damage in the normal appearing white matter of the spinal cord has been shown to be associated with inflammation in the meninges (95) and a similar process may trigger neuronal loss in the normal appearing cortex. In addition, age related neurodegeneration and comorbidities, such as vascular pathology and subsequent diffuse hypoxia are likely to be additional factors, driving diffuse neurodegeneration in the brain of patients with progressive MS (50).

Some studies have shown profound diffuse myelin lipid changes in the normal appearing white matter of patients with progressive MS. This can be visualized by myelin imaging in MRI as well as by neuropathological or biochemical analysis (96, 97). Overall, these changes consist of diffuse myelin abnormalities and diffuse alterations in phospholipids, and it was suggested that these changes reflect a metabolic disturbance of myelin, which may be the primary cause of MS or amplify myelin damage (98). An alternative explanation is that these changes reflect Wallerian degeneration, since they are associated with diffuse axonal injury in pathology.

All these diffuse changes in the normal appearing white and gray matter are increasing with age and disease duration of the patients and are, thus, most pronounced in patients with progressive disease. So far, however, they have been seen in similar extent in patients with PPMS and SPMS.

PATHOGENETIC IMPLICATIONS

All the data discussed above show that there are differences in clinical disease, pathology and immunology between the relapsing and the progressive stage of MS. However, when primary and secondary progressive MS are compared with each other no qualitative differences become apparent, but there are some quantitative differences in the presence of focal and active classical white matter lesions and the global degree of inflammation, being lower in PPMS compared to SPMS. The key issue, however, is to explain the difference between early acute and relapsing MS and the progressive disease stage.

Overall these differences could be explained by acknowledging that there are two different types of inflammation in MS patients (**Figures 1–3**). The first, which is associated with the formation of new focal lesions mainly in the white matter, is the focal bulk invasion of inflammatory cells into the brain, which is associated with a major disturbance of the blood brain barrier. Like in experimental models of brain inflammation, such as for instance autoimmune encephalomyelitis, lymphocytes enter the brain in the course of immune surveillance, and when they recognize their cognate antigen within the central nervous system, they may become activated, produce a variety of pro-inflammatory mediators and recruit additional cells and serum components through the impaired blood brain barrier (99). It has originally been thought that this process is mediated by MHC Class II antigen restricted $CD4^+$ T-lymphocytes. However, as discussed above, more recent neuropathological data and experience from therapeutic trials do not support their dominant role in patients with established disease. Instead, $CD8^+$ T-cells or $CD20^+$ B-cells may be more important at least at the stage, when the lesions arise or expand in the brain and spinal cord.

The mere presence of T- and B-cells in the brain of MS patients alone does not allow conclusions regarding their potential involvement in the disease process. The $CD8^+$ T-cells in the MS brain show the phenotype of tissue resident memory cells. They could have entered the brain and spinal cord as disease-unrelated bystander cells during disease activity and persist as tissue resident memory cells without any direct involvement in the disease process. Support for this view comes from a recent study, showing that similar $CD8^+$ tissue resident memory T-cells without signs of activation also populate in small numbers the brain of normal controls and patients with neurodegenerative disease (100). Similarly, a major component of the intrathecal antibody response in MS patients is directed against measles, rubella and varicella zoster virus (101), possibly reflecting the B-cell repertoire at the time of their recruitment into the inflammatory brain lesions. However, in contrast to controls the $CD8^+$ T-cells in the MS brain focally proliferate and show signs of activation (37, 57) or clonal expansion (102), indicating local antigen recognition. Such cells could either promote disease or have regulatory function. Although they do not express interleukin 10 or TGF-ß, a regulatory function through interferon-γ of perforin mediated mechanisms, as suggested to operate in a mouse model of EAE cannot be excluded (103, 104). However, in the MS brain these cells are associated with active demyelination and neurodegeneration, indicating a disease promoting role in the lesions (37, 57). Regarding B-cells the therapeutic effect of anti-CD20 antibodies supports their pathogenetic role in MS patients. However, plasmablasts and plasma cells within the MS lesions highly express interleukin 10 (37) suggesting that these cells may ameliorate inflammation. Thus, the role of cells derived from the B-cell lineage in MS lesion may depend upon their stage of differentiation in different types or activity stages of the lesions (105, 106).

The acute inflammatory process may lead to focal areas of primary demyelination with variable axonal injury, mainly accomplished by activated microglia and macrophages and possibly also by specific antibodies and may give rise to the appearance of different types of active focal MS plaques (107). One possible pathogenic demyelinating autoantibody is directed against myelin oligodendrocyte glycoprotein (MOG), which, however, is present in patients with a disease that turned out to be different from MS (108). In addition, antibodies binding to the surface of oligodendrocytes and astrocytes (109, 110) have been found in MS patients, but the molecular nature of the target antigen is so far undefined. The acutely recruited and activated lymphocytes are in part destroyed by programed cell death (37) and microglia and macrophages are transformed in part into an anti-inflammatory phenotype (38). Thus, these lesions may become inactive and a subset of them may even be repaired by remyelination (53). New bouts of the disease (also termed disease activity in clinical terms) will then be induced by new waves of T-cells and B-cells, focally entering the brain in association with blood brain barrier damage, a process termed "disease activity" in clinical and imaging studies (2).

The second pattern of inflammation in the MS brain is an inflammatory reaction, which accumulates in the large connective tissue spaces of the brain and spinal cord, dominantly affecting the meninges (111) and the large periventricular Virchow Robin spaces (63). Clearance of T- and B-cells from the central nervous system by apoptosis is highly effective for those cells, which penetrate the brain tissue, but is only minor or absent in lymphocytes present in the perivascular and meningeal connective tissue (112). The phenotype of $CD8^+$ T-cells in these chronic lesions is similar to that of tissue resident memory T-cells, which are largely present in an inactive stage, but show focal spots of activation (37, 57). Regarding cells of the B-cell lineage, CD20 positive cells are most frequent in active lesions, but the majority of cells present in chronic lesions are plasmablasts and plasma cells (37). In the meninges and perivascular space this inflammatory reaction is present diffusely but it may form focal aggregates or structures, which resemble tertiary lymph follicles with clearly separated T-cell, B-cell and plasma cells areas (111). In contrast to the inflammatory reaction in classical active white matter lesions blood brain barrier damage is minor or absent in this compartmentalized inflammatory reaction in chronic MS (48). The meningeal and perivascular infiltrates are associated with slow expansion of pre-existing focal white matter lesions, with subpial cortical demyelination and with diffuse damage of the normal appearing white and gray matter, which are the changes typically found in the brain and spinal cord of patients with active demyelination and neurodegeneration in the progressive stage of the disease (113). Tissue injury may at least in be part mediated by a cascade involving microglia and macrophage activation, oxidative injury and mitochondrial damage (5). All these data indicate that demyelination and neurodegeneration in MS is driven by the inflammatory process in all disease stages. However, it is unlikely that inflammatory T- and B-cells interact by direct contact with the specific target cells. More likely, soluble factors, produced by the inflammatory cells, may exert tissue damage either directly or indirectly by the activation of microglia or macrophages (84, 85).

These two types of inflammation occur in parallel in patients with relapsing as well as progressive disease. However, classical active plaques with inflammation and leaky blood brain barrier are most frequent in the early disease stages and then decline with age and disease duration in patients with progressive disease and are even less frequent in particular in patients with primary progressive disease (46, 69, 73). It is so far not clear, whether these two different types of inflammation reflect immune reactions to different target antigens within the brain or just represent inflammatory reactions to a single antigen. To answer this question, knowledge on the specific target antigens for T-cells and B-cells in the MS brain is required, but so far lacking (6, 7).

In summary, inflammation in the brain and spinal cord is present in all patients with active disease, reflected by classical active lesions in the early disease stages and by slowly expanding lesions in the white and gray matter and ongoing neurodegeneration in the progressive stage of the disease. The dominant inflammatory cells are CD8+ T-cells with proliferenation and activation in early stages of classical active lesions and a phenotype of tissue resident memory cells with focal activation in lesions with ongoing demyelination and neurodegeneration in the progressive stage. Numerous CD20+ B-cells are found in perivascular and meningeal inflammatory aggregates in relation to lesion activity in all disease stages, but they apparently transform into plasmablasts and plasma cells in the course of lesion maturation. Depending on the lesion stage lymphocytes may play a role in the induction of tissue damage or have regulatory function. Demyelination and neurodegeneration takes place at a distance from the T- and B-lymphocytes and is associated with activated microglia and macrophages. The structure of active lesions suggests that tissue damage is driven by a soluble factor, produced by lymphocytes. Neither the molecular nature of the soluble factor nor the antigen specificity of the infiltrating T- and B-cells has been identified so far.

ARE DIFFERENT COURSES OF MS REPRODUCED IN EXPERIMENTAL AUTOIMMUNE ENCEPHALOMYELITIS?

Experimental autoimmune encephalomyelitis (EAE) is an acute or chronic neuro-inflammatory disease of the brain and spinal cord, induced by sensitization of animals with tissue or specific antigens of the central nervous system. The value and limits of different EAE models for MS research has recently been reviewed in detail (99), and therefore only few points directly related to the current topic are mentioned here. EAE can be induced in most, if not all, mammalian species including humans and leads to an inflammatory disease, which, depending upon the model, is associated with focal plaques of demyelination and/or diffuse neurodegeneration. The respective experimental models provide excellent tools to elucidate basic mechanisms of brain inflammation and immune mediated tissue injury in the central nervous system, mediated by different T-cell populations and components of the innate immune system. Most importantly, many anti-inflammatory or immunomodulatory therapies, which have been proven effective in MS patients, have been developed with the help of EAE models. However, the value of these treatments in patients, who have reached the progressive stage of MS, is limited. In addition, effective anti-inflammatory treatments in MS so far target many different immune cells simultaneously, including different T-cell populations, B-lymphocytes and in part also macrophages, while treatments selectively directed against the MHC Class II restricted CD4+ T-cell population, which drives inflammation in most EAE models, have so far not provided significant beneficial effects (99). Furthermore, the nature of the inflammatory response and the mechanisms of demyelination and neurodegeneration in the lesions are different between MS and EAE, and so far no EAE model is available, which reproduces the specific clinical and neuropathological features of progressive MS (99). Thus, despite the undisputed value of EAE for basic research related to mechanisms of brain inflammation and immune mediated tissue injury, their value as models for MS is limited and the elucidation of specific mechanisms related to MS pathogenesis depends on the analysis of the human disease itself. However, EAE models induced by sensitization with myelin oligodendrocyte glycoprotein (MOG) in rats and primates are perfect models for MOG auto-antibody associated inflammatory demyelinating disease (99), which however is a disease distinctly different from MS (108).

FUTURE PERSPECTIVES OF MS RESEARCH

There are at present a number of key questions, which require focused attention:

1) One key point is to elucidate the function of tissue resident memory CD8+ T-cells, which are the most abundant inflammatory cells in MS lesions. Further studies are necessary to define their activation stages, their molecular profiles and their functional role in MS lesions in relation to active tissue damage, clearance of tissue debris and tissue repair. CD8+ resident memory cells have originally been defined and functionally characterized in experimental models of virus induced disease (114, 115). It is unlikely that such cells will develop in a condition of classical autoimmunity, when they are directed against an antigen, which is ubiquitously present within the target tissue and is not eliminated in the course of the inflammatory response. Thus, it will be of critical importance to identify the specific antigen(s), which are recognized by tissue infiltrating T- and B-lymphocytes within MS lesions at different stages of lesion formation and disease development (7).
2) Accumulating evidence supports an important role of CD20 positive B-lymphocytes in MS pathogenesis. Although their role may in part be related to the augmentation of T-cell mediated inflammatory responses (116), for instance through effective antigen presentation, an (additional) more direct involvement in the inflammatory process is likely (see above). In addition, they may have disease promoting or regulatory functions, dependent on their differentiation stage in the evolution of the brain lesions. Functional studies so far have concentrated on the production and pathogenic involvement of (auto) antibodies, but little is known regarding the role of B-cells themselves in the process of immune surveillance of the normal brain, in brain inflammation and in immune mediated tissue injury.
3) Another key feature, which is not well-reproduced in models of EAE is cortical demyelination, associated with meningeal inflammation. The only EAE models, which show MS like cortical demyelination are those, which are mediated by a combination of an encephalitogenic T-cell response in concert with a demyelinating antibody response against myelin

oligodendrocyte glycoprotein [MOG, (99, 117)]. Despite extensive search the identification of MS-specific target antigens for demyelinating antibodies was not convincingly successful up to now.

4) Most evidence from pathological studies suggests that demyelination and neurodegeneration in MS is driven by the inflammatory cells, but that these processes are not directly induced by cellular contacts. In addition, plaque like primary demyelination is a specific feature of MS, not seen in other inflammatory conditions of the brain and spinal cord with the exception of diseases with viral infection of oligodendrocytes (89). Evidence from expanding cortical lesions and slowly expanding white matter lesions suggest that demyelination and neurodegeneration is driven by an MS specific soluble factor, produced by inflammatory cells, which induces tissue damage either directly or indirectly through microglia activation (83), and that this soluble factor may be produced by B-cells from MS patients, but not from controls (60). To identify the molecular nature of this soluble factor will be instrumental for our understanding of MS pathogenesis.

AUTHOR CONTRIBUTIONS

The author confirms being the sole contributor of this work and has approved it for publication.

REFERENCES

1. Lassmann H, Brück W, Lucchinetti C. The immunopathology of multiple sclerosis: an overview. *Brain Pathol.* (2007) 17:210–8. doi: 10.1111/j.1750-3639.2007.00064.x
2. Lublin FD, Reingold SC, Cohen JA, Cutter GR, Sørensen PS, Thompson AJ, et al. Defining the clinical course of multiple sclerosis. The 2013 revision. *Neurology* (2014) 83:1–9. doi: 10.1212/WNL.0000000000000560
3. Trapp BD, Nave KA. Multiple sclerosis: an immune or neurodegenerative disorder? *Ann Rev Neurosci.* (2008) 31:247–2696. doi: 10.1146/annurev.neuro.30.051606.094313
4. Antel J, Antel S, Caramanos Z, Arnold DL, Kuhlmann T. Promary progressive multiple sclerosis: part of the MS disease spectrum or separate disease entity?- *Acta Neuropathol.* (2012) 123:627–38. doi: 10.1007/s00401-012-0953-0
5. Mahad DH, Trapp BD, Lassmann H. Pathological mechanisms in progressive multiple sclerosis. *Lancet Neurol.* (2015) 14:183–93. doi: 10.1016/S1474-4422(14)70256-X
6. Hohlfeld R, Dornmair K, Meinl E, Wekerle H. The search for the target antigens of multiple sclerosis, part 1: autoreactive CD4+ T lymphocytes as pathogenic effectors and therapeutic targets. *Lancet Neurol.* (2016) 15:198–209. doi: 10.1016/S1474-4422(15)00334-8
7. Hohlfeld R, Dornmair K, Meinl E, Wekerle H. The search for the target antigens of multiple sclerosis, part 2: CD8+ T cells, B cells, and antibodies in the focus of reverse-translational research. *Lancet Neurol.* (2016) 15:317–31. doi: 10.1016/S1474-4422(15)00313-0
8. Claes N, Fraussen J, Stinissen P, Hupperts R, Somers V. B cells are multifunctional players in multiple sclerosis pathogenesis: insights from therapeutic interventions. *Front Immunol.* (2015) 6:642. doi: 10.3389/fimmu.2015.00642
9. Dargahi N, Katsara M, Tselios T, Androutsou ME, de Courten M, Matsoukas J, et al. Multiple sclerosis: immunopathology and treatment update. *Brain Sci.* (2017) 7:E78. doi: 10.3390/brainsci7070078
10. Rice CM, Cottrell D, Wilkins A, Scolding NJ. Primary progressive multiple sclerosis: progress and chalenges. *J Neurol Neurosurg Psychiat.* (2013) 84:1100–6. doi: 10.1136/jnnp-2012-304140
11. Abdelhack A, Weber MS, Tumani H. Primary progressive multiple sclerosis: putting together the puzzle. *Front Neurol.* (2017) 8:234. doi: 10.3389/fneur.2017.00234
12. Confafreux C, Vukusic S, Moreau T, Adeleine P. Relapses and progression of disability in multiple sclerosis. *N Engl J Med.* (2000) 343:1430–8. doi: 10.1056/NEJM200011163432001
13. Leray E, Yaouang J, Le Page E, Coustans M, Laplaud D, Oger J, et al. Evidence of a two stage disability progression in multiple sclerosis. *Brain* (2010) 133:1900–13. doi: 10.1093/brain/awq076
14. Kuchling J, Ramien C, Bozin I, Dörr J, Harms L, Rosche B, et al. Identical lesions morphology in primary progressive and relapsing-remitting MS. An ultrahigh filed MRI study. *Mult Scler.* (2014) 20:1866–71. doi: 10.1177/1352458514531084
15. Scalfari A, Lederer C, Daumer M, Nicholas R, Ebers GC, Muraro PA. The relationship of age with the clinical phenotype in multiple sclerosis. *Mult Scler.* (2016) 22:1750–8. doi: 10.1177/1352458516630396
16. Zeydan B, Kantarci OH. Progressive forms of multiple sclerosis: distinct entity of age dependent phenomena. *Neurol Clin.* (2018) 36:163–72. doi: 10.1016/j.ncl.2017.08.006
17. Ebers GC. Natural history of primary progressive multiple sclerosis. *Mult Scler.* (2004) 10(Suppl. 1):S8–13. doi: 10.1191/1352458504ms1025oa
18. Sadovnick AD. Differential effects of genetic susceptibility factors in males and females with multiple sclerosis. *Clin Immunol.* (2013) 149:170–5. doi: 10.1016/j.clim.2013.05.002
19. International Multiple Sclerosis Genetcis Consortium. Analysis of immune-related loci identifies 48 new susceptibility variants for multiple sclerosis. *Nat. Genet.* (2013) 45:1353–60. doi: 10.1038/ng.2770
20. International Multiple Sclerosis Genetcis Consortium. Low-frequency abd rare-coding variation contributes to multiple sclerosis risk. *Cell* (2018) 175:1679–87.e7. doi: 10.1016/j.cell.2018.09.049
21. Chataway J, Mander A, Robertson N, Sawcer S, Deans J, Fraser M, et al. Multiple sclerosis in sibling pairs: an analysis of 250 families. *J Neurol Neurosurg Psychiatr.* (2001) 71:757–61. doi: 10.1136/jnnp.71.6.757
22. Oturai AB, Ryder LP, Fredrickson S, Myhr KM, Celius EG, Harbo HF, et al. Concordance of disease course and age of onset in Scandinavian multiple sclerosis co-affected sib pairs. *Mult Scler.* (2004) 10:5–8. doi: 10.1191/1352458504ms975oa
23. Jia X, Madireddy L, Caillier S, Santaniello A, Esposito F, Comi G, et al. Genomic sequencing uncovers phenocopies in primary progressive multiple sclerosis. *Ann Neurol.* (2017) 84:51–63. doi: 10.1002/ana.25263
24. Pan G, Simpson S, van der Mei I, Charlesworth JC, Lucas R, Ponsonby AL, et al. Role of genetic susceptibility variants in predicting clinical course in multiple sclerosis: a cohort study. *J Neuro Neurosurg Psychiat.* (2016) 87:1204–11. doi: 10.1136/jnnp-2016-313722
25. Wang Z, Sadovnick AD, Traboulsee AL, Ross JP, Bernales CQ, Encarnacion M, et al. Nuclear receptor NR1H3 in familial multiple sclerosis. *Neuron* (2016) 90:948–54. doi: 10.1016/j.neuron.2016.04.039
26. International Multiple Sclerosis Genetcis Consortium. NR1H3 p.Arg415Gln is not associated to multiple sclerosis risk. *Neuron*(2016) 92:333–5. doi: 10.1016/j.neuron.2016.09.052
27. Sawcer S, Hellenthal G, Pirinen M, Spencer CC, Patsopoulos NA, Moutsianas L, et al. Genetic risk and a primary role for cell-mediated immune mechanisms in multiple sclerosis. *Nature* (2011) 476:214–9. doi: 10.1038/nature10251
28. Housley WJ, Pitt D, Hafler DA. Biomarkers in multiple sclerosis. *Clin Immunol.* (2015) 161:51–8. doi: 10.1016/j.clim.2015.06.015
29. Paul A, Comabella M, Gandhi R. Biomarkers in multiple sclerosis. *Cold Spring Harb Perspect Med.* (2018) a029058. doi: 10.1101/cshperspect.a029058
30. Abdelhak A, Hottenrott T, Mayer C, Hintereder G, Zettl U, Stich O, et al. CSF profile in primary progressive multiple sclerosis; reexploring the basics. *PLoS ONE* (2017) 12:e0182647. doi: 10.1371/journal.pone.0182647

31. Thompson AJ, Reingold SC, Cohen JA. Applying the 2017 McDonald diagnostic criteria for multiple sclerosis - Authors' reply. *Lancet Neurol.* (2018) 17:499–500. doi: 10.1016/S1474-4422(18)30168-6
32. Hohlfeld R. Immunologic factors in primary progressive multiple sclerosis. *Mult Scler.* (2004) 10:S16–22. doi: 10.1191/1352458504ms1026oa
33. Bielekova B, Komori M, Xu Q, Reich DS, Wu T. Cerebrospinal fluid Il12p40, CXCL13 and Il-8 as a combinatorial biomarker of active intrathecal inflammation. *PLoS ONE* (2012) 7:e48370. doi: 10.1371/journal.pone.0048370
34. Han S, Lin YC, Wu T, Salgado AD, Mexhitaj I, Wuest SC, et al. Comprehensive immunophenotyping of cerebrospinal fluid cells in patients with neuroimmunological disease. *J Immunol.* (2014) 192:2551–63. doi: 10.4049/jimmunol.1302884
35. Barbour C, Kosa P, Komori M, Tanigawa M, Masvekar R, Wu T, et al. Molecular-based diagnosis of multiple sclerosis and ist progressive stage. *Ann Neurol.* (2017) 82:795–812. doi: 10.1002/ana.25083
36. Wurth S, Kuenz B, Bsteh G, Ehling R, DiPauli F, Heegen H, et al. Cerebrospinal fluid B cells and disease progression in multiple sclerosis - a longitudinal study. *PLoS ONE* (2017) 12:e0182462. doi: 10.1371/journal.pone.0182462
37. Machado-Santos J, Saji E, Tröscher A, Paunovic M, Liblau R, Gabriely G, et al. The compartmentalized inflammatory response in the multiple sclerosis brain is composed of tissue-resident CD8+ T lymphocytes and B cells. *Brain* (2018) 141:2066–82. doi: 10.1093/brain/awy151
38. Zrzavy T, Hametner S, Wimmer I, Butovsky O, Weiner H, Lassmann H. Loss of 'homeostatic' microglia and patterns of their activation in active multiple sclerosis. *Brain* (2017) 140:1900–13. doi: 10.1093/brain/awx113
39. Thompson EJ, Keir G. Laboratory investigation of cerebrospinal fluid proteins. *Ann Clin Biochem.* (1990) 27:425–35. doi: 10.1177/000456329002700503
40. Cepok S, Zhou D, Vogel F, Rosche B, Grummel V, Sommer N, et al. The immune response at onset and during recovery from Borrelia buf'rgdorferi meningoradiculitis. *Arch Neurol.* (2003) 60:849–55. doi: 10.1001/archneur.60.6.849
41. Cepok S, Rosche B, Brummel V, Vogel F, Zhou D, Sayn J, et al. Short-lived plasma blasts are the main B-cell effector subset during the course of multiple sclerosis. *Brain* (2005) 128:1667–76. doi: 10.1093/brain/awh486
42. Magliozzi R, Howell OW, Nicholas R, Cruciani C, Castellaro M, Romualdi C, et al. Inflammatory intrathecal profiles and cortical damage in multiple sclerosis. *Ann Neurol.* (2018) 83:739–55. doi: 10.1002/ana.25197
43. Mane-Martinez MA, Olsson B, Bau L, Matas E, Cobo-Calvo A, Andreasson U, et al. Glial and neuronal markers in cerebrospinal fluid in different types of multiple sclerosis. *J Neuroimmunol.* (2016) 299:112–7. doi: 10.1016/j.jneuroim.2016.08.004. [Epub ahead of print].
44. Barro C, Benkert P, Disanto G, Tsagkas C, Amann M, Naegelin Y, et al. Serum neurofilament as a predictor of disease worsening and brain and spinal cord atrophy in multiple sclerosis. *Brain* (2018) 141:2382–91. doi: 10.1093/brain/awy154
45. Stoessel D, Stellmann JP, Willimg A, Behrens B, Rosenkranz SC, Hodecker SC, et al. Metabolomic profiles for primary progressive multiple sclerosis stratification and disease course monitoring. *Front Hum Neurosci.* (2018) 12:226. doi: 10.3389/fnhum.2018.00226
46. Frischer JM, Weigand SD, Guo Y, Kale N, Parisi JE, Pirko I, et al. Clinical and pathological insights into the dynamic nature of the white matter multiple sclerosis plaque. *Ann Neurol.* (2015) 78:710–21. doi: 10.1002/ana.24497
47. Frischer JM, Bramow S, Dal Bianco A, Lucchinetti CF, Rauschka H, Schmidbauer M, et al. The relation between inflammation and neurodegeneration in multiple sclerosis brains. *Brain* (2009) 132:1175–89. doi: 10.1093/brain/awp070
48. Hochmeister S, Grundtner R, Bauer J, Engelhardt B, Lyck R, Gordon G, et al. Dysferlin is a new marker for leaky brain blood vessels in multiple sclerosis. *J Neuropathol Exp Neurol.* (2006) 65:855–65. doi: 10.1097/01.jnen.0000235119.52311.16
49. Kutzelnigg A, Lucchinetti CF, Stadelmann C, Bruck W, Rauschka H, Bergmann M, et al. Cortical demyelination and diffuse white matter injury in multiple sclerosis. *Brain* (2005) 128(Pt 11):2705–12. doi: 10.1093/brain/awh641
50. Haider L, Simeonidou C, Steinberger G, Hametner S, Grigoriadis N, Deretzi G, et al. Multiple sclerosis deep grey matter: the relation between demyelination, neurodegeneration, inflammation and iron. *J Neurol Neurosurg Psychiatry* (2014) 85:1386–95. doi: 10.1136/jnnp-2014-307712
51. Schmierer K, Miquel ME. Magnetic resonance imaging correlates of neuro-axonal pathology in the MS spinal cord. *Brain Pathol.* (2018) 28:765–72. doi: 10.1111/bpa.12648
52. Bjartmar C, Kidd G, Mork S, Rudick R, Trapp BD. Neurological disability correlates with spinal cord axonal loss and reduced N-acetyl aspartate in chronic multiple sclerosis patients. *Ann-Neurol.* (2000) 48:893–901. doi: 10.1002/1531-8249(200012)48:6<893::AID-ANA10>3.0.CO;2-B
53. Patrikios P, Stadelmann C, Kutzelnigg A, Rauschka H, Schmidbauer M, Laursen H, et al. Remyelination is extensive in a subset of multiple sclerosis patients. *Brain* (2006) 129:3165–72. doi: 10.1093/brain/awl217
54. Patani R, Balaratnam M, Vora A, Reynolds R. Remyelination can be extensive in multiple sclerosis despite a long disease course. *Neuropath Appl Neurobiol.* (2007) 33:277–87. doi: 10.1111/j.1365-2990.2007.00805.x
55. Hayashi T, Morimoto C, Burks JS, Kerr C, Hauser SL. Dual-label immunocytochemistry of the active multiple sclerosis lesion: major histocompatibility complex and activation antigens. *Ann Neurol.* (1988) 24:523–31. doi: 10.1002/ana.410240408
56. Booss J, Esiri MM, Tourtellotte WW, Mason DY. Immunohistological analysis of T lymphocyte subsets in the central nervous system in chronic progressive multiple sclerosis. *J Neurol Sci.* (1983) 62:219–32. doi: 10.1016/0022-510X(83)90201-0
57. van Nierop GP, van Luijn MM, Michels SS, Melief MJ, Janssen M, Langerak AW, et al. Phenotypic and functional characterization of T cells in white matter lesions of multiple sclerosis patients. *Acta Neuropathol.* (2017) 134:383–401. doi: 10.1007/s00401-017-1744-4
58. Hauser SL, Waubant E, Arnold DL, Vollmer T, Antel J, Fox RJ, et al. B-cell depletion with rituximab in relapsing-remitting multiple sclerosis. *N Engl J Med.* (2008) 358:676–88. doi: 10.1056/NEJMoa0706383
59. Montalban X, Hauser SL, Kappos L, Arnold DL, Bar-Or A, Comi G, et al. Ocrelizumab versus placebo in primary progressive multiple sclerosis. *N Engl J Med.* (2017) 376:209–20. doi: 10.1056/NEJMoa1606468
60. Lisak RP, Benjamins JA, Nedelkoska L, Barger JL, Ragheb S, Fan B, et al. Secretory products of multiple sclerosis B cells are cytotoxic to oligodendroglia *in vitro*. *J Neuroimmunol.* (2012) 246:85–95. doi: 10.1016/j.jneuroim.2012.02.015
61. Lisak RP, Nedelkoska L, Benjamins JA, Schalk D, Bealmear B, Touil H, et al. B cells from patients with multiple sclerosis induce cell death via apoptosis in neurons *in vitro*. *J Neuroimmunol.* (2017) 309:88–99. doi: 10.1016/j.jneuroim.2017.05.004
62. Revesz T, Kidd D, Thompson AJ, Barnard RO, McDonals WI. A comparison of the pathology of primary and secondary progressive multiple sclerosis. *Brain* (1994) 117:759–65. doi: 10.1093/brain/117.4.759
63. Esiri MM, Gay D. Immmunological and neuropathological significance of the Virchow-Robin space. *J Neurol Sci.* (1990) 100:3–8. doi: 10.1016/0022-510X(90)90004-7
64. Serafini B, Rosicarelli B, Magliozzi R, Stigliano E, Aloisi F. Detection of ectopic B-cell follicles with germinal centers in the meninges of patients with secondary progressive multiple sclerosis. *Brain Pathol.* (2004) 14:164–74. doi: 10.1111/j.1750-3639.2004.tb00049.x
65. Howell OW, Reeves CA, Nicholas R, Carassiti D, Radotra B, Gentleman SM, et al. Meningeal inflammation is widespread and linked to cortical pathology in multiple sclerosis. *Brain* (2011) 134(Pt 9):2755–71. doi: 10.1093/brain/awr182
66. Choi S, Howell OW, Carassiti D, Magliozzi R, Gveric D, Muraro PA, et al. Meningeal inflammation plays a role in the pathology of primary progressive multiple sclerosis. *Brain* (2012) 135:2925–37. doi: 10.1093/brain/aws189
67. Haider L, Zrzavy T, Hametner S, Höftberger R, Bagnato F, Grabner G, et al. The topograpy of demyelination and neurodegeneration in the multiple sclerosis brain. *Brain* (2016) 139:807–15. doi: 10.1093/brain/awv398
68. Kuhlmann T, Ludwin S, Prat A, Antel J, Bruck W, Lassmann H. An updated histological classification system for multiple sclerosis lesions. *Acta Neuropathol.* (2017) 133:13–24. doi: 10.1007/s00401-016-1653-y

69. Luchetti S, Fransen NL, van Eden CG, Ramaglia V, Mason M, Huitinga I. Progressive multiple sclerosis patients show substantial lesion activity that correlates with clinical disease severity and sex. A retrospective autopsy cohort analysis. *Acta Neuropathol.* (2018) 135:511–28. doi: 10.1007/s00401-018-1818-y
70. Dal-Bianco A, Grabner G, Kronnerwetter C, Weber M, Höftberger R, Berger T, et al. Slow expansion of multiple sclerosis iron rim lesions: pathology and 7 T magnetic resonance imaging. *Acta Neuropathol.* (2017) 133:25–42. doi: 10.1007/s00401-016-1636-z
71. Thompson AJ, Kermode AG, Wicks D, MacManus DG, Kendall BE, Kingsley DP, et al. Major differences in the dynamics of primary and secondary progressive multiple sclerosis. *Ann Neurol.* (1991) 29:53–62. doi: 10.1002/ana.410290111
72. Thompson AJ, Polamn CH, Miller DH, McDonals WI, Brochet B, Filippi M, et al. Primary progressive multiple sclerosis. *Brain* (1997) 120:1085–96. doi: 10.1093/brain/120.6.1085
73. Bramow S, Frischer JM, Lassmann H, Koch-Henriksen N, Lucchinetti CF, Sørensen PS, et al. Demyelination versus remyelination in progressive multiple sclerosis. *Brain* (2010) 133:2983–98. doi: 10.1093/brain/awq250
74. Trapp DB, Vignos M, Dudman J, Chang A, Fisher E, Staugaitis SM, et al. Cortical neuronal densities and cerebral white matter demyelination in multiple sclerosis: a retrospective study. *Lancet Neurol.* (2018) 17:870–84. doi: 10.1016/S1474-4422(18)30245-X
75. Zarei M, Chandran S, Compston A, Hodges J. Cognitive presentation of multiple sclerosis: evidence for a cortical variant. *J Neurol Neurosurg Psychiatr.* (2003) 74:872–7. doi: 10.1136/jnnp.74.7.872
76. Kutzelnigg A, Faber-Rod JC, Bauer J, Lucchinetti CF, Sorensen PS, Laursen H, et al. Widespread demyelination in the cerebellar cortex in multiple sclerosis. *Brain Pathol.* (2007) 17:38–44. doi: 10.1111/j.1750-3639.2006.00041.x
77. Howell OW, Schulz-Trieglaff EK, Carassiti D, Gentleman SM, Nicholas R, Roncaroli F, et al. Extensive grey matter pathology in the cerebellum in multiple sclerosis is linked to inflammation in the subarachnoid space. *Neuropath Appl Neurobiol.* (2015) 41:798–813. doi: 10.1111/nan.12199
78. Geurts JJ, Bo L, Roosendaal SD, Hazes T, Daniels R, Barkhof F, et al. Extensive hippocampal demyelination in multiple sclerosis. *J Neuropath Exp Neurol.* (2007) 66:819–27. doi: 10.1097/nen.0b013e3181461f54
79. Pitt D, Boster A, Pei W, Wohleb E, Jasne A, Zachariah CR, et al. Imaging cortical lesions in multiple sclerosis with ultra-high-filed magnetic resonance imaging. *Arch Neurol.* (2010) 67:812–8. doi: 10.1001/archneurol.2010.148
80. Schmierer K, Parkes HG, So PW, So PW, Brandner A, Ordidge RJ, et al. High field (9.4 Tesla) magnetic resonance imaging of cortical grey matter lesions in multiple sclerosis. *Brain* (2010) 133:858–67. doi: 10.1093/brain/awp335
81. Hametner S, Bianco AD, Trattnig S, Lassmann H. Iron related changes in MS lesions and their validity to characterize MS lesion types and dynamics with ultra-high filed magnetic resonance imaging. *Brain Pathol.* (2018) 28:743–9. doi: 10.1111/bpa.12643
82. Lucchinetti CF, Popescu BF, Bunyan RF, Moll NM, Roemer SF, Lassmann H, et al. Inflammatory cortical demyelination in early multiple sclerosis. *N Engl J Med.* (2011) 365:2188–97. doi: 10.1056/NEJMoa1100648
83. Magliozzi R, Howell O, Vora A, et al. Meningeal B-cell follicles in secondary progressive multiple sclerosis associate with early onset of disease and severe cortical pathology. *Brain* (2007) 130:1089–104. doi: 10.1093/brain/awm038
84. Magliozzi R, Howell OW, Reeves C, Roncaroli F, Nicholas R, Serafini B, et al. A Gradient of neuronal loss and meningeal inflammation in multiple sclerosis. *Ann Neurol.* (2010) 68:477–93. doi: 10.1002/ana.22230
85. Kutzelnigg A, Lassmann H. Cortical demyelination in multiple sclerosis: a substrate for cognitive deficits ? *J Neurol Sci.* (2006) 245:123–6. doi: 10.1016/j.jns.2005.09.021
86. Bornstein MB, Appel SH. Tissue culture studies of demyelination. *Ann N Y Acad Sci.* (1965) 122:280–6. doi: 10.1111/j.1749-6632.1965.tb20212.x
87. Vidaurre OG, Haines JD, Katz Sand I, Adula KP, Huynh JL, McGraw CA, et al. Cerebrospinal fluid ceramides from patents with multiple sclerosis impair neuronal bioenergetics. *Brain* (2014) 137:2271–86. doi: 10.1093/brain/awu139
88. Chiou B, Lucassen E, Sather M, Kallianpur A, Connor J. Semaphorin 4A and H-Ferritin utilize Tim-1 on human oligodendrocytes: a novel neuro-immune axis. *Glia* (2018) 66:1317–30. doi: 10.1002/glia.23313
89. Fischer MT, Wimmer I, Hoftberger R, Gerlach S, Haider L, Zrzavy T, et al. Disease-specific molecular events in cortical multiple sclerosis lesions. *Brain* (2013) 136:1799–815. doi: 10.1093/brain/awt110
90. Vercellino M, Masera S, Lorenzatti M, Condello C, Merola A, Mattioda A, et al. Demyelination, inflammation, and neurodegeneration in multiple sclerosis deep grey matter. *J Neuropath Exp Neurol.* (2009) 68:489–502. doi: 10.1097/NEN.0b013e3181a19a5a
91. Huitinga I, De Groot CJ, van der Valk P, Kamphorst W, Tilders FJ, Swaab DF. Hypothalamic lesions in multiple sclerosis. *J Neuropath Exp Neurol.* (2001) 60:1208–18. doi: 10.1093/jnen/60.12.1208
92. Mews I, Bergmann M, Bunkowski S, Gullotta F, Brück W. Oligodendrocyte and axon pathology in clinically silent multiple sclerosis lesions. *Mult Scler.* (1998) 4:55–62. doi: 10.1177/135245859800400203
93. Kornek B, Storch M, Weissert R, Wallstroem E, Stefferl A, Olsson T, et al. Multiple sclerosis and chronic autoimmune encephalomyelitis: a comparative quantitative study of axonal injury in active, inactive and remyelinated lesions. *Amer J Pathol.* (2000) 157:267–76. doi: 10.1016/S0002-9440(10)64537-3
94. Singh S, Dallenga T, Winkler A, Roemer S, Maruschak B, Siebert H, et al. Relationship of acute axonal damage, Wallerian degeneration and clinical disability in multiple sclerosis. *J Neurinflammation* (2017) 14:57. doi: 10.1186/s12974-017-0831-8
95. Androdias G, Reynolds R, Chanal M, Ritleng C, Confavreux C, Nataf S. Meningeal T cells associate with diffuse axonal loss in multiple sclerosis spinal cords. *Ann Neurol.* (2010) 68:465–76. doi: 10.1002/ana.22054
96. Moore GR, Laule C, Mackay A, Leung E, Li DK, Zhao G, et al. Dirty-appearing white matter in multiple sclerosis: preliminary observations of myelin phospholipid and axonal loss. *J Neurol.* (2008) 255:1802–11. doi: 10.1007/s00415-008-0002-z
97. Laule C, Vavasour IM, Leung E, Li DK, Kozlowski P, Traboulsee AL, et al. Pathological basis of diffusely abnormal white matter: insights from magnetic resonance imaging and histology. *Mult Scler.* (2011) 17:144–50. doi: 10.1177/1352458510384008
98. Laule C, Pavlova V, Leung E, Zhao G, MacKay AL, Kozlowski P, et al. Diffusely abnormal white matter in multiple sclerosis; further histologic studies provide evidence for a primary lipid abnormality with neurodegeneration. *J Neuropath Exp Neurol.* (2013) 72:42–52. doi: 10.1097/NEN.0b013e31827bced3
99. Lassmann H, Bradl M. Multiple sclerosis: experimental models and reality. *Acta Neuropathol.* (2017) 133:223–44. doi: 10.1007/s00401-016-1631-4
100. Smolders J, Heutinck KM, Fransen NL, Remmerswaal EBM, Hombrink P, Ten Berge IJM, et al. Tissue-resident memory T cells populate the human brain. *Nat Commun.* (2018) 9:4593. doi: 10.1038/s41467-018-07053-9
101. Jarius S, Eichhorn P, Franciotta D, Petereit HF, Akman-Demir G, Wich M, et al. The MRZ reaction as a highly specific marker of multiple sclerosis: re-evaluation and structures review of the literature. *J Neurol.* (2017) 264:453–66. doi: 10.1007/s00415-016-8360-4
102. Babbe H, Roers A, Waisman A, Lassmann H, Goebels N, Hohlfeld R, et al. Clonal expansions of CD8(+) T cells dominate the T cell infiltrate in active multiple sclerosis lesions as shown by micromanipulation and single cell polymerase chain reaction. *J Exp Med.* (2000) 192:393–404. doi: 10.1084/jem.192.3.393
103. Sinha S, Boyden AW, Itani FR, Crawford MP, Karandikar NJ. CD8(+) T-cells as immune regulators pf multiple sclerosis. *Front Immunol.* (2015) 6:619. doi: 10.3389/fimmu.2015.00619
104. Boyden AW, Brate AA, Karandikar NJ. Early IFNg-mediated and late perforin mediated suppression of pathogenic CD4 T cell responses are both required for inhibition of demyelinating disease by CNS-specific autoregulatory CD8 cells. *Front Immunol.* (2018) 9:2336. doi: 10.3389/fimmu.2018.02336
105. Lehmann-Horn K, Kinzel S, Weber MS. Deciphering the role of B cells in multiple sclerosis. Towards specific targeting of pathogenic functions. *Int J Mol Sci.* (2017) 18:E2048. doi: 10.3390/ijms18102048
106. Li R, Patterson KR, Bar-Or A. Reassessing B cell contributions in multiple sclerosis. *Nat Immunol.* (2018) 19:696–707. doi: 10.1038/s41590-018-0135-x
107. Lucchinetti C, Brück W, Parisi J, Scheithauer B, Rodriguez M, Lassmann H. Heterogeneity of multiple sclerosis lesions: implications for the pathogenesis

of demyelination. *Ann Neurol.* (2000) 47:707–17. doi: 10.1002/1531-8249(200006)47:6<707::AID-ANA3>3.0.CO;2-Q

108. Jarius S, Ruprecht K, Kleiter I, Borisow N, Asgari N, Pitarokoili K, et al. MOG-IgG in NMO and related disorders: a multicenter study of 50 patients. Part 2: Epidemiology, clinical presentation, radiological and laboratory features, treatment responses, and long-term outcome. *J Neuroinflammation* (2016) 13:280. doi: 10.1186/s12974-016-0718-0
109. Lily O, Palace J, Vincent A. Serum antibodies to sell surface determinants in multiple sclerosis: a flow cytometric study. *Brain* (2004) 127:269–79. doi: 10.1093/brain/awh031
110. Blauth K, Soltys J, Matschulat A, Reiter CR, Ritchie A, Baird NL, et al. Antibodies produced by clonally expanded plasma cells in multiple sclerosis cerebrospinal fluid cause demyelination of spinal cord explants. *Acta Neuropathol.* (2015) 130:765–81. doi: 10.1007/s00401-015-1500-6
111. Aloisi F, Pujol-Borrell R. Lymphoid neogenesis in chronic inflammatory diseases. *Nat Rev Immunol.* (2006) 6:205–17. doi: 10.1038/nri1786
112. Schmied M, Breitschopf H, Gold R, Zischler H, Rothe G, Wekerle H, et al. Apoptosis of T lymphocytes in experimental autoimmune encephalomyelitis. Evidence for programmed cell death as a mechanism to control inflammation in the brain. *Am J Pathol.* (1993) 143:446–52.
113. Lassmann H, van Horssen J, Mahad D. Progressive multiple sclerosis: pathology and pathogenesis. *Nat Rev Neurol.* (2012) 8:647–56. doi: 10.1038/nrneurol.2012.168
114. Schenkel JM, Masopust D. Tissue-resident memory T cells. *Immunity* (2014) 41:886–97. doi: 10.1016/j.immuni.2014.12.007
115. Steinbach K, Vincenti I, Kreutzfeldt M, Page N, Muschaweckh A, Wagner I, et al. Brain-resident memory T cells represent an autonomous cytotoxic barrier to viral infection. *J Exp Med.* (2016) 213:1571–87. doi: 10.1084/jem.20151916
116. Hauser SL. The Charcot Lecture / Beating MS: a story of B cells, with twists and turns. *Mult Scler J.* (2015) 21:8–21. doi: 10.1177/1352458514561911
117. Storch MK, Bauer J, Linington C, Olsson T, Weissert R, Lassmann H. Cortical demyelination can be modeled in specific rat models of autoimmune encephalomyelitis and is major histocompatibility complex (MHC) haplotype-related. *J Neuropathol Exp Neurol.* (2006) 65:1137–42. doi: 10.1097/01.jnen.0000248547.13176.9d

10

The MRZ-Reaction and Specific Autoantibody Detection for Differentiation of ANA-Positive Multiple Sclerosis From Rheumatic Diseases With Cerebral Involvement

Nils Venhoff[1†], Jens Thiel[1†], Marta Rizzi[1], Ana Venhoff[1], Sebastian Rauer[2], Dominique Endres[3], Carolin Hentze[1], Julian Staniek[1], Daniela Huzly[4], Reinhard E. Voll[1], Ulrich Salzer[1†] and Tilman Hottenrott[2†]*

[1] Department of Rheumatology and Clinical Immunology, Faculty of Medicine, Medical Center – University of Freiburg, Freiburg im Breisgau, Germany, [2] Department of Neurology and Neurophysiology, Faculty of Medicine, Medical Center – University of Freiburg, Freiburg im Breisgau, Germany, [3] Department of Psychiatry and Psychotherapy, Faculty of Medicine, Medical Center – University of Freiburg, Freiburg im Breisgau, Germany, [4] Faculty of Medicine, Institute of Virology, Medical Center – University of Freiburg, Freiburg im Breisgau, Germany

***Correspondence:**
Nils Venhoff
nils.venhoff@uniklinik-freiburg.de

†These authors have contributed equally to this work

Objective: Rheumatic diseases with involvement of the central nervous system (RDwCNS) may mimic multiple sclerosis (MS). Inversely, up to 60% of MS-patients have antinuclear autoantibodies (ANAs) and may be misdiagnosed as RDwCNS. The detection of antibodies against extractable nuclear antigens (ENA) and oligoclonal bands (OCB) are established valuable diagnostic tools in the differential diagnosis of RDwCNS and MS. The MRZ-reaction (MRZR) is defined by three antibody indices (AIs) against neurotropic viruses and is frequently positive in MS. To investigate the added value of MRZR combined with testing for antibodies against ENAs and OCB detection to distinguish RDwCNS from ANA positive MS.

Methods: MRZR was evaluated in RDwCNS ($n = 40$) and 68 ANA positive MS-patients. Two stringency levels, MRZR-1 and MRZR-2 (at least one respectively two of three AIs positive) were applied. Autoantibody testing included ANA plus ENA and anti-dsDNA antibodies, antiphospholipid antibodies, and anti-neutrophil cytoplasmic antibodies.

Results: Most of the RDwCNS patients ($n = 32$; 80%) suffered from systemic lupus erythematosus. Within the RDwCNS group 20% had a positive MRZR-1 and 8.5% a positive MRZR-2 compared to 80.9 and 60%, respectively within the MS-group ($p < 0.0001$ for both comparisons). Oligoclonal bands were found in 28.6% of the RDwCNS patients and 94.3% of the MS-patients ($p < 0.0001$). Conversely, autoantibodies to specific nuclear antigens or phospholipids were found more frequently in RDwCNS. A positive MRZR in conjunction with the absence of ENA autoantibodies distinguished MS from RDwCNS with high specificity (97.5%).

Conclusions: We suggest combining MRZR, OCBs, and specific autoantibody diagnostics to differentiate RDwCNS from MS.

Keywords: anti-nuclear antibodies, systemic lupus erythematosus (SLE), multiple sclerosis (MS), intrathecal polyspecific antiviral immune response, MRZ-reaction (MRZR)

INTRODUCTION

Multiple sclerosis (MS) is an immune-mediated inflammatory disease of the central nervous system (CNS). MS and rheumatic diseases show several commonalities. Between 20 and 60% of MS-patients have a positive immunofluorescence testing for anti-nuclear antibodies (ANAs) (1, 2) and in rheumatic diseases such as systemic lupus erythematosus (SLE) or anti-neutrophil cytoplasmic-antibodies (ANCA) associated small vessel vasculitides, neuropsychiatric manifestations are common and may mimic magnetic resonance imaging (MRI), and cerebrospinal fluid (CSF) findings of MS (3, 4). As neuropsychiatric symptoms may be the first clinical manifestation of rheumatic diseases with involvement of the central nervous system (RDwCNS) and inflammatory CSF alterations and MS-like lesions in MRI are frequent, the differential diagnosis between RDwCNS and ANA-positive MS is difficult. Moreover, differentiating RDwCNS from ANA-positive MS is essential for adequate treatment. Also the coexistence of both a systemic inflammatory rheumatic disease and MS in the same patient has to be considered since both entities are of autoimmune origin and occur predominantly in female patients. One essential diagnostic procedure in these patients is the analysis of CSF which requires lumbar puncture. The MRZ-reaction (MRZR) is a polyspecific, intrathecal humoral immune response directed against three neurotropic viruses: measles (M), rubella (R), and varicella zoster (Z), assessed using the three respective antibody indices (AIs) (5). The AI is a calculated parameter to assess whether the antibodies measured in the CSF are produced intrathecally or whether they are originally blood derived. A high AI ($\geq$1.5) is an indicator for antibody production within the CNS whereas an AI $<$ 1.5 is indicative for an antibody synthesis in plasma cells that are not located within the CNS. In MS studies frequently two thresholds defining a positive AI ($\geq$1.5 and $>$2.0) are assessed (6). Furthermore, it is common to distinguish a positive MRZR-1 and a positive MRZR-2. A positive MRZR-1 is defined by at least one positive AI and a positive MRZR-2 by at least two positive AIs out of the three calculated AIs. Very likely the positive MRZR represents a polyspecific B-cell-activation within the CNS. Also the detection of oligoclonal bands (OCB), a very sensitive but compared to the MRZR less specific marker for MS, is an indicator for the involvement B-cells in the pathogenesis of MS.

A high prevalence of positive MRZR has been described in patients with relapsing remitting MS and with primary progressive MS (6), while the significance of positive MRZR in RDwCNS has not yet been explored in larger cohorts. Since ANA can be detected also in healthy individuals, a positive ANA-screening should lead to an analysis of extractable nuclear antigens (ENA). Certain antibodies to ENA are highly specific for connective tissue diseases (CTD), whereas the absence of ENA or exclusive detection of DFS70-autoantibodies in ANA-positive individuals does not further support the diagnosis of an underlying CTD (7). Therefore, the MRZR together with ANA and ENA testing might represent a valuable diagnostic procedure to separate MS from RDwCNS. This is the first report on the diagnostic value of the MRZR in combination with ENA-autoantibody diagnostics to differentiate RDwCNS-patients from ANA-positive MS in the largest cohort of RDwCNS-patients published so far.

MATERIALS AND METHODS

Patients participating in this retrospective study were treated at the University Medical Centre Freiburg and were identified by an electronic database search. Routine medical diagnostic workup included lumbar puncture in all patients and the storage (-80°C) of paired CSF and serum samples according to local biobanking protocols. Informed consent was obtained from all patients. All experiments were carried out in accordance with the Declaration of Helsinki. This study was approved by the ethics committee of the University Medical Centre Freiburg (EK-Fr489/14, EK-Fr507/16). Diagnoses of the rheumatic diseases were made by board certified rheumatologists according to current classification criteria (8–11). CNS-involvement of RDwCNS was diagnosed based on clinical signs, and the presence of at least one of the following findings: (A) inflammatory CSF (intrathecal immunoglobulin synthesis, increased cell-count, positive CSF specific oligoclonal bands (OCB), or disturbance in the blood-CSF barrier indicated by an increased albumin quotient) or (B) inflammation in brain or spinal MRI compatible with RDwCNS as assessed by board-certified neuroradiologists. MS-diagnosis was made according to the 2010 revised McDonald criteria (12). Total immunoglobulin concentrations (IgG_{total}) were measured by nephelometry (BN-ProSpec System, Siemens, Germany). Measles-, rubella-, and varicella zoster-specific IgG concentrations (IgGspec) were measured using ELISA (Serion *classic* ELISA, Germany). MRZR was calculated from the virus-specific antibody index (AI) $= QIgG_{spec}/QIgG_{total}$, if QIgG[total]<Qlim, and AI = QIgG[spec]/Qlim, if QIgG[total]>Qlim (13). The upper reference range of QIgG, Qlim, was calculated according to Reiber's formula (13). Two thresholds for a positive AI indicating specific intrathecal IgG-production ($\geq$1.5 and $>$2.0) were analyzed (6, 14). MRZR-1 and MRZR-2 were positive when at least one respectively two of the three calculated AIs were positive. ANA-staining pattern was assessed using indirect immunofluorescence (IIF) on HEp-2000® cells (Immuno Concepts, Sacramento, CA, USA). Patients with positive IIF were screened for autoantibodies against ENA using a lineblot assay including nRNP/Sm, Sm, SS-A, Ro-52, SS-B, Scl-70, PM-Scl,Jo-1, CENP-B, PCNA, dsDNA, nucleosomes, histones, ribosomal-P-proteins, AMA-M2, and DFS70 (ANA-Profile3plusDFS70, Euroimmun, Luebeck, Germany) and an anti-dsDNA-IgG-ELISA (Euro-Diagnostica, Malmö, Sweden). Anti-phospholipid-antibodies (Cardiolipin-IgG-ELISA, Euro-Diagnostica, Malmö, Sweden) and anti-proteinase-3 (Orgentec Diagnostika, Mainz, Germany) or myeloperoxidase (Euroimmun, Luebeck, Germany) was measured using ELISA. Two or more OCB detected by an isoelectric focusing technique (Hydragel Isofocusing, Sebia, France) were regarded as positive (15). Statistical analyses were performed using Fisher's exact test (two-sided) and Student's

TABLE 1 | Patient characteristics, serological findings, and MRZ-reaction.

	RDwCNS ($n = 40$)		**MS ($n = 68$)**		**Statistics (p-value)**	
Gender, female, *n* (%)	30 (75)		48 (71)		n.s.	
Mean age years (range, SD)	45.7 (19–79, 19.1)		44.9 (23–73, 12.3)		n.s.	
CEREBROSPINAL FLUID ANALYSIS RESULTS						
Increased total CSF cell count (>5/μl), *n* (%)	15 (37.5)		20 (29.4)		n.s.	
Mean cell count/μl in CSF, (range, SD)	31 (1–433, 84)		6 (1–44, 8)		$p = 0.0176$	
Cell count >50/μl, *n* (%)	4 (10)		0 (0)		$p = 0.0171$	
Intrathecal synthesis of IgG, IgM, or IgA, *n* (%)	11 (27.5)		43 (63.2)		$p = 0.0006$	
Oligoclonal bands, *n* (%)	13 (32.5)		61 (89.7)		$p < 0.0001$	
SEROLOGICAL FINDINGS						
Autoantibody positive, *n* (%)	38 (95)		68 (100)		n.s.	
IIF ANA positive, *n* (%)	33 (82.5)		68 (100)		n.s.	
Median ANA titer (IQR, range)	800 (400–3200; 200–6400)		400 (200–700; 100–3200)		$p = 0.0035$	
Anti-dsDNA, *n* (%)	22 (55)		3 (3.8)		$p < 0.0001$	
Anti-nucleosome/anti-PCNA-antibodies, *n* (%)	13 (32.5)		0 (0)		$p < 0.0001$	
Anti-SS-A/Ro, SS-B/La-antibodies, *n* (%)	6 (15)		0 (0)		$p < 0.0001$	
Anti-centromere, anti-Scl70 antibodies, *n* (%)	3 (7.5)		0 (0)		$p = 0.0352$	
DFS70-antibodies, *n* (%)	0 (0)		2 (2.9)		n.s.	
ANCA, *n* (%)	5 (12.5)		1 (1.5)		$p = 0.0254$	
APA, *n* (%)	12 (30)		2 (2.9)		$p < 0.0001$	
MEASLES-RUBELLA-ZOSTER-(MRZ)-REACTION						
Mean AI for M (range, SD)	1.2 (0.6–4.9; 0.7)		3.1 (0.5–22.7; 3.3)		$p = 0.0007$	
Mean AI for R (range, SD)	1.2 (0.6–5.4; 0.8)		3.3 (0.5–22.7; 4.1)		$p = 0.0021$	
Mean AI for Z (range, SD)	1.3 (0.6–4.2; 0.8)		2.3 (0.7–11.9; 2.3)		$p = 0.008$	
FREQUENCY OF POSITIVE ANTIBODY INDECES (AIs) FOR MEASLES, RUBELLA, ZOSTER						
Applied threshold defining a positive AI	**≥1.5**	**>2.0**	**≥1.5**	**>2.0**	**≥1.5**	**>2.0**
Positive AIs (**M**easles), *n* (%)	4 (10)	2 (5)	40 (58.8)	31 (45.6)	$p < 0.0001$	$p < 0.0001$
Positive AIs (**R**ubella), *n* (%)	4 (10)	2 (5)	33 (48.5)	27 (39.7)	$p < 0.0001$	$p < 0.0001$
Positive AIs (**Z**oster), *n* (%)	5 (12.5)	3 (7.5)	30 (44.1)	21 (30.9)	$p = 0.0006$	$p = 0.0043$
FREQUENCY OF PATIENTS WITH 0, 1, 2, 3 POSITIVE ANTIBODY INDECES (AI)						
Applied threshold defining a positive AI	**≥1.5**	**>2.0**	**≥1.5**	**>2.0**	**≥1.5**	**>2.0**
0 positive AI, *n* (%)	32 (80)	35 (88)	13 (19.1)	21 (30.9)	$p < 0.0001$	$p < 0.0001$
1 positive AI, *n* (%)	3 (7.5)	3 (7.5)	18 (26.5)	22 (32.4)	$p = 0.0221$	$p = 0.0039$
2 positive AIs, *n* (%)	3 (7.5)	1 (2.5)	19 (27.9)	16 (23.5)	$p = 0.0128$	$p = 0.0048$
3 positive AIs, *n* (%)	2 (5)	1 (2.5)	18 (26.5)	9 (13.2)	$p = 0.0049$	n.s.

AI, antibody index; ANA, antinuclear antibody; ANCA, anti-neutrophil cytoplasmic antibodies; APA, antiphospholipid antibodies; dsDNA, double stranded DNA; IIF, indirect immunofluorescence; M, measles; MS, multiple sclerosis; n, number of patients; n.s., not significant; RDwCNS, rheumatic diseases with involvement of the central nervous system; R, rubella; SD, standard deviation; Z, varicella zoster. The bold values are the applied thresholds (>1.5 or >2.0) defining a positive AI for the calculation of the MRZR.

t-test (two-sided) with a $p < 0.05$ regarded as statistically significant (Graphpad Prism version 7.01).

RESULTS

ANAs were assessed by IIF in a cohort of 149 MS-patients. We found 68 MS-patients (45.6%) with positive ANA and we compared them with 40 RDwCNS-patients. The RDwCNS-group consisted of 32 patients with SLE (80%), six with ANCA-associated vasculitis (15%), one with Cogan's syndrome and one with Behcet's disease. All RDwCNS patients fulfilled the classification criteria for their underlying rheumatic disease and showed signs of CNS involvement (definition see above). Except for the patients with Cogan's syndrome, Behcet's disease and one patient with ANCA-associated vasculitis all had at least one specific autoantibody supporting the diagnosis of the rheumatic disease. The diagnosis was also supported by concomitant non-neurological manifestations at the skin/mucosa ($n = 34$), joints ($n = 26$), blood/cytopenia ($n = 15$), peripheral nervous system ($n = 7$), ear-nose-throat-involvement ($n = 5$), pericarditis/pleuritis ($n = 5$), or lung-involvement ($n = 4$). Both groups were similar regarding age and sex (**Table 1**). In both, the MS- and the RDwCNS-group, <40% of patients had total CSF cell-counts above 5/μl. The RDwCNS-group though showed higher mean CSF cell-count (cells/μl) and higher frequency of patients with high CSF cell counts (>50 cells/μl) ($p < 0.05$ for both comparisons). The proportion of patients with increased intrathecal immunoglobulin synthesis (IgG, IgM, or IgA) and positive OCBs, both used as diagnostic parameters for MS, was significantly higher in MS-patients ($p < 0.001$ for both comparisons). Within the MS-group positive OCBs were found in 89.7% which was more frequent than a positive MRZR-1 (80.1%). Nevertheless positive OCBs and intrathecal immunoglobulin synthesis were also found in approximately 30% of our RDwCNS-patients. With respect to serological findings ANA-positive MS-patients had a lower median ANA serum titer compared to RDwCNS. Correspondingly, specific autoantibodies directed against nuclear antigens (ENA-analysis) were more frequent in RDwCNS (see **Table 1**).

Mean AIs for measles, rubella, and zoster were significantly higher in MS-patients compared to RDwCNS-patients (**Table 1**). Positive AIs, irrespectively of the thresholds used for definition (>1.5 and >2.0) were found with a higher frequency in ANA-positive MS compared to RDwCNS for all three specificities. Within the MS-group AIs were most frequently positive for measles, followed by rubella and varicella zoster. This AI-distribution pattern was not found within the RDwCNS-group. The MRZR-1 (AI positive when ≥1.5) was positive in 80.9% of ANA-positive MS-patients and 20% of RDwCNS-patients ($p < 0.0001$), the MRZR-2 was positive in 54.4% compared to 12.5% in RDwCNS ($p < 0.0001$) (**Figure 1**). By using the higher threshold of >2.0 for a positive AI, the prevalence of a positive MRZR-2 dropped to 2.5% ($n = 1$) within the RDwCNS-group compared to 36.8% within the MS-group ($p < 0.0001$).

Within the ANA-positive MS-group 55 of the 68 patients (80.9%) had a positive MRZR-1 but only seven MS-patients (10.3%) had specific autoantibodies. When combining both biomarkers, a positive MRZR-1 and the absence of autoantibodies against specific autoantigens, statistical analysis showed an increased specificity of 97.5% and an only slightly decreased sensitivity of 75% for the diagnosis of MS.

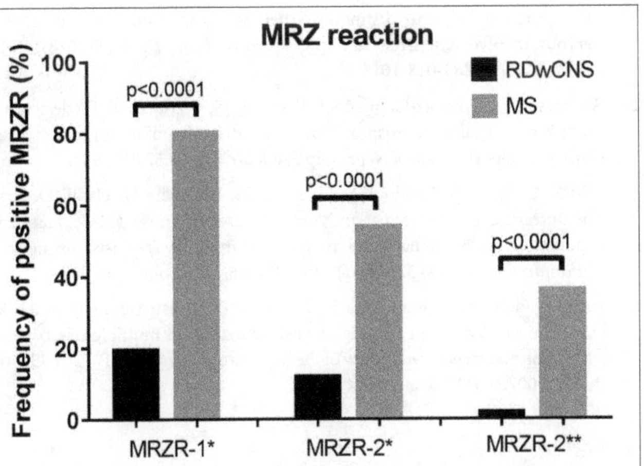

FIGURE 1 | MRZ reaction in RDwCNS patients compared to MS patients. Illustrated is the frequency of a positive MRZR-1 and MRZR-2 calculated with an AI defined positive when ≥1.5 (*) or >2.0 (**). MRZR, MRZ reaction; MS, multiple sclerosis; RDwCNS, rheumatic disease with CNS involvement.

DISCUSSION

Rheumatic diseases with involvement of the central nervous system are a diagnostic challenge, especially if CNS-involvement is the first or only manifestation. Furthermore, RDwCNS has to be distinguished from rheumatic diseases with co-manifestation of MS. Not only clinically, but also by using imaging diagnostics and CSF analyses it is often difficult to distinguish RDwCNS clearly from MS, especially within the early disease course of MS and when autoantibodies like ANA are present in MS-patients (1–3).

Antinuclear antibodies, which are the hallmark of connective tissue diseases, were found in nearly half of our MS-cohort, a frequency within the published range between 20 and 60% (1, 2). Also ANCA, crucial in the diagnostics of ANCA-associated vasculitides were found to be present in a small proportion of MS-patients. Since testing for specific autoantibodies (extractable nuclear antigens, dsDNA, anti-phospholipid-antibodies, anti-proteinase 3- or anti-myeloperoxidase-antibodies) was positive in only 10% of the ANA-positive MS-patients, ANA-diagnostics should always comprise both, indirect immunofluorescence for screening and immunoblot/ELISA for differentiation of antibodies against nuclear antigens, to distinguish RDwCNS from ANA-positive MS. ANA-differentiation should include DFS70-antibodies. If DFS70-antibodies are detected exclusively in an ANA-positive patient, the positive ANA-test does not increase the likelihood for a CTD (7). We found statistically significant differences between RDwCNS and MS regarding CSF cell count, the presence of OCBs and the production of intrathecal immunoglobulins, but none of these parameters was able to reliably differentiate ANA-positive MS from RDwCNS, when used exclusively. It has already been shown that a positive MRZR has a higher specificity than the presence of OCBs for the diagnosis of MS, while positive OCBs have a high sensitivity but quite low specificity. In line with these data we found OCBs more frequent than a positive MRZR-1 in our MS-group but also in a relatively high frequency in our RDwCNS-cohort. Even when combining MRI, CSF and clinical findings it can be difficult to differentiate MS from RDwCNS. Therefore, only the combination of several diagnostic parameters established for MS and for RDwCNS, may result in a diagnostic algorithm with sufficient sensitivity and specificity to distinguish between both disease entities. MRZR is already established as a valuable diagnostic tool in MS, but to date it is not used to differentiate RDwCNS from ANA-positive MS. Therefore, we aimed to include MRZR in the diagnostic algorithm in addition to already established diagnostic procedures (e.g., OCBs). MRZR was found positive more frequently in MS than in RDwCNS, despite a high frequency of autoantibodies, hypergammaglobulinemia and positive OCBs in RDwCNS. This is in accordance with findings described before in MS-patients independently of their ANA-status (14, 16, 17). Especially in combination with the absence of specific autoantibodies to nuclear antigens or lack of ANCA-reactivity against PR3 or MPO, MRZR-1 yielded a high specificity and a good sensitivity for diagnosis of MS. Since DFS70-autoantibodies, which help to exclude CTDs, were positive in only 2.5% of the MS-group, this test was of no further diagnostic value in ANA-positive MS-patients (7).

Three female patients in our RDwCNS-group had a positive MRZR-2 reaction (threshold $\geq$1.5). In one of these the MRZR remained positive even when a threshold >2.0 was applied, making it difficult to exclude the coexistence of both SLE and MS. Unfortunately, CSF diagnostics, electrophysiological tests, MRI, and the pattern of non-neurological clinical manifestations were not sufficient to exclude MS in this patient. In conclusion, we found a positive MRZR in a large proportion of ANA-positive MS-patients but in very few RDwCNS-patients. MRZR seems to be less sensitive but more specific than OCBs for the diagnosis of MS. Especially, when specific autoantibodies are absent, a positive MRZR yields a high specificity with good sensitivity. Therefore, we recommend including both, the MRZR and autoantibody screening for ENA, as parameters additionally to the established parameters like OCB in the diagnostic algorithm for differentiation of RDwCNS from ANA-positive MS.

AUTHOR CONTRIBUTIONS

NV, JT, US, DE, and TH designed and initiated this study. TH and SR identified the enrolled MS patients. NV, JT, CH, and RV identified the RDwCNS patients enrolled in this study. NV, TH, US, and JT performed the statistical analysis and drafted the manuscript. RV, MR, JS, DE, AV, and US helped in interpretation of the data and in drafting the manuscript. US and AV supervised the measurements of the rheumatic antibodies. DH supervised the performance of the immunoassays in the Institute of Virology. All authors have read the manuscript, contributed to manuscript revision, and approved the submitted version.

ACKNOWLEDGMENTS

Special thanks to the staff of the Institute of Virology who performed the immunoassays for MRZ; to the staff of the CSF laboratory at the Department of Neurology who analyzed the CSF/serum samples; and to the staff of the laboratory at the Clinic for Rheumatology and Clinical Immunology who helped in performing the measurements of the autoantibodies. This research received no specific financial or material support from any funding agency of the public, commercial, or not-for-profit sectors.

REFERENCES

1. Szmyrka-Kaczmarek M, Pokryszko-Dragan A, Pawlik B, Gruszka E, Korman L, Podemski R, et al. Antinuclear and antiphospholipid antibodies in patients with multiple sclerosis. *Lupus*. (2012) 21:412–20. doi: 10.1177/0961203311427550
2. Collard RC, Koehler RP, Mattson DH. Frequency and significance of antinuclear antibodies in multiple sclerosis. *Neurology*. (1997) 49:857–61. doi: 10.1212/WNL.49.3.857
3. Govoni M, Bortoluzzi A, Padovan M, Silvagni E, Borrelli M, Donelli F, et al. The diagnosis and clinical management of the neuropsychiatric manifestations of lupus. *J Autoimmun*. (2016) 74:41–72. doi: 10.1016/j.jaut.2016.06.013
4. Harirchian MH, Saberi H, Najafizadeh SR, Hashemi SA. Evaluation of brain and cervical MRI abnormality rates in patients with systemic lupus erythematosus with or without neurological manifestations. *Iran J Radiol*. (2011) 8:157–60. doi: 10.5812/kmp.iranjradiol.17351065.3138
5. Felgenhauer K, Reiber H. The diagnostic significance of antibody specificity indices in multiple sclerosis and herpes virus induced diseases of the nervous system. *Clin Investig*. (1992) 70:28–37. doi: 10.1007/BF00422934
6. Hottenrott T, Dersch R, Berger B, Rauer S, Huzly D, Stich O. The MRZ reaction in primary progressive multiple sclerosis. *Fluids Barriers CNS*. (2017) 14:2. doi: 10.1186/s12987-016-0049-7
7. Seelig CA, Bauer O, Seelig HP. Autoantibodies against DFS70/LEDGF exclusion markers for Systemic Autoimmune Rheumatic Diseases (SARD). *Clin Lab*. (2016) 62:499–517. doi: 10.7754/Clin.Lab.2015.150905
8. Hochberg MC. Updating the American College of Rheumatology revised criteria for the classification of systemic lupus erythematosus. *Arthritis Rheum*. (1997) 40:1725. doi: 10.1002/art.1780400928
9. Leavitt RY, Fauci AS, Bloch DA, Michel BA, Hunder GG, Arend WP, et al. The American College of Rheumatology 1990 criteria for the classification of Wegener's granulomatosis. *Arthritis Rheum*. (1990) 33:1101–7. doi: 10.1002/art.1780330807
10. Jennette JC, Falk RJ, Bacon PA, Basu N, Cid MC, Ferrario F, et al. 2012 revised International Chapel Hill Consensus Conference Nomenclature of Vasculitides. *Arthritis Rheum*. (2013) 65:1–11. doi: 10.1002/art.37715
11. Evaluation of diagnostic ('classification') criteria in Behçet's disease–towards internationally agreed criteria. The International Study Group for Behçet's disease. *Br J Rheumatol*. (1992) 31:299–308.
12. Polman CH, Reingold SC, Banwell B, Clanet M, Cohen JA, Filippi M, et al. Diagnostic criteria for multiple sclerosis: 2010 revisions to the McDonald criteria. *Ann Neurol*. (2011) 69:292–302. doi: 10.1002/ana.22366
13. Reiber H. Cerebrospinal fluid-physiology, analysis and interpretation of protein patterns for diagnosis of neurological diseases. *Mult Scler*. (1998) 4:99–107.
14. Hottenrott T, Dersch R, Berger B, Endres D, Huzly D, Thiel J, et al. The MRZ reaction helps to distinguish rheumatologic disorders with central nervous involvement from multiple sclerosis. *BMC Neurol*. (2018) 18:14. doi: 10.1186/s12883-018-1018-3
15. Andersson M, Alvarez-Cermeño J, Bernardi G, Fredman P, Frederiksen J, Fredrikson S, et al. Cerebrospinal fluid in the diagnosis of multiple sclerosis: a consensus report. *J Neurol Neurosurg Psychiatr*. (1994) 57:897–902.
16. Feki S, Gargouri S, Mejdoub S, Dammak M, Hachicha H, Hadiji O, et al. The intrathecal polyspecific antiviral immune response (MRZ reaction): a potential cerebrospinal fluid marker for multiple sclerosis diagnosis. *J Neuroimmunol*. (2018) 321:66–71. doi: 10.1016/j.jneuroim.2018.05.015
17. Jarius S, Eichhorn P, Franciotta D, Petereit HF, Akman-Demir G, Wick M, et al. The MRZ reaction as a highly specific marker of multiple sclerosis: re-evaluation and structured review of the literature. *J Neurol*. (2017) 264:453–66. doi: 10.1007/s00415-016-8360-4

11

Seizure and Myelin Oligodendrocyte Glycoprotein Antibody-Associated Encephalomyelitis in a Retrospective Cohort of Chinese Patients

Xiaonan Zhong [1†], Yifan Zhou [1†], Yanyu Chang [1], Jingqi Wang [1], Yaqing Shu [1], Xiaobo Sun [1], Lisheng Peng [1], Alexander Y. Lau [2], Allan G. Kermode [1,3,4,5] and Wei Qiu [1]*

[1] Department of Neurology, The Third Affiliated Hospital of Sun Yat-sen University, Guangzhou, China, [2] Department of Medicine and Therapeutics, The Chinese University of Hong Kong, Shatin, China, [3] Centre for Neuromuscular and Neurological Disorders, University of Western Australia, Perth, WA, Australia, [4] Department of Neurology, Sir Charles Gairdner Hospital, Queen Elizabeth II Medical Centre, Perth, WA, Australia, [5] Institute of Immunology and Infectious Diseases, Murdoch University, Perth, WA, Australia

***Correspondence:**
Wei Qiu
qiuwei120@vip.163.com

† These authors have contributed equally to this work

Background: Myelin oligodendrocyte glycoprotein (MOG) antibody associated encephalomyelitis is increasingly being considered a distinct disease entity, with seizures and encephalopathy commonly reported. We investigated the clinical features of MOG-IgG positive patients presenting with seizures and/or encephalopathy in a single cohort.

Methods: Consecutive patients with suspected idiopathic inflammatory demyelinating diseases were recruited from a tertiary University hospital in Guangdong province, China. Subjects with MOG-IgG seropositivity were analyzed according to whether they presented with or without seizure and/or encephalopathy.

Results: Overall, 58 subjects seropositive for MOG-IgG were analyzed, including 23 (40%) subjects presenting with seizures and/or encephalopathy. Meningeal irritation ($P = 0.030$), fever ($P = 0.001$), headache ($P = 0.001$), nausea, and vomiting ($P = 0.004$) were more commonly found in subjects who had seizures and/or encephalopathy, either at presentation or during the disease course. Nonetheless, there was less optic nerve (4/23, 17.4%, $P = 0.003$) and spinal cord (6/16, 37.5%, $P = 0.037$) involvement as compared to subjects without seizures or encephalopathy. Most MOG encephalomyelitis subjects had cortical/subcortical lesions: 65.2% (15/23) in the seizures and/or encephalopathy group and 50.0% (13/26) in the without seizures or encephalopathy group. Cerebrospinal fluid (CSF) leukocytes were elevated in both groups. Subgroup analysis showed that 30% (7/23) MOG-IgG positive subjects with seizures and/or encephalopathy had been misdiagnosed for central nervous system infection on the basis of meningoencephalitis symptoms and elevated CSF leukocytes ($P = 0.002$).

Conclusions: Seizures and encephalopathy are not rare in MOG encephalomyelitis, and are commonly associated with cortical and subcortical brain lesions. MOG-encephalomyelitis often presents with clinical meningoencephalitis symptoms and abnormal CSF findings mimicking central nervous system infection in pediatric and young adult patients.

Keywords: MOG-IgG, MOG antibody-associated encephalomyelitis, seizures, encephalopathy, demyelinating disease

BACKGROUND

Immunoglobulin-G against myelin oligodendrocyte glycoprotein (MOG-IgG) is considered a potential demyelinating disease-associated autoantibody. Previous experimental studies have established MOG-IgG as a pathogenic antigen rather than an epiphenomenal bystander or a secondary immune reaction caused by previous demyelination (1–4). Although some cases of MOG-IgG positive patients fulfill the diagnostic criteria of neuromyelitis optica spectrum disorders (NMOSD), multiple sclerosis (MS), acute disseminated encephalomyelitis (ADEM), or other idiopathic inflammatory demyelinating diseases (IIDDs), there are no distinct types of IIDDs that can explain all presentations of MOG-IgG positive patients. Currently, most experts consider MOG-IgG-associated demyelination as an isolated disease entity distinct from both classic MS and aquaporin-4 (AQP4)-IgG-positive NMOSD (5–7).

MOG encephalomyelitis is associated with a wide spectrum of symptoms, including seizure and encephalopathy. Of note, seizure and encephalopathy have been recommended recently as typical clinical findings of MOG encephalomyelitis (8). In several case reports, MOG-IgG positive patients, who initially presented with optic neuritis (ON) (9) or ADEM (10), developed seizures in subsequent disease course. MOG-IgG positive patients often had an aggressive disease course with residual cognitive dysfunction (11). Several observational studies with small sample sizes reported the presence of seizures ranged from 14.70 to 36.36% in MOG-IgG positive patients (12, 13), and the main symptoms were generalized seizure with or without encephalopathy (12, 14). Nevertheless, studies with detailed description of the clinical, radiological, laboratory characteristics, and disease course of MOG-IgG positive patients with seizures and/or encephalopathy are lacking.

In our registry of patients with IIDDs, MOG-IgG positive patients with seizures and/or encephalopathy were also observed. In the present study, we investigated the clinical profiles of MOG-IgG positive patients with seizures and/or encephalopathy.

Abbreviations: ADEM, acute disseminated encephalomyelitis AQP4, aquaporin-4; ATM, acute transverse myelitis; CNS, central nervous system; CSF, cerebrospinal fluid; EDSS, expanded disability status scale; IIDDs, idiopathic inflammatory demyelinating diseases; MOG, myelin oligodendrocyte glycoprotein; MOG-IgG, immunoglobulin G against myelin oligodendrocyte glycoprotein; MRI, magnetic resonance imaging; MS, multiple sclerosis; NMOSD, neuromyelitis optica spectrum disorders; OCB, oligoclonal bands; ON, optic neuritis; LEON, Longitudinally extensive optic neuritis; LETM, Longitudinally extensive transverse myelitis.

METHODS

Subjects

Consecutive MOG encephalomyelitis patients who were seropositive for MOG-IgG and seronegative for AQP4-IgG were recruited from the Third Affiliated Hospital of Sun Yat-sen University in Guangzhou, China, between June 2015 and December 2017. These patients were prospectively enrolled and followed up for at least 1 year after diagnosis. Our hospital is a tertiary general hospital with a demyelinating disease center. Over 2,000 IIDDs patients, such as patients with MS, NMOSD, and ADEM and so on, are follow-up in outpatient per year, and about 300 newly diagnosed IIDDs patients attended every year. This study was approved by the Ethics Committees of the Third Affiliated Hospital of Sun Yat-sen University. Written informed consent was obtained from each participant.

We diagnosed MS, NMOSD, and ADEM according to the 2010 McDonald diagnostic criteria for MS (15), the 2015 Wingerchuk criteria for NMOSD (16), and the 2012 criteria for ADEM (17), respectively. Data of clinical presentation, initial clinical diagnosis, MOG-IgG serum titer, cerebrospinal fluid characteristics, MRI characteristics, treatments and prognosis were collected. A clinical relapse was defined as a sudden appearance of new symptoms lasting for at least 24 h, with an increase in the Expanded Disability Status Scale (EDSS) score over 1.0 and magnetic resonance imaging (MRI) showing the presence of enhanced lesions or new T2 lesions. The remission phase was defined as a period when the neurological condition of the patient had been stable for more than 3 months and the next relapse did not occur for at least a further 3 months. The EDSS score was evaluated at the nadir of disease recurrence when the patient first came to our hospital and at the last follow-up.

Detection of MOG-IgG and AQP4-IgG

All subjects were tested for serum MOG-IgG and AQP4-IgG. Serum was collected at the nadir of clinical relapse when the subjects first came to one of our academic centers. MOG-IgG in serum was tested by an in-house, cell-based assay using live cells transfected with full-length human MOG, as we described in other published articles (18, 19). Full-length human MOG was subcloned into the pIRES2-EGFP plasmid. The purified plasmids were DNA sequenced and they were used to transiently transfect HEK293T cells using Lipofectamine2000 reagent, according to the manufacturer's instructions (Thermo Scientific, USA). Thirty-six hours after transfection, live cells were incubated at room temperature with centrifuged serum [1:50, diluted in

Dulbecco's modified Eagle's medium (DMEM)] from patients and the control group for 30 min. After removing the media and washing with PBS, the HEK293T cells were fixed with 4% paraformaldehyde for 20 min and blocked with 5% goat serum for 30 min. Cells were then immunolabeled with an AlexaFluor 546 secondary antibody against human IgG (1:1,000; Thermo Scientific) for 1 h at room temperature. Images were acquired using a Zeiss Axiovert A1 fluorescence microscope (**Supplement**). Indirect immunofluorescence test systems for detecting human AQP4-IgG (Euroimmun Medizinische Labordiagnostika, Lübeck, Germany) were used according to the manufacturer's instructions.

Study of Cerebrospinal Fluid (CSF) Samples

Lumbar puncture was performed in the acute phase of the disease. Cerebrospinal fluid (CSF) leukocyte count, total protein, and absence/presence of oligoclonal bands (OCB) were determined by the hospital laboratories.

Magnetic Resonance Imaging Scanning

Brain and spinal cord MRI scans of subjects were performed for routine clinical diagnostic purposes using a 1.5 or 3.0 T Siemens system (Siemens). All MRI were performed using T1 with and without gadolinium enhancement and T2. In brain MRI scans T2 were also performed with T2 fluid-attenuated inversion recovery sequences. Lesions in the brain and spinal cord were scanned sagittally and axially, and the results were analyzed anonymously by two independent radiologists who were blinded to the subjects' clinical features. Lesions were scored as "large" if their size exceeded 2 cm in any plane.

Statistical Analysis

For continuous variables, the data were reported as mean ± standard deviation or median with range. The Mann–Whitney *U*-test and chi-square test were used to compare clinical, laboratory and MRI data between subjects in different groups or subgroups. The Wilcoxon test was used to compare MOG-IgG titers at relapse and at remission within a group. Correlations between MOG-IgG titers and clinical data were analyzed using Spearman's correlation coefficient. All statistical analyses were performed using SPSS 23.0 software (SPSS Inc., Chicago, IL, USA) for Windows. Differences with $P < 0.05$ were considered statistically significant.

RESULTS

Clinical Presentation

Overall, we recruited 58 subjects seropositive for MOG-IgG and seronegative for AQP4-IgG, including 23 (39.7%, 23/58) subjects with seizures and/or encephalopathy and 35 subjects without seizures or encephalopathy. The demographic and clinical features of the subjects were shown in **Table 1**.

Subjects with seizures and/or encephalopathy had a younger onset age and a higher EDSS score at the nadir stage of disease

TABLE 1 | Comparison of clinical features between MOG-IgG positive subjects with or without seizures and/or encephalopathy.

	Subjects with seizures or encephalopathy (*n* = 23)	Subjects without seizures or encephalopathy (*n* = 35)
Sex, male, N(%)	12 (52%)	17 (49%)
Onset age, years (range)	12 (3–56)*	26 (3–63)
Disease duration, months (range)	34 (9–85)	22 (8–120)
Follow-up, months (range)	13 (5–85)	15 (4–50)
Multiphasic disease course, N(%)	18 (78%)*	16 (46%)
Number of attacks, N (range)	3 (2–8)	3 (2–5)
Time to second attack, months, median (range)	5 (1–48)	3 (1–48)
Annualized relapse rate, ARR median (range)	1.16 (0.67–2.77)	1.42 (0.38–3.75)
With prodromal symptoms, N (%)	7 (30%)	6 (17%)
Manifestations at onset, N(%)		
Seizures	11 (48%)*	0 (0%)
Disturbance of consciousness	6 (26%)*	0 (0%)
Psychiatric symptoms	2 (9%)	0 (0%)
Cognitive disorders	3 (13%)*	0 (0%)
Meningeal symptoms	3 (13%)*	0 (0%)
Optic nerve symptoms	4 (17%)*	21 (60%)
Spinal symptoms	5 (22%)	10 (29%)
Brainstem symptoms	2 (9%)	2 (6%)
Diencephalon	2 (9%)	0 (0%)
Cerebrum symptoms	5 (22%)	3 (9%)
Cerebellar symptoms	0 (0%)	0 (0%)
Fever	13 (57%)*	4 (11%)
Headache	13 (57%)*	4 (11%)
Dizziness	4 (17%)	3 (9%)
Nausea and Vomiting	5 (22%)*	0 (0%)
Ever manifestations of full course, N(%)		
Seizures	14 (61%)*	0 (0%)
Disturbance of consciousness	9 (39%)*	0 (0%)
psychiatric symptoms	4 (17%)*	0 (0%)
Cognitive disorders	4 (17%)*	0 (0%)
Meningeal symptoms	4 (17%)*	0 (0%)
Optic nerve symptoms	11 (48%)	24 (69%)
Spinal symptoms	7 (30%)	15 (43%)
Brainstem symptoms	4 (17%)	6 (17%)
Diencephalon	4 (17%)*	0 (0%)
Cerebrum symptoms	9 (39%)*	5 (14%)
Cerebellar symptoms	2 (9%)	0 (0%)
Fever	14 (61%)*	4 (11%)
Headache	14 (61%)*	4 (11%)
Dizziness	6 (26%)	3 (9%)
Nausea and Vomiting	11 (48%)*	1 (3%)
EDSS score		
EDSS score at peak stage (range)	5 (2–8) *	3 (1–8.5)
EDSS score at last follow up (range)	0 (0–2) *	1 (0–5)

(Continued)

TABLE 1 | Continued

	Subjects with seizures or encephalopathy ($n = 23$)	Subjects without seizures or encephalopathy ($n = 35$)
Autoantibody, *N* (%)		
Concomitant autoantibody	3 (13%)	5 (14%)
Coexisting autoimmune disease#	1 (4%)	1 (3%)
MOG-Ab titer, *N* (%)		
1:25-1:100	10 (43%)	16 (46%)
1:320-1:640	9 (39%)	14 (40%)
≧ 1:1280	4 (17%)	5 (14%)
AQP4-IgG, *N* (%)	0(0%)	0(0%)

Time to second attack and annualized relapse rate refers to multiphasic patients.
EDSS, expanded disability status scale.
NA, not available.
#Coexisting autoimmune disease refers to autoimmune disease other than IIDDs.
**P < 0.05.*

compared to those without seizure and/or encephalopathy. At disease onset, the percentages of meningeal irritation (including nuchal rigidity, Brudzinski sign, or Kerning sign), fever, headache, nausea and vomiting were significantly higher in subjects who experienced seizures and/or encephalopathy. But there was less optic nerve involvement in the patients had seizures and/or encephalopathy.

Seizures and Encephalopathy in MOG-IgG Positive Subjects

During the course of the disease, seizure was observed in 14 subjects among the whole 58 patients recruited in our study (all in the MOG encephalomyelitis with seizures and/or encephalopathy group): 11 (79%) subjects had seizure as the first symptom, and 3 (21%) developed seizure during the subsequent relapse at 5, 29, and 42 months, respectively after the disease onset. The types of seizure were generalized tonic-clonic seizure ($n = 7$, 50%), focal seizure with secondary generalization ($n = 5$, 36%), complex partial seizure with alternated conscious and facial twitching ($n = 1$, 7%), and simple partial seizure with focal left arm twitching ($n = 1, 7\%$).

Encephalopathy was observed in 13 subjects during the period of the disease. This symptom was the first symptom in 10 (77%) subjects; subjects had disturbance of consciousness with varying degrees of somnolence and stupor, psychiatric symptoms including hallucinations, confused speech and apathy, and, cognitive disorders including memory impairment and acalculia.

Electroencephalogram (EEG) was abnormal among 15 (25.9%) subjects, including slowed background (theta to delta rhythm), intermittent low amplitude fast waves, focal sharp-wave complex and asymmetry focal slow waves.

Initial Clinical Diagnosis

A significantly higher proportion of subjects suffered from seizures and/or encephalopathy were diagnosed as non-specific IIDDs, while NMOSD was a common diagnosis in the patients who did not subject from seizures or encephalopathy (**Figure 1**).

MOG-IgG Serum Titer

The median serum MOG-IgG titer at the nadir stage of disease was 1:320 (range 1:25–1:1280). There was no difference in the MOG-IgG titer between subjects with and without seizure and/or encephalopathy (**Table 1, Figure 2**).

In the seizures and/or encephalopathy group, the MOG-IgG titer at the peak stage was positive related with EDSS score at last follow-up (**Table 2**).

Other Autoantibodies and Autoimmune Disease

Rheumatoid and thyroid autoantibodies were found in a small number of subjects, including antinuclear antibody (3/58, 5%), anti-Sjogren syndrome A antibody (SSA) (2/58, 3%), anti-thyroid peroxidase antibodies (aTPO) and/or antithyroglobulin antibodies (aTG) (5/58, 9%). Concurrent systemic autoimmune diseases were found in 2 subjects; one had systemic vasculitis and the other has autoimmune hyperthyroidism (**Table 1**).

CSF Investigation

Records of CSF were available for analysis in 45 (78%, 45/58) subjects, including 18 (78%, 18/23) subjects in the seizures and/or encephalopathy group and 27 (77%, 27/35) subjects in the without seizures or encephalopathy group. Some CSF data in remaining 13 (22%, 13/58) subjects were examined in the local hospitals which the patients had visited before they came to our hospital and were not offered to us. CSF leukocytosis was noted in 61% (11/18) subjects subjected from seizures and/or encephalopathy and 41% (11/27) subjects who did not have seizures or encephalopathy, and there was no statistical significance in the levels of CSF leukocytosis between these groups. No difference was found in the CSF protein concentration between the two groups. Oligoclonal band was present in 7 (12%, 7/58) subjects, and no difference was noted among those with or without seizure and/or encephalopathy (**Table 3**).

MRI Findings

Brain MRI was performed in 46 (79%, 46/58) subjects. In MOG-IgG positive subjects with seizures and/or encephalopathy, the lesions in cortical/subcortical (15/23, 65%), white matter (including periventricular and corpus callosum, 21/23, 91%), deep gray matter (including thalamus and basal ganglia, 13/23, 57%), and infratentorial (including cerebral peduncle, brain stem and cerebellum, 14/23, 60.9%) areas were involved (**Figure 3**). There was a higher proportion of deep white matter and cerebral peduncle in the seizures and/or encephalopathy group.

Spinal MRI was performed in 40 (69%, 40/58) subjects, including 16 subjects with seizures and/or encephalopathy and 24 subjects without seizures or encephalopathy. Less involvement of the spinal cord was found in the seizures and/or encephalopathy group (**Table 4**).

Clinical Course Over Time

After followed up for at least 1 year, subjects suffered from seizures and/or encephalopathy had more multiphasic disease course compared to those without seizure and/or

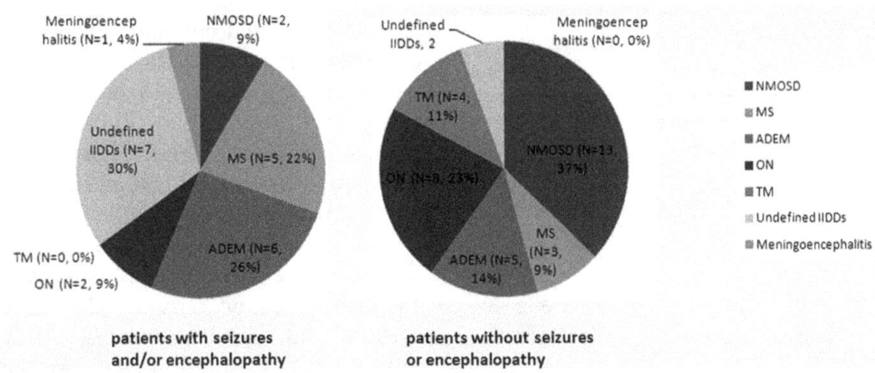

FIGURE 1 | Initial clinical diagnosis in MOG-IgG positive patients with or without seizures and/or encephalopathy. A significantly higher proportion of subjects with seizures and/or encephalopathy were diagnosed as non-specific IIDDs ($P = 0.030$), while NMOSD were commonly diagnosed among subjects without seizures or encephalopathy ($P = 0.035$).

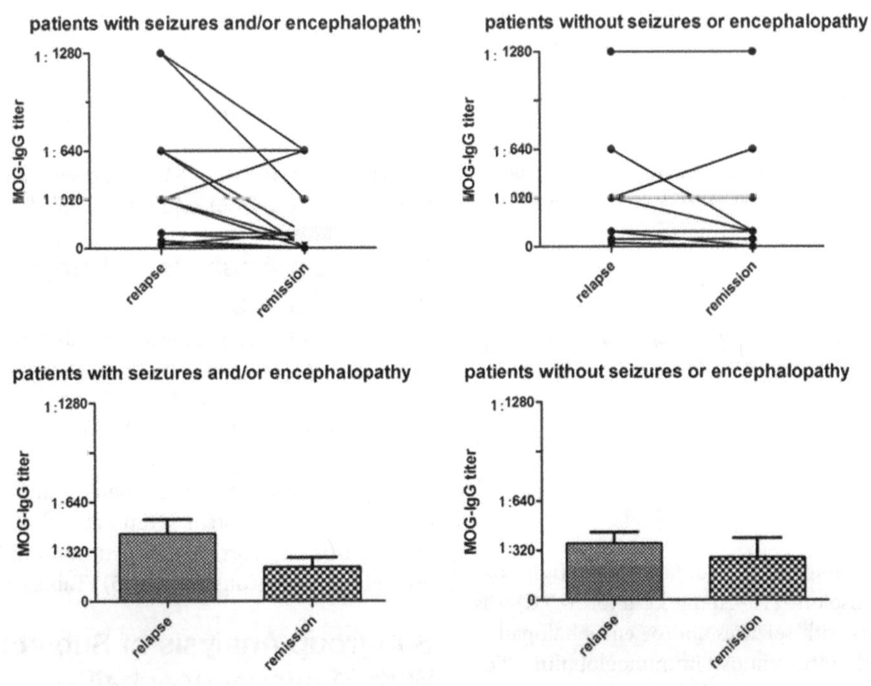

FIGURE 2 | Serum MOG-IgG titers in MOG-IgG positive patients with or without seizures and/or encephalopathy. In the seizure and/or encephalopathy group, MOG-IgG titers were significantly higher at the nadir stage of relapse when compared with titers at last follow-up ($P = 0.021$), although there was no difference in serum MOG-IgG titers between relapses and remission in the without seizures or encephalopathy group ($P = 0.080$).

encephalopathy. At the last follow-up, complete recovery (EDSS 0) was noted in over half ($n = 14$, 61%) of the subjects who had seizures and/or encephalopathy, and a smaller proportion of benign prognosis was observed in the counterparts without seizures and/or encephalopathy ($n = 13$, 37%). Throughout the period of the disease, the percentages of meningeal irritation, fever, headache, nausea and vomiting, diencephalon, and cerebrum symptoms were significantly higher in subjects with seizures and/or encephalopathy than those without. The proportions of number of attacks, time to the second attack and annual relapse rate were not significantly different between the two groups.

We evaluated the longitudinal changes in serum MOG-IgG titres during the remission phase at the last follow-up in 17 (73.9%) subjects who had seizure and/or encephalopathy and 14 (40.0%) subjects not experiencing these symptoms; MOG-IgG titer decreased 65% and 57% in the two groups, respectively. In the seizures and/or encephalopathy group, MOG-IgG titers

TABLE 2 | Correlations between MOG-IgG titers at relapse and clinical features in MOG-IgG positive patients.

	Patients with seizures and encephalopathy (n = 23)	Patients without seizures or encephalopathy (n = 35)
	r value	*r* value
MOG-IgG titers at last follow up	0.558*	0.921*
EDSS score at peak stage	0.150	0.415*
EDSS score at last follow up	0.494*	−0.188
Annual relapse rate	−0.020	−0.024
CSF leukocyte	−0.134	0.368
CSF total protein	−0.188	0.462*

r: correlation coefficient.
CSF: cerebrospinal fluid; EDSS, expanded disability status scale; MOG-IgG, immunoglobulin G against myelin oligodendrocyte glycoprotein.
NA, not available.
$^{*}P < 0.05$.

TABLE 3 | Comparison of CSF features between MOG-IgG positive patients with or without seizures and/or encephalopathy.

	Patients with seizures or encephalopathy (n = 18)	Patients without seizures or encephalopathy (n = 27)
Presence of oligoclonal bands, N (%)	3 (16.7%)	4 (14.8%)
Leukocyte count, x10^6/L, median (range)	21 (0–457)	2 (0–314)
Total protein (mg/L), median (range)	0.25 (0.09–1.06)	0.28 (0.07–0.99)

were significantly higher at the nadir stage compared with last follow-up (**Figure 2**).

Treatments

All subjects received treatment for acute attacks. High-dose intravenous methylprednisolone (10–20 mg/kg/d for 3–5 d) was used in 22 (96%) subjects with seizures and/or encephalopathy, and 5 (22%) received intravenous immunoglobulin. For subjects without seizure and/or encephalopathy, intravenous methylprednisolone was used in 35 (100%) subjects, and 3 (9%) received intravenous immunoglobulin. Low-dose oral glucocorticoid (4–8 mg qd/qod) for maintenance was used in 10 (44%) subjects suffered from seizures and/or encephalopathy and 20 (57%) subjects who did not have seizure and/or encephalopathy. Long-term immunosuppressive or immunomodulatory treatments were used in 7 (30%) of subjects with seizures and/or encephalopathy: rituximab (n = 3, 13%), azathioprine (n = 2, 9%), mycophenolate mofetil (n = 1, 4%), and tacrolimus (n = 1, 4%). For subjects without seizure and/or encephalopathy, 12 (34%) subjects were treated with immunosuppressive or immunomodulatory treatments: azathioprine (n = 7, 20%), mycophenolate mofetil (n = 2, 6%), rituximab (n = 1, 3%), tacrolimus (n = 1, 3%), and cyclophosphamide (n = 1, 3%).

The two subgroups have similar response to the corticosteroids and immunosuppression. In the seizure and/or encephalopathy group, 18 subjects had multiphasic disease course. And 10 of these 18 subjects were treated by low-dose oral glucocorticoid at the early stage of disease, but 40% (4/10) of them were suffered from relapse and started the combination therapy of oral glucocorticoid and immunosuppressive; however, 1 of the patients receive combination therapy still experienced treatment failure. Another 3 subjects with a high relapse rate did not recurrence after immunosuppressive treatment. Among the 16 subjects without seizure and/or encephalopathy, low-dose corticoid was utilized in 9 subjects, and 33.3% (3/9) of them relapse but refuse to immunosuppression, with 2 of these 3 subjects experienced recurrence after steroid withdrawal. No relapse was observed after immunosuppression was used in 7 subjects.

In the seizures and/or encephalopathy group, antiviral drugs were used in 4 (17%) subjects who were initially suspected to have CNS viral infection, antibiotics were used in 5 (22%) subjects initially suspected to have a CNS bacterial infection, and 1 (4%) subject initially diagnosed as tuberculosis meningoencephalitis was treated with anti-tuberculosis drugs.

Some subjects (10/14, 71%) with seizure were treated with anti-epileptic drugs, including levetiracetam (n = 4, 29%), oxcarbazepine (n = 3, 21%), carbamazepine (n = 2, 14%), sodium valproate (n = 2, 14%), and nitrazepam (n = 1, 7%).

Subgroup Analysis of Subjects With Seizures

Among the 14 (24%) subjects who developed seizure, 11 (79%) subjects had seizure as their first symptoms. These subjects were younger ($P < 0.001$) and were associated with more clinical relapses ($P = 0.007$). In addition to seizure, these subjects commonly presented with disturbance of consciousness, meningism, fever, headache, nausea and vomiting, as well as cognitive and brainstem symptoms ($P < 0.05$) (**Table 1**). CSF leukocytosis and cortical/subcortical brain lesions on MRI were noted in this subgroup ($P < 0.05$) (**Tables 3, 4**).

Subgroup Analysis of Subjects With Meningoencephalitis

A small subgroup of subjects (n = 7, 12%) presented with symptoms suggesting CNS infection, including fever, headache, nausea, meningism, seizures, and encephalopathy. Antiviral or antibacterial treatments were prescribed. The CSF showed raised opening pressure (median 205 mm) and marked leukocytosis (median 177 × 10^6/L), and raised total protein (median 0.49 mg/L).

DISCUSSION

We have presented the clinical features of a cohort of Chinese patients with MOG-associated encephalomyelitis from Guangdong, China. We found that seizures and/or encephalopathy were commonly seen in pediatric and young adult patients with MOG-IgG, often complicating with a

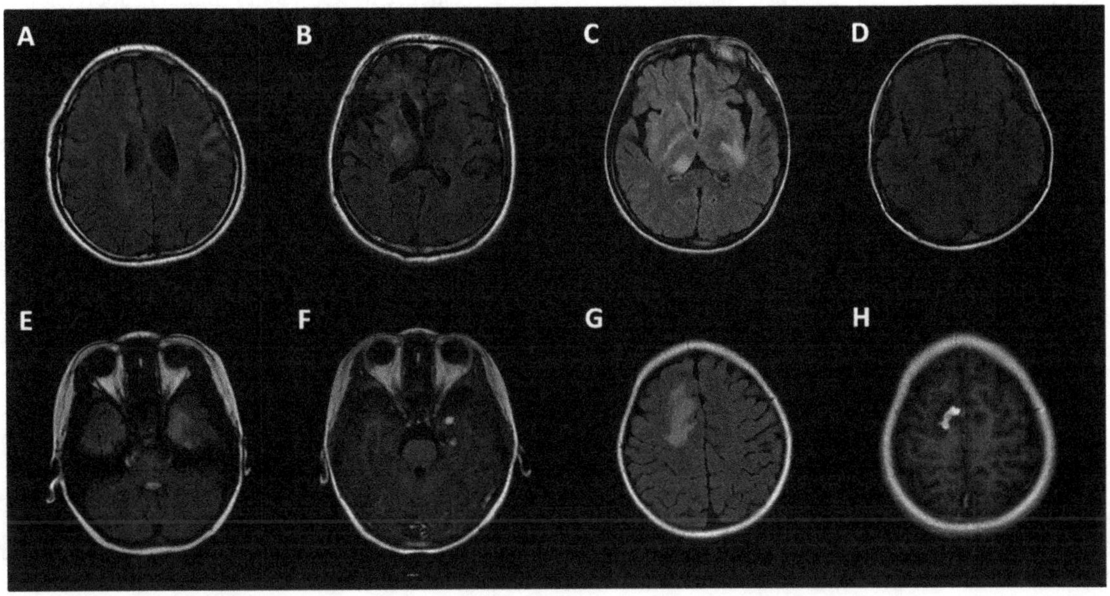

FIGURE 3 | Brain MRI of MOG-IgG positive patients with seizures and/or encephalopathy. **(A)** Cortical and subcortical lesions; **(B)** Deep white matter lesions and periventricular lesions; **(C)** Thalamus lesions; **(D)** Cerebral peduncle lesions; **(E,G)** Large white matter lesions of a patient in temporal lobe and parietal lobe, with prominent gadolinium enhancement **(F,H)**.

relapsing disease course. Unlike older patients with classical optic neuritis, myelitis, or brainstem syndromes, these patients were often diagnosed as CNS infection due to clinical, radiological, and CSF findings. MOG encephalomyelitis should be considered to be a differential diagnosis in these patients.

Consistent with previous studies, ON, myelitis, and/or brainstem symptoms were the predominant clinical features in most adult MOG-encephalomyelitis patients, whilst in children and younger adults there was a shift toward ADEM imitation (8, 18, 20–22), with encephalopathy as a clinical characteristic.

In our study, the percentage of subjects with seizures and/or encephalopathy was 40%, which is higher than most of the previous studies, and is more consistent with a recent study by Gutman et al. (13). However, our study had a much larger sample size ($n = 58$). Therefore, we speculate that the proportion of seizures and encephalopathy in MOG encephalomyelitis patients is higher than originally thought, but in the past, these patients might be diagnosed as CNS infection rather than immune mediated encephalomyelitis. Moreover, most of these patients had seizures (79%) and/or encephalopathy (77%) as their first symptoms. Furthermore, generalized seizure was the main type of seizure in our study, which is consistent with a study by Ogawa et al. (14). In our cohort, 42% subjects had focal seizure with secondary generalization, suggesting that epileptogenic regions, such as the cortex and temporal lobe, may be affected. This was supported by the finding of cortical lesions on MRI brain in 40% of our cohort.

In addition, we added further knowledge to previous studies by showing that meningoencephalitis symptoms, including fever, headache, nausea/vomiting, meningeal irritation, and CSF leukocytosis were common in MOG encephalomyelitis patients who were suffered from seizures and/or encephalopathy. Some of these symptoms had been noticed in various previous studies; however, most of the studies did not discuss the symptoms with seizures and/or encephalopathy meanwhile (23). Often, these patients may have delayed immunosuppressive treatment because of being misdiagnosed as CNS infection. Therefore, young patients with fever and meningoencephalitis should also be evaluated for possible MOG encephalomyelitis. Immunosuppressive treatment could be commenced if CSF microbiological results were negative and MOG-IgG was positive, which may improve clinical prognosis.

Another finding was the multiphasic course of patients who were subjected to seizures and/or encephalopathy. Similarly, disease relapse was reported in all 5 MOG-IgG positive patients with seizures in a study by Hamid et al. (12). Yet our patients who had not experienced seizures or encephalopathy had a lower multiphase ratio which were analogous to the previous researches (23–25). Thus, maintenance immunomodulation treatment should be used to prevent relapse in MOG encephalomyelitis patients who had seizures and/or encephalopathy.

From another perspective, part of the clinical features of our MOG encephalomyelitis patients with seizures and/or encephalopathy was close to that of MOG encephalomyelitis patients without seizures or encephalopathy, suggesting that these two subgroups were the same disease. For instance, our MOG encephalomyelitis patients who were suffered from seizures and/or encephalopathy also had a less female dominance, a relative lower coexisting autoimmunity rate, a

TABLE 4 | Comparison of MRI features between MOG-IgG positive patients with or without seizures and/or encephalopathy.

	Patients with seizures and encephalopathy	Patients without seizures or encephalopathy
BRAIN MRI, *N* (%)		
Total abnormal	21 (91%)	22 (85%)
Frontal lobe	18 (86%)	12 (55%)
Parietal lobe	13 (62%)	12 (55%)
Temporal lobe	11 (52%)	7 (32%)
Hippocampus	3 (14%)	1 (5%)
Occipital lobe	7 (33%)	5 (23%)
Insula	7 (33%)	2 (9%)
Meninges	3 (14%)	2 (9%)
Cortical	7 (33%)	4 (18%)
Subcortical	14 (67%)	12 (55%)
Deep white matter	20 (95%)*	10 (45%)
Periventricular	14 (67%)	9 (41%)
Corpus callosum	7 (33%)	4 (18%)
Thalamus	7 (33%)	5 (23%)
Hypothalamus	0 (0%)	1 (5%)
Basal ganglia	8 (38%)	6 (27%)
Internal capsule	1 (5%)	2 (9%)
cerebral peduncle	7 (33%)*	0 (0%)
Midbrain	4 (19%)	3 (14%)
Pons	6 (29%)	4 (18%)
Medulla	4 (19%)	2 (9%)
Cerebellum	7 (33%)	2 (9%)
Extensive white matter lesions	8 (38%)	3 (14%)
SPINAL MRI, *N* (%)		
Total abnormal	6 (37.5%)*	17 (71%)
LETM	4 (67%)	8 (47%)
Distribution		
Cervical	5 (83%)	16 (94%)
Thoracic	4 (67%)	11 (65%)
Lumbar	1 (17%)	2 (12%)
OPTIC NERVE MRI, *N* (%)		
Total abnormal	6 (75%)	9 (69%)
Bilateral ON	2 (33%)	7 (78%)
LEON	2 (33%)	4 (44%)

LEON, Longitudinally extensive optic neuritis; LETM, Longitudinally extensive transverse myelitis.
NA, not available.
**$P < 0.05$.*

better response to steroid and immunosuppression and a more benign prognosis compared with NMOSD and other IIDDs (21, 23–26). Moreover, these patients had a correlation between disease condition and MOG-IgG antibody titer which was the same as the counterparts who did not experience seizures or encephalopathy (27).

Seizures and encephalopathy, which suggest neuronal damage on top of demyelinating disease affecting the white matter, further support MOG encephalomyelitis as a broader disease entity. The observations in the present study suggest that MOG encephalomyelitis with seizures and/or encephalopathy may be a distinct clinical disease entity in addition to commonly recognized demyelinating diseases.

CONCLUSIONS

Seizures and encephalopathy are common among subjects with MOG-associated encephalomyelitis, and may be associated with cortical and subcortical brain lesions. Young subjects with high titers of MOG-IgG may present with meningoencephalitis mimicking CNS infection.

AUTHOR CONTRIBUTIONS

XZ, WQ, LP, AL, and AK determined the study design and performed the study. XZ, YZ, and YC were responsible for data collection. XZ, JW, YS, and XS analyzed the data. XZ and WQ drafted the manuscript. All authors read, critically revised, and approved the final manuscript.

FUNDING

This work was supported by grants from the National Natural Science Foundation of China (grant number 81771300) and the Natural Science Foundation of Guangdong Province, China (grant number 2017A030313853).

ACKNOWLEDGMENTS

We thank Prof. Min Dong (Department of Microbiology and Immunobiology, Harvard Medical School), for critically reading the manuscript and useful comments.

REFERENCES

1. Sakuma H, Kohyama K, Park IK, Miyakoshi A, Tanuma N, Matsumoto Y. Clinicopathological study of a myelin oligodendrocyte glycoprotein-induced demyelinating disease in LEW.1AV1 rats. *Brain.* (2004) 127(Pt 10):2201–13. doi: 10.1093/brain/awh260
2. Bettelli E, Baeten D, Jäger A, Sobel RA, Kuchroo VK. Myelin oligodendrocyte glycoprotein-specific T and B cells cooperate to induce a Devic-like disease in mice. *J Clin Invest.* (2006) 116:2393–402. doi: 10.1172/JCI 28334
3. Krishnamoorthy G, Lassmann H, Wekerle H, Holz A. Spontaneous opticospinal encephalomyelitis in a double-transgenic mouse model of autoimmune T cell/B cell cooperation. *J Clin Invest.* (2006) 116:2385–92. doi: 10.1172/JCI28330
4. Peschl P, Bradl M, Höftberger R, Berger T, Reindl M. Myelin oligodendrocyte glycoprotein: deciphering a target in inflammatory demyelinating diseases. *Front Immunol.* (2017) 8:529. doi: 10.3389/fimmu.2017.00529
5. Reindl M, Rostasy K. MOG antibody-associated diseases. *Neurol Neuroimmunol Neuroinflamm.* (2015) 2:e60. doi: 10.1212/NXI.0000000000000060

6. Ramanathan S, Dale RC, Brilot F. Anti-MOG antibody: The history, clinical phenotype, and pathogenicity of a serum biomarker for demyelination. *Autoimmun Rev.* (2016) 15:307–24. doi: 10.1016/j.autrev.2015.12.004
7. Zamvil SS, Slavin AJ. Does MOG Ig-positive AQP4-seronegative opticospinal inflammatory disease justify a diagnosis of NMO spectrum disorder? *Neurol Neuroimmunol Neuroinflamm.* (2015) 2:e62. doi: 10.1212/NXI.0000000000000062
8. Jarius S, Paul F, Aktas O, Asgari N, Dale RC, de Seze J, et al. MOG encephalomyelitis: international recommendations on diagnosis and antibody testing. *J Neuroinflammation.* (2018) 15:134. doi: 10.1186/s12974-018-1144-2
9. Tsuburaya RS, Miki N, Tanaka K, Kageyama T, Irahara K, Mukaida S, et al. Anti-myelin oligodendrocyte glycoprotein (MOG) antibodies in a Japanese boy with recurrent optic neuritis. *Brain Dev.* (2015) 37:145–8. doi: 10.1016/j.braindev.2014.02.002
10. Fukushima N, Suzuki M, Ogawa R, Hayashi K, Takanashi JI, Ohashi T. A case of anti-MOG antibody-positive multiphasic disseminated encephalomyelitis co-occurring with unilateral cerebral cortical encephalitis. *Rinsho Shinkeigaku.* (2017) 57:723–8. doi: 10.5692/clinicalneurol.cn-001078
11. Pandit L, Nakashima I, Mustafa S, Takahashi T, Kaneko K. Anti myelin oligodendrocyte glycoprotein associated immunoglobulin G (AntiMOG-IgG)-associated neuromyelitis optica spectrum disorder with persistent disease activity and residual cognitive impairment. *Ann Indian Acad Neurol.* (2017) 20:411–3. doi: 10.4103/aian.AIAN_250_17
12. Hamid SHM, Whittam D, Saviour M, Alorainy A, Mutch K, Linaker S, et al. Seizures and encephalitis in myelin oligodendrocyte glycoprotein IgG disease vs aquaporin 4 IgG disease. *JAMA Neurol.* (2018) 75:65–71. doi: 10.1001/jamaneurol.2017.3196
13. Gutman JM, Kupersmith M, Galetta S, Kister I. Anti-myelin oligodendrocyte glycoprotein (MOG) antibodies in patients with optic neuritis and seizures. *J Neurol Sci.* (2018) 387:170–3. doi: 10.1016/j.jns.2018.01.042
14. Ogawa R, Nakashima I, Takahashi T, Kaneko K, Akaishi T, Takai Y, et al. MOG antibody-positive, benign, unilateral, cerebral cortical encephalitis with epilepsy. *Neurol Neuroimmunol Neuroinflamm.* (2017) 4:e322. doi: 10.1212/NXI.0000000000000322
15. Polman CH, Reingold SC, Banwell B, Clanet M, Cohen JA, Filippi M, et al. Diagnostic criteria for multiple sclerosis: 2010 revisions to the McDonald criteria. *Ann Neurol.* (2011) 69:292–302. doi: 10.1002/ana.22366
16. Wingerchuk DM, Banwell B, Bennett JL, International Panel for NMO Diagnosis. International consensus diagnostic criteria for neuromyelitis optica spectrum disorders. *Neurology.* (2015) 85:177–89. doi: 10.1212/WNL.0000000000001729
17. Krupp LB, Tardieu M, Amato MP, Banwell B, Chitnis T, Dale RC, et al. International Pediatric Multiple Sclerosis Study Group criteria for pediatric multiple sclerosis and immune-mediated central nervous system demyelinating disorders: revisions to the 2007 definitions. *Mult Scler.* (2013) 19:1261–7. doi: 10.1177/1352458513484547
18. Chen L, Chen C, Zhong X, Sun X, Zhu H, Li X, et al. Different features between pediatric-onset and adult-onset patients who are seropositive for MOG-IgG: A multicenter study in South China. *J Neuroimmunol.* (2018) 321:83–91. doi: 10.1016/j.jneuroim.2018.05.014
19. Zhou Y, Jia X, Yang H, Chen C, Sun X, Peng L, et al. Myelin oligodendrocyte glycoprotein antibody-associated demyelination: comparison between onset phenotypes. *Eur J Neurol.* (2019) 26:175–83. doi: 10.1111/ene.13791
20. Hacohen Y, Mankad K, Chong WK, Barkhof F, Vincent A, Lim M, et al. Diagnostic algorithm for relapsing acquired demyelinating syndromes in children. *Neurology.* (2017) 89:269–78. doi: 10.1212/WNL.0000000000004117
21. Ramanathan S, Mohammad S, Tantsis E, Nguyen TK, Merheb V, Fung VSC, et al. Clinical course, therapeutic responses and outcomes in relapsing MOG antibody-associated demyelination. *J Neurol Neurosurg Psychiatry.* (2018) 89:127–37. doi: 10.1136/jnnp-2017-316880
22. Hyun JW, Woodhall MR, Kim SH, Jeong IH, Kong B, Kim G, et al. Longitudinal analysis of myelin oligodendrocyte glycoprotein antibodies in CNS inflammatory diseases. *J Neurol Neurosurg Psychiatry.* (2017) 88:811–7. doi: 10.1136/jnnp-2017-315998
23. Jarius S, Ruprecht K, Kleiter I, Borisow N, Asgari N, Pitarokoili K, et al. MOG-IgG in NMO and related disorders: a multicenter study of 50 patients. Part 2: Epidemiology, clinical presentation, radiological and laboratory features, treatment responses, and long-term outcome. *J Neuroinflammation.* (2016) 13:280. doi: 10.1186/s12974-016-0718-0
24. Jurynczyk M, Messina S, Woodhall MR, Raza N, Everett R, Roca-Fernandez A, et al. Clinical presentation and prognosis in MOG-antibody disease: a UK study. *Brain.* (2017) 140:3128–38. doi: 10.1093/brain/awx276
25. Spadaro M, Gerdes LA, Krumbholz M, Ertl-Wagner B, Thaler FS, Schuh E, et al. Autoantibodies to MOG in a distinct subgroup of adult multiple sclerosis. *Neurol Neuroimmunol Neuroinflamm.* (2016) 3:e257. doi: 10.1212/NXI.0000000000000257
26. Borisow N, Mori M, Kuwabara S, Scheel M, Paul F. Diagnosis and treatment of NMO spectrum disorder and MOG-encephalomyelitis. *Front Neurol.* (2018) 9:888. doi: 10.3389/fneur.2018.00888
27. Jarius S, Ruprecht K, Kleiter I, Borisow N, Asgari N, Pitarokoili K, et al. MOG-IgG in NMO and related disorders: a multicenter study of 50 patients. Part 1: Frequency, syndrome specificity, influence of disease activity, long-term course, association with AQP4-IgG, and origin. *J Neuroinflammation.* (2016) 13:279. doi: 10.1186/s12974-016-0717-1

12

Salivary IL-1ß as an Objective Measure for Fatigue in Multiple Sclerosis?

Katrin Hanken [1], *Carina Sander* [2,3], *Lara Qaiser* [2], *Hans-Peter Schlake* [3], *Andreas Kastrup* [1], *Michael Haupts* [4,5], *Paul Eling* [6] *and Helmut Hildebrandt* [1,2*]

[1] Klinikum Bremen-Ost, Department of Neurology, Bremen, Germany, [2] Department of Psychology, Carl von Ossietzky Universität Oldenburg, Oldenburg, Germany, [3] Rehabilitationszentrum Oldenburg GmbH, Oldenburg, Germany, [4] Augustahospital Anholt, Clinic for Neurology, Anholt, Germany, [5] Department of Neurology, Heinrich-Heine-Uni, Dusseldorf, Germany, [6] Donders Institute for Brain, Cognition and Behaviour, Radboud University Nijmegen, Nijmegen, Netherlands

Correspondence:
Helmut Hildebrandt
helmut.hildebrandt@uni-oldenburg.de

Background: The causes of fatigue in multiple sclerosis (MS) and other inflammatory disorders are not well understood. One possible cause that might explain fatigue in inflammatory disorders appears to be the immunological process itself, triggering neural activity that is experienced as fatigue.

Objectives: To investigate whether salivary IL-1ß concentration, associated with systemic inflammation, is related to subjective fatigue in MS.

Methods: 116 MS patients (62 relapsing remitting MS, 54 secondary progressive MS) and 51 healthy controls participated in this study. Salivary concentration of IL-1ß was determined using a commercially available enzyme-linked immunosorbent assay (ELISA) kit. Fatigue was assessed using various fatigue scales. We compared IL-1ß concentration between groups and performed regression analyses to investigate which variables best predict fatigue scores.

Results: We found that the IL-1ß concentration best predicts fatigue scores in relapsing remitting MS patients, even though the IL-1ß concentration did not differ significantly between relapsing remitting MS patients and healthy controls. Secondary progressive MS patients showed a somewhat elevated IL-1ß concentration compared to relapsing remitting MS patients and healthy controls. Furthermore, disease modifying treatment had a significant effect on the IL-1ß concentration, with treated patients showing a lower IL-1ß concentration than non-treated patients.

Conclusions: The present study points to a significant relation between the proinflammatory cytokine IL-1ß and fatigue in relapsing remitting MS patients. It also suggests a potential effect of disease modifying treatment on the peripheral IL-1ß concentration.

Keywords: multiple sclerosis, disease course, fatigue, inflammation, proinflammatory cytokines, IL-1ß

INTRODUCTION

Fatigue arguably presents the most challenging symptom for a majority of multiple sclerosis (MS) patients (1). Its prevalence ranges from 65 to 97% and it tends to seriously impair approximately one-third of all MS patients (1–3). Apart from having negative effects on a patient's social and private life, fatigue imposes significant socioeconomic consequences and is a major reason for the reduction of working hours and early retirement (4–6). Despite this serious negative impact on daily life activities, fatigue is still poorly understood and often under-estimated. That is why we recently developed a model explaining the origin and consequences of MS-related fatigue (7). According to our model, subjective fatigue in MS patients is related to peripheral inflammation. The feeling of fatigue in MS patients is considered a form of sickness behavior, resulting from cytokine-mediated activity changes within brain areas involved in interoception such as the hypothalamus, the amygdala, the insula and the anterior cingulate. Looking at proinflammatory cytokines, IL-1ß is one of the main mediators of sickness behavior. IL-1ß activates afferent vagal neurons and it has been strongly and consistently linked to symptoms of sickness behavior including fatigue (8–11).

To date, only few studies have investigated the association between subjective fatigue in MS patients and systemic inflammation (12–18). Studies investigating the characteristics of peripheral T lymphocytes frequently found increased production capacities for proinflammatory cytokines such as IFN-γ and TNF-α in fatigued MS patients (14, 15, 17). Other studies reported a higher serum concentration of proinflammatory cytokines (IL-6, IL-1ß) in patients with high levels of self-reported fatigue (13, 16). It has been argued that increased peripheral inflammatory processes cannot explain fatigue in progressive MS patients since progressive MS is characterized by diffuse central nervous system atrophy and new inflammatory lesions are rare in these disease stages (19). In our view, the fact that there are no relapses any more does not necessarily imply that there are no underlying inflammatory processes in the body periphery (19). Hardly any study investigated the relation between proinflammatory cytokines and fatigue in chronic disease stages of MS, or compared the proinflammatory cytokine concentration of MS patients with relapsing-remitting (rr) and secondary progressive (sp) MS. Hence, we wanted to investigate whether there is a difference in the concentration of proinflammatory cytokines between rrMS and spMS patients and whether proinflammatory cytokines may predict fatigue scores in MS patients suffering from different clinical disease courses. Furthermore, few studies indicate that a disease modifying therapy alters cytokine production in MS patients (20–23). Thus, we also aimed to investigate whether disease modifying drugs have an effect on peripheral markers of inflammation.

Most biomarkers that are present in blood and urine can also be detected in a sample of saliva. Several inflammatory markers have been reliably determined from saliva and some studies reported even higher levels of inflammatory markers in saliva than in blood (24–27). Riis et al. (26) detected higher levels of the proinflammatory cytokine IL-1ß in saliva than in blood serum, and they also found a moderate correlation between these two measures in healthy adolescent girls. Hence, saliva, a non-invasive method for measuring salivary concentration of IL-1ß, may be a promising tool for monitoring patients with systemic inflammatory diseases.

Because we assume that systemic inflammation contributes to fatigue in rrMS as well as in spMS patients, we compared the salivary IL-1ß concentration and investigated which variables best predict fatigue for rrMS and spMS patients.

MATERIALS AND METHODS

Study Population

From August 2015 till the end of June 2017, inpatients of the Klinikum Bremen-Ost, Bremen, Germany, the Augusta Hospital Anholt, Anholt, Germany and patients from the Median Clinic Wilhelmshaven, Wilhelmshaven, Germany were asked to participate in the study. Additionally, MS patients were recruited from MS support groups in Bremen and surroundings. A total of 116 patients with rrMS ($n = 62$) and spMS ($n = 54$) participated in this multi-center study. Pregnant patients or individuals with an MS relapse or using corticosteroids during the last 4 weeks before assessment, under legal care and/or with a diagnosis of any other neurodegenerative disease were excluded from the study. Additionally, 51 healthy controls participated. The study was approved by the ethical board of the German Society of Psychology (DGP) and written informed consent was obtained from participants.

Clinical Investigation

Clinical status of all patients was assessed with the Expanded Disability Status Scale [EDSS; (28)]. Fatigue was assessed with two self-reported questionnaires, the Fatigue Severity Scale [FSS; (29)] and the Fatigue Scale for Motor and Cognitive Functions [FSMC; (30)]. The FSS consists of nine items assessing severity and frequency of fatigue, with higher scores representing stronger fatigue. The FSMC evaluates two main components of fatigue, namely cognitive and motor fatigue. It is composed of 20 items. The cut-off score between normal and mild pathological fatigue is 43 for the total scale and 22 for the cognitive and motor scale.

Depressive mood was investigated using the Beck Depression Inventory Scale [BDI; (31)]. The items A-O, the psychological items, were used to calculate the score for mood impairment whereas items P-U (sleep, tiredness, body weight, loss of sexual interest, somatic concerns) reflect the somatic score and were excluded from further analysis (32, 33).

Saliva Collection

Participants were asked not to drink, eat, brush their teeth, smoke or chew gum at least for 1 h prior to the examination on the day of saliva collection. Whole unstimulated saliva was collected using standard techniques according to Navazesh (34). Participants were asked to swallow first, tilt their head forward and then letting saliva pool in their mouth for 5 min. Each minute, participants were instructed to gently spit their saliva into a sterile 100 ml container. Saliva samples were immediately refrigerated and stored at −20°C.

Salivary IL-1ß Analysis

The analysis of the saliva samples was performed at the Department of Biochemistry of the Carl von Ossietzky University Oldenburg. On the day of the analysis, samples were stored for approx. 30 min at room temperature to defrost. 1000 μl of each sample was pipetted into a tube and centrifuged for 15 min at 1000 × g. IL-1ß levels in salivary supernatants were determined using a commercially available enzyme-linked immunosorbent assay (ELISA) kit (Quantikine® ELISA Human IL-1β/IL-1F2 Immunoassay, R&D Systems, Inc., Minneapolis, MN, USA) according to the manufacturer's instructions for serum/plasma samples. The minimum detectable dose of human IL-1β is typically less than 1 pg/ml. Samples were analyzed in duplicate and the absorbance was measured at 450 nm (wavelength correction was set at 620 nm). The concentration of the samples was calculated from the standard curve. The results are presented in picogram per milliliter (pg/ml).

Statistical Analysis

We first checked whether the IL-1ß scores deviated from a normal distribution using the Kolmogorov-Smirnov Test. As they were not normally distributed and since the manufacturer of the ELISA kit recommends laboratory based cut-off values, we performed an outlier analysis on the IL-1ß results to exclude possibly spoiled samples from further analyses. This outlier analysis was based on a boxplot for the healthy control samples and determined the 1.5 * interquantile score, considering an IL-1ß concentration beyond 1,200 pg/ml as an outlier (see **Figure 1**).

We subsequently compared IL-1ß concentration between rrMS patients, spMS patients and healthy controls, controlling for age, gender, depressive mood (psychological item score of the BDI) and disease modifying drugs using an univariate analysis of covariance (ANCOVA).

In a final step, we performed separate linear forward regression analyses for the three groups to check which variables best predict the variance in the fatigue scores of rrMS patients, spMS patients and healthy controls. The fatigue scores were defined as dependent variables. IL-1ß concentration, age, gender, number of completed school years, the psychological BDI score and status on disease modifying treatment were defined as independent variables.

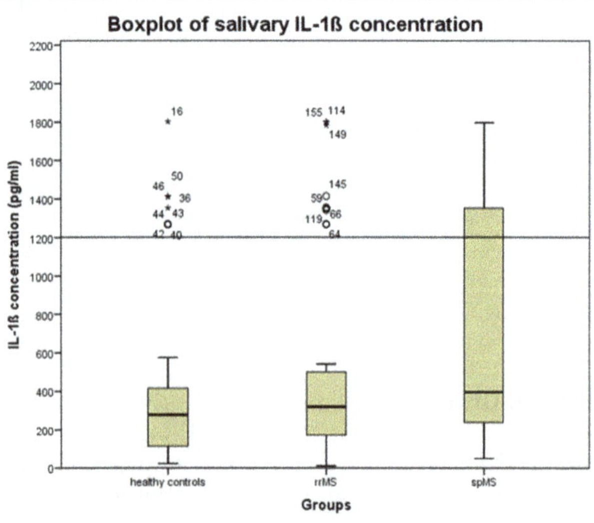

FIGURE 1 | Boxplot of the salivary concentration of IL-1ß in the whole sample to determine the upper cut-off scores for excluding possibly spoiled samples. The error bars reflect the standard deviation. Stars, circles, and numbers display IL-1β concentration of study participants. rrMS, relapsing remitting multiple sclerosis; spMS, secondary progressive multiple sclerosis.

RESULTS

After applying the cut-off score of IL-1ß concentration <1.200 pg/ml, the salivary IL-1ß concentration showed a normal distribution. Applying the cut-off score reduced the groups to 45 rrMS patients (73% of the original sample), 35 spMS patients (65% of the original sample) and 41 healthy controls (80% of the original sample). **Table 1** presents the characteristics and mean scores of the groups.

There was no significant difference in gender distribution between the three groups. As expected, spMS patients were significantly older than rrMS patients and healthy controls, and they had a longer disease duration and a higher EDSS score than rrMS patients. Significantly more rrMS patients received a disease modifying therapy than spMS patients (76 vs. 31%, $p < 0.001$). 70% of MS patients suffered from moderate cognitive fatigue and 83% suffered from moderate motor fatigue. 64% had a FSS score higher or equal than 4 indicating pathological fatigue. RrMS and spMS patients did not differ significantly in the cognitive fatigue score of the FSMC and the FSS score. Only on the motor score of the FSMC, spMS patients scored significantly higher than rrMS patients. 94% of spMS and 76% of rrMS patients suffered from moderate motor fatigue. Overall, rrMS and spMS scored significantly higher on all fatigue scores than healthy controls. RrMS patients and healthy controls did not differ significantly in age. RrMS patients did not differ significantly on the psychological items score of the BDI between spMS and healthy controls. But spMS patients scored significantly higher on the psychological items of the BDI than healthy controls. There was no significant difference in the IL-1ß concentration between rrMS patients and healthy controls or between rrMS and spMS patients. But, spMS patients presented a significantly higher IL-1ß concentration than healthy controls.

The ANCOVA on the IL-1ß concentration, controlling for age, gender, the psychological symptom BDI score and a disease modifying therapy, revealed a significant Group effect ($F = 4.037$, $p = 0.020$) and a significant effect of a disease modifying therapy ($F = 5.498$, $p = 0.021$). In absolute terms, spMS patients showed the highest IL-1ß concentration, but *post-hoc* Bonferroni corrected *t*-tests revealed no significant differences between the groups. Further, MS patients with a disease modifying therapy had a significantly lower IL-1ß concentration than MS patients without disease modifying therapy (222.9 vs. 319.9 pg/ml, $p = 0.008$). The difference in IL-1ß concentration between treated and non-treated patients was larger in the group of spMS patients

(164.8 vs. 353.4 pg/ml, $p = 0.001$) than in the group of rrMS patients (241.7 vs. 246.7 pg/ml, $p = 0.9$; see **Figure 2**).

The results of the linear forward regression analyses, separate for groups, are presented in **Table 2**. The results revealed that the cognitive fatigue score of the FSMC of rrMS patients is best predicted by the IL-1ß concentration. The model explains a significant percentage of the variance of the cognitive fatigue score ($R^2 = 0.108$, $F = 5.223$, $p = 0.027$). The motor fatigue score of the rrMS patients can be best predicted by a model including the psychological BDI score, disease modifying therapy and the concentration of IL-1ß ($R^2 = 0.438$, $F = 10.657$, $p < 0.001$). The FSS score of rrMS patients can be best predicted by a model including disease modifying therapy, the IL-1ß concentration, the psychological BDI score and a patient's age ($R^2 = 0.439$, $F = 7.828$, $p < 0.001$). In all models, the IL-1ß concentration positively correlated with the fatigue scores (see **Figures 3, 4**). For spMS patients, none of the independent variables significantly predicted fatigue scores of the Fatigue Scale for Motor and Cognition. The FFS of spMS patients was best predicted by a model including age ($R^2 = 0.147$, $F = 4.294$, $p = 0.049$). For

TABLE 1 | Group characteristics.

	rrMS Male: 7, female: 38 DMT: 34 (76%)		spMS Male: 6, female: 29 DMT: 11 (31%)		Healthy controls Male: 10, female: 31	
	Mean	*SD*	Mean	*SD*	Mean	*SD*
Age (years)[a,c]	44.0	10.9	52.1	10.6	41.8	16.2
Time since diagnosis (months)[a]	111.0	84.8	228.7	103.5		
EDSS[a]	3.4	2.0	5.8	1.5		
Cognitive fatigue score (FSMC)[b,c]	31.8	9.9	33.8	9.7	18.2	7.8
Motor fatigue score (FSMC)[a,b,c]	34.1	9.2	38.3	6.1	18.5	7.5
Total fatigue score (FSMC)[b,c]	65.9	17.2	72.1	14.5	36.7	14.8
Fatigue severity scale score[b,c]	42.0	15.6	41.8	15.9	24.4	11.3
Psychological item score (BDI)[c]	5.2	4.1	6.5	5.2	3.6	4.2
IL-1beta (pg/ml)[c]	242.9	126.6	294.1	168.1	222.7	138.0

[a]significant difference (p < 0.05) between rrMS and spMS.
[b]significant difference (p < 0.05) between rrMS and healthy controls.
[c]significant difference (p < 0.05) between spMS and healthy controls.
BDI, beck depression inventory; DMT, disease modifying therapy; EDSS, expanded disability status scale; FSMC, fatigue scale for motor and cognition; rrMS, relapsing remitting multiple sclerosis; SD, standard deviation; spMS, secondary progressive multiple sclerosis.

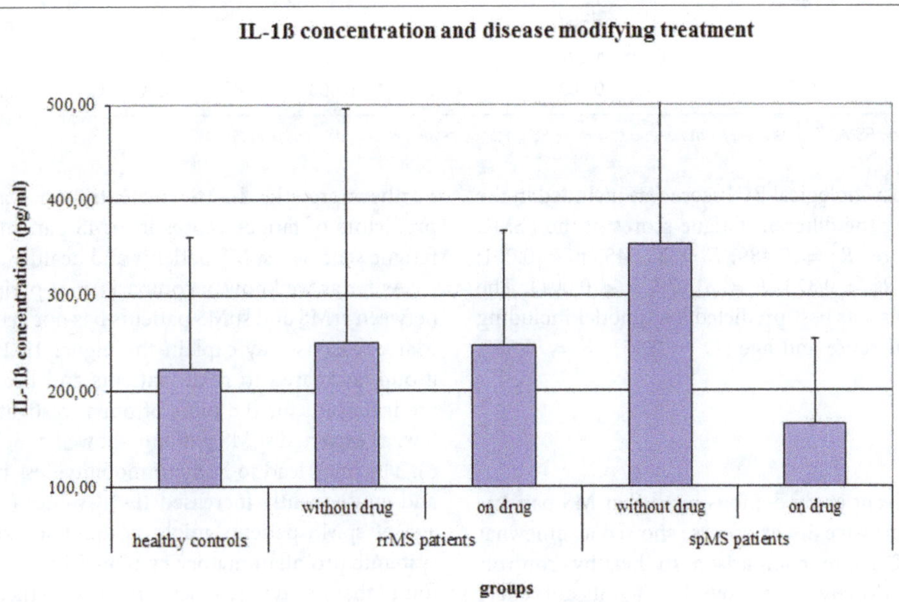

FIGURE 2 | Salivary IL-1ß concentration (pg/ml) of healthy controls and of rrMS and spMS patients with and without a disease modifying therapy. Error bars present the standard deviation. rrMS, relapsing remitting multiple sclerosis; spMS, secondary progressive multiple sclerosis.

TABLE 2 | Results of the forward regression analyses with the different fatigue scores described as dependent variables.

Model	Regression coefficient B	*SD*	Beta	*T*	*p*
Relapsing remitting MS patients					
DEPENDENT VARIABLE: COGNITIVE FATIGUE SCORE OF THE FSMC					
(Constant)	25.558	3.072		8.320	0.000
IL-1ß concentration	0.026	0.011	0.329	2.285	0.027
DEPENDENT VARIABLE: MOTOR FATIGUE SCORE OF THE FSMC					
(Constant)	17.941	3.226		5.561	0.000
Psychological BDI score	0.957	0.266	0.424	3.597	0.001
Disease modifying drugs	8.821	2.484	0.416	3.551	0.001
IL-1ß concentration	0.018	0.009	0.254	2.153	0.037
DEPENDENT VARIABLE: FSS SCORE					
(Constant)	31.825	9.598		3.316	0.002
Disease modifying drugs	11.939	4.354	0.334	2.742	0.009
IL-1ß concentration	0.051	0.015	0.415	3.398	0.002
Psychological BDI score	1.018	0.454	0.267	2.242	0.031
Age	−0.376	0.178	−0.263	−2.113	0.041
Secondary progressive MS patients					
DEPENDENT VARIABLE: FSS SCORE					
(Constant)	72.421	14.856		4.875	0.000
Age	−0.575	0.278	−0.383	−2.072	0.049
Healthy controls					
DEPENDENT VARIABLE: COGNITIVE FATIGUE SCORE OF THE FSMC					
(Constant)	13.500	1.162		11.637	0.000
Psychological BDI score	1.288	1.288	0.699	6.111	0.000
DEPENDENT VARIABLE: MOTOR FATIGUE SCORE OF THE FSMC					
(Constant)	14.548	1.250		11.642	0.000
Psychological BDI score	1.091	0.227	0.611	4.814	0.000
DEPENDENT VARIABLE: FSS SCORE					
(Constant)	28.387	4.415		6.430	0.000
Psychological BDI score	1.227	0.380	0.460	3.227	0.003
Age	−0.202	0.099	−0.291	−2.044	0.048

BDI, beck depression inventory; FSMC, fatigue scale for motor and cognition; FSS, fatigue severity scale; MS, multiple sclerosis.

healthy controls, the psychological BDI score was included in the models best predicting the different fatigue scores of the FSMC (cognitive fatigue score: $R^2 = 0.489$, $F = 37.345$, $p < 0.001$; motor fatigue score: $R^2 = 0.373$, $F = 23.179$, $p < 0.001$). The FSS of healthy controls was best predicted by a model including the psychological BDI score and age ($R^2 = 0.251$, $F = 6.365$, $p = 0.004$).

DISCUSSION

The results of the present study demonstrated that MS patients with a secondary progressive disease course showed a somewhat increased level of IL-1ß in comparison to healthy controls and rrMS patients. Moreover, we found a significant effect of disease modifying treatment on the IL-1ß concentration. Patients receiving such a therapy showed a significantly lower IL-1ß concentration than patients not receiving such a therapy. Furthermore, the IL-1ß concentration was one of the main predictors of fatigue scores in rrMS patients. It did not predict fatigue scores of spMS patients and healthy controls.

As far as we know, a comparison of peripheral inflammation between rrMS and spMS patients has not been performed before. Many reasons may explain the higher IL-1ß level in the spMS group compared to rrMS patients and healthy controls, which are irrelevant for the topic of our investigation. To name just a few: as expected spMS patients showed a high EDSS score (about 6). This may lead to body immobility, less immune competence and consequently increased IL-1ß values (35). Also, the higher age of spMS patients might account for an increased level of systemic proinflammatory cytokines in this group (36). We also found that receiving a disease modifying therapy has a significant effect on the IL-1ß concentration. This finding stands in line with previous studies demonstrating a potential effect of a disease modifying therapy on cytokine production (20–23). The fact

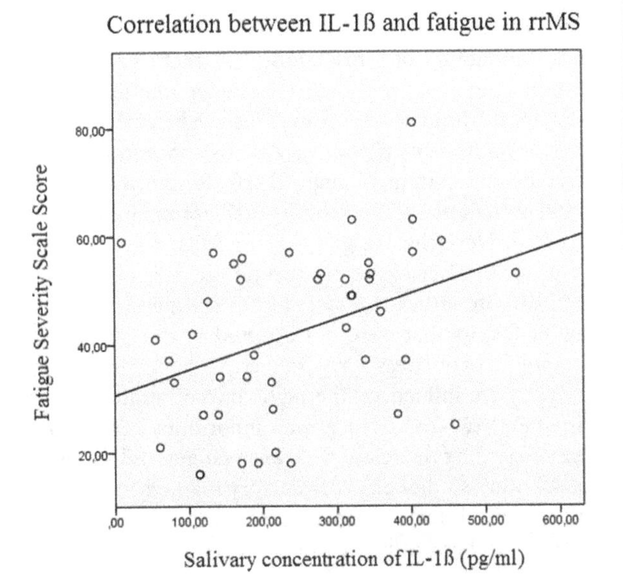

FIGURE 3 | Correlation between the salivary IL-1ß concentration (pg/ml) and the Fatigue Severity Scale Score in relapsing remitting MS patients (Beta = 0.382, $F = 7.3$, $p = 0.010$). rrMS, relapsing remitting multiple sclerosis.

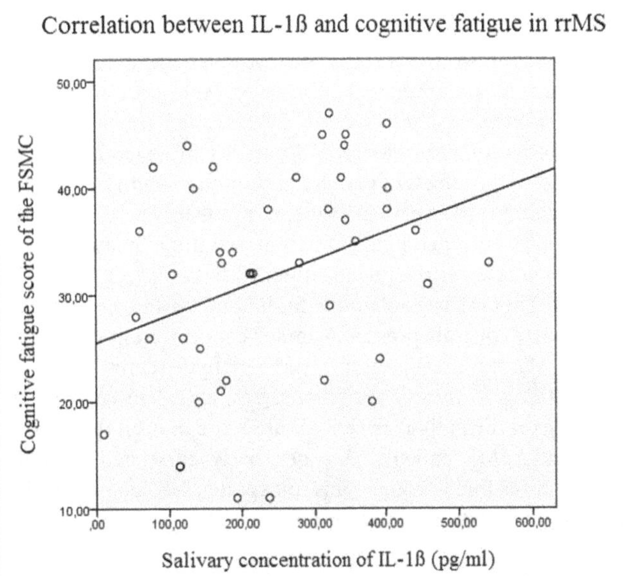

FIGURE 4 | Correlation between the salivary IL-1ß concentration (pg/ml) and the Cognitive Fatigue Score of the Fatigue Scale for Motor and Cognition in relapsing remitting MS patients (Beta = 0.329, $F = 5.2$, $p = 0.027$). FSMC, Fatigue Scale for Motor and Cognition, rrMS, relapsing remitting multiple sclerosis.

that less spMS patients than rrMS patients received a disease modifying therapy may also be relevant for the higher IL-1ß concentration in spMS patients as compared to rrMS patients and healthy controls. Irrespectively of the underlying causes for the increased IL-1ß concentration in spMS patients, the finding that spMS patients had a somewhat elevated concentration of IL-1ß might indicate that even in spMS patients there may be a link between inflammatory activity and the feeling of fatigue.

The findings of the regression analyses point to a relationship between the proinflammatory cytokine IL-1ß and fatigue only in MS patients suffering from a relapsing remitting disease course. The salivary concentration of IL-1ß was included in all models best predicting fatigue scores in rrMS patients. This finding stands in contrast to two previous studies that did not find a relation between fatigue and blood levels of IL-1ß in MS patients (16, 37). This difference might be due to the fact that Akali and colleagues did not use regression analyses to investigate the relation between fatigue and the IL-1ß concentration. They did not control for factors such as depression, MS type or disease modifying drugs (37). Also Malekzadeh et al. did not consider depressive symptoms in their statistical analysis (16). We did control for an effect of depressive symptoms on the IL-1ß concentration. Furthermore, we included a larger amount of MS patients than the two previous studies and we divided patients into rrMS and spMS patients and checked for a relationship between IL-1ß and fatigue in the separate groups. Our results suggest that especially in the early disease stages of MS, bodily inflammation may be one dominant cause for fatigue. However, the relatively low R^2 scores indicate that IL-1ß alone may explain only a limited part of the variance in experienced fatigue. Other cytokines like TNF-α, IL-6, IL-12, or IL-17 may have an additional impact on subjective fatigue (7).

Overall, fatigue seems to be a multi-factorial symptom resulting from different causes. Besides immunological abnormalities, also structural brain changes may contribute to fatigue. Several studies found a relation between fatigue and gray matter atrophy within specific brain areas such as frontal motor areas and subcortical areas such as the thalamus and basal ganglia (38). Nevertheless, it is noteworthy that in rrMS patients IL-1ß best predicted fatigue scores, whereas in healthy controls the psychological items of the BDI appeared to best predict the variance of the different fatigue scores. Hence, the level of IL-1ß seems to play an important role in fatigue in rrMS patients, whereas—as shown in healthy controls—fatigue might also be related to depressive symptoms as argued in many prior investigations (39–41).

The absence of a significant difference in IL-1ß concentration between rrMS patients and healthy controls raises some questions. One may argue that the peripheral level of IL-1ß cannot explain subjective fatigue, because then rrMS patients should show a higher IL-1ß concentration than healthy controls. The lack of a significant difference in the IL-1ß concentration between rrMS patients and healthy controls may be due to the small group sizes. Furthermore, the majority of rrMS patients received a disease modifying therapy. We found that patients receiving such a therapy had a significantly lower IL-1ß concentration. Hence, the lack of a difference may also be due to fact that most rrMS patients received a disease modifying therapy. Nevertheless, several studies show that chronic neuroinflammation sensitizes the brain to produce an exaggerated response to peripheral inflammation resulting in prolonged sickness behavior and increased cytokine induction within the central nervous system (42, 43). MS is a chronic inflammatory disease of the central nervous system which is characterized by chronic peripheral and central inflammation. Hence, MS patients in general might be sensitized to the effects of peripheral proinflammatory cytokines. Consequently, MS patients might produce an exaggerated response to peripheral inflammation resulting in exaggerated fatigue, whereas peripheral inflammation has no effect on healthy controls. This might explain the finding that even though rrMS and healthy controls present a similar concentration of salivary IL-1ß, rrMS present significantly higher fatigue scores.

According to the regression analyses, age seems to have an influence on the Fatigue Severity Scale Score in healthy controls, rrMS and spMS patients. Age negatively correlated with the fatigue scores in all groups. This unexpected finding contradicts the assumption that increased age is related to higher fatigue scores.

Additional evidence for a relationship between fatigue and bodily inflammation in MS patients comes from recent studies in which we demonstrated the importance of inflammation-induced vagal nerve activity for the generation of fatigue. In a previous study (44), we found that fatigue severity predicts future relapses in MS patients, additionally pointing to a relation between bodily inflammation and fatigue severity in rrMS patients. We also showed that fatigue in MS patients is associated with afferent vagal nerve signaling. A disruption of afferent interoceptive signaling is related to the absence of fatigue in MS patients (45, 46). Furthermore, fatigue correlates with autonomic symptoms (47), especially with those that strongly depend on vagal nerve signaling such as bladder dysfunctions, orthostatic intolerance and pupillomotor dysfunctions.

Given that an elevated systemic concentration of IL-1ß causes fatigue in rrMS patients, anti-inflammatory interventions should have a positive effect on fatigue in this patient population. Recent studies did show that aerobic exercise and resistance training have a combined positive effect on proinflammatory cytokine concentration and on fatigue in mildly impaired MS patients (48–53). Moreover, substances with anti-inflammatory properties such as Alfacalcidol, vitamin A or coenzyme Q10 seem to have the potential to reduce subjective fatigue in MS patients (54–57). Other studies showed that blocking IL-1ß signaling via Anakinra, an IL-1ß receptor antagonist exerts a positive effect on fatigue in patients suffering from inflammatory diseases such as rheumatoid arthritis or Sjögren's syndrome (58, 59).

There is another finding of our study, not directly related to the question of IL-1ß level and fatigue, that should be mentioned. As expected, rrMS and spMS patients differed in age, disease duration and EDSS, but not in their total and cognitive fatigue level. Consequently, the argument that fatigue results from a loss of function and a compensatory effort to solve everyday problems is less likely. Only the motor fatigue score showed a significant difference between the groups. Motor fatigue is strongly associated to muscle strength and motor impairment and might reflect the impact of motor impairment rather than the actual feeling of fatigue (60, 61). If the compensatory effort model of fatigue is correct, then it will concern motor fatigue more than cognitive fatigue.

One limitation of this study is that salivary IL-1ß concentration may not only reflect systemic immune responses but also local immune responses. This might explain the high number of outliers for the salivary IL-1ß concentration scores. To exclude an extremely high IL-1ß concentration due to local inflammation in the mouth, oral examinations need to be included. Nevertheless, gingival crevicular fluid is not only the result of local cytokine production but it is also a fluid of systemic origin indicating systemic inflammation. Moreover, also other factors that were not assessed in this study such as obesity, smoking or stress may also increase bodily inflammation and might have influenced the high concentration of IL-1ß in spMS patients (62–64). Hence, we cannot draw conclusions on causality regarding the relation between fatigue and IL-1ß in MS patients. Future studies on inflammatory markers in MS patients should also check for a potential effect of the above mentioned factors on peripheral inflammation.

CONCLUSION

We recently developed a model for MS-related fatigue arguing that the feeling of fatigue is caused by systemic inflammation, resulting from inflammation-induced activity changes within interoceptive brain areas (7). The present study points to an association between the salivary concentration of the proinflammatory cytokine IL-1ß and subjective fatigue in rrMS patients. We also found that a disease modifying therapy significantly lowered the IL-1ß concentration. Future studies combining immunological and radiological measures are needed for a better understanding of the relation between subjective fatigue scores, peripheral immune markers and structural and functional changes in the central nervous system.

AUTHOR CONTRIBUTIONS

KH: elaboration of study design, data collection, saliva analysis, writing of manuscript. CS and LQ: data collection, saliva analysis. H-PS and AK: help on patient recruitment, facilitation of examination room and materials. MH: help on patient recruitment, data collection, facilitation of examination room and materials. PE: writing of manuscript. HH: elaboration of study design, writing of manuscript.

FUNDING

The study was sponsored by Merck KGaA, Darmstadt, Germany: (MS200136-0058 Fatigue__IST, July 2016–October 2017).

ACKNOWLEDGMENTS

We would like to thank the Department of Biochemistry of the Carl von Ossietzky University Oldenburg for providing us with the necessary equipment for the salivary analysis. A special thanks goes to Michael Müller for his helpful instructions and the time he spent on familiarizing us with the ELISA analysis.

REFERENCES

1. Freal JE, Kraft GH, Coryell JK. Symptomatic fatigue in multiple sclerosis. *Arch Phys Med Rehabil.* (1984) 65:135–8.
2. Bakshi R. Fatigue associated with multiple sclerosis: diagnosis, impact and management. *Mult Scler.* (2003) 9:219–27. doi: 10.1191/1352458503ms904oa
3. Krupp LB, Alvarez LA, LaRocca NG, Scheinberg LC. Fatigue in multiple sclerosis. *Arch Neurol.* (1988) 45:435–7. doi: 10.1001/archneur.1988.00520280085020
4. Coyne KS, Boscoe AN, Currie BM, Landrian AS, Wandstrat TL. Understanding drivers of employment changes in a multiple sclerosis population. *Int J MS Care.* (2015) 17:245–52. doi: 10.7224/1537-2073.2014-051
5. Smith MM, Arnett PA. Factors related to employment status changes in individuals with multiple sclerosis. *Mult Scler.* (2005) 11:602–9. doi: 10.1191/1352458505ms1204oa
6. Simmons RD, Tribe KL, McDonald EA. Living with multiple sclerosis: longitudinal changes in employment and the importance of symptom management. *J Neurol.* (2010) 257:926–36. doi: 10.1007/s00415-009-5441-7
7. Hanken K, Eling P, Hildebrandt H. The representation of inflammatory signals in the brain – a model for subjective fatigue in multiple sclerosis. *Front Neurol.* (2014) 5:264. doi: 10.3389/fneur.2014.00264
8. Gaykema RPA, Goehler LE, Tilders FJH, Bol JGJM, McGorry M, Fleshner M, et al. Bacterial endotoxin induces Fos immunoreactivity in primary afferent neurons of the vagus nerve. *Neuroimmunomodulation* (1998) 5:234–40. doi: 10.1159/000026343
9. Harboe E, Tjensvoll AB, Vefring HK, Gøransson LG, Kvaløy JT, Omdal R. Fatigue in primary Sjögren's syndrome–a link to sickness behaviour in animals? *Brain Behav Immun.* (2009) 23:1104–8. doi: 10.1016/j.bbi.2009.06.151
10. Lampa J, Westman M, Kadetoff D, Agréus AN, Le Maître E, Gillis-Haegerstrand C, et al. Peripheral inflammatory disease associated with centrally activated IL-1 system in humans and mice. *Proc Natl Acad Sci USA.* (2012) 109:12728–33. doi: 10.1073/pnas.1118748109
11. Vollmer-Conna U, Fazou C, Cameron B, Li H, Brennan C, Luck L, et al. Production of pro-inflammatory cytokines correlates with the symptoms of acute sickness behaviour in humans. *Psychol Med.* (2004) 34:1289–97. doi: 10.1017/S0033291704001953
12. Flachenecker P, Bihler I, Weber F, Gottschalk M, Toyka KV, Rieckmann P. Cytokine mRNA expression in patients with multiple sclerosis and fatigue. *Mult Scler.* (2004) 10:165–9. doi: 10.1191/1352458504ms991oa
13. Bertolone K, Coyle PK, Krupp LB, Doscher CA. Cytokine correlates of fatigue in multiple sclerosis. *Neurology* (1993) 43:A356.
14. Heesen C, Nawrath L, Reich C, Bauer N, Schulz KH, Gold SM. Fatigue in multiple sclerosis: an example of cytokine mediated sickness behaviour? *J Neurol Neurosurg Psychiatry.* (2006) 77:34–9. doi: 10.1136/jnnp.2005.065805
15. Gold SM, Krüger S, Ziegler KJ, Krieger T, Schulz KH, Otte C, et al. Endocrine and immune substrates of depressive symptoms and fatigue in multiple sclerosis patients with comorbid major depression. *J Neurol Neurosurg Psychiatry.* (2011) 82:814–8. doi: 10.1136/jnnp.2010.230029
16. Malekzadeh A, Van de Geer-Peeters W, De Groot V, Teunissen CE, Beckerman H, TREFAMS-ACE Study Group. Fatigue in patients with multiple sclerosis: is it related to pro- and anti-inflammatory cytokines? *Dis Markers.* (2015) 2015:758314. doi: 10.1155/2015/758314
17. Pokryszko-Dragan A, Frydecka I, Kosmaczewska A, Ciszak L, Bilinska M, Gruszka E, et al. Stimulated peripheral production of interferon-gamma is related to fatigue and depression in multiple sclerosis. *Clin Neurol Neurosurg.* (2012) 114:1153–8. doi: 10.1016/j.clineuro.2012.02.048
18. Rudick RA, Barna BP. Serum interleukin 2 and soluble interleukin 2 receptor in patients with multiple sclerosis who are experiencing severe fatigue. *Arch Neurol.* (1990) 47:254–5. doi: 10.1001/archneur.1990.00530030018008
19. Hanken K, Eling P, Hildebrandt H. Is there a cognitive signature for MS-related fatigue? Response to Feinstein. *Mult Scler.* (2016) 22:575–6. doi: 10.1177/1352458515595133
20. Lalive PH, Neuhaus O, Benkhoucha M, Burger D, Hohlfeld R, Zamvil SS, et al. Glatiramer acetate in the treatment of multiple sclerosis: emerging concepts regarding its mechanism of action. *CNS Drugs.* (2011) 25:401–14. doi: 10.2165/11588120-000000000-00000
21. Limone P, Ferrero B, Calvelli P, Del Rizzo P, Rota E, Berardi C, et al. Hypothalamic-pituitary-adrenal axis function and cytokine production in multiple sclerosis with or without interferon-beta treatment. *Acta Neurol Scand.* (2002) 105:372–7. doi: 10.1034/j.1600-0404.2002.01155.x
22. Reske D, Thomas AV, Petereit HF, Fink GR, Schroeter M. Impact of immunomodulatory treatment on leukocyte cytokine production in multiple sclerosis patients and healthy donors. Author information. *Neuroimmunomodulation* (2009) 16:385–91. doi: 10.1159/000228913
23. Sega S, Wraber B, Mesec A, Horvat A, Ihan A. IFN-beta1a and IFN-beta1b have different patterns of influence on cytokines. *Clin Neurol Neurosurg.* (2004) 106:255–8. doi: 10.1016/j.clineuro.2004.02.010
24. Byrne ML, O'Brien-Simpson NM, Reynolds EC, Walsh KA, Laughton K, Waloszek JM, et al. Acute phase protein and cytokine levels in serum and saliva: a comparison of detectable levels and correlations in a depressed and healthy adolescent sample. *Brain Behav Immun.* (2013) 34:164–75. doi: 10.1016/j.bbi.2013.08.010
25. Khan A. Detection and quantitation of forty eight cytokines, chemokines, growth factors and nine acute phase proteins in healthy human plasma, saliva and urine. *J Proteomics.* (2012) 75:4802–19. doi: 10.1016/j.jprot.2012.05.018
26. Riis JL, Out D, Dorn LD, Beal SJ, Denson LA, Pabst S, et al. Salivary cytokines in healthy adolescent girls: intercorrelations, stability, and associations with serum cytokines, age, and pubertal stage. *Dev Psychobiol.* (2014) 56:797–811. doi: 10.1002/dev.21149
27. Williamson S, Munro C, Pickler R, Grap MJ, Elswick RK Jr. Comparison of biomarkers in blood and saliva in healthy adults. *Nurs Res Pract.* (2012) 2012:246178. doi: 10.1155/2012/246178
28. Kurtzke JF. Rating neurologic impairment in multiple sclerosis: an expanded disability status scale (EDSS). *Neurology* (1983) 33:1444–52. doi: 10.1212/WNL.33.11.1444
29. Krupp LB, LaRocca NG, Muir-Nash J, Steinberg AD. The fatigue severity scale. Application to patients with multiple sclerosis and systemic lupus erythematosus. *Arch Neurol.* (1989) 46:1121–3. doi: 10.1001/archneur.1989.00520460115022
30. Penner IK, Raselli C, Stöcklin M, Opwis K, Kappos L, Calabrese P, et al. The fatigue scale for motor and cognitive functions (FSMC): validation of a new instrument to assess multiple sclerosis-related fatigue. *Mult Scler.* (2009) 15:1509–17. doi: 10.1177/1352458509348519
31. Beck AT, Steer RA, Garbin MG. Psychometric properties of the beck depression inventory: twenty five years of evaluation. *Clin Psychol Rev.* (1988) 8:77–100. doi: 10.1016/0272-7358(88)90050-5
32. Brokate B, Reimer J, Hildebrandt H. Charakteristik depressiver Symptome bei psychischen Erkrankungen und Multipler Sklerose-eine retrospektive Datenanalyse. *Z Neuropsychol.* (2017) 28:197–205. doi: 10.1024/1016-264X/a000203
33. Delisle VC, Abbey SE, Beck AT, Dobson KS, Dozois DJ, Grace SL, et al. The influence of somatic symptoms on beck depression inventory scores in hospitalized postmyocardial infarction patients. *Can J Psychiatry.* (2012) 57:752–8. doi: 10.1177/070674371205701207
34. Navazesh M. Methods for collecting saliva. *Ann N Y Acad Sci.* (1993) 20:72–7. doi: 10.1111/j.1749-6632.1993.tb18343.x
35. Skinner GW, Mitchell D, Harden LM. Avoidance of physical activity is a sensitive indicator of illness. *Physiol Behav.* (2009) 96:421–7. doi: 10.1016/j.physbeh.2008.11.004
36. Gomez CR, Boehmer ED, Kovacs EJ. The aging innate immune system. *Curr Opin Immunol.* (2005) 17:457–62. doi: 10.1016/j.coi.2005.07.013
37. Akcali A, Zengin F, Aksoy SN, Zengin O. Fatigue in multiple sclerosis: is it related to cytokines and hypothalamic-pituitary-adrenal axis? *Mult Scler Relat Disord.* (2017) 15:37–41. doi: 10.1016/j.msard.2017.03.004
38. Induruwa I, Constantinescu CS, Gran B. Fatigue in multiple sclerosis–a brief review. *J Neurol Sci.* (2012) 323:9–15. doi: 10.1016/j.jns.2012.08.007
39. Simpson S Jr, Tan H, Otahal P, Taylor B, Ponsonby AL, Lucas RM, et al. Anxiety, depression and fatigue at 5-year review following CNS demyelination. *Acta Neurol Scand.* (2016) 134:403–13. doi: 10.1111/ane.12554

40. Schreiber H, Lang M, Kiltz K, Lang C. Is personality profile a relevant determinant of fatigue in multiple sclerosis? *Front Neurol.* (2015) 6:2. doi: 10.3389/fneur.2015.00002
41. Feinstein A, Magalhaes S, Richard JF, Audet B, Moore C. The link between multiple sclerosis and depression. *Nat Rev Neurol.* (2014) 10:507–17. doi: 10.1038/nrneurol.2014.139
42. Hennessy E, Gormley S, Lopez-Rodriguez AB, Murray C, Murray C, Cunningham C. Systemic TNF-α produces acute cognitive dysfunction and exaggerated sickness behavior when superimposed upon progressive neurodegeneration. *Brain Behav Immun.* (2017) 59:233–44. doi: 10.1016/j.bbi.2016.09.011
43. Sparkman NL, Johnson RW. Neuroinflammation associated with aging sensitizes the brain to the effects of infection or stress. *Neuroimmunomodulation* (2008) 15:323–30. doi: 10.1159/000156474
44. Sander C, Eling P, Hanken K, Klein J, Kastrup A, Hildebrandt H. The impact of MS-related cognitive fatigue on future brain parenchymal loss and relapse: a 17-month follow-up study. *Front Neurol.* (2016) 7:155. doi: 10.3389/fneur.2016.00155
45. Hanken K, Eling P, Kastrup A, Klein J, Hildebrandt H. Integrity of hypothalamic fibers and cognitive fatigue in multiple sclerosis. *Mult Scler Relat Disord.* (2015) 4:39–46. doi: 10.1016/j.msard.2014.11.006
46. Hanken K, Manousi A, Klein J, Kastrup A, Eling P, Hildebrandt H. On the relation between self-reported cognitive fatigue and the posterior hypothalamic-brainstem network. *Eur J Neurol.* (2015) 0:1–9. doi: 10.1111/ene.12815
47. Sander C, Hildebrandt H, Schlake HP, Eling P, Hanken K. Subjective cognitive fatigue and autonomic abnormalities in multiple sclerosis patients. *Front Neurol.* (2017) 8:475. doi: 10.3389/fneur.2017.00475
48. Alvarenga-Filho H, Sacramento PM, Ferreira TB, Hygino J, Abreu JE, Carvalho SR, et al. Combined exercise training reduces fatigue and modulates the cytokine profile of T-cells from multiple sclerosis patients in response to neuromediators. *J Neuroimmunol.* (2016) 293:91–9. doi: 10.1016/j.jneuroim.2016.02.014
49. Golzari Z, Shabkhiz F, Soudi S, Kordi MR, Hashemi SM. Combined exercise training reduces IFN-γ and IL-17 levels in the plasma and the supernatant of peripheral blood mononuclear cells in women with multiple sclerosis. *Int Immunopharmacol.* (2010) 10:1415–9. doi: 10.1016/j.intimp.2010.08.008
50. Kierkegaard M, Lundberg IE, Olsson T, Johansson S, Ygberg S, Opava C, et al. High-intensity resistance training in multiple sclerosis–an exploratory study of effects on immune markers in blood and cerebrospinal fluid, and on mood, fatigue, health-related quality of life, muscle strength, walking and cognition. *J Neurol Sci.* (2016) 362:251–7. doi: 10.1016/j.jns.2016.01.063
51. Kjølhede T, Vissing K, Dalgas U. Multiple sclerosis and progressive resistance training: a systematic review. *Mult Scler.* (2012) 18:1215–28. doi: 10.1177/1352458512437418
52. Mokhtarzade M, Ranjbar R, Majdinasab N, Patel D, Molanouri Shamsi M. Effect of aerobic interval training on serum IL-10, TNFα, and adipokines levels in women with multiple sclerosis: possible relations with fatigue and quality of life. *Endocrine* (2017) 57:262–71. doi: 10.1007/s12020-017-1337-y
53. Mostert S, Kesselring J. Effects of a short-term exercise training program on aerobic fitness, fatigue, health perception and activity level of subjects with multiple sclerosis. *Mult Scler.* (2002) 8:161–8. doi: 10.1191/1352458502ms779oa
54. Achiron A, Givon U, Magalashvili D, Dolev M, Liraz Zaltzman S, Kalron A, et al. Effect of alfacalcidol on multiple sclerosis-related fatigue: a randomized, double-blind placebo-controlled study. *Mult Scler.* (2015) 21:767–75. doi: 10.1177/1352458514554053
55. Bitarafan S, Saboor-Yaraghi A, Sahraian MA, Soltani D, Nafissi S, Togha M, et al. Effect of vitamin A supplementation on fatigue and depression in multiple sclerosis patients: a double-blind placebo-controlled clinical trial. *Iran J Allergy Asthma Immunol.* (2016) 15:13–9. Available online at: http://ijaai.tums.ac.ir/index.php/ijaai/article/view/692
56. Sanoobar M, Dehghan P, Khalili M, Azimi A, Seifar F. Coenzyme Q10 as a treatment for fatigue and depression in multiple sclerosis patients: a double blind randomized clinical trial. *Nutr Neurosci.* (2016) 19:138–43. doi: 10.1179/1476830515Y.0000000002
57. Sanoobar M, Eghtesadi S, Azimi A, Khalili M, Khodadadi B, Jazayeri S, et al. Coenzyme Q10 supplementation ameliorates inflammatory markers in patients with multiple sclerosis: a double blind, placebo, controlled randomized clinical trial. *Nutr Neurosci.* (2015) 18:169–76. doi: 10.1179/1476830513Y.0000000106
58. Norheim KB, Harboe E, Gøransson LG, Omdal R. Interleukin-1 inhibition and fatigue in primary Sjögren's syndrome–a double blind, randomised clinical trial. *PLoS ONE* (2012) 7:e30123. doi: 10.1371/journal.pone.0030123
59. Omdal R, Gunnarsson R. The effect of interleukin-1 blockade on fatigue in rheumatoid arthritis–a pilot study. *Rheumatol Int.* (2005) 25:481–4. doi: 10.1007/s00296-004-0463-z
60. Penner IK, Bechte IN, Raselli C, Söcklin M, Opwis K, Kappos L, et al. Fatigue in multiple sclerosis: relation to depression, physical impairment, personality and action control. *Mult Scler.* (2007) 13:1161–7. doi: 10.1177/1352458507079267
61. Rietberg MB, van Wegen EE, Uitdehaag BM, Kwakkel G. The association between perceived fatigue and actual level of physical activity in multiple sclerosis. *Mult Scler.* (2011) 17:1231–7. doi: 10.1177/1352458511407102
62. Javed F, Al-Kheraif AA, Al Amri MD, Alshehri M, Vohra F, Al-Askar M, et al. Periodontal status and whole salivary cytokine profile among smokers and never-smokers with and without prediabetes. *J Periodontol.* (2015) 86:890–8. doi: 10.1902/jop.2015.140593
63. Kitahara CM, Trabert B, Katki HA, Chaturvedi AK, Kemp TJ, Pinto LA, et al. Body mass index, physical activity, and serum markers of inflammation, immunity, and insulin resistance. *Cancer Epidemiol Biomarkers Prev.* (2014) 23:2840–9. doi: 10.1158/1055-9965.EPI-14-0699-T
64. Slavish DC, Graham-Engeland JE, Smyth JM, Engeland CG. Salivary Markers of inflammation in response to acute stress. *Brain Behav Immun.* (2015) 0:253–69. doi: 10.1016/j.bbi.2014.08.008

13

Computational Intelligence Technique for Prediction of Multiple Sclerosis Based on Serum Cytokines

Mehendi Goyal[1], Divya Khanna[2], Prashant Singh Rana[2], Timur Khaibullin[3], Ekaterina Martynova[4], Albert A. Rizvanov[4], Svetlana F. Khaiboullina[4,5] and Manoj Baranwal[1]*

[1] Department of Biotechnology, Thapar Institute of Engineering and Technology, Patiala, India, [2] Department of Computer Science and Engineering, Thapar Institute of Engineering and Technology, Patiala, India, [3] Republican Clinical Neurological Canter, Republic of Tatarstan, Russian Federation, Kazan, Russia, [4] Institute of Fundamental Medicine and Biology, Kazan Federal University, Kazan, Russia, [5] Department of Microbiology and Immunology, University of Nevada, Reno, NV, United States

***Correspondence:**
Manoj Baranwal
manoj.baranwal@thapar.edu;
baranwal.manoj@gmail.com

Multiple sclerosis (MS) is a neurodegenerative disease characterized by lesions in the central nervous system (CNS). Inflammation and demyelination are the leading causes of neuronal death and brain lesions formation. The immune reactivity is believed to be essential in the neuronal damage in MS. Cytokines play important role in differentiation of Th cells and recruitment of auto-reactive B and T lymphocytes that leads to neuron demyelination and death. Several cytokines have been found to be linked with MS pathogenesis. In the present study, serum level of eight cytokines (IL-1β, IL-2, IL-4, IL-8, IL-10, IL-13, IFN-γ, and TNF-α) was analyzed in USA and Russian MS to identify predictors for the disease. Further, the model was extended to classify MS into remitting and non-remitting by including age, gender, disease duration, Expanded Disability Status Scale (EDSS) and Multiple Sclerosis Severity Score (MSSS) into the cytokines datasets in Russian cohorts. The individual serum cytokines data for the USA cohort was generated by Z score percentile method using R studio, while serum cytokines of the Russian cohort were analyzed using multiplex immunoassay. Datasets were divided into training (70%) and testing (30%). These datasets were used as an input into four machine learning models (support vector machine, decision tree, random forest, and neural networks) available in R programming language. Random forest model was identified as the best model for diagnosis of MS as it performed remarkable on all the considered criteria i.e., Gini, accuracy, specificity, AUC, and sensitivity. RF model also performed best in predicting remitting and non-remitting MS. The present study suggests that the concentration of serum cytokines could be used as prognostic markers for the prediction of MS.

Keywords: multiple sclerosis, cytokines, serum, machine learning, prediction

INTRODUCTION

Multiple sclerosis (MS) is a chronic disease of the central nervous system (CNS) caused by chronic inflammation and autoimmune response. MS can be classified on the basis of onset of symptoms and their progression into relapsing remitting (symptoms appearing and disappearing), primary progressive (progressive symptom elevation), and secondary progressive (relapse-remitting MS development to progressive MS) multiple sclerosis. The disease is characterized by demyelinating areas in the brain and spinal cord which appear as plaques or lesions in the white and gray matter (1, 2). Blood Brain Barrier (BBB) was shown to be affected, which explains the presence of circulating leukocytes into the brain matter (3). The auto-reactive T lymphocytes penetrating BBB could target neuroglia leading to more damage within the brain and thus exposing myelin antigens. These auto-reactive T cells can cause deterioration of the myelin sheath, which is essential for signal transmission within the brain (4). Depending on the varied locations of lesions in brain, clinical symptoms of MS may vary including vision loss, numbness, fatigue, movement difficulties, and many more (5).

Neuronal damage and neuroglial activation could cause the secretion of various cytokines which are involved in differentiation of Th1, Th2, Th9, and Th17 lymphocytes (6). Studies have shown changes in various cytokines level in serum and cerebrospinal fluid (CSF) of MS patients as compared to controls (7–9). These cytokines are associated with Th1 (IFN-γ, TNF-α, IL-2) and Th2 (IL-4, IL-5, IL-13, IL-6) type immune responses. Also, activation of Th17 and Th9, secreting IL-17 and IL-9, respectively, was shown to play role in the progression of MS (10). Interestingly, loss of the natural regulatory T cells (T_{reg}) function was demonstrated as one of the factors leading to MS (11, 12). It is believed that suppression of the T_{reg} population can lead to proliferation of auto-reactive T cells in MS (11).

The analysis of body fluids such as blood, saliva, cerebrospinal fluid, and urine is often used to diagnose various diseases at the early stage. This analysis can be highly accurate and cost effective than the conventional diagnostic techniques such as computed tomography (CT), magnetic resonance imaging (MRI) scans, and tissue biopsies. The body fluids are commonly analyzed to determine changes in biomolecules which are either directly or indirectly associated with the disease progression. Since, blood cytokines is known to be affected in MS, hence we propose that changes in cytokine could be used as a prognostic markers for MS diagnosis.

Machine learning approaches were successfully employed for prediction of Alzheimer's disease, diabetes, inflammatory bowel disease, and diagnosis of glaucoma (13–16). Recently, machine learning approach was applied into demographic dataset to predict MS disease course (17). Martins et al. analyzed thirteen inflammatory cytokines in 833 MS patients and 117 controls of USA population (18). Eight out of thirteen cytokines were found to differ significantly in MS as compared to controls (18). These eight cytokines were also analyzed in MS patients and controls of Russian cohort. In current study, four machine learning models were applied to predict MS using these eight cytokines (IL-1β, IL-2, IL-4, IL-8, IL-10, IL-13, IFN-γ, and TNF-α) data of USA and Russian cohorts. Further, machine learning models were also used to classify MS into remitting and non-remitting based on eight cytokine serum level, age, gender, disease duration, Expanded Disability Status Scale (EDSS) and Multiple Sclerosis Severity Score (MSSS).

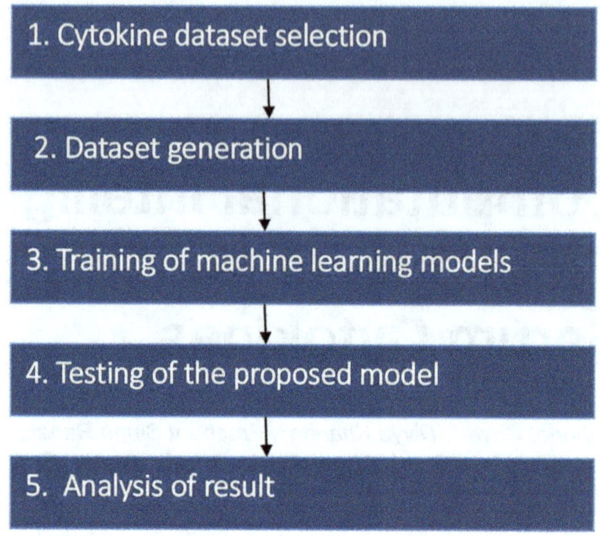

FIGURE 1 | Methodology of the proposed work.

MATERIALS AND METHODS

The research strategy of the proposed model was divided into the five stages: (1) Dataset selection, (2) Dataset generation, (3) Training of machine learning models (4) Testing of the proposed model, and (5) Analysis of the result. The methodology of proposed work and details of each stage are summarized in **Figure 1**.

Dataset Selection

Concentration data of eight cytokines (IL-1β, IL-2, IL-4, IL-8, IL-10, IL-13, IFN-γ, and TNF-α) in serum of MS patients and controls was selected from two different studies of USA and Russian population. Out of the two independent USA studies, one analyzed the concentration of serum cytokines in 833 MS patients and 117 healthy volunteers using multiplex immunoassay (18) while the other group analyzed the concentrations of serum cytokines in 26 MS patients and 11 controls (19). Data on eight serum cytokines (IL-1β, IL-2, IL-4, IL-8, IL-10, IL-13, IFN-γ, and TNF-α) in 97 MS patients and 71 controls in Russian cohort was also included into the analysis. There were 53 females and 18 males average age 28.6 ± 8.8 years, in Russian control cohort. The demographic and clinical features of 97 Russian MS patients are summarized in **Table 1**.

TABLE 1 | Demographic and clinical details of MS patients from Russian cohort.

Characteristic		Number or mean ± SD
Age		39.1 ± 13.4
Gender	Female	67
	Male	30
MS types	Relapsing remitting	46
	Secondary progressive	31
	Primary progressive	20
Disease duration		3.9 ± 2.2
EDSS		2.6 ± 1.5
MSSS		4.9 ± 2.3
Patients on treatment		22
Not on treatment		75

Dataset Generation

Dataset containing USA populations was generated using Z score percentile based method while Russian cytokine data was analyzed using multiplex magnetic bead-based antibody detection assays.

Z Score Percentile Method

Cytokine data from two previously published USA studies was reported in the mean ± standard deviation (SD)/standard error of mean (SEM) format. To convert SEM into SD, the SEM was multiplied by square root of total number (n). One of the major challenges was to generate the individual cytokines data from reported values as the data was mostly available as mean ± SD/SEM. Data was generated by two methods: solving the series of non-linear equations and Z score percentile based approach. To choose best method for data analysis, random values of 50 cytokines were taken, and the actual values were compared with the generated values from Z score method and non-linear systems equations (data not shown). The data generated by Z score method was found to be more accurate. Hence, to generate the raw data from mean ± SD/SEM, Z score percentile method was used, where the population was presumed to follow the normal distribution (20). The Z score percentile method was implemented in R (an open source software licensed under GNU GPL) to calculate individual data. In this method, 99.7% of the total population was included and the remaining 0.3% was considered outliers and was excluded from the analysis (**Supplementary Figure 1**).

Cytokine Analysis

Ninety seven MS patients, admitted to the Republican Clinical Neurological Center, Republic of Tatarstan, Russian Federation were recruited into the study. MS diagnosis was based upon clinical presentation and brain MRI results. Serum samples were collected from each patient and control. Informed consent was obtained from each subject according to the clinical and experimental research protocol, approved by the Biomedicine Ethic Expert Committee of Republican Clinical Neurological Center, Republic of Tatarstan, Russian Federation (No.218; 11.15.2012).

TABLE 2 | Tuning parameters of machine learning models.

Model	Method	Required package	Tuning parameter
SVM	Ksvm	Kernlab	Kernel radial basis
DT	Rpart	rpart	Min split = 20, Max depth = 30
RF	Rf	Random forest	mtry = 2, number of tree = 500
NN	nn.train	Deepnet	hidden layer = 5

SVM, Support vector machine; DT, Decision tree; RF, Random forest; NN, Neural network.

Serum cytokines (IL-1β, IL-2, IL-4, IL-8, IL-10, IL-13, IFN-γ, and TNF-α) were analyzed using Pro Human Cytokine 27-plex Bio-Plex (Bio-Rad, Hercules, CA, USA) multiplex magnetic bead-based antibody detection kits following the manufacturer's instructions. Serum aliquots (50 μl) were used for the analysis with a minimum of 50 beads per analyte acquired. Median fluorescence intensities were measured using a Luminex 200 analyzer. Data collected was analyzed with MasterPlex CT control software and MasterPlex QT analysis software (Hitachi Software, San Bruno, CA, USA). Standard curve for each analyte was generated using standards provided by the manufacturer.

Machine Learning Methods

Four machine learning models, Random Forest (RF) (21), Decision Tree (DT), Support Vector Machine (SVM) (22), and Neural Network (NN) (23) were used in the study. The required packages and tuning parameters to obtain the optimum results using these models are summarized in **Table 2**. The models were trained based on equation which includes factors required to predict the target 1 (MS vs. control) or classify target 2 (remitting vs. non-remitting MS).

$$\begin{aligned} Target\ 1.1 &\sim f(IL1\beta + IL2 + IL4 + IL8 + IL10 + IL13 \\ &\quad + IFN\gamma + TNF\alpha) \\ Target\ 1.2 &\sim f(IL1\beta + IL2 + IL4 + IL8 + IL10 \\ &\quad + IL13 + IFN\gamma + TNF\alpha + Age + Gender) \\ Target\ 2 &\sim f(IL1\beta + IL2 + IL4 + IL8 + IL10 \\ &\quad + IL13 + IFN\gamma, + TNF\alpha + Age + Gender \\ &\quad + EDSS + MSSS + Disease\ duration) \end{aligned}$$

Model Evaluation

The performance of models was evaluated using various parameters such as Gini, AUC, accuracy, specificity, and sensitivity (24). The following equations were used to calculate these parameters:

$$Gini = 2 \times AUC - 1$$

$$Accuracy = \frac{TP + TN}{TP + TN + FN + FP} \times 100$$

$$Sensitivity = \frac{TP}{TP + FN}$$

$$Specificity = \frac{TN}{TN + FP}$$

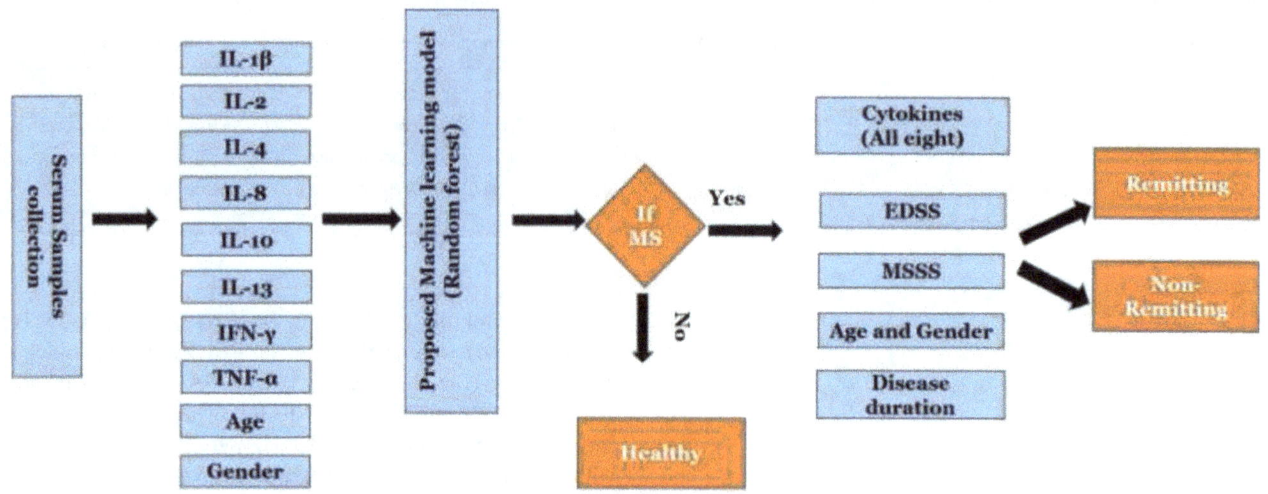

FIGURE 2 | Work flow of the proposed scheme. EDSS, Expanded Disability Status Scale; MSSS, Multiple Sclerosis Severity Score.

TABLE 3 | Performance of machine learning models based on evaluation parameters.

Model name	Gini	Accuracy	AUC	Sensitivity	Specificity
SVM	0.862	87.56	0.931	0.5	0.633
DT	0.715	83.73	0.858	0.069	0.541
RF	**0.914**	**90.91**	**0.957**	**0.756**	**0.857**
NN	0.566	45.45	0.783	0.456	0.082

SVM, Support vector machine; DT, Decision tree; RF, Random forest; NN, Neural network. The bold values suggests that Random Forest (RF) was selected as the best predictive model based on the listed evaluation parameters.

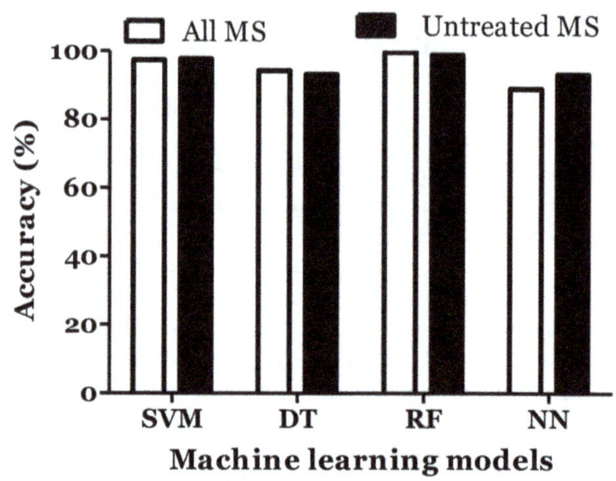

FIGURE 3 | Prediction accuracy of different models to diagnose MS in Russian cohort. All MS: MS patients which includes the patients undergoing and not on treatment when serum samples was collected. Untreated MS: MS patients which includes the patients which were not on treatment when serum samples was collected.

Where,

TN: True negative; TP: True positive; FP: False positive; FN: False negative. AUC: AUC (Area under Curve) is area under Receiver Operating Characteristics (ROC) curve which is calculated to measure the quality of model. Higher AUC value depicts a good quality model.

Repeated K-Fold Cross Validation

K-fold cross validation was done to test the robustness of proposed model by increasing the number of runs in model. In this method, K-folds are repeated n times to trace out the fluctuations in the model accuracy. If low variation in accuracy is identified, the model is identified as robust and the predictions to be reliable. In the present study, the dataset was divided into six equal portions and 6-fold cross validation was repeated three times to avoid discrepancies.

RESULTS

The Proposed Predictive Model

The proposed algorithm to predict and classify MS is summarized in **Figure 2**. The model is based on eight cytokines level in serum for MS and control. Datasets of cytokine levels, age and gender were used as input for machine learning model to predict if a person is having MS or not. Once MS is diagnosed, the model will be able to classify MS into remitting and non-remitting MS based on serum cytokines, age, gender, disease duration, EDSS, and MSSS.

Four machine learning models were employed to predict MS using dataset including 910 MS patients and 199 controls. The dataset was prepared by random shuffling of USA and Russian cohorts and then the data was divided into training (70%) and testing (30%) subsets. The data was divided as follows: 900 (training dataset) and 209 (testing dataset). The training dataset consisted of unbalanced data on MS patients (750) and controls (150) which was further distributed by

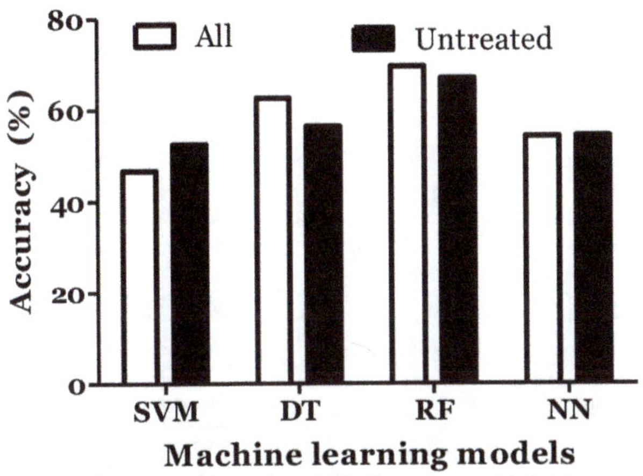

FIGURE 4 | Prediction accuracy of different models to classify MS types in Russian cohort. All MS: MS patients which includes the patients undergoing treatment and not on treatment when serum samples was collected. Untreated MS: MS patients which includes the patients which were not on treatment when serum samples was collected.

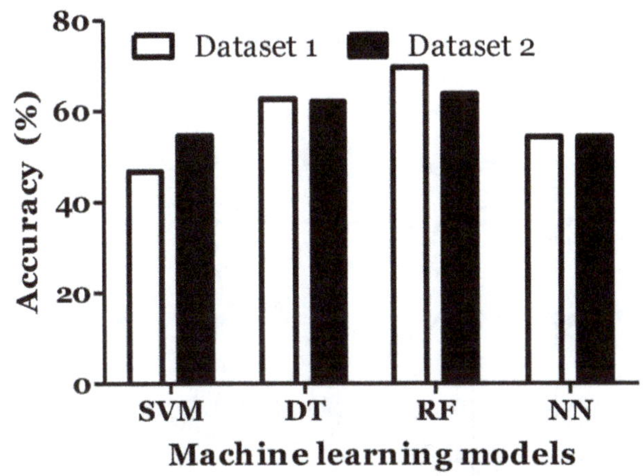

FIGURE 6 | Prediction accuracy of different models of different datasets to classify MS types in Russian cohort. Dataset 1: IL1-β + IL-2 + IL-4 + IL-8 + IL-10 + IL-13 + IFN-γ + TNF-α + Age + Gender + Disease duration + EDSS + MSSS. Dataset 2: IL1-β + IL-2 + IL-4 + IL-6 + IL-8 + IL-10 + IL-13 + IFN-α + IFN-γ + TNF-α + Age + Gender + Disease duration + EDSS + MSSS.

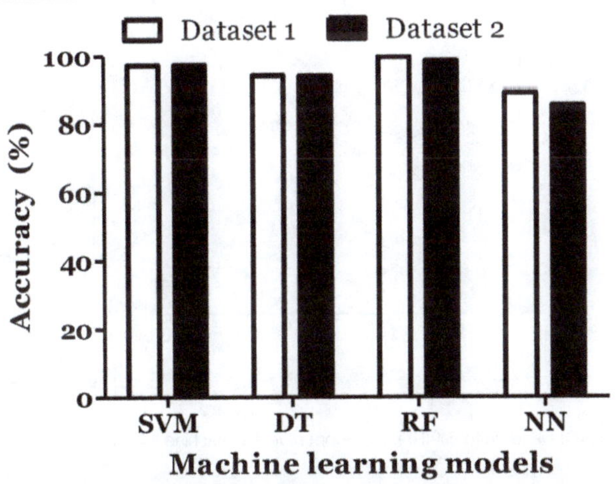

FIGURE 5 | Prediction accuracy of different models of different datasets to diagnose MS in Russian cohort. Dataset 1: IL1-β + IL-2 + IL-4 + IL-8 + IL-10 + IL-13 + IFN-γ + TNF-α + Age + Gender. Dataset 2: IL1-β + IL-2 + IL-4 + IL-6 + IL-8 + IL-10 + IL-13 + IFN-α + IFN-γ + TNF-α + Age + Gender.

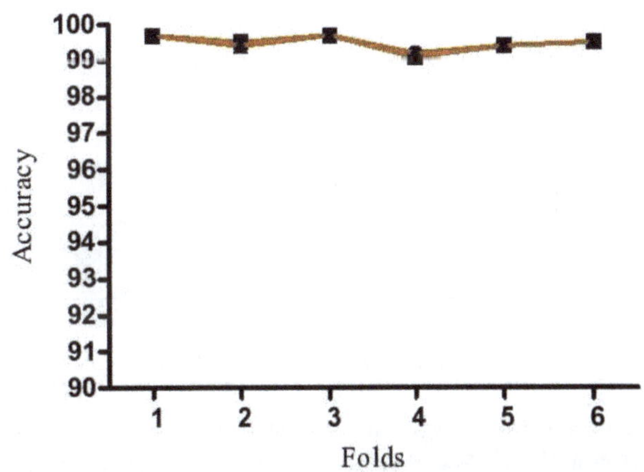

FIGURE 7 | Repeated K-fold validation of the proposed model. Data is mean of three independent runs.

dividing patient data into five subsets to create a balance between the patient and control datasets. All four machine learning models were trained separately using each balanced dataset. All five trained models were then tested by using test dataset. Predictions generated via five trained models were combined using majority voting ensemble technique. Using SVM, DT, and RF, fare accuracy of MS prediction was demonstrated (83–91%). When additional parameters used for the analysis (Gini, AUC, specificity, and sensitivity) were looked, RF model demonstrated the best performance as compared to other models. Therefore, RF was selected as model for the prediction of MS and used for validation (**Table 3**).

The prediction of MS was also done with inclusion of age and gender along with cytokine values in Russian cohort where datasets were divided into training (70%) and testing (30%). The accuracy of MS diagnosis for different models was within the range of 89–99% (**Figure 3**). RF model demonstrated 70% accuracy in classifying remitting and non-remitting MS while the percentage accuracy for DT, NN, and SVM models was 63, 54, and 47, respectively (**Figure 4**). In the Russian MS cohort, 97 patients, consisting of 22 patients taking medication, were included. Therefore, to compare the effect of MS treatment on MS prediction accuracy, 97 MS patients were compared with 75 MS patients without treatment. Data analysis did not reveal difference between these two groups (**Figures 3, 4**). Thus, it was

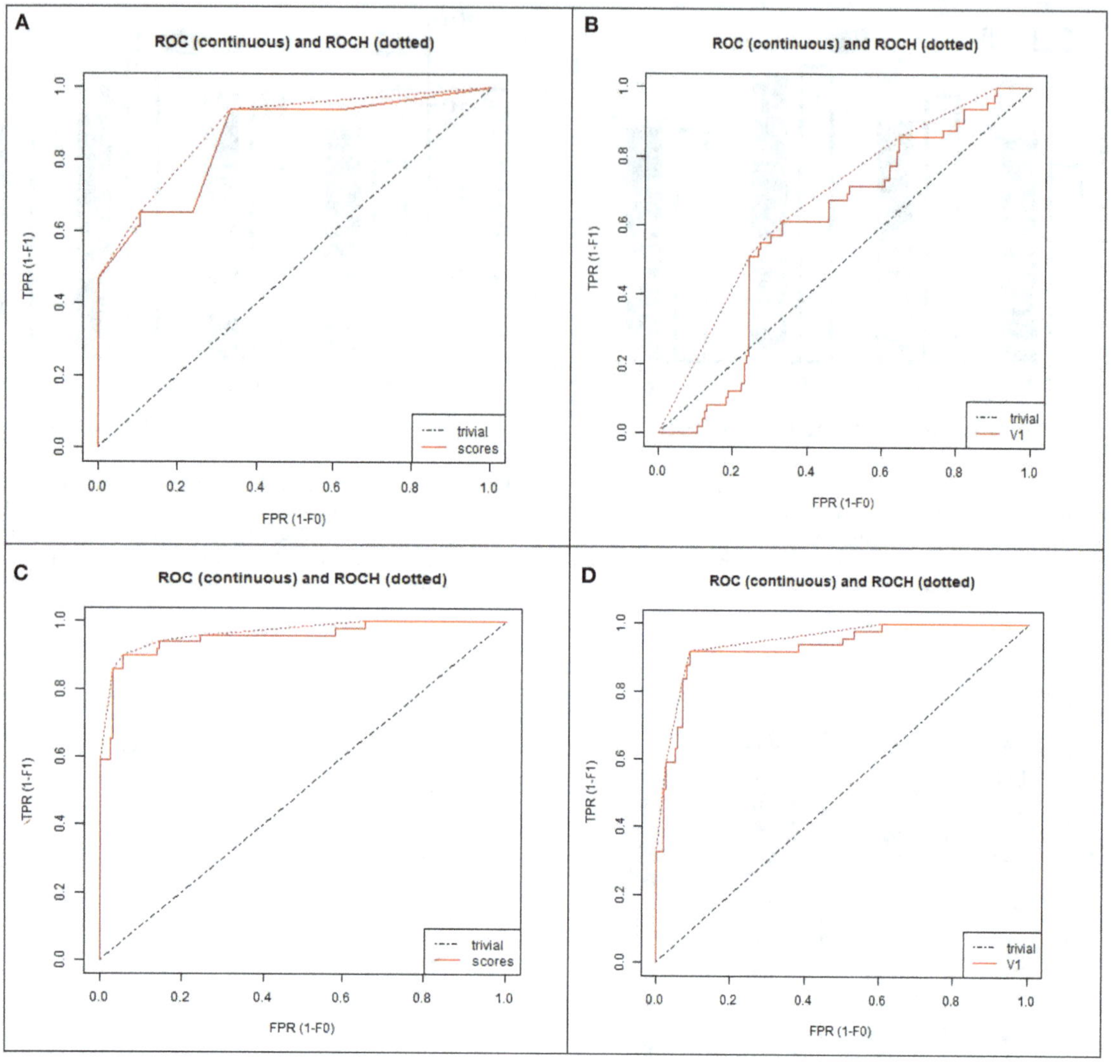

FIGURE 8 | ROC curve plot of four models: **(A)** Decision tree (DT), **(B)** Neural network (NN), **(C)** Random forest (RF), **(D)** Support vector machine (SVM). TPR, True positive rate; FPR, False positive rate.

concluded that, the MS prediction accuracy is not affected by inclusion of patients undergoing treatment.

IL-6 and IFN-α were shown to play role in MS pathogenesis (25, 26). Therefore, we included these cytokines in dataset and calculated the MS prediction accuracy. We have found that inclusion of these cytokines did not improve the accuracy of MS prediction and classification (**Figures 5, 6**).

Validation of the Proposed Model

To demonstrate that the trained model is not overfitted, underfitted or biased, repeated 6-fold cross validation was performed. The accuracy of the proposed model was evaluated by repeated K-fold cross validation (**Figure 7**). The Receiver operating Characteristic (ROC) is the representation of the true positive rate (sensitivity) and false positive rate (1 specificity) of the models where for each data point, the sensitivity and specificity are calculated to plot the graph. The area under the curve (AUC) can be considered as the criterion for the measurement of the discriminative ability of the model to distinguish well-among the patients and controls. Receiver operating Characteristic (ROC) curve plots for each model were generated to demonstrate the performance of each model (**Figure 8**). It was observed that the RF model is performing well as compared with other models (**Figure 8**).

DISCUSSIONS

The pathogenesis of MS is complex and involves multiple factors which makes prediction and early diagnosis of the disease challenging. Recently, different computational methods were applied to develop interactive design and optimisation of the synthetic biological system to study pathogenesis of diabetes

(27). This study was designed to develop novel approaches for diagnosis of the disease; because, early diagnosis of the disease could significantly increase the success rate of the current treatment. Artificial intelligence holds a great potential for early diagnosis and prediction of the treatment outcome. Several machine learning models have been developed to predict development of the heart diseases, Parkinson's disease and breast cancers (28–30). In this study, RF model was identified as the best to predict MS based on eight cytokine levels in serum. RF model has also shown good accuracy in classifying MS into remitting and non-remitting.

MS is a neurological disease highly prevalent in many European countries, USA, Canada and Australia (31). Clinically, MS is characterized by neurological dysfunction which often leads to a disability (32). Despite the advances made in our understanding of MS pathogenesis, prognostic markers for prediction of the disease remain largely unknown. Cytokines were shown to be consistently affected in serum of MS (18). Also, multiple studies have demonstrated that cytokines play a crucial role in the pathogenesis of MS (33, 34). For example, Martins et al have shown that seven cytokines (IL-2, IL-4, IL-10, IL-13, IL1β, IFN-γ, and TNF-α) were significantly elevated in MS patients while IL-8 was significantly lower in MS as compared to controls (18). Interestingly, IL-2, IL-4, IL-10, IL-13, IL1β, IFN-γ, and TNF-α serum level was found elevated in Russian MS as compared to controls, which was similar to that found in USA cohort. These data suggest that the pathogenesis of MS in Russian and USA could be similar. The only exception was changes in serum level of IL8, which was lower in USA and higher in Russian MS as compared to the respective controls. IL-8 is polypotent cytokine involved in regulation of inflammation, recruiting neutrophils, basophils, T lymphocytes, NK cells as well as enhancing the permeability of endothelial barrier (35–38). Difference in IL-8 serum level in Russian and USA MS cohort could reflect the dissimilarities in the disease pathogenesis which could be related to the genetic predisposition, sun exposure, vitamin D production, smoking, etc.

We suggest that changes in serum cytokine levels could be used as predictors or diagnostic biomarkers for MS. Data on serum cytokine level in USA MS cohort was used in our study to develop the machine learning model. To increase the number of samples, data from another report on USA MS serum cytokine levels was included into the analysis (19). The raw data from these two studies was calculated via Z score percentile method. In the resulting synthetic data, the real experimental data obtained by multiplex immunoassay from Russian cohort was included to have high quality prediction. Four machine learning models were trained to predict MS where prediction was based on combined effect of level of eight cytokines in serum. Three models (SVM, DT, and RF) showed good accuracy for MS prediction. The model performance was further evaluated using additional factors (Gini, AUC, specificity and sensitivity). RF model has shown the best performance in each evaluation parameters. This data suggest that RF analysis of eight cytokine (IL-1β, IL-2, IL-4, IL-8, IL-10, IL-13, IFN-γ, and TNF-α) levels in serum could be used to predict MS. RF model has shown the accuracy of 70% to classify MS into remitting vs. non-remitting where age, gender, disease duration, EDSS, and MSSS in addition to cytokines levels were included as classification parameters. This data corroborates previous report where the accuracy of MS disease course was 60–70% when demographic (age, disease onset, gender, and smoking history) and clinical factors (expanded disability status scale, visual disability score, and mental disability score) were included into the prediction model (17).

IL-6 and IFN-α are the inflammatory cytokines which also affected in MS (25, 26). Therefore, prediction and classification of MS algorithm was designed including these cytokines. Interestingly, adding IL-6 and INF-α did not improve the accuracy of MS diagnosis and classification. This suggests that although IL-6 and INF-α contribute into MS pathogenesis, data on level of eight cytokines (IL-1β, IL-2, IL-4, IL-8, IL-10, IL-13, IFN-γ, and TNF-α) in serum provides sufficient input data to diagnose and classify MS.

Analysis of Cerebrospinal fluid (CSF) demonstrated association between cytokines and MS pathogenesis; however, data remains inconsistent (39). In our previous report, ten (IL-2RA, CCL5, CCL11, CXCL1, CXCL10, CXCL12, MIF, IFN-γ, TRAIL, and SCF) out of forty eight cytokines were found elevated in MS as compared to non-MS controls (40). IFN-γ level was only found to be increased in CSF of MS in this study, while the remaining cytokines (IL-1β, IL-2, IL-4, IL-8, IL-10, IL-13, IFN-γ, and TNF-α), used in our prediction model, did not change significantly as compared to controls. Therefore, we did not include CSF cytokine data into our prediction model. Additionally, CSF collection painful and invasive procedure requiring highly trained personnel. Also, CSF analysis is not always required for MS diagnosis. In contrast, MS serum samples are often collected for routine clinical analysis, making them readily available for cytokine detection. Current approach could also be applied to differentiate MS from other neuro-inflammatory diseases.

CONCLUSION

Early diagnosis of MS remains a challenge since the disease develops slowly and clinical symptoms are often identified when brain tissue is already damaged. In the present study, RF model was found to have an accuracy of 91% which suggests that it could be applied to predict MS using serum level of eight cytokines (IL-1β, IL-2, IL-4, IL-8, IL-10, IL-13, IFN-γ, and TNF-α). Further, the accuracy of MS classification into remitting vs. non-remitting was observed to 70% by RF with inclusion of age, gender, diseases duration, EDSS and MSSS in addition to serum cytokines. This is the first study where eight cytokine levels in serum was used to predict MS in two distinct cohorts of patients.

AUTHOR CONTRIBUTIONS

MG: original idea generation, literature reviews for MS cytokines data, computational work that includes generation of USA MS cytokines data, compilation of results and figures, manuscript writing. DK: running of machine learning models and results generation of the models. PR: supervised the research work of machine learning models. TK and EM: involved in collection of MS and control samples and MS clinical data. SK: cytokines analysis of Russian population and manuscript editing. AR: arranging the work of Russian cytokines data analysis that includes the MS and control samples. MB: formulation of idea, overall responsible for coordinating the research project and managing multisite collaboration, writing the manuscript.

ACKNOWLEDGMENTS

AR and SK were supported by the Russian Government Program of Competitive Growth of Kazan Federal University. AR was personally supported by state assignments 20.5175.2017/6.7 and 17.9783.2017/8.9 of the Ministry of Science and Higher Education of Russian Federation.

REFERENCES

1. Ruuls SR, Sedgwick JD. Cytokine-directed therapies in multiple sclerosis and experimental autoimmune encephalomyelitis. *Immunol Cell Biol.* (1998) 76:65–73. doi: 10.1046/j.1440-1711.1998.00715.x
2. Kantarci OH. A new dawn for genetic association studies in multiple sclerosis. *Neurol Genet.* (2016) 2:e93. doi: 10.1212/NXG.00000000000 00093
3. Dendrou CA, Fugger L, Friese MA. Immunopathology of multiple sclerosis. *Nat Rev Immunol.* (2015) 15:545–8. doi: 10.1038/nri3871
4. Goverman J. Autoimmune T cell responses in the central nervous system. *Nat Rev Immunol.* (2009) 9:393. doi: 10.1038/nri2550
5. Vellinga M, Geurts J, Rostrup E, Uitdehaag B, Polman C, Barkhof F, et al. Clinical correlations of brain lesion distribution in multiple sclerosis. *J Mag Reson Imaging.* (2009) 29:768–3. doi: 10.1002/jmri.21679
6. Trenova A, Slavov G. Cytokines in multiple sclerosis–possible targets for immune therapies. *J Neurol Exp Neurosci.* (2016) 1:25–9. doi: 10.17756/jnen.2016-006
7. Kallaur AP, Oliveira SR, Delicato de Almeida ER, Kaminami Morimoto H, Lopes J, de Carvalho Jennings Pereira WL, et al. Cytokine profile in relapsing remitting multiple sclerosis patients and the association between progression and activity of the disease. *Mol Med Rep.* (2013) 7:1010–20. doi: 10.3892/mmr.2013.1256
8. Taşdemir N, Karaca EE, Ece A, Yücel Y, Dikici S, Taşdemir MS. Multiple sclerosis: relationships between cytokines, MRI lesion burden, visual evoked potentials and disability scores. *Eur J Gen Med.* (2010) 7:167–73. doi: 10.29333/ejgm/82845
9. Khaiboullina SF, Gumerova AR, Khafizova IF, Martynova EV, Lombardi VC, Bellusci S, et al. CCL27: novel cytokine with potential role in pathogenesis of multiple sclerosis. *BioMed Res Int.* (2015) 2015:189638. doi: 10.1155/2015/189638
10. Amedei A, Prisco D, D'elios MM. Multiple sclerosis: the role of cytokines in pathogenesis and in therapies. *Int J Mol Sci.* (2012) 13:13438–60. doi: 10.3390/ijms131013438
11. Kumar M, Putzki N, Limmroth V, Remus R, Lindemann M, Knop D, et al. CD4+ CD25+ FoxP3+ T lymphocytes fail to suppress myelin basic protein-induced proliferation in patients with multiple sclerosis. *J Neuroimmunol.* (2006) 180:178–84. doi: 10.1016/j.jneuroim.2006.08.003
12. Putzki N, Kumar M, Kreuzfelder E, Grosse-Wilde H, Diener H, Limmroth V. Mitoxantrone does not restore the impaired suppressive function of natural regulatory T cells in patients suffering from multiple sclerosis. *Eur Neurol.* (2009) 61:27–32. doi: 10.1159/000165346
13. Mossotto E, Ashton J, Coelho T, Beattie R, MacArthur B, Ennis S. Classification of paediatric inflammatory bowel disease using machine learning. *Sci Rep.* (2017) 7:2427. doi: 10.1038/s41598-017-02606-2
14. Dagliati A, Marini S, Sacchi L, Cogni G, Teliti M, Tibollo V, et al. Machine learning methods to predict diabetes complications. *J Diabetes Sci Technol.* (2017) 12:295–302. doi: 10.1177/1932296817706375
15. Abós A, Baggio HC, Segura B, García-Díaz AI, Compta Y, Martí MJ, et al. Discriminating cognitive status in Parkinson's disease through functional connectomics and machine learning. *Sci Rep.* (2017) 7:45347. doi: 10.1038/srep45347
16. Kim SJ, Cho KJ, Oh S. Development of machine learning models for diagnosis of glaucoma. *PLoS ONE.* (2017) 12:e0177726. doi: 10.1371/journal.pone.0177726
17. Zhao Y, Healy BC, Rotstein D, Guttmann CR, Bakshi R, Weiner HL, et al. Exploration of machine learning techniques in predicting multiple sclerosis disease course. *PLoS ONE.* (2017) 12:e0174866. doi: 10.1371/journal.pone.0174866
18. Martins TB, Rose JW, Jaskowski TD, Wilson AR, Husebye D, Seraj HS, et al. Analysis of proinflammatory and anti-inflammatory cytokine serum concentrations in patients with multiple sclerosis by using a multiplexed immunoassay. *Am J Clin Pathol.* (2011) 136:696–704. doi: 10.1309/AJCP7UBK8IBVMVNR
19. Cala CM, Moseley CE, Steele C, Dowdy SM, Cutter GR, Ness JM, et al. T cell cytokine signatures: biomarkers in pediatric multiple sclerosis. *J Neuroimmunol.* (2016) 297:1–8. doi: 10.1016/j.jneuroim.2016.04.015
20. Wang Y, Chen HJ. Use of percentiles and z-scores in anthropometry. In: Preedy VR, editor. *Handbook of Anthropometry.* New York, NY: Springer (2012). p. 29–48. doi: 10.1007/978-1-4419-1788-1_2
21. RColorBrewer S, Liaw A, Wiener M, Liaw MA. *Package 'randomForest'* (2015). Available online at: https://cran.r-project.org/web/packages/randomForest/randomForest.pdf
22. Karatzoglou A, Smola A, Hornik K, Karatzoglou MA. *Package 'kernlab'* (2016). Available online at: http://cran.rediris.es/web/packages/kernlab/kernlab.pdf
23. Rong X. *Deepnet: Deep Learning Toolkit in R. R Package Version 0.2.* (2014). Available online at: http://CRAN.R-project.org/package=deepnet
24. Khanna D, Rana PS. Multilevel ensemble model for prediction of IgA and IgG antibodies. *Immunol Lett.* (2017) 184:51–60. doi: 10.1016/j.imlet.2017.01.017
25. Göbel K, Ruck T, Meuth SG. Cytokine signaling in multiple sclerosis: lost in translation. *Mult Scler J.* (2018) 24:432–9. doi: 10.1177/1352458518763094
26. Reder AT, Feng X. How type I interferons work in multiple sclerosis and other diseases: some unexpected mechanisms. *J Interferon Cytokine Res.* (2014) 34:589–99. doi: 10.1089/jir.2013.0158
27. Miller M, Hafner M, Sontag E, Davidsohn N, Subramanian S, Purnick PE, et al. Modular design of artificial tissue homeostasis: robust control through synthetic cellular heterogeneity. *PLoS Comput Biol.* (2012) 8:e1002579. doi: 10.1371/journal.pcbi.1002579
28. Nikhar S, Karandikar A. Prediction of heart disease using machine learning algorithms. *Int J Eng Technol.* (2018) 7:363–6. doi: 10.14419/ijet.v7i2.32.15714
29. Bind S, Tiwari AK, Sahani AK. A survey of machine learning based approaches for Parkinson disease prediction. *Int J Comp Sci Inform Technol.* (2015) 6:1648–55.
30. Ahmad L, Eshlaghy A, Poorebrahimi A, Ebrahimi M, Razavi A. Using three machine learning techniques for predicting breast cancer recurrence. *J Health Med Inform.* (2013) 4:124. doi: 10.4172/2157-7420.10 00124
31. Leray E, Moreau T, Fromont A, Edan G. Epidemiology of multiple sclerosis. *Rev Neurol.* (2016) 172:3–13. doi: 10.1016/j.neurol.2015.10.006
32. Frohman EM, Racke MK, Raine CS. Multiple sclerosis—the plaque and its pathogenesis. *New Engl J Med.* (2006) 354:942–55. doi: 10.1056/NEJMra052130
33. Becher B, Spath S, Goverman J. Cytokine networks in neuroinflammation. *Nat Rev Immunol.* (2017) 17:49–59. doi: 10.1038/nri.2016.123
34. Codarri L, Fontana A, Becher B. Cytokine networks in multiple sclerosis: lost in translation. *Curr Opin Neurol.* (2010) 23:205–11. doi: 10.1097/WCO.0b013e3283391feb

35. Fogh K, Larsen C, Iversen L, Kragballe K. Interleukin-8 stimulates the formation of 15-hydroxy-eicosatetraenoic acid by human neutrophils *in vitro*. *Agents Actions*. (1992) 35:227–31. doi: 10.1007/BF01997504
36. Nourshargh S, Perkins J, Showell H, Matsushima K, Williams T, Collins P. A comparative study of the neutrophil stimulatory activity *in vitro* and pro-inflammatory properties *in vivo* of 72 amino acid and 77 amino acid IL-8. *J Immunol.* (1992) 148:106–11.
37. Baggiolini M, Dewald B, Moser B. lnterleukin-8 and related chemotactic cytokines—CXC and CC chemokines. *Adv Immunol.* (1993) 55:97–179. doi: 10.1016/S0065-2776(08)60509-X
38. Mukaida N, Harada A, Matsushima K. Interleukin-8 (IL-8) and monocyte chemotactic and activating factor (MCAF/MCP-1), chemokines essentially involved in inflammatory and immune reactions. *Cytokine Growth F R.* (1998) 9:9–23. doi: 10.1016/S1359-6101(97)00022-1
39. Kothur K, Wienholt L, Brilot F, Dale RC. CSF cytokines/chemokines as biomarkers in neuroinflammatory CNS disorders: a systematic review. *Cytokine.* (2016) 77:227–37. doi: 10.1016/j.cyto.2015.10.001
40. Khaibullin T, Ivanova V, Martynova E, Cherepnev G, Khabirov F, Granatov E, et al. Elevated levels of proinflammatory cytokines in cerebrospinal fluid of multiple sclerosis patients. *Front immunol.* (2017) 8:531. doi: 10.3389/fimmu.2017.00531

14

Impact of Disease-Modifying Treatments on the Longitudinal Evolution of Anti-JCV Antibody Index in Multiple Sclerosis

*Harald Hegen[1], Janette Walde[2], Gabriel Bsteh[1], Michael Auer[1], Sebastian Wurth[1], Anne Zinganell[1], Franziska Di Pauli[1], Florian Deisenhammer[1] and Thomas Berger[1]**

[1] Department of Neurology, Medical University of Innsbruck, Innsbruck, Austria, [2] Department of Statistics, Faculty of Economics and Statistics, University of Innsbruck, Innsbruck, Austria

***Correspondence:**
Thomas Berger
thomas.berger@i-med.ac.at

Background: Risk of natalizumab-related progressive multifocal leukoencephalopathy is associated with the presence of anti-JC-virus (JCV) antibodies.

Objective: To investigate the impact of disease-modifying treatments (DMT) on the longitudinal evolution of anti-JCV antibody index.

Methods: Patients with multiple sclerosis who had serum sampling at intervals of 6 ± 3 months over up to 6 years and who either started DMT (interferon-β, glatiramer acetate or natalizumab) during the observation period with at least one serum sample available before and after treatment initiation or received no DMT during the observation period were included. Anti-JCV antibody serological status and index were determined by 2-step second-generation anti-JCV antibody assay.

Results: A total of 89 patients were followed for a median time of 55.2 months. Of those, 62 (69.7%) started DMT and 27 (30.3%) were without therapy during the observation period. Variation of longitudinal anti-JCV antibody index ranged from 9 to 15% and was similar in patients with and without DMT. Applying a mixed model considering the combined effects of treatment and time as well as individual heterogeneity did not show a significant change of anti-JCV antibody index by the start of treatment with interferon-β, glatiramer acetate, or natalizumab.

Conclusion: Evaluated DMTs do not impact longitudinal anti-JCV antibody index evolution.

Keywords: JC virus, anti-JCV antibody index, natalizumab, interferon beta, glatiramer acetate, multiple sclerosis, seroconversion, longitudinal

INTRODUCTION

Natalizumab (NTZ) treatment in multiple sclerosis (MS) patients is associated with the risk of progressive multifocal leukoencephalopathy (PML), an opportunistic infection of the brain caused by John Cunningham virus (JCV) (1). PML risk is determined by the prior use of immunosuppressants, duration of NTZ treatment and presence of serum anti-JCV antibodies (2). In seropositive patients, anti-JCV antibody index (AI) correlates with PML risk (3). In seronegative patients, seroconversion might occur with a rate of approximately 2–6% per year (4, 5). Previous studies evaluating the impact of DMT on anti-JCV antibodies yielded conflicting results, some of them claiming an increase of anti-JCV AI by NTZ treatment (6, 7).

Here, we aimed to investigate the impact of different DMTs on anti-JCV AI evolution in a cohort of MS patients using—in contrast to earlier studies—a longitudinal study design with high frequency sampling over a long observation time and with several samples available before and after start of the respective treatment.

METHODS

Patients and Samples

Out of a previously published cohort of MS patients who had serum sampling over 4–6 years at intervals of 6 ± 3 months (4), patients fulfilling one of the following (additional) criteria were included: (A) start with interferon-β (IFN-β) or glatiramer acetate (GLAT) therapy during the observation period with at least one serum sample available before and after treatment initiation (the sample immediately before treatment begin had to be off any prior treatment) *or* (B) start with NTZ therapy during the observation period with at least one serum sample available before and after treatment initiation, *or* (C) no DMT administration within the observation period. In groups A and B, all serum samples after treatment initiation were obtained while the patient was still on the same therapy.

Anti-JCV Antibody Assay

Anti-JCV AI (and serological status) were determined at Unilabs (Copenhagen, Denmark) by a two-step enzyme-linked immunosorbent assay (STRATIFY JCV DxSelect; Focus Diagnostics, Cypress; CA, USA) as previously described (3, 8).

An anti-JCV AI >0.40 denoted anti-JCV antibody positivity and an index <0.20 denoted anti-JCV antibody negativity. For samples with an index ≥0.20 but ≤0.40 (intermediate response) further evaluation in the confirmation test was required. In the confirmation test, patient sample is pre-inhibited with the coating antigen in solution and, then, the pre-inhibited and non-inhibited aliquots of patient serum are tested. The results of the confirmation assay are reported as percentage inhibition, calculated as 100 × [1-(optical density of pre-inhibited/non-inhibited sample)]. Samples were scored eventually positive when inhibition was >45% (3, 8).

Definition of Seroconversion and Seroreversion

Seroconversion was defined as occurrence of a positive anti-JCV antibody result at least once during follow-up, if baseline serostatus was negative. Seroreversion was defined as occurrence of a negative anti-JCV antibody testing at least once during the observation period in case of baseline positive serostatus. Hence, stable anti-JCV antibody status was defined by the same serological result obtained in all longitudinal samples per patient.

Statistical Analysis

Coefficient of variation (CV) of anti-JCV AI is displayed as the median of the CVs calculated for each patient by using all longitudinal anti-JCV AI. To test for statistical difference of the CV between each treatment group (IFN-β, GLAT, NTZ) and the no DMT group, a permutation test was applied for the median difference (10,000 runs).

In order to investigate a possible increase of the anti-JCV AI after treatment a mixed model was employed (**Figure 1**). The variable *patient group* indicating the specific treatment (IFN-β, GLAT, NTZ, no DMT) and the variable *time* denoting two periods before treatment and four after treatment and their interaction were included in the regression equation. This time period was chosen as the dataset within these periods was almost balanced. The individual heterogeneity was modeled via the variables age, sex and random effects. Additionally, due to the time structure the within variance structure was assumed to follow an autoregressive process of order one. Furthermore, also an unstructured within-subject covariance was employed. Since the findings did not change quantitatively, we present the results of the approach with more degrees of freedom. Using joint tests the main effects (i.e., *patient group* and *time*) and the interaction effects were investigated. A power analysis was conducted regarding the combined effects of *time and patient group* considering repeated measurements and unequal sample sizes of employed patient groups (significance level = 5%, power = 80%, increase of anti-JCV antibody index after treatment = 0.2 per year).

P values were considered statistically significant at the level of 5%. Statistical analysis was done using Stata/MP 15.0 (StataCorp LLC, College Station, TX, USA). Permutation test and graphs were done in R system for statistical computing (9).

Ethics

The study was approved by the ethics committee of Medical University of Innsbruck (approval number AN2014-0347 344/4.8). Written informed consent was obtained from all patients.

RESULTS

A total of 89 patients with a mean age of 36.6 years (SD 11.0) and a female predominance of 76.4% were included into the study, had median of 9 longitudinally collected serum samples and were followed for a median time of 55.2 months. Of those, 62 (69.7%) started DMT and 27 (30.3%) were without therapy during the observation period. None of the patients who started a DMT switched therapy and none of the untreated patients started any DMT during the observation period. Overall, 75 (84.3%) patients showed stable anti-JCV antibody status during the observation period.

Longitudinal Evolution of Anti-JCV Antibody Index in Untreated MS Patients

Twenty-seven patients without DMT were followed for median 53.9 months. Demographic and clinical data are shown in **Table 1**. Of those, 25 (92.6%) showed stable anti-JCV antibody

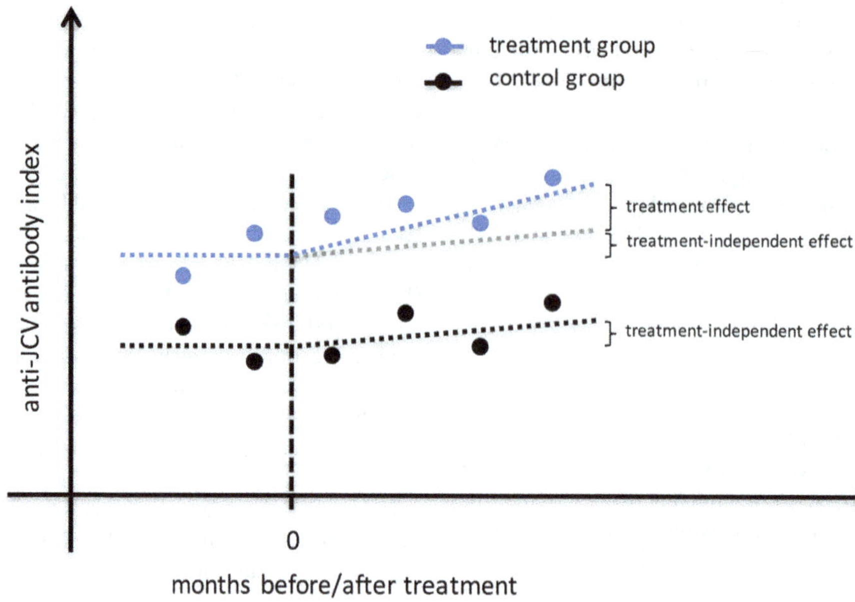

FIGURE 1 | Study design for identification of treatment effect on anti-JCV antibody index. The illustrated estimation approach shows anti-JCV AI evolution for the no DMT group that may change (e.g., increase) over time, as well as anti-JCV AI evolution for a treatment group that may change (e.g., increase) due to the same effect as in the no DMT group plus a possible treatment effect. To correctly estimate the treatment effect, a mixed model is employed that considers any effect that appears also in the no DMT group independent of the applied treatment. Therefore, several samples before and after start of treatment per patient are required. AI, antibody index; DMT, disease modifying treatment; JCV, John Cunningham virus.

TABLE 1 | Demographic and clinical characteristics of the study cohort.

	No DMT	IFN-β	GLAT	NTZ
Number of patients	27	25	9	28
Sex (female), *n* (%)	21 (77.8)	20 (80)	7 (77.8)	20 (71.4)
Age (years), mean (SD)	46.5 (10.9)	34.4 (8.5)	28.1 (8.6)	30.9 (7.1)
Disease duration (years), median (IQR)	9.0 (4.0–16.8)	3.6 (1.2–7.2)	4.9 (3.3–8.0)	5.4 (1.6–9.3)
Prior DMT, *n* (%)	11 (40.7)[a]	0	6 (66.7)[b]	27 (96.4)[c]
Time period between end of prior and begin of current DMT (months), median (IQR)	8.1 (2.7–89.4)[d]	n.a.	20.7 (13.8–48.2)	1.4 (0.7–2.3)
Number of longitudinal samples per patient, median	9	7	9	11
Observation period (months), median	53.9	49.3	65.1	64.2

[a] *Prior to the observation period, six patients received IFN-β, one GLAT and four patients immunosuppressive therapy (azathioprine and/ or cyclophosphamide).*
[b] *Five patients were treated with IFN-β before starting GLAT therapy, one patient had already received GLAT once before.*
[c] *A total of 22 patients were on IFN-β and five patients on GLAT before switching to NTZ.*
[d] *In this patient group, time period between end of prior DMT and baseline visit is given.*
DMT, disease-modifying treatment; GLAT, glatiramer acetate; IFN-β, interferon-β; IQR, interquartile range; n.a., not applicable; NTZ, natalizumab; SD, standard deviation.

status during the observation period. Anti-JCV AI did not significantly change over time neither including all patients (**Table S1**) nor patients with stable anti-JCV antibody status (**Figure 2A**, **Table S2**) or stable positive anti-JCV antibody status (**Table S3**). The median CV of anti-JCV AI in patients with stable anti-JCV antibody status was 14.4% (**Table 2**).

Longitudinal Evolution of Anti-JCV Antibody Index Before and After Start of DMT

Out of 62 patients, who were followed for median 55.9 months, 25 (40.3%) started treatment with IFN-β, 9 (14.5%) with GLAT and 28 (45.2%) with NTZ. Demographic and clinical data are shown in **Table 1**.

Interferon-Beta

All patients starting IFN-β were treatment-naïve before. Twenty (80%) patients did not change their initial anti-JCV antibody status during the observation period. Using the mixed model, there was no statistically significant change of anti-JCV AI by the start of IFN-β therapy regardless of including all patients (**Table S1**), patients with stable anti-JCV antibody status (**Figure 2B**, **Table S2**) or stable positive anti-JCV antibody status (**Table S3**). Median CV of anti-JCV AI in patients with

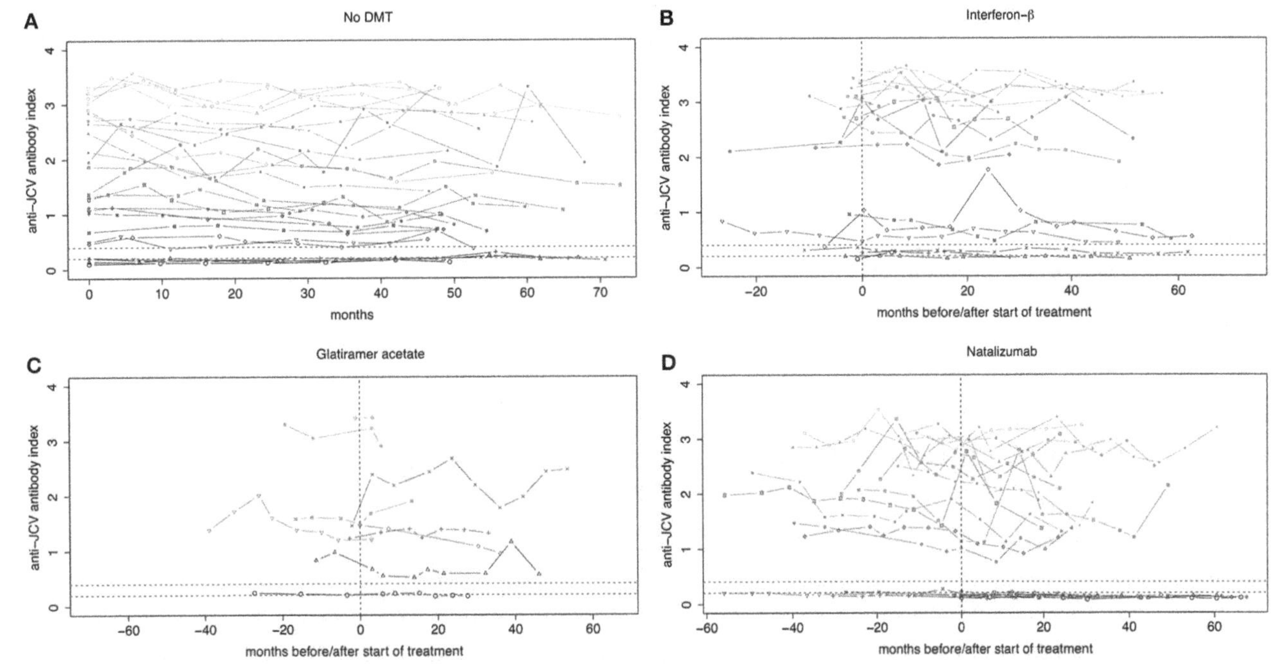

FIGURE 2 | Longitudinal evolution of anti-JCV antibody index in patients with stable anti-JCV antibody status. **(A)** Serial anti-JCV antibody indices in patients without any disease-modifying treatment. **(B)** Serial anti-JCV antibody indices in patients before and after start of IFN-β therapy. Before, all patients were treatment-naïve. Afterwards, index values are shown as long as IFN-β was administered. **(C)** Serial anti-JCV antibody indices in patients before and after start of GLAT therapy. After treatment begin, index values are shown as long as GLAT was administered. **(D)** Serial anti-JCV antibody indices in patients before and after start of NTZ therapy. All but one patient received prior treatment. Afterwards, index values are shown as long as NTZ was applied. For building this graph, only patients with stable anti-JCV antibody status (i.e., without seroconversion/-reversion) during the observation period were included. Using a mixed model, there was no statistically significant change of anti-JCV antibody index before and after initiation of the respective treatment. *Vertical dashed line* indicates start of treatment. *Upper horizontal dashed line* indicates an anti-JCV antibody index of 0.4. Index values >0.4 are denoted anti-JCV antibody positive. *Lower horizontal dashed line* indicates an anti-JCV antibody index of 0.2. Index values <0.2 are denoted anti-JCV antibody negative. Samples with an index ≥0.20 but ≤0.40 (intermediate response) are classified as anti-JCV antibody positive or negative based on confirmation test (second step of the enzyme-linked immunosorbent assay), i.e., the displayed index values within this range might be classified as positive or negative. For further details see (3, 8). DMT, disease-modifying treatment; GLAT, glatiramer acetate; IFN-β, interferon-beta; JCV, John Cunningham virus; NTZ, natalizumab.

stable anti-JCV antibody status was 9.4% (**Table 2**) and did not statistically significantly differ from the no DMT group ($p = 0.127$).

Glatiramer Acetate

Three of nine (33.3%) patients starting GLAT were treatment-naïve before. In the remaining six patients, prior DMT was stopped median 20.7 months before. In all patients, at least the sample immediately before start of GLAT therapy was collected while being off any prior DMT. During the observation period, none of the patients showed seroconversion or seroreversion. As determined by the mixed model, there was no change of anti-JCV AI by the start of GLAT therapy including all (and therefore also serostable) patients (**Figure 2C**, **Tables S1**, **S2**) or patients with stable positive anti-JCV antibody status only (**Table S3**). Median CV of anti-JCV AI was 13.5% (**Table 2**) and did not significantly differ from the no DMT group ($p = 0.449$).

Natalizumab

All but one patient, who switched to NTZ treatment during the observation period, received prior DMT and stopped it median 1.4 months before NTZ initiation. Twenty-one (75%) patients showed stable anti-JCV antibody status during follow-up. There was no statistically significant change in anti-JCV AI due to start of NTZ therapy including all patients (**Table S1**), patients with stable anti-JCV antibody status (**Figure 2D**, **Table S2**) or stable positive anti-JCV antibody status (**Table S3**). Median CV of anti-JCV AI in the serostable group was 14.8% (**Table 2**) and was similar as compared to the no DMT group ($p = 0.699$).

Patients With Seroconversion or Seroreversion

Longitudinal evolution of anti-JCV AI in those 14 (15.7%) patients who showed either seroconversion ($n = 6$, 42.9%) or seroreversion ($n = 8$, 57.1%) is shown in **Figure 3**. Five patients started treatment with IFN-β and seven with NTZ, while two patients where without any DMT during the observation period. Out of the 12 patients receiving treatment, seven patients changed anti-JCV antibody status while on treatment, the remaining five before treatment initiation.

TABLE 2 | Variability of longitudinal anti-JCV antibody index in patients with stable anti-JCV antibody status.

	No DMT	IFN-β	GLAT	NTZ
ALL PATIENTS WITH STABLE ANTI-JCV ANTIBODY STATUS				
CV of anti-JCV antibody index, (%) median (IQR)[a]	14.4 (7.2–19.7)	9.4 (7.0–16.3)	13.5 (5.7–18.8)	14.8 (9.8–21.0)
Anti-JCV antibody index, median	1.32	2.67	1.38	1.60
Number of patients	25	20	9	21
Number of longitudinal samples per patient, median	8	7.5	9	10
PATIENTS WITH STABLE NEGATIVE ANTI-JCV ANTIBODY STATUS				
CV of anti-JCV antibody index, (%) median (IQR)[a]	18.2 (16.6–19.7)	16.5 (13.0–23.9)	10.9	15.4 (14.2–20.6)
Anti-JCV antibody index, median	0.18	0.21	0.22	0.14
Number of patients	4	4	1	8
Number of longitudinal samples per patient, median	11.5	11.5	9	9.5
PATIENTS WITH STABLE POSITIVE ANTI-JCV ANTIBODY STATUS				
CV of anti-JCV antibody index, (%) median (IQR)[a]	12.1 (6.8–15.5)	7.6 (6.0–13.0)	15.1 (5.6–19.4)	10.9 (8.0–21.0)
Anti-JCV antibody index, median	1.85	2.84	1.48	2.18
Number of patients	21	16	8	13
Number of longitudinal samples per patient, median	8	7.5	8.5	10

[a]*Coefficient of variation (CV) is displayed as the median of the CVs calculated for each patient using all longitudinally determined anti-JCV antibody indices. Only patients with stable JCV serostatus during the observation period were included.*

DMT, disease modifying treatment; GLAT, glatiramer acetate; IFN-β, interferon-β; JCV, John Cunningham virus; IQR, interquartile range; n.a., not applicable; NTZ, natalizumab.

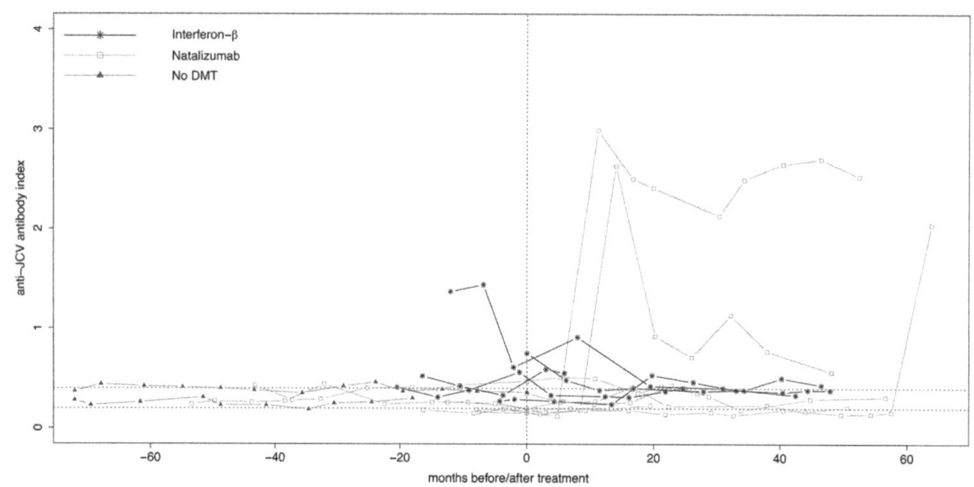

FIGURE 3 | Longitudinal evolution of anti-JCV antibody index in patients with changing anti-JCV antibody status. Serial anti-JCV antibody indices in patients before and after start of interferon-β or natalizumab therapy, as well as in patients without DMT are shown. For building this graph, only patients with changing anti-JCV antibody status (i.e., with either seroconversion or seroreversion) during the observation period were included. Patients without DMT appear per definition left of the vertical dashed line, as in this group no treatment is commenced. *Vertical dashed line* indicates start of treatment. *Upper horizontal dashed line* indicates an anti-JCV antibody index of 0.4. Index values >0.4 are denoted anti-JCV antibody positive. *Lower horizontal dashed line* indicates an anti-JCV antibody index of 0.2. Index values <0.2 are denoted anti-JCV antibody negative. Samples with an index ≥0.20 but ≤0.40 (intermediate response) are classified as anti-JCV antibody positive or negative based on confirmation test (second step of the enzyme-linked immunosorbent assay), i.e., the displayed index values within this range might be classified as positive or negative. For further details see (3, 8). DMT, disease-modifying treatment; JCV, John Cunningham virus.

DISCUSSION

Here we observed that evolution of anti-JCV AI is not influenced by the administration of DMT using—for the first time—a longitudinal study design with samples available before and after start of therapy.

To date, several studies have investigated the influence of different variables on serum anti-JCV antibodies. In this context, it has to be distinguished whether the influence of the variable of interest (e.g., age) on either anti-JCV antibody status or index was investigated, and it has to be distinguished whether a cross-sectional study design (establishing an association between the variable of interest and anti-JCV antibody status or index) or a longitudinal study design (assessing the change over time, i.e., seroconversion/-reversion or change in anti-JCV AI) was applied. By cross-sectional design, higher anti-JCV antibody prevalence (5, 10–17) and indices (4, 6) were observed with increasing patients' age, as well as in most studies higher antibody prevalence in males (5, 10–12, 14, 16, 18). Prior use of DMTs had no impact on anti-JCV antibody positivity (11–14, 16, 17) and index (10). By longitudinal design, age (4) and baseline anti-JCV AI (4, 19) were predictors of later anti-JCV antibody serostatus change, whereas no influence of prior and current DMTs on seroconversion rate were observed (14, 17). One study reported an increase in the annual rate of seroconversion with NTZ treatment duration, however, these higher rates were observed at the end of follow-up when the number of patients were small due to high drop-outs (e.g., only 20 of 85 patients remained in the study at year 5) (18). With respect to longitudinal anti-JCV AI evolution, two recent studies observed an increase of anti-JCV AI while on NTZ therapy (6, 7). Both studies compared anti-JCV AI of two consecutive samples that were both collected while patients received treatment with NTZ with a time period of approximately 1 year in between (6, 7). The first study found that the observed increase of anti-JCV AI (of ~0.1 per year) was higher than expected and explainable by the effect of age (7). However, the effect of age was estimated by correlation of anti-JCV AI and age at baseline, and then extrapolated over time. The second study focused on anti-JCV antibody positive patients and reported an increase of anti-JCV AI in this subgroup of patients. The authors argued that the increase of anti-JCV AI would go beyond an age effect, as there was no statistically significant correlation of age with anti-JCV AI in the anti-JCV antibody positive patient group (but in the whole cohort that also includes seroconverters) (6).

From a methodological point of view, the bivariate (cross-sectional) correlation between anti-JCV AI and baseline age cannot be estimated without bias (when no control variables are included or heterogeneity is not considered). Furthermore, it seems obvious that samples are needed before and after start of treatment to reliably assess the impact of treatment on anti-JCV AI evolution, and/ or to include a control group. Using a control allows the consideration of treatment-independent effects on anti-JCV AI evolution (**Figure 1**). Also, several sampling time points are required in order to minimize the possibility that a change in anti-JCV AI is artificially observed when comparing only two measurements against the background of a certain variability in anti-JCV AI over time.

Here, we applied a design that encounters the above-mentioned problems in assessing whether DMTs impact on anti-JCV AI. Even though the requirement of study design to include patients with long follow-up (median 5 years) and multiple consecutive samples (median 9 samples; available before as well as after start of therapy) resulted in a moderate total number of patients, especially compared to other previous studies, we still had a statistical power for our hypothesis (tested with the mixed model) of 80%. Power calculation was based on the decision to consider an increase in anti-JCV AI of 0.2 per year as relevant. This magnitude was based on our observation of the CV of anti-JCV AI over time, that in case of a statistically significant finding by the model, this would mean a true change in anti-JCV AI that goes beyond the "natural" fluctuation. Accordingly, the maximum increase of anti-JCV AI per year that has been reported by previous studies (6, 7) is within this variability, as e.g., a variability of 10% at an anti-JCV AI of 2.0 might result in an index of 2.2. Whereas reproducibility of the anti-JCV antibody assay has been shown to be high (6, 8), there has been so far no analysis of the "natural" long-term variation of anti-JCV AI over time [besides the longitudinal assessment of e.g., (bi-) annual anti-JCV antibody prevalence (4) and median anti-JCV AI (4, 16)].

There are some limitations of our study. First, we used a subgroup ($n = 89$) of a previously published cohort ($n = 154$) that was based on the availability of samples (before as well as after treatment initiation). Nevertheless, we are confident that the presented results are reliable, as the demographic characteristics (such as age and sex) as well as the clinical variables of interest (such as rate of seroconversion/ -reversion) are similar compared to the original cohort. Furthermore, the rate of seroconversion of ~3% per year is realistic (4). Higher conversion rates that were published by some prior studies [mostly between 10 to 15% per year, determined already within a relatively short observation period of approximately 1 year (3, 6, 10)] seem in our opinion somehow unrealistic, owing to the fact that anti-JCV antibody prevalence in MS patients is at least 50% (11), and applying these high seroconversion rates (of up to 15%) would implicate that after several years all patients have converted to anti-JCV antibody positivity. Secondly, to test our hypothesis we had a statistical power of 80%. Although this value is considered as a standard type II error and indeed a high number of samples were included, the number of patients was moderate. To further strengthen our findings, a higher statistical power (e.g., 90%) and thus a higher number of patients is desirable—an aim which has to be addressed by further studies. Another limitation of our study is that samples before start of NTZ were not treatment naïve, but on first-line treatment, in the majority of cases with IFN-β. This is because samples were collected during routine clinical visits and usually NTZ is used as second-line treatment. However, as IFN-β did not show an impact on anti-JCV AI over time (this group was therapy-naïve before), we hypothesize that pre-treatment with IFN-β will also have no impact on the analysis of NTZ samples. It seems indispensable that further studies should again not only address the impact of NTZ on longitudinal anti-JCV AI evolution, but also the impact of the various baseline DMT such as IFN-β so that the above drawn conclusion, that is starting of NTZ does not influence anti-JCV AI as assessed in pre-treated patients because the use of these pre-treatments has no impact on anti-JCV AI as well, can be confirmed.

AUTHOR CONTRIBUTIONS

HH has participated in the conception and design of the study, acquisition, and statistical analysis of the data, and in drafting the manuscript. JW has participated in statistical analysis of the data and reviewing the manuscript for intellectual content. GB and MA has participated in data acquisition and reviewing the manuscript for intellectual content. SW, AZ, FDP, and FD have participated in reviewing the manuscript for intellectual content. TB has participated in the conception and design of the study and reviewing the manuscript for intellectual content.

REFERENCES

1. Tan CS, Koralnik IJ. Progressive multifocal leukoencephalopathy and other disorders caused by JC virus: clinical features and pathogenesis. *Lancet Neurol.* (2010) 9:425–37. doi: 10.1016/S1474-4422(10)70040-5
2. Bloomgren G, Richman S, Hotermans C, Subramanyam M, Goelz S, Natarajan A, et al. Risk of natalizumab-associated progressive multifocal leukoencephalopathy. *N Engl J Med.* (2012) 366:1870–80. doi: 10.1056/NEJMoa1107829
3. Plavina T, Subramanyam M, Bloomgren G, Richman S, Pace A, Lee S, et al. Anti-JC virus antibody levels in serum or plasma further define risk of natalizumab-associated progressive multifocal leukoencephalopathy. *Ann Neurol.* (2014) 76:802–12. doi: 10.1002/ana.24286
4. Hegen H, Auer M, Bsteh G, Di Pauli F, Plavina T, Walde J, Deisenhammer F, Berger T. Stability and predictive value of anti-JCV antibody index in multiple sclerosis: a 6-year longitudinal study. *PLoS ONE* (2017) 12:e0174005. doi: 10.1371/journal.pone.0174005
5. Gorelik L, Lerner M, Bixler S, Crossman M, Schlain B, Simon K, et al. Anti-JC virus antibodies: implications for PML Risk Stratification. *Ann Neurol.* (2010) 68:295–303. doi: 10.1002/ana.22128
6. Schwab N, Schneider-Hohendorf T, Pignolet B, Breuer J, Gross CC, Göbel K, et al. Therapy with natalizumab is associated with high JCV seroconversion and rising JCV index values. *Neurology Neuroimmunol Neuroinflam.* (2016) 3:e195. doi: 10.1212/NXI.0000000000000195
7. Raffel J, Gafson AR, Malik O, Nicholas R. Anti-JC virus antibody titres increase over time with natalizumab treatment. *Multiple Scler.* (2015) 21:1833–8. doi: 10.1177/1352458515599681
8. Lee P, Plavina T, Castro A, Berman M, Jaiswal D, Rivas S, et al. A second-generation ELISA (STRATIFY JCV^{TM} DxSelect^{TM}) for detection of JC virus antibodies in human serum and plasma to support progressive multifocal leukoencephalopathy risk stratification. *J Clin Virol.* (2013) 57:141–6. doi: 10.1016/j.jcv.2013.02.002
9. R Core Team. *R: A Language and Environment for Statistical Computing.* Available online at: www.R-project.org
10. Trampe AK, Hemmelmann C, Stroet A, Haghikia A, Hellwig K, Wiendl H, et al. Anti-JC virus antibodies in a large German natalizumab-treated multiple sclerosis cohort. *Neurology* (2012) 78:1736–42. doi: 10.1212/WNL.0b013e3182583022
11. Olsson T, Achiron A, Alfredsson L, Berger T, Brassat D, Chan A, et al. Anti-JC virus antibody prevalence in a multinational multiple sclerosis cohort. *Mult Scler.* (2013) 19:1533–8. doi: 10.1177/1352458513477925
12. Bozic C, Richman S, Plavina T, Natarajan A, Scanlon JV, Subramanyam M, et al. Anti-John Cunnigham virus antibody prevalence in multiple sclerosis patients: baseline results of STRATIFY-1. *Ann Neurol.* (2011) 70:742–50. doi: 10.1002/ana.22606
13. Salmen A, Ahsen von N, Trampe AK, Hoepner R, Plavina T, Subramanyam M, et al. Longitudinal analyses of anti-JCV antibody index for risk assessment of progressive multifocal leukoencephalopathy. *Multiple Scler. J.* (2016) 2:2055217316630008. doi: 10.1177/2055217316630008
14. Alroughani R, Akhtar S, Ahmed SF, Khoury SJ, Al-Hashel JY, Sahraian MA, et al. JC virus seroprevalence and seroconversion in multiple sclerosis cohort: a Middle-Eastern study. *J Neurol Sci.* (2016) 360:61–5. doi: 10.1016/j.jns.2015.11.044
15. Aladro Y, Terrero R, Cerezo M, Ginestal R, Ayuso L, Meca-Lallana V, et al. Anti-JC virus seroprevalence in a Spanish multiple sclerosis cohort. *J Neurol Sci.* (2016) 365:16–21. doi: 10.1016/j.jns.2016.03.050
16. Kolasa M, Hagman S, Verkkoniemi-Ahola A, Airas L, Koivisto K, Elovaara I. Anti-JC virus seroprevalence in a Finnish MS cohort. *Acta Neurol Scand.* (2016) 133:391–7. doi: 10.1111/ane.12475
17. Dominguez-Mozo MI, Rus M, Santiago JL, Izquierdo G, Casanova I, Galan V, et al. Study of the anti-JCV antibody levels in a Spanish multiple sclerosis cohort. *Eur J Clin Invest.* (2017) 47:158–66. doi: 10.1111/eci.12721
18. Correia I, Jesus-Ribeiro J, Batista S, Martins AI, Nunes C, Macário MC, et al. Anti-JCV antibody serostatus and longitudinal evaluation in a Portuguese Multiple Sclerosis population. *J Clin Neurosci.* (2017) 45:257–60. doi: 10.1016/j.jocn.2017.08.006
19. Vennegoor A, van Rossum JA, Leurs C, Wattjes MP, Rispens T, Murk JLAN, et al. High cumulative JC virus seroconversion rate during long-term use of natalizumab. *Eur J Neurol.* (2016) 23:1079–85. doi: 10.1111/ene.12988

15

Vaccination in Multiple Sclerosis: Friend or Foe?

Tobias Zrzavy [1], Herwig Kollaritsch [2], Paulus S. Rommer [1,3], Nina Boxberger [3], Micha Loebermann [4], Isabella Wimmer [1], Alexander Winkelmann [5] and Uwe K. Zettl [3,5]*

[1] Department of Neurology, Medical University of Vienna, Vienna, Austria, [2] Institute of Specific Prophylaxis and Tropical Medicine, Medical University of Vienna, Vienna, Austria, [3] Department of Neurology, Neuroimmunological Section, University of Rostock, Rostock, Germany, [4] Department of Tropical Medicine and Infectious Diseases, University of Rostock, Rostock, Germany, [5] Department of Neurology, University of Rostock, Rostock, Germany

***Correspondence:**
Uwe K. Zettl
Uwe.zettl@med.uni-rostock.de

Multiple sclerosis (MS) is a debilitating disease of the central nervous systems (CNS). Disease-modifying treatments (including immunosuppressive treatments) have shown positive effects on the disease course, but are associated with systemic consequences on the immune system and may increase the risk of infections and alter vaccine efficiency. Therefore, vaccination of MS patients is of major interest. Over the last years, vaccine hesitancy has steadily grown especially in Western countries, partly due to fear of sequelae arising from vaccination, especially neurological disorders. The interaction of vaccination and MS has been discussed for decades. In this review, we highlight the immunology of vaccination, provide a review of literature and discuss the clinical consideration of MS, vaccination and immunosuppression. In conclusion, there is consensus that MS cannot be caused by vaccines, neither by inactivated nor by live vaccines. However, particular attention should be paid to two aspects: First, in immunocompromised patients, live vaccines may lead to a stronger immune reaction with signs of the disease against which the patients have been vaccinated, albeit in weakened form. Second, protection provided by vaccination should be controlled in patients who have been vaccinated while receiving immunomodulatory or immunosuppressive treatment. In conclusion, there is evidence that systemic infections can worsen MS, thus vaccination will lower the risk of relapses by reducing the risk of infections. Therefore, vaccination should be in general recommended to MS patients.

Keywords: multiple scleorsis (MS), immunology, vaccination, disease modifying therapy (DMT), vaccination immunology

INTRODUCTION

Over the last years, especially in Western countries, vaccine hesitancy has steadily grown and poses an increasing health concern (1). The recent upsurge of measles in Europe is an impressive example. Anti-vaccinationists argue that possible side effects weigh out the benefits (2). Especially sequelaes such as autism, multiple sclerosis (MS) and various neurological syndromes have been emphasized by the anti-vaccination lobby (3, 4). This alarming development is even partly supported by health-care providers including some MS neurologists, who are afraid of iatrogenic deterioration of pre-existing MS. Indeed, studies linking vaccination and disease onset have been published. Although these studies were often underpowered and lacked an adequate design in order to provide evidence of the suspected link, they caught public awareness leading to a drop of public vaccination coverage rates (5, 6).

Epidemiological studies and pharmacovigilance data have repeatedly demonstrated safety for the vast majority of vaccines. Lately, a review concluded that there is no significant evidence for a causal relationship between the onset or deterioration of MS and vaccination against measles, mumps and rubella (MMR), influenza, hepatitis A, hepatitis B, human papilloma virus (HPV), diphtheria, tetanus, acellular pertussis, or meningococcal disease (7). Some studies have even indicated a decreased risk for MS and reduced disease activity in preexisting MS (8).

The aim of this review is to summarize data on vaccination and disease activity of both MS and acute disseminated encephalomyelitis (ADEM). Moreover, vaccination-induced effects on the immune system are presented and potential interactions between MS and immunizations are discussed.

BASIC IMMUNOLOGY OF VACCINATION

Vaccine-induced protection is a complex issue and depends on a cascade of mechanisms and mediators (**Figure 1**). Eventually, protection is accomplished either by antibodies or T cell-dependent factors or by a combination of both including neutralizing or antitoxic antibodies, $CD8^+$ T cells, $CD4^+$ T cells and corresponding cytokines (e.g., interleukin (IL)-2, 3, 4, 5, 9, 13, 17, 21, 22, and 26) (9). Generally, vaccines have to be capable of activating antigen-presenting cells (APCs) of the innate immune system, which subsequently present the vaccine epitope(s) to T cells—the so-called 'immunogenic potential' (10). In this context, dendritic cells play a pivotal role due to their enhanced capability to stimulate naïve T cells (11).

The nature of vaccine-induced immunity depends on several parameters, of which the biological properties of the vaccine's epitope are of high importance (9). Live vaccines are attenuated variants of pathogens that still can activate APCs, especially immature dendritic cells, patrolling through the body. This immunogenic potential is often lost by subcellular- or subunit-based vaccines (12), which is why these inactivated vaccine antigens are usually combined with so-called adjuvants to increase and modulate the vaccine's immunogenicity via a longer lasting and more effective activation of immune cells.

One of the most widely used adjuvants are aluminum salts, which were originally thought to create a long-lasting depot of the antigen in order to provide its slow release, but have instead been shown to act on dendritic cells via PRRs (pattern recognition receptors) leading to the secretion of pro-inflammatory cytokines (13). Similarly, novel adjuvants like squalens or monophosphoryl lipid A (MPLA—a detoxified lipopolysaccharide) aim to enhance the innate immune response, but never reach the immunogenic potential of live attenuated vaccines (14). Adjuvants have been added to vaccines for more than 90 years and over the last decades, considerable progress has been made in understanding their mode of action and to improve safety (15). Besides the above mentioned aluminum salts, squalene and MPLA, oil emulsions, saponin, Toll-like receptor (TLR) agonists, enterotoxins, polysaccharides, and glycolipid adjuvants (16) are used, all of which stimulate the immune system as well.

Aluminum adjuvants have now been used for decades and lots of experience has been gained on its use, effectiveness, and safety and they still remain the most frequently used adjuvants. Their effects on the immune system comprise stimulation of macrophages and dendritic cells via PRRs, inflammasome activation, IL-1β release and activation of Th2 lymphocytes (15, 16). However, besides increased immunogenicity, aluminum adjuvants also increase reactogenicity and based on data from animal models and reports on narcolepsy, silicosis, Guillain-Barré-syndrome (GBS) and macrophagic myofasciitis, they are also discussed to induce autoimmunity (17). The second most commonly and long used adjuvants are oil emulsions. They have a strong reactogenic potential and can cause severe inflammatory local reactions such as ulceration and granulomas. The most well-known oil emulsion is complete Freund's adjuvant. However, due to its potent reactogenicity, it is not suitable for human use. A possible association between oil emulsions and autoimmunity disorders has been hypothesized from animal models. Oil emulsions are potent inducers of IL-1β and IL-17 (18, 19). IL-17 plays a major role in autoimmunity and MS and may trigger the migration of peripheral lymphocytes into the CNS across the BBB (20, 21). Frequently, a combination of adjuvants is used to increase immunogenicity of vaccines. AS03 is an adjuvant emulsion containing squalene, DL-α-tocopherol, and polysorbate 80. It is e.g., used for the pandemic swine flu vaccine Pandemrix® (15) or the FDA-licensed H5N1 monovalent influenza vaccine. In animal studies, autoimmunity was observed in connection with AS03 (22) and in humans, cases of narcolepsy have been reported (23). Oil emulsions are often combined with TLR agonists such as MPLA. Generally, TLR agonist adjuvants activate the inflammatory transcription factor NFκB AS04 is a combination of MPLA and aluminum salts and is used as adjuvant in vaccines against hepatitis B (Fendrix®) and HPV, as well as in the new recombinant vaccine against Herpes zoster. Most polysaccharide adjuvants activate NFκB to induce immune processes (e.g., dextran, zymosan) (24). However, delta-inulin for instance, a polysaccharide adjuvant used for Advax®, acts via NFκB-independent mechanisms to enhance humoral and cellular immune responses. Although the mechanisms are not yet fully understood, Advax® has so far not shown inflammatory side effects and has proven safety in hepatitis B vaccination and influenza (16).

After activation of the immune cascade and stimulation of dendritic cells, the latter increase their expression of MHC molecules and chemokine receptors such as CCR7 leading to their migration toward the draining lymph nodes in order to provide co-stimulatory signals for the differentiation of naïve T cells into immune effector cells (25). The activation of the immune cascade has various effects on T and B cells. In short, antigen-recognition by B cells leads to their activation and migration toward the T-B cell border of the lymph node, where they can subsequently receive additional stimuli by activated T helper (TH) cells. These signals include CD40 interaction, secretion of cytokines by TH1 or TH2 cells, and finally the transformation of B cells into plasma cells predominantly secreting low affinity antibodies (26). Later, the

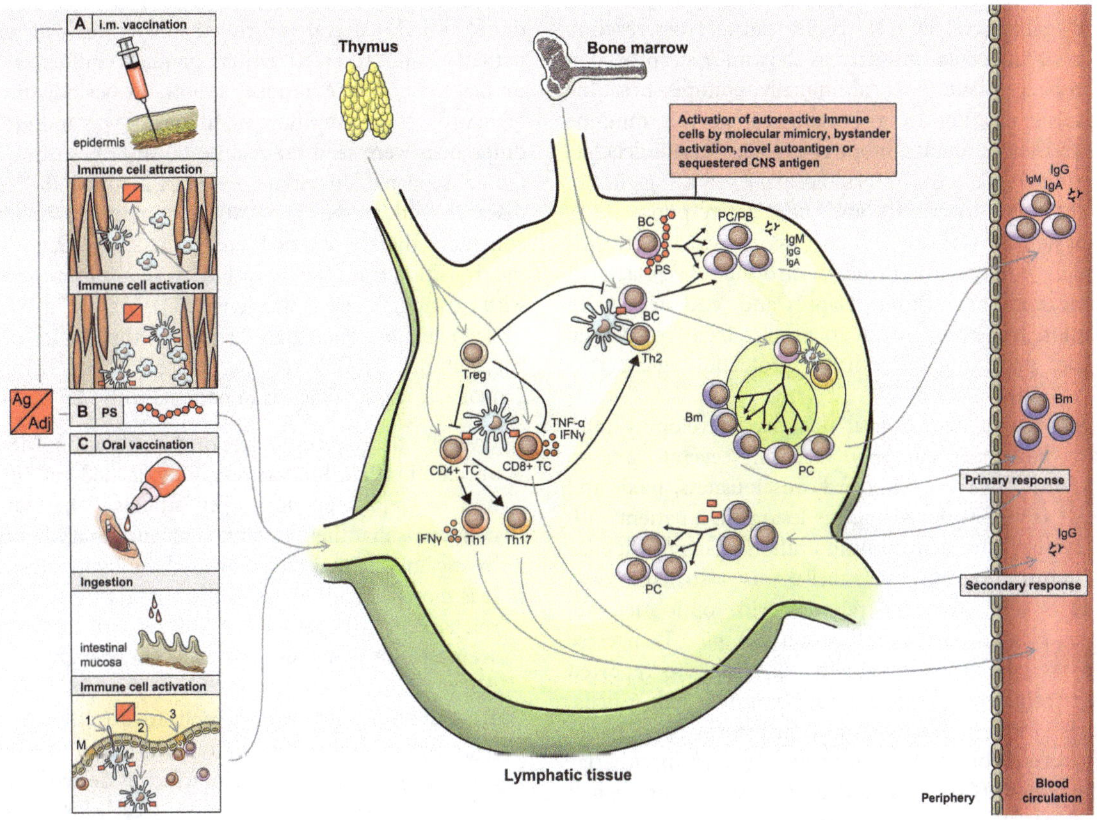

FIGURE 1 | Immunology of vaccination. Routes of vaccine administration include: Injection of vaccine into muscle tissue (A) leading to attraction, activation, uptake and processing (B) in APCs (antigen-presenting cells), which then migrate to lymphatic tissue. Similarly, oral or nasal administration (C) leads to activation and migration of innate immune cells into the lymphatic tissue. APCs activate lymphocytes leading to a T cell immune response and activation of B cells, which receive additional stimuli by activated T helper cells. The primary immune response is short-lived and associated with the early appearance of low affinity antibodies, which are later replaced by high affinity antibodies generated via the germinal center reaction. PS, polysaccharide; PC, Plasma cell; PB, plasma blast; BC, B-cell; Bm, memory B cells; Treg, Regulatory T Cells.

germinal center response contributes via affinity maturation (somatic hypermutation and affinity-based selection) and isotype switch to a sustained production of high affinity antibodies by predominantly plasma cells but also memory B cells. Basically, in the lymph nodes, numerous B cells with various affinity compete for the antigens presented by follicular dendritic cells. These antigens are processed and further presented via MHC II to follicular TH cells, which provide costimulatory signals (e.g., CD40, ICOS, and IL-21) leading to survival and further proliferation of B cells with highest affinity for the antigen (27).

In conclusion, vaccination-induced immune responses, including employed cell types and mediators, vary depending on the type of vaccine administration, kind of vaccine and choice of adjuvant. While antibodies will directly prevent and reduce infections, $CD4^+$ and $CD8^+$ T cells rather support the organism eventually reducing, controlling and clearing the pathogens. Antibodies bind to their antigen, neutralize pathogens, activate macrophages and neutrophils as well as the complement system, while $CD4^+$ and $CD8^+$ T cells secrete cytokines, perforins, and granzymes (9). The choice of adjuvant seems to be critical, since some may cause problems in autoimmune diseases. Thus, monitoring side effects regarding autoimmunity is essential.

Vaccination and MS

In the early days of vaccine development, Louis Pasteur used nerve tissue of infected animals to obtain a rabies virus vaccine (28). Although saving countless lives it was recognized that active sensitization with neuronal tissue could occasionally lead to neuroparalytic autoimmune complications (29) with self-limiting autoimmune encephalomyelitis that fulfilled the pathological criteria of MS (29, 30). Advances in processing techniques and increasing insights in immunology led to modern vaccines devoid of neuronal tissue. MS is a chronic disease thought to be caused by immune-mediated mechanisms. Thus, immune responses caused by vaccinations will affect the immune system. However, their effects on immunology *per se*, but especially those in MS patients, are scarcely understood.

The same means by which infections can induce autoimmunity also apply for vaccination-induced immune activation. Possible structural similarities between microbial epitopes and epitopes of the CNS could lead to cross-reaction of antibodies via molecular mimicry as shown for streptococcal antibodies in heart tissue (31). Additionally, epitope spreading is a mechanism leading to a broadening of the immune response from the dominant epitope to cryptic (intramolecular) or neighboring molecules (intermolecular) resulting in an increased antibody repertoire and cellular response (32). Moreover, bystander activation, a process in which activated APCs stimulate autoreactive T cells, can occur (33). Bacterial and viral infections can trigger relapses and MRI activity in MS; vaccination has been proven to protect from or weaken infections, thus providing an "indirect" protection against MS disease activity (34).

Several reports on neurological disorders developing after immunization have been published including several cases on encephalomyelitic disorders (impaired consciousness, ataxia and optic neuritis) as well as demyelinating lesions in a patient with transverse myelitis after active immunization against influenza (35–38). Immunization against rubella was associated with diffuse myelitis and recurrent relapses with optic neuritis, paraparesis and impaired motor function (39, 40). Transverse myelitis (41) as well as optic neuritis (42, 43) were reported in patients vaccinated against measles, mumps and rubella. Further cases with symptoms suggestive for disseminated encephalitis were reported after vaccination against diphtheria-tetanus-poliomyelitis (DTP) (44) and after immunization against smallpox, rabies or typhus (45). Exacerbations of MS and demyelinating lesions were reported in MS patients and patients without a history of neurological conditions after immunization against hepatitis B (46). Similarly, Tourbah reported on 8 patients with demyelinating lesions and clinical symptoms after vaccination against hepatitis B (47).

In contrast to these case series, a case-control study (evidence class II) (48) including more than 440 patients with MS or optic neuritis and 950 controls without any underlying neuroimmunological disorder did not reveal an elevated risk for the development of MS or optic neuritis after immunization against hepatitis B, tetanus, influenza, measles/mumps/rubella, measles, or rubella (49). While Hernan came to same results for immunization against influenza or tetanus in a case-control study (evidence class II), active immunization against hepatitis B was reported to pose a higher risk for MS (50). The latter finding could, however, not be confirmed by Confavreux in a large case-crossover study. Additionally, no increased risk was seen for vaccination against tetanus and influenza as well (51). Similarly, other class II case-control studies did not report on an increased risk for MS after hepatitis B vaccination (52–54). An even decreased risk for MS was reported after tetanus immunization (8). In a large class I study, a patient register including 789,082 females vaccinated with the quadrivalent HPV vaccine was analyzed. Thereof, 4,322 patients with MS and 3,300 patients with other demyelinating disorders were studied and no increased risk for CNS manifestations was seen in this large cohort (55).

Miller et al. performed a prospective class II, randomized, double-blind, placebo-controlled study, which included 104 MS patients, who received either standard influenza vaccination or placebo. For a 6 months follow-up period, the occurrence of neurological symptoms or influenza was monitored and no differences were seen for relapse rates (56). A study by Langer-Gould reported on an increased risk for CNS demyelinating diseases within the first 30 days after vaccination. It was concluded that there is no increased risk for MS, but it seems that the transition from subclinical to overt autoimmunity in patients with existing disease is shortened (53).

Two major questions arise on the topic of "MS and vaccination": (i) Can vaccines cause MS and (ii) can vaccines provoke or trigger relapses in patients with MS?

(i) Overall, the anecdotal reports associating MS onset and vaccination had limited reliability, lacked validity and could not be replicated in larger studies. Therefore, there is consensus that there is yet no evidence that MS can be caused by vaccines neither by inactivated nor by live vaccines (57).
(ii) It is more difficult to assess the potency of vaccines to trigger relapses in MS patients. With respect to live vaccines it seems to be plausible that they may be able to provoke a deterioration of the disease, since they fulfill the criteria of an active infection with a replicative (although attenuated) organism. There is class IV evidence that at least the yellow fever (YF) 17D vaccine strain, which is derived from a natural occurring YF-virus and hasn't completely lost its neurotoxicity even after numerous passages, is able to provoke relapses in MS patients. However, it has to be kept in mind that the patient cohort had received immunomodulatory treatment and the sample size of this self-controlled case series study was rather small (58). The underlying potential immunologic mechanisms, which are responsible for this elevated relapse rate, are not understood yet and larger studies are necessary to confirm this association. Hypotheses may be generated based on observations after infections with helminths, mycobacteria and Epstein-Barr virus, or by the immunologic properties of this particular vaccine strain (59). Immunological analyzes showed that after immunization against YF, MS patients had a significantly increased MBP- and MOG-specific response shown by increased numbers of cells secreting interferon, IL-1α, IL-1β and tumor necrosis factor compared to unvaccinated MS patients or MS patients vaccinated against influenza (58).

Still, there is no evidence for other live vaccines such as MMR to deteriorate MS (57, 60). For inactivated vaccines, there is already more evidence available that an association between MS relapses and different kinds of vaccines does not exist (7). Even for vaccines, which were publicly accused to be associated with MS disease or relapse rate, like HPV or hepatitis B vaccines, there is no evidence to support any association between vaccination and clinical course of MS, as well as for vaccines containing inactivated neurotropic viruses like TBE (53, 61). It still remains unclear if inactivated vaccines may accelerate an upcoming relapse in patients with active MS by non-specific stimulation

TABLE 1 | Overview of standard vaccination in the general population and MS patients.

Vaccine		USA (CDC/ACIP) (66)	Germany (STIKO) (67)	Recommendation for multiple sclerosis
Diphteria	Toxoid	All individuals	All individuals	Considered safe
Human papilloma virus	recombinant vaccine	All individuals 11-12a	All individuals 9-14a	Probably safe
Measles, mumps and rubella	live attenuated vaccine	All children and at-risk adults	Unprotected individuals and children exposed to kids	Probably safe, CAVE: Immunosuppression
Meningococcal A,C,W,Y	inactivated vaccine	At-risk individuals	At-risk individuals	Probably safe
Meningococcal B	recombinant vaccine	At-risk individuals	At-risk individuals	Probably safe
Pertussis	Toxoid	All individuals	All individuals	Probably safe
Pneumococcus	polysaccharide vaccine	All individuals > 65a and individuals at risk	All individuals > 60a and individuals at risk	Insufficient data
Tetanus	Toxoid	All individuals	All individuals	Considered safe
Varicella	live attenuated vaccine	Individuals lacking evidence of immunity	Seronegative individuals at risk	Probably safe, CAVE: Immunosuppression
Zoster	recombinant vaccine	All individuals > 50a	All individuals > 60a and individuals > 50 at risk	Insufficient data
Zoster	live attenuated vaccine	All individuals > 60a, recombinant preferred	Not recommended	Insufficient data, CAVE: Immunosuppression
Hepatitis B	recombinant vaccine	All children, individuals not at risk but who want protection from hepatitis B	All children, individuals at risk	Considered safe
Hepatitis A	inactivated vaccine	All children, individuals not at risk but who want protection from hepatitis A	All children, individuals at risk	Considered safe
Poliomyelitis	inactivated vaccine	All children	All children, individuals at risk	Considered safe
Haemophilus influenzae type b	Conjugate vaccine	All children, individuals at risk	All children, individuals at risk	Insufficient data
Tick-borne encephalitis	Inactivated vaccine	not available	Endemic areas and tick exposure	Probably safe
Yellow fever	live attenuated vaccine	endemic areas	endemic areas	Probably increased risk, CAVE: Immunosuppression
Rabies	inactivated vaccine	People at high risk of exposure	People at high risk of exposure	Considered safe
Influenza	inactivated vaccine	All individuals > 6 months	Individuals >65 years old, those with chronic diseases, and pregnant women	Considered safe
Influenza	live attenuated vaccine	Individuals 2a-49a with restrictions	Individuals w/ chronic disease 2-17a, inac. preferred	Not recommended

of cytokine production. However, data are scanty and most studies are underpowered leaving an uncertainty about very small risks (62).

Adjuvants and MS

Besides effects of vaccines on induction and the disease course of MS, potential immunological effects of adjuvants have to be considered as well. Most experience on the possible induction of autoimmunity following administration of adjuvant-containing vaccines has been gained from animal models. However, results from experimental studies cannot be transferred to humans without reservation. First, the dose ratios tested in animal models are not the same as in humans and second, human immunology differs from animals. Indeed, oil emulsions, aluminum salts and squalene have shown severe side effects in animal models, while they are considered to be safe in humans (17).

An analysis performed by the European Medicines Agency (EMA) (63) investigated autoimmune disorders following vaccination against pandemic influenza A/H1N1 between October 2009 and December 2010 (64). Thirty percent of the 150 million doses of the distributed vaccines contained aluminum salts and squalene-based adjuvants. Overall, the study did not suggest a significant difference in the risk for autoimmune disorders for adjuvant and non-adjuvant vaccinations. ADEM was reported for 10 people (adjuvant vaccines: 7, non-adjuvant vaccines: 3), MS for 21 people (adjuvant vaccines: 20, non-adjuvant vaccines: 1), MS relapses for 24 patients (adjuvant vaccines: 21, non-adjuvant vaccines: 3), and one case of relapsing remitting MS was reported for adjuvant-containing vaccination (64). Statistical analysis revealed only a non-significantly increased risk for GBS (15). Also, a favorable benefit-risk profile of the vaccines was demonstrated (15, 65).

In conclusion, following the reports from literature, all of the EMA/FDA-approved vaccines (with exception for Yellow Fever) and adjuvants do not show a significantly increased risk for MS and ADEM. Constant improvement of basic immunological knowledge and technology will further improve the safety of adjuvants. **Table 1** gives an overview of the recommendations of standard vaccinations in the general population and in MS patients.

Vaccination and ADEM

While there is a lot of literature on vaccination and risk for MS or MS relapses available, reports on vaccination and ADEM are scarce. Yet, ADEM has been discussed to be a sequelae of vaccinations (68) as well as to be preceded by infections. Several cases of ADEM have been reported to be timely related to vaccinations against rabies (69), HPV (70, 71), hepatitis A and B, diphtheria, tetanus and poliovirus (72), measles, rubella and booster immunization for Japanese encephalitis (73). ADEM has been reported following vaccination against influenza, including eight cases after vaccination against H1N1. Also, four ADEM cases after vaccination against YF can be found in literature (74, 75). Besides case reports, there have been some observational studies, albeit all having their limitations. In 26 out of 35 reported cases of ADEM, patients had infections or vaccinations prior to disease onset (76). Also, Pellegrino et al. concluded a possible relation between post-vaccination ADEM in children and adults. Four hundred four cases of ADEM were analyzed based on the data of the Vaccine Adverse Event Reporting System (VAERS) database and the EudraVigilance post-authorization module (EVPM) (77). About 60% of the cases occurred between 2 and 30 days after vaccination, most commonly against influenza and HPV. A case-control study on vaccination against hepatitis B, influenza, polio, diphtheria, pertussis, tetanus, measles, mumps, rubella, Japanese encephalitis, meningitis, hepatitis A, varicella and rabies did not reveal an increased risk for the onset of ADEM in the time spans of 0–30 days and 61–180 days after vaccination, but between 31 and 60 days (78). Based on these reports, the risk for ADEM after vaccination cannot be completely ruled out.

Effective Vaccination in MS Treatment

Considerations on MS exacerbation and vaccination apply only for MS patients receiving no immunomodulatory/immunosuppressive treatment. If any kind of immunosuppression is used for MS therapy, this choice of treatment will dominate the decision whether to vaccinate or not (79). In recent years, consensus statements on vaccinations during immunosuppressive treatments were published by various national and international societies and expert panels (80–84). There is consensus that inactivated vaccines will do no harm (85) even in immunosuppressed patients. However, data on the efficacy of vaccinations in combination with the various available MS medications are missing. Thus, for patients either receiving more than one immunomodulatory treatment or having underlying immunomodulating condition, the outcome is difficult to predict (86). Therefore, the success of vaccination should be verified by antibody testing if a valid test is available.

Except for a few treatments, which only lead to mild immunosuppression, live vaccines are contraindicated under immunosuppressive treatment. In some situations, risks and benefits of a live vaccine have to be weighed against each other, e.g., in varicella zoster virus (VZV)-negative MS patients under fingolimod treatment, varicella vaccination may be considered, since severe complications from natural varicella infection may outweigh the risk from this live vaccine. However, recommendations vary between different institutions even within the same country (80, 82, 83). A recent case report on a lethal VZV infection in an immunocompromised patient after VZV live vaccination drives the discussion on this issue (87).

There is consensus about the timing of vaccination in patients, who will undergo immunosuppressive treatment: Vaccinations should be given well in advance to the start of treatment (at least 2 weeks for inactivated and $\geq$ 4 weeks for live vaccines) and should be distinguished between primo-vaccinations and boosters. Importantly, the refractory period after immunosuppression has to be considered as well, which may be up to 1 year depending on the type of medication (e.g., rituximab or alemtuzumab) (81). Vaccines will have various effects on the immune system, which greatly depend on the cell types typically engaged by the respective vaccines. The impact of immunosuppression on the various cell types (and possible mitigation of effects) should be taken into consideration. Protective efficacy is mostly mediated by antibodies for the following vaccines: cholera, diphtheria toxoid, hepatitis A and B, haemophilus influenzae type b, influenza, Japanese encephalitis, meningococcal PS and conjugates, papillomavirus, pneumococcal PS and conjugates, polio (Sabin and Salk), rabies, rotavirus, rubella, tetanus toxoid, typhoid PS, and YF. Effects are solely born by T cells for tuberculosis (BCG), or by a combination of antibodies and T cells for measles and intranasal influenza vaccination. Besides antibody-mediated protection, effects of T cells are discussed for pertussis (9).

For patients receiving immunosuppressive treatment, vaccination control should be performed. For diphtheria, TBE (with caution), hepatitis A, B, haemophilus influenzae type b, measles, mumps, pneumococcus, polio, rubella, tetanus, rabies and varicella, standards are available and recommended to be tested. In general, to increase the validity of vaccination control, titers should be assessed in paired samples (before and after immunization) via the same method and at high-quality standards (81). In general, patients should have received their recommended standard vaccines according to their region-specific vaccine guidelines. Before certain

TABLE 2 | Recommended vaccination in MS patients in dependency of treatment.

	FDA/EMA vaccination	FDA/EMA screening	Extended vaccination
GLAT			
IFN beta			
Cladribin	VZV	Screen for HBV, HCV	
Teriflunomid			
Fingolimod	VZV		HBV, HPV
DMF			
Rituximab	n.a.	n.a.	HBV, Pneumococcal
Ocrelizumab		Screen for HBV, HCV	HBV, Pneumococcal
Natalizumab			VZV
Alemtuzumab	VZV	Screen for HBV, HCV	HBV, Influenza, HPV and Pneumococcal

GLAT, glatiramer acetate; IFN beta, interferon beta; DMF, dimethyl fumarate; HBV, hepatitis B; HCV, hepatitis C; VZV, varicella-zoster virus; HPV, human papillomavirus; n.a., not applicable.

immunosuppressive treatments are initiated, it is mandatory to exclude former infections and if necessary, vaccination should be considered according to the regulatory agencies. **Table 2** provides an overview on necessary vaccinations according to FDA/EMA guidelines (extended vaccination reflects the authors' suggestion). For many immunotherapies, a prior exclusion of an ongoing VZV infection is required and vaccination should be offered to those, who haven't gained any immunity yet. Additionally, VZV-seropositive patients undergoing immunotherapy should be offered vaccination as well to prevent zoster reactivation and late effects. Recently, a non-live subunit vaccine has been authorized for VZV-seropositive patients. It possesses a better risk-benefit profile compared to the live vaccine and has already been approved by many countries (88).

Additionally, it should be considered to offer patients with upcoming fingolimod or alemtuzumab treatment the option of vaccination against HPV, as post-market surveillance showed increased reports of warts and cervical dysplasia due to these two MS therapies [EMA; (89)]. Furthermore, pneumococcal vaccine might be considered in patients receiving B cell-depleting therapies, as severe respiratory infections during Phase III studies were seen (90, 91).

DISCUSSION

Vaccine hesitancy is a major problem nowadays. The usefulness of active immunization is undisputed and has saved numerous lives. However, fear of possible, but also often unconfirmed, side effects has fostered this anti-vaccine sentiment. This has led to a recent outbreak of measles (2) and curiously some viruses and disorders, which have been assumed to be eradicated, seem to become a hot topic for Western health systems again.

Indeed, side effects upon vaccination may occur in rare cases, however, the benefits for individual people as well as the whole population will generally outweigh adverse effects. Vaccine hesitancy results in a twofold problem: (1) The missing protection for the unvaccinated people themselves but also (2) a risk for people, who are not able to get vaccinated. The missing herd immunity poses a major problem for a group of patients with fragile health. For MS patients receiving immunosuppressive treatment, an acute infection can have dangerous sequelae. Thus, if possible, MS patients should be vaccinated beforehand. The possible benefits outweigh—dependent on the individual case—the possible risks.

An additional perspective raises the possibility of vaccination against MS. Indeed, early approaches exploring vaccination with synthetic peptides in experimental animal models were successful, but translation into clinical treatment was so far unsatisfying (92–94).

Interestingly, it was recently shown that an anti-typhus vaccination (Typhim vaccine) might have the potential to ameliorate the disease course of MS by targeting prohibitins on TH17 cells. Tested in an experimental MS model it led to decreased levels of IL17 and increased numbers of $FOXp3^{+}$ regulatory T cells (95). Further investigations are needed before studies should investigate treatment options for MS patients. Still, it is a good example, how immunology of vaccination might overlap with and modulate the immunology of MS.

CONCLUSION

Theoretically, an increased immune response against different types of vaccines, such as live attenuated viruses, inactive attenuated viruses, or portions of bacteria and viruses, could trigger increased immune response to self-antigens (45, 58, 96), but an increased risk for MS itself or increased relapse rates after vaccination have not been show (with exception for YF) in case-control studies (7). There is, however, evidence that infections can trigger relapses in MS (96–104), which is why vaccination of MS patients should be pursued in order to reduce the risk of infections. To assure the best vaccination success, immunization and immunosuppressive treatments have to be well timed.

AUTHOR CONTRIBUTIONS

All authors listed have made a substantial, direct and intellectual contribution to the work, and approved it for publication.

REFERENCES

1. Macdonald NE, Hesitancy SWGOV. Vaccine hesitancy: definition, scope and determinants. *Vaccine*. (2015) 33:4161–4. doi: 10.1016/j.vaccine.2015.04.036
2. WHO. *Global Measles and Rubella Update* (2018). Available online at: http://www.who.int/immunization/monitoring_surveillance/burden/vpd/surveillance_type/active/Global_MR_Update_August_2018.pdf (accessed July 30, 2019).
3. Kata A. A postmodern Pandora's box: anti-vaccination misinformation on the internet. *Vaccine*. (2010) 28:1709–16. doi: 10.1016/j.vaccine.2009.12.022
4. Gasparini R, Panatto D, Lai PL, Amicizia D. The "urban myth" of the association between neurological disorders and vaccinations. *J Prevent Med Hyg*. (2015) 56:E1.
5. Denis F, Levy-Bruhl D. Mass vaccination against hepatitis B: the French example. In: Plotkin SA, editor. *Mass Vaccination: Global Aspects—Progress and Obstacles*. Berlin; Heidelberg: Springer (2006). p. 115–29. doi: 10.1007/3-540-36583-4_7
6. Martinez-Sernandez V, Figueiras A. Central nervous system demyelinating diseases and recombinant hepatitis B vaccination: a critical systematic review of scientific production. *J Neurol*. (2013) 260:1951–9. doi: 10.1007/s00415-012-6716-y
7. Mailand MT, Frederiksen JL. Vaccines and multiple sclerosis: a systematic review. *J Neurol*. (2017) 264:1035–50. doi: 10.1007/s00415-016-8263-4
8. Hernan MA, Alonso A, Hernandez-Diaz S. Tetanus vaccination and risk of multiple sclerosis: a systematic review. *Neurology*. (2006) 67:212–5. doi: 10.1212/01.wnl.0000225079.51201.f9
9. Siegrist CA. *Vaccine Immunology In:* SPWOPOKM, editor. *Plotkin's Vaccines*. 7th ed. Edwards: Elsevier (2018).
10. Coffman RL, Sher A, Seder RA. Vaccine adjuvants: putting innate immunity to work. *Immunity*. (2010) 33:492–503. doi: 10.1016/j.immuni.2010.10.002
11. Jenkins MK, Khoruts A, Ingulli E, Mueller DL, Mcsorley SJ, Reinhardt RL, et al. *In vivo* activation of antigen-specific CD4 T cells. *Annu Rev*. (2001) 19:23–45. doi: 10.1146/annurev.immunol.19.1.23
12. Geeraedts F, Goutagny N, Hornung V, Severa M, De Haan A, Pool J, et al. Superior immunogenicity of inactivated whole virus H5N1 influenza vaccine

is primarily controlled by Toll-like receptor signalling. *PLoS Pathog.* (2008) 4:e1000138. doi: 10.1371/journal.ppat.1000138
13. Li H, Nookala S, Re F. Aluminum hydroxide adjuvants activate caspase-1 and induce IL-1beta and IL-18 release. *J Immunol.* (2007) 178:5271–6. doi: 10.4049/jimmunol.178.8.5271
14. Pulendran B, Ahmed R. Immunological mechanisms of vaccination. *Nat Immunol.* (2011) 12:509–17. doi: 10.1038/ni.2039
15. Di Pasquale A, Preiss S, Tavares Da Silva F, Garcon N. Vaccine adjuvants: from 1920 to 2015 and beyond. *Vaccines.* (2015) 3:320–43. doi: 10.3390/vaccines3020320
16. Petrovsky N. Comparative safety of vaccine adjuvants: a summary of current evidence and future needs. *Drug Saf.* (2015) 38:1059–74. doi: 10.1007/s40264-015-0350-4
17. Van Der Laan JW, Gould S, Tanir JY, *Vaccines* IH, Adjuvants Safety Project C. Safety of vaccine adjuvants: focus on autoimmunity. *Vaccine.* (2015) 33:1507–14. doi: 10.1016/j.vaccine.2015.01.073
18. Morel S, Didierlaurent A, Bourguignon P, Delhaye S, Baras B, Jacob V, et al. Adjuvant System AS03 containing α-tocopherol modulates innate immune response and leads to improved adaptive immunity. *Vaccine.* (2011) 29:2461–73. doi: 10.1016/j.vaccine.2011.01.011
19. Vitoriano-Souza J, Das Dores Moreira N, Teixeira-Carvalho A, Carneiro CM, Siqueira FAM, et al. Cell recruitment and cytokines in skin mice sensitized with the vaccine adjuvants: saponin, incomplete Freund's adjuvant, and monophosphoryl lipid A. *PLoS ONE.* (2012) 7:e40745. doi: 10.1371/journal.pone.0040745
20. Kebir H, Kreymborg K, Ifergan I, Dodelet-Devillers A, Cayrol R, Bernard M, et al. Human T H 17 lymphocytes promote blood-brain barrier disruption and central nervous system inflammation. *Nat Med.* (2007) 13:1173. doi: 10.1038/nm1651
21. Huppert J, Closhen D, Croxford A, White R, Kulig P, Pietrowski E, et al. Cellular mechanisms of IL-17-induced blood-brain barrier disruption. *FASEB J.* (2010) 24:1023–34. doi: 10.1096/fj.09-141978
22. Satoh M, Kuroda Y, Yoshida H, Behney KM, Mizutani A, Akaogi J, et al. Induction of lupus autoantibodies by adjuvants. *J Autoimmun.* (2003) 21:1–9. doi: 10.1016/S0896-8411(03)00083-0
23. Partinen M, Saarenpaa-Heikkila O, Ilveskoski I, Hublin C, Linna M, Olsen P, et al. Increased incidence and clinical picture of childhood narcolepsy following the 2009 H1N1 pandemic vaccination campaign in Finland. *PLoS ONE.* (2012) 7:e33723. doi: 10.1371/journal.pone.0033723
24. Petrovsky N, Cooper PD. Carbohydrate-based immune adjuvants. *Expert Rev Vacc.* (2011) 10:523–37. doi: 10.1586/erv.11.30
25. Siegrist C-A. Vaccine immunology. *Vaccines.* (2008) 5:17–36.
26. Maclennan IC, Toellner KM, Cunningham AF, Serre K, Sze DM, Zuniga E, et al. Extrafollicular antibody responses. *Immunol Rev.* (2003) 194:8–18. doi: 10.1034/j.1600-065X.2003.00058.x
27. Goodnow CC, Vinuesa CG, Randall KL, Mackay F, Brink R. Control systems and decision making for antibody production. *Nat Immunol.* (2010) 11:681–8. doi: 10.1038/ni.1900
28. Plotkin SA. Rabies vaccine prepared in human cell cultures: progress and perspectives. *Rev Infect Dis.* (1980) 2:433–48. doi: 10.1093/clinids/2.3.433
29. Stuart G, Krikorian K. The neuro-paralytic accidents of anti-rabies treatment. *Ann Trop Med Parasitol.* (1928) 22:327–77. doi: 10.1080/00034983.1928.11684582
30. Höftberger R, Leisser M, Bauer J, Lassmann H. Autoimmune encephalitis in humans: how closely does it reflect multiple sclerosis? *Acta Neuropathol Commun.* (2015) 3:80. doi: 10.1186/s40478-015-0260-9
31. Zabriskie JB, Freimer EH. An immunological relationship between the group A streptococcus and mammalian muscle. *J Exp Med.* (1966) 124:661–78. doi: 10.1084/jem.124.4.661
32. Lehmann PV, Forsthuber T, Miller A, Sercarz EE. Spreading of T-cell autoimmunity to cryptic determinants of an autoantigen. *Nature.* (1992) 358:155–7. doi: 10.1038/358155a0
33. Munz C, Lunemann JD, Getts MT, Miller SD. Antiviral immune responses: triggers of or triggered by autoimmunity? *Nat Rev Immunol.* (2009) 9:246–58. doi: 10.1038/nri2527
34. Correale J, Fiol M, Gilmore W. The risk of relapses in multiple sclerosis during systemic infections. *Neurology.* (2006) 67:652–9. doi: 10.1212/01.wnl.0000233834.09743.3b
35. Yahr MD, Lobo-Antunes J. Relapsing encephalomyelitis following the use of influenza vaccine. *Arch Neurol.* (1972) 27:182–3. doi: 10.1001/archneur.1972.00490140086012
36. Bienfang DC, Kantrowitz FG, Noble JL, Raynor AM. Ocular abnormalities after influenza immunization. *Arch Ophthalmol.* (1977) 95:1649. doi: 10.1001/archopht.1977.04450090171018
37. Bakshi R, Mazziotta JC. Acute transverse myelitis after influenza vaccination: magnetic resonance imaging findings. *J Neuroimaging.* (1996) 6:248–50. doi: 10.1111/jon199664248
38. Hull TP, Bates JH. Optic neuritis after influenza vaccination. *Am J Ophthalmol.* (1997) 124:703–4. doi: 10.1016/S0002-9394(14)70918-3
39. Holt S, Hudgins D, Krishnan KR, Critchley EM. Diffuse myelitis associated with rubella vaccination. *Br Med J.* (1976) 2:1037–8. doi: 10.1136/bmj.2.6043.1037
40. Behan PO. Diffuse myelitis associated with rubella vaccination. *Br Med J.* (1977) 1:166. doi: 10.1136/bmj.1.6054.166-b
41. Joyce KA, Rees JE. Transverse myelitis after measles, mumps, and rubella vaccine. *BMJ.* (1995) 311:422. doi: 10.1136/bmj.311.7002.422a
42. Kazarian EL, Gager WE. Optic neuritis complicating measles, mumps, and rubella vaccination. *Am J Ophthalmol.* (1978) 86:544–7. doi: 10.1016/0002-9394(78)90304-5
43. Stevenson VL, Acheson JF, Ball J, Plant GT. Optic neuritis following measles/rubella vaccination in two 13-year-old children. *Br J Ophthalmol.* (1996) 80:1110–1. doi: 10.1136/bjo.80.12.1110
44. Mancini J, Chabrol B, Moulene E, Pinsard N. Relapsing acute encephalopathy: a complication of diphtheria-tetanus-poliomyelitis immunization in a young boy. *Eur J Pediatr.* (1996) 155:136–8. doi: 10.1007/BF02075768
45. Miller H, Cendrowski W, Shapira K. Multiple sclerosis and vaccination. *Br Med J.* (1967) 2:210–3. doi: 10.1136/bmj.2.5546.210
46. Herroelen L, De Keyser J, Ebinger G. Central-nervous-system demyelination after immunisation with recombinant hepatitis B vaccine. *Lancet.* (1991) 338:1174–5. doi: 10.1016/0140-6736(91)92034-Y
47. Tourbah A, Gout O, Liblau R, Lyon-Caen O, Bougniot C, Iba-Zizen MT, et al. Encephalitis after hepatitis B vaccination: recurrent disseminated encephalitis or MS? *Neurology.* (1999) 53:396–401. doi: 10.1212/WNL.53.2.396
48. Ashman EJ, Gronseth GS. Level of evidence reviews: three years of progress. *Neurology.* (2012) 79:13–4. doi: 10.1212/WNL.0b013e31825dce83
49. Destefano F, Verstraeten T, Jackson LA, Okoro CA, Benson P, Black SB, et al. Vaccinations and risk of central nervous system demyelinating diseases in adults. *Arch Neurol.* (2003) 60:504–9. doi: 10.1001/archneur.60.4.504
50. Hernan MA, Jick SS, Olek MJ, Jick H. Recombinant hepatitis B vaccine and the risk of multiple sclerosis: a prospective study. *Neurology.* (2004) 63:838–42. doi: 10.1212/01.WNL.0000138433.61870.82
51. Confavreux C, Suissa S, Saddier P, Bourdes V, Vukusic S, Vaccines in Multiple Sclerosis Study G. Vaccinations and the risk of relapse in multiple sclerosis. *Vacc Multiple Scler Study Group N Engl J Med.* (2001) 344:319–26. doi: 10.1056/NEJM200102013440501
52. Ascherio A, Zhang SM, Hernan MA, Olek MJ, Coplan PM, Brodovicz K, et al. Hepatitis B vaccination and the risk of multiple sclerosis. *N Engl J Med.* (2001) 344:327–32. doi: 10.1056/NEJM200102013440502
53. Langer-Gould A, Qian L, Tartof SY, Brara SM, Jacobsen SJ, Beaber BE, et al. Vaccines and the risk of multiple sclerosis and other central nervous system demyelinating diseases. *JAMA Neurol.* (2014) 71:1506–13. doi: 10.1001/jamaneurol.2014.2633
54. Eftekharian MM, Mousavi M, Hormoz MB, Roshanaei G, Mazdeh M. Multiple sclerosis and immunological-related risk factors: results from a case-control study. *Hum Antibod.* (2015) 23:31–6. doi: 10.3233/HAB-150281
55. Scheller NM, Svanstrom H, Pasternak B, Arnheim-Dahlstrom L, Sundstrom K, Fink K, et al. Quadrivalent HPV vaccination and risk of multiple sclerosis and other demyelinating diseases of the central nervous system. *JAMA.* (2015) 313:54–61. doi: 10.1001/jama.2014.16946
56. Miller AE, Morgante LA, Buchwald LY, Nutile SM, Coyle PK, Krupp LB, et al. A multicenter, randomized, double-blind, placebo-controlled trial of influenza immunization in multiple sclerosis. *Neurology.* (1997) 48:312–4. doi: 10.1212/WNL.48.2.312

57. Vaccines CTRaEO. *Adverse Effects of Vaccines: Evidence and Causality.* Washington, DC: The National Academies Press (2012). doi: 10.17226/13164
58. Farez MF, Correale J. Yellow fever vaccination and increased relapse rate in travelers with multiple sclerosis. *Arch Neurol.* (2011) 68:1267–71. doi: 10.1001/archneurol.2011.131
59. De Menezes Martins R, Fernandes Leal Mda L, Homma A. Serious adverse events associated with yellow fever vaccine. *Hum Vaccin Immunother.* (2015) 11:2183–7. doi: 10.1080/21645515.2015.1022700
60. Langer-Gould A, Wu J, Lucas R, Smith J, Gonzales E, Amezcua L, et al. Epstein-Barr virus, cytomegalovirus, and multiple sclerosis susceptibility: a multiethnic study. *Neurology.* (2017) 89:1330–7. doi: 10.1212/WNL.0000000000004412
61. Baumhackl U, Franta C, Retzl J, Salomonowitz E, Eder G. A controlled trial of tick-borne encephalitis vaccination in patients with multiple sclerosis. *Vaccine.* (2003) 21 (Suppl 1):S56–61. doi: 10.1016/S0264-410X(02)00815-0
62. Frederiksen JL, Topsoe Mailand M. Vaccines and multiple sclerosis. *Acta Neurol Scand.* (2017) 136 (Suppl 20) 1:49–51. doi: 10.1111/ane.12837
63. EMA LEMTRADA. *Summary of Product Characteristics.* European Medicines Agency (2018).
64. Isai A, Durand J, Le Meur S, Hidalgo-Simon A, Kurz X. Autoimmune disorders after immunisation with Influenza A/H1N1 vaccines with and without adjuvant: EudraVigilance data and literature review. *Vaccine.* (2012) 30:7123–9. doi: 10.1016/j.vaccine.2012.09.032
65. Paul-Ehrlich-Institute (2014). Available online at: https://www.pei.de/DE/arzneimittelsicherheit-vigilanz/archiv-sicherheitsinformationen/2014/ablage2014/2014-01-21-sicherheitsbewertung-von-aluminium-in-therapieallergenen.html (accessed July 30, 2019).
66. Kim DK, Hunter P. Recommended adult immunization schedule, United States, 2019. *Ann Int Med.* (2019) 170:182–92. doi: 10.7326/M18-3600
67. Stiko SI. Ständige Impfkommission: Empfehlungen der Ständigen Impfkommission (STIKO) am Robert Koch-Institut. In: *Ständige Impfkommission: Empfehlungen der Ständigen Impfkommission (STIKO) Epid Bull.* Vol. 34. Berlin: Robert Koch-Institu (2018). p. 335–82.
68. Menge T, Hemmer B, Nessler S, Wiendl H, Neuhaus O, Hartung HP, et al. Acute disseminated encephalomyelitis: an update. *Arch Neurol.* (2005) 62:1673–80. doi: 10.1001/archneur.62.11.1673
69. Kulkarni V, Nadgir D, Tapiawala S, Malabari A, Kalgikar A, Kela R, et al. Biphasic demyelination of the nervous system following anti-rabies vaccination. *Neurol India.* (2004) 52:106–8.
70. Wildemann B, Jarius S, Hartmann M, Regula JU, Hametner C. Acute disseminated encephalomyelitis following vaccination against human papilloma virus. *Neurology.* (2009) 72:2132–3. doi: 10.1212/WNL.0b013e3181aa53bb
71. Sekiguchi K, Yasui N, Kowa H, Kanda F, Toda T. Two cases of acute disseminated Encephalomyelitis following vaccination against human papilloma virus. *Intern Med.* (2016) 55:3181–4. doi: 10.2169/internalmedicine.55.5472
72. Rogalewski A, Kraus J, Hasselblatt M, Kraemer C, Schäbitz W-R. Improvement of advanced postvaccinal demyelinating encephalitis due to plasmapheresis. *Neuropsychiatr Dis Treat.* (2007) 3:987. doi: 10.2147/NDT.S2024
73. Azumagawa K, Nomura S, Shigeri Y, Jones LS, Sato DK, Nakashima I, et al. Post-vaccination MDEM associated with MOG antibody in a subclinical Chlamydia infected boy. *Brain Dev.* (2016) 38:690–3. doi: 10.1016/j.braindev.2016.02.004
74. Mcmahon AW, Eidex RB, Marfin AA, Russell M, Sejvar JJ, Markoff L, et al. Neurologic disease associated with 17D-204 yellow fever vaccination: a report of 15 cases. *Vaccine.* (2007) 25:1727–34. doi: 10.1016/j.vaccine.2006.11.027
75. Chaves M, Riccio P, Patrucco L, Rojas JI, Cristiano E. Longitudinal myelitis associated with yellow fever vaccination. *J Neurovirol.* (2009) 15:348–50. doi: 10.1080/13550280903062805
76. De Seze J, Debouverie M, Zephir H, Lebrun C, Blanc F, Bourg V, et al. Acute fulminant demyelinating disease: a descriptive study of 60 patients. *Arch Neurol.* (2007) 64:1426–32. doi: 10.1001/archneur.64.10.1426
77. Pellegrino P, Carnovale C, Perrone V, Pozzi M, Antoniazzi S, Clementi E, et al. Acute disseminated encephalomyelitis onset: evaluation based on vaccine adverse events reporting systems. *PLoS ONE.* (2013) 8:e77766. doi: 10.1371/annotation/1d544202-04f5-4848-83f1-696c2de4221e
78. Chen Y, Ma F, Xu Y, Chu X, Zhang J. *Vaccines* and the risk of acute disseminated encephalomyelitis. *Vaccine.* (2018) 36:3733–9. doi: 10.1016/j.vaccine.2018.05.063
79. Winkelmann A, Loebermann M, Reisinger EC, Hartung HP, Zettl UK. Disease-modifying therapies and infectious risks in multiple sclerosis. *Nat Rev Neurol.* (2016) 12:217–33. doi: 10.1038/nrneurol.2016.21
80. Rubin LG, Levin MJ, Ljungman P, Davies EG, Avery R, Tomblyn M, et al. 2013 IDSA clinical practice guideline for vaccination of the immunocompromised host. *Clin Infect Dis.* (2014) 58:e44–100. doi: 10.1093/cid/cit816
81. Wiedermann U, Sitte HH, Burgmann H, Eser A, Falb P, Holzmann H, et al. [Guidelines for vaccination of immunocompromised individuals]. *Wien Klin Wochenschr.* (2016) 128 Suppl 4:337–76. doi: 10.1007/s00508-016-1033-6
82. Kroger AT, Duchin J, Vázquez M. *General Best Practice Guidelines for Immunization. Best practices guidance of the Advisory Committee on Immunization Practices (ACIP)*Atlanta, GA: US Department of Health and Human Services, CDC (2017).
83. Niehues T, Bogdan C, Hecht J, Mertens T, Wiese-Posselt M, Zepp F. Impfen bei Immundefizienz. *Bundesgesundheitsblatt-Gesundheitsforschung-Gesundheitsschutz.* (2017) 60:674–84. doi: 10.1007/s00103-017-2555-4
84. Martire B, Azzari C, Badolato R, Canessa C, Cirillo E, Gallo V, et al. Vaccination in immunocompromised host: recommendations of italian primary immunodeficiency network centers (IPINET). *Vaccine.* (2018) 36:3541–54. doi: 10.1016/j.vaccine.2018.01.061
85. Loebermann M, Winkelmann A, Hartung HP, Hengel H, Reisinger EC, Zettl UK. Vaccination against infection in patients with multiple sclerosis. *Nat Rev Neurol.* (2012) 8:143–51. doi: 10.1038/nrneurol.2012.8
86. Hertzell KB, Pauksens K, Rombo L, Knight A, Vene S, Askling HH. Tick-borne encephalitis (TBE) vaccine to medically immunosuppressed patients with rheumatoid arthritis: a prospective, open-label, multi-centre study. *Vaccine.* (2016) 34:650–5. doi: 10.1016/j.vaccine.2015.12.029
87. Alexander KE, Tong PL, Macartney K, Beresford R, Sheppeard V, Gupta M. Live zoster vaccination in an immunocompromised patient leading to death secondary to disseminated varicella zoster virus infection. *Vaccine.* (2018) 36:3890–3. doi: 10.1016/j.vaccine.2018.05.078
88. Heineman TC, Cunningham A, Levin M. Understanding the immunology of Shingrix, a recombinant glycoprotein E adjuvanted herpes zoster vaccine. *Curr Opin Immunol.* (2019) 59:42–8. doi: 10.1016/j.coi.2019.02.009
89. Triplett J, Kermode AG, Corbett A, Reddel SW. Warts and all: Fingolimod and unusual HPV-associated lesions. *Multiple Scler J.* (2018) doi: 10.1177/1352458518807088. [Epub ahead of print].
90. Cohen JA, Coles AJ, Arnold DL, Confavreux C, Fox EJ, Hartung HP, et al. Alemtuzumab versus interferon beta 1a as first-line treatment for patients with relapsing-remitting multiple sclerosis: a randomised controlled phase 3 trial. *Lancet.* (2012) 380:1819–28. doi: 10.1016/S0140-6736(12)61769-3
91. Hauser SL, Bar-Or A, Comi G, Giovannoni G, Hartung HP, Hemmer B, et al. Ocrelizumab versus Interferon Beta-1a in relapsing multiple sclerosis. *N Engl J Med.* (2017) 376:221–34. doi: 10.1056/NEJMoa1601277
92. Howell MD, Winters ST, Olee T, Powell HC, Carlo DJ, Brostoff SW. Vaccination against experimental allergic encephalomyelitis with T cell receptor peptides. *Science.* (1989) 246:668–70. doi: 10.1126/science.2814489
93. Hohlfeld R, Wiendl H. The ups and downs of multiple sclerosis therapeutics. *Ann Neurol.* (2001) 49:281–4. doi: 10.1002/ana.61
94. Lutterotti A, Martin R. Antigen-specific tolerization approaches in multiple sclerosis. *Expert Opin Investig Drugs.* (2014) 23:9–20. doi: 10.1517/13543784.2014.844788
95. Buehler U, Schulenburg K, Yurugi H, Šolman M, Abankwa D, Ulges A, et al. Targeting prohibitins at the cell surface prevents Th17-mediated autoimmunity. *EMBO J. (2018)* 37:e99429. doi: 10.15252/embj.201899429
96. Cahill JF, Izzo A, Garg N. Immunization in patients with multiple sclerosis. *Neurol Bull.* (2010) 2:17–21. doi: 10.7191/neurol_bull.2010.1020
97. Sriram S, Stratton CW, Yao S, Tharp A, Ding L, Bannan JD, et al. Chlamydia pneumoniae infection of the central nervous system in multiple sclerosis. *Ann Neurol.* (1999) 46:6–14.

98. Ascherio A, Munch M. Epstein-Barr virus and multiple sclerosis. *Epidemiology*. (2000) 11:220–4. doi: 10.1097/00001648-200003000-00023
99. Dessau RB, Lisby G, Frederiksen JL. Coronaviruses in brain tissue from patients with multiple sclerosis. *Acta Neuropathol.* (2001) 101:601–4. doi: 10.1007/s004010000331
100. Alvarez-Lafuente R, Martin-Estefania C, De Las Heras V, Castrillo C, Picazo JJ, Varela De Seijas E, et al. Active human herpesvirus 6 infection in patients with multiple sclerosis. *Arch Neurol.* (2002) 59:929–33. doi: 10.1001/archneur.59.6.929
101. Contini C, Cultrera R, Seraceni S, Castellazzi M, Granieri E, Fainardi E. Cerebrospinal fluid molecular demonstration of Chlamydia pneumoniae DNA is associated to clinical and brain magnetic resonance imaging activity in a subset of patients with relapsing-remitting multiple sclerosis. *Multiple Sclerosis J.* (2004) 10:360–9. doi: 10.1191/1352458504ms1049oa
102. Ebringer A, Rashid T, Wilson C, Tiwana H, Green A, Thompson E, et al. Multiple sclerosis, sporadic creutzfeldt–jakob disease and bovine spongiform encephalopathy: are they autoimmune diseases evoked by acinetobacter microbes showing molecular mimicry to brain antigens? *J Nutr Environ Med.* (2004) 14:293–302. doi: 10.1080/13590840500088131
103. Kriesel JD, SibleyW.A. *The Case for Rhinoviruses in the Pathogenesis of Multiple Sclerosis.* Sage Publications Sage CA: Thousand Oaks, CA (2005).
104. Ascherio A, Munger KL. Epstein-barr virus infection and multiple sclerosis: a review. *J Neuroimmune Pharmacol.* (2010) 5:271–7. doi: 10.1007/s11481-010-9201-3

16

Sex-Specific Gene-by-Vitamin D Interactions Regulate Susceptibility to Central Nervous System Autoimmunity

Dimitry N. Krementsov[1], Loredana Asarian[2], Qian Fang[2], Mahalia M. McGill[1] and Cory Teuscher[2,3]**

[1] Department of Biomedical and Health Sciences, University of Vermont, Burlington, VT, United States, [2] Department of Medicine, University of Vermont, Burlington, VT, United States, [3] Department of Pathology, University of Vermont, Burlington, VT, United States

***Correspondence:**
Dimitry N. Krementsov
dkrement@uvm.edu;
Cory Teuscher
c.teuscher@uvm.edu

Vitamin D3 (VitD) insufficiency is postulated to represent a major modifiable risk factor for multiple sclerosis (MS). While low VitD levels strongly correlate with higher MS risk in white populations, this is not the case for other ethnic groups, suggesting the existence of a genetic component. Moreover, VitD supplementation studies in MS so far have not shown a consistent benefit. We sought to determine whether direct manipulation of VitD levels modulates central nervous system autoimmune disease in a sex-by-genotype-dependent manner. To this end, we used a dietary model of VitD modulation, together with the autoimmune animal model of MS, experimental autoimmune encephalomyelitis (EAE). To assess the impact of genotype-by-VitD interactions on EAE susceptibility, we utilized a chromosome substitution (consomic) mouse model that incorporates the genetic diversity of wild-derived PWD/PhJ mice. High VitD was protective in EAE in female, but not male C57BL/6J (B6) mice, and had no effect in EAE-resistant PWD/PhJ (PWD) mice. EAE protection was accompanied by sex- and genotype-specific suppression of proinflammatory transcriptional programs in CD4 T effector cells, but not CD4 regulatory T cells. Decreased expression of proinflammatory genes was observed with high VitD in female CD4 T effector cells, specifically implicating a key role of MHC class II genes, interferon gamma, and Th1 cell-mediated neuroinflammation. In consomic strains, effects of VitD on EAE were also sex- and genotype dependent, whereby high VitD: (1) was protective, (2) had no effect, and (3) unexpectedly had disease-exacerbating effects. Systemic levels of 25(OH)D differed across consomic strains, with higher levels associated with EAE protection only in females. Analysis of expression of key known VitD metabolism genes between B6 and PWD mice revealed that their expression is genetically determined and sex specific and implicated *Cyp27b1* and *Vdr* as candidate genes responsible for differential EAE responses to VitD modulation. Taken together, our results support the observation that the association between VitD status and MS susceptibility is genotype dependent and suggest that the outcome of VitD status in MS is determined by gene-by-sex interactions.

Keywords: vitamin D, multiple sclerosis, CD4 T cells, genetic variation, experimental autoimmune encephalomyelitis (EAE), sex differences, gene–environment interactions, wild-derived inbred strains

INTRODUCTION

Multiple sclerosis (MS) is a multifactorial autoimmune disease, in which an immune-initiated attack on the central nervous system (CNS) results in demyelination, axonal loss, and eventual neurological dysfunction. Genetics contribute to a significant portion of MS risk, with estimates ranging from 20 to 30% (1). The primary genetic risk factor lies in the major histocompatibility complex class II locus, with up 200 other minor risk loci identified by recent genome-wide association studies (2).

The remainder of MS risk is thought to come from environmental factors or gene-by-environment interactions. A number of different environmental risk factors have been associated with MS susceptibility. The most prominent of these are Epstein–Barr virus (EBV) infection, low sunlight/ultraviolet (UV) radiation exposure, vitamin D3 (VitD) deficiency, and cigarette smoking (3, 4). In addition, over the past 100 years, MS incidence has remained stable in men, but has tripled in women, suggesting the existence of sex/gender-specific risk factors and/or behavioral changes (3).

Vitamin D3 is one of the best-studied MS risk factors. Early epidemiologic studies documented a gradient of increasing MS incidence with increasing distance from the equator, which in later studies was attributed to decreased exposure to sunlight/UV radiation (3). This protective effect of sunlight in MS has long been thought to be mediated by the immunomodulatory effects of VitD. Photoconversion of 7-dehydrocholesterol to VitD (cholecalciferol) in the skin is catalyzed by UV-B radiation. VitD from the skin and dietary VitD (absorbed in the intestine) enters the circulation and is subsequently converted in the liver to calcidiol [$25(OH)D_3$], and then in the kidney or in target tissues to calcitriol [$1,25(OH)_2D_3$], the hormonally active form which can bind and activate the nuclear vitamin D receptor (VDR) in many different target tissues, including bone, kidneys, intestine, and the immune system (5). Calcitriol-mediated activation of VDR in different immune cells is thought to generally result in immunoregulatory transcriptional responses (5). With regard to MS, low systemic VitD levels [typically measured using the most stable VitD metabolite $25(OH)D_3$ as a surrogate] are associated with increased disease risk (6), relapse rate, and disease progression (7, 8). A number of MS susceptibility genes are predicted to be regulated by VitD (9, 10), but the underlying *in vivo* mechanisms contributing to the etiopathogenesis of MS remain unclear. In addition, recent Mendelian randomization studies have shown that genetic variants that are associated with reduced circulating $25(OH)D_3$ levels also predict increased risk of MS (11–13). There are ongoing clinical trials to test the benefits of dietary VitD supplementation as a preventative or therapeutic strategy, but to date no clear beneficial effect has been reported (14–17). Importantly, the immunosuppressive effects of UV radiation independent of VitD are also well documented (18, 19). In fact, the results of recent epidemiological studies suggest that VitD and UV radiation can exert independent effects on MS risk (20–22), and data from animal models support this concept (19, 23–25).

Intriguingly, while low VitD levels are strongly associated with MS risk in white populations, a number of studies have shown that this is not the case in blacks and Hispanics (6, 26–30). This is surprising, since these populations typically have darker skin pigmentation and thus lower VitD levels compared with whites living at the same latitude (31), and it demonstrates that the association between VitD and MS risk is modified by unidentified genetic factors. This also suggests that any benefits of VitD supplementation for MS would be genotype dependent.

Effects of VitD have also been explored in animal models of MS. Experimental autoimmune encephalomyelitis (EAE), the principal autoimmune model used to study the pathogenesis of MS, can be induced by immunization with CNS homogenate or specific myelin proteins/peptides, or by transfer of CD4 T cells reactive to these antigens (32). As in MS, autoreactive CD4 T cells enter the CNS to initiate inflammation and pathology, culminating in neurologic disability. Treatment of adult animals with the hormone calcitriol has long been known to suppress EAE in mice (33, 34). More recent mechanistic studies have shown that this suppression requires VDR signaling in T cells and the expression of interferon gamma (IFNγ) (35, 36), thus likely acting directly to inhibit T helper (Th)-1 effector functions. In addition, calcitriol-mediated suppression of EAE is associated with induction of regulatory T cells (Tregs) (37), and hence it has been proposed that VDR signaling may act as a switch between Th1 effector and regulatory CD4 T cells (38). However, the physiologic validity of this approach has been called into question, as treatment with calcitriol can cause hypercalcemia, which itself can suppress EAE (39, 40), although this point remains controversial (38). As a more physiologically relevant approach, dietary supplementation with VitD during adolescence also inhibited EAE in mice (41, 42) and rats (43, 44). Strikingly, this effect was observed only in female, but not male mice, and was dependent on the presence of estrogen (41, 42).

The EAE model is an attractive approach to directly test hypotheses generated from epidemiologic studies on MS risk factors (45). However, one of the common limitations of this approach is that the immense genetic diversity of human populations is not represented among standard inbred laboratory strains of mice (46, 47). We and others have attempted to more closely model human genetic diversity by incorporating into the experimental design wild-derived inbred strains of mice, such as PWD/PhJ (PWD), or chromosome substitution (consomic) strains that carry individual PWD chromosomes on the common B6 background (B6.Chr^{PWD}) (48, 49). We have shown that compared with B6 mice, a classical inbred laboratory strain, wild-derived inbred PWD mice have widely divergent immune cell transcriptomes, which result in differential expression of MS relevant genes and reduced susceptibility to EAE (50). We have also used the B6.Chr^{PWD} consomic model to identify multiple EAE susceptibility loci, many of which were sex specific (51).

In this study, we combined the physiologically relevant dietary approach to manipulate VitD levels (41–43), with the genetic diversity of B6.Chr^{PWD} consomic model, to examine gene-by-sex interactions on the effects of VitD in CNS autoimmune disease. In agreement with previous reports, we show that the effects of VitD supplementation on EAE susceptibility in B6 mice are female specific. This was associated with induction of sex- and genotype-specific transcriptional responses in effector and regulatory CD4 T cells. Strikingly, the EAE response to VitD supplementation varied widely across B6.Chr^{PWD} consomic strains, suggesting that, as in MS, genotype modifies the outcome of VitD status in EAE.

RESULTS

Dietary Manipulation of VitD Levels Modulates Systemic VitD Levels and EAE Severity

To directly manipulate systemic VitD levels in a controlled fashion, we adopted a previously described dietary paradigm initiated during adolescence, which has been shown to modulate EAE in the mouse (41, 42) and rat (43, 44). Briefly, 3-week-old B6 and PWD mice were randomized to either a VitD-low diet or a VitD-high diet, as described in Section "Materials and Methods" (see Figure S1 in Supplementary Material for a diagrammatic overview of the experimental design). Serum samples were collected at 3 and 5 weeks post-dietary intervention, and analyzed for the levels of 25(OH)D, the most abundant and stable metabolite of VitD that is typically used as an indicator of VitD status in clinical studies (6). The dietary regimen induced rapid and sustained changes that appeared to plateau at approximately 3 weeks post-intervention (**Figure 1A**). PWD mice exhibited significantly lower baseline 25(OH)D levels compared with B6 (**Figure 1B**). These differences disappeared on the VitD-low diet (**Figures 1C,D**). Interestingly, on the VitD-high diet, female B6 mice reached higher levels of 25(OH) D compared with B6 males at both time points (**Figures 1E,F**), which were also significantly higher than PWD females at 5 weeks (**Figure 1F**).

Having established the dietary paradigm, we tested whether the robust differences in systemic VitD levels achieved by VitD-high and VitD-low diets impacted clinical progression of EAE. Female and male B6 mice were subjected to the dietary paradigm above, followed by EAE induction at 5 weeks post-dietary intervention. Exposure to the VitD-high diet resulted in lower EAE severity compared with VitD-low diet in female B6 mice (**Figure 2A**). By contrast, no significant difference in EAE clinical course on the two diets was observed in male B6 mice (**Figure 2B**). DeLuca and colleagues have observed that suppression of EAE in mice by treatment with the bioactive VitD metabolite, calcitriol, is associated with and dependent on hypercalcemia, questioning the physiological relevance of that approach (39, 40). Hence, we tested whether our dietary paradigm affected systemic Ca^{2+} levels and found that EAE suppression was not accompanied by significant changes in Ca^{2+} levels (**Figure 2C**), suggesting that our dietary model influences EAE susceptibility independent of Ca^{2+}.

We have previously shown that PWD mice are almost completely resistant to EAE (50). To test whether this resistance

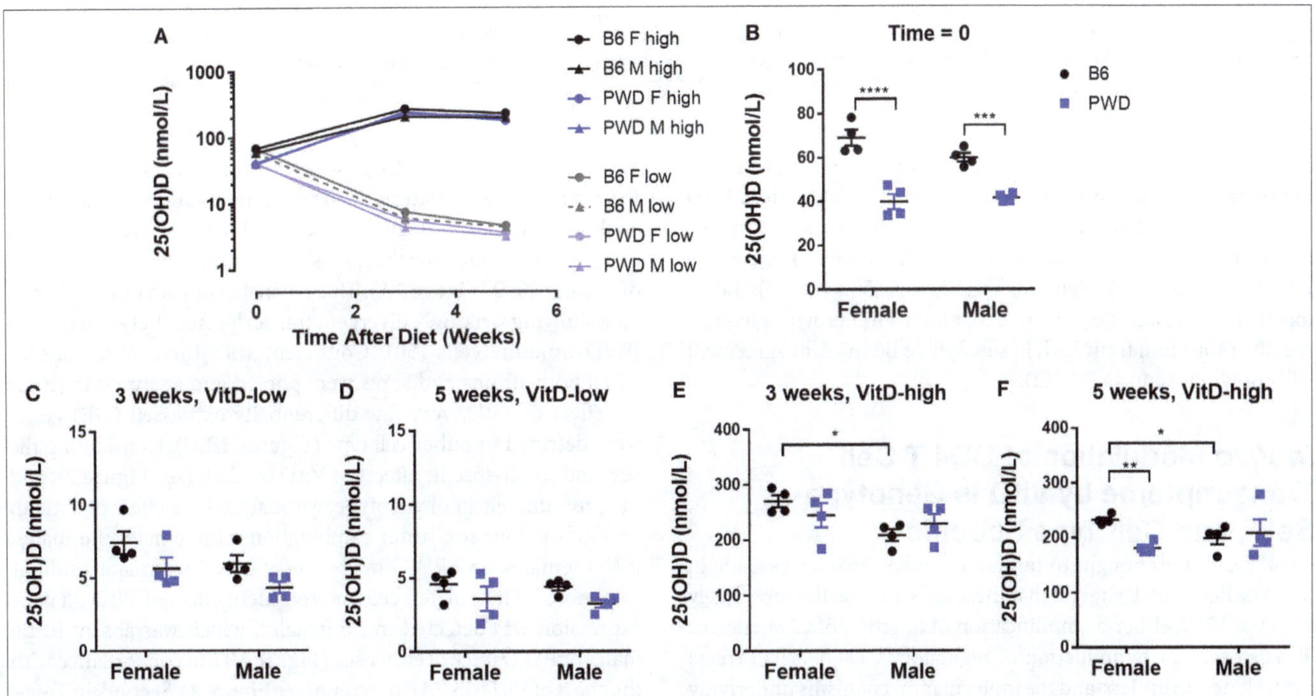

FIGURE 1 | Manipulation of dietary vitamin D3 (VitD) results in robust changes in systemic VitD levels that are sex- and genotype dependent. Female and male B6 and PWD mice (*N* = 4 for each sex/strain combination) were assigned to VitD-high and VitD-low diets at 3 weeks of age. Serum samples were collected at the outset (Time = 0), and at 3 and 5 weeks post-treatment. 25(OH)D levels were measured by enzyme-linked immunoassay (see Materials and Methods). An overview of kinetic data is shown in **(A)**, followed by comparisons at individual time points in **(B–F)**, segregated by diet. The significance of the observed differences in **(B–F)** was assessed by two-way ANOVA, with Holm–Sidak's *post hoc* comparisons: B6 vs. PWD (within sex), and female vs. male (within strain). Symbols indicate a significant difference between the indicated groups, as follows: $^*p < 0.05$; $^{**}p < 0.01$; $^{***}p < 0.001$; $^{****}p < 0.0001$.

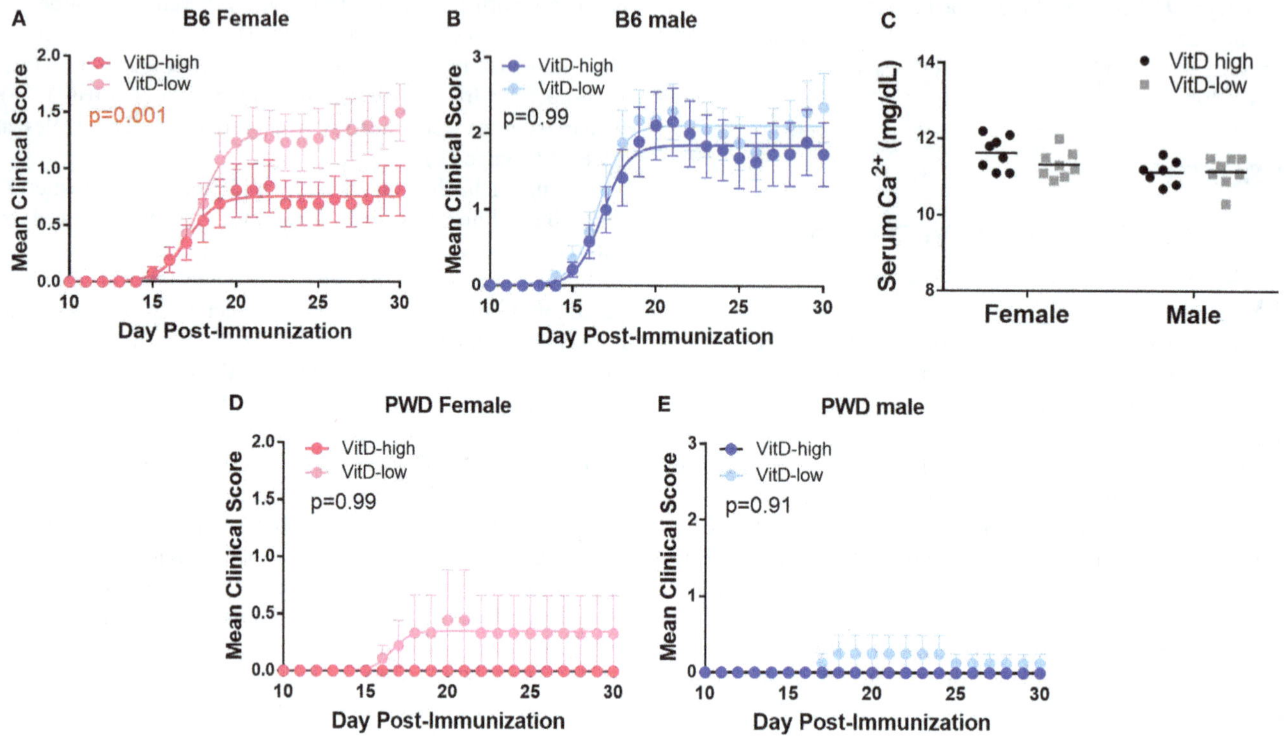

FIGURE 2 | Strain- and sex-specific suppression of EAE by vitamin D3 (VitD). B6 **(A–C)** and PWD **(D,E)** mice were maintained on VitD-high and VitD-low diets as in **Figure 1**, followed by EAE induction after 5 weeks post-dietary intervention. Mice were maintained on the respective diets until the end of the experiment. **(C)** B6 serum Ca^{2+} levels were measured for the indicated groups, and the significance of the observed differences assessed by two-way ANOVA, followed by Holm–Sidak's *post hoc* comparisons. The significance of the observed differences in the severity of the clinical disease course was assessed as described in Section "Materials and Methods." *p*-Values for the effect of diet on overall disease course (representing the interaction term for treatment × time, repeated measures two-way ANOVA) are shown. The numbers of animals for each group are provided in Table S1 in Supplementary Material.

could be affected by VitD status, PWD mice were subjected to the dietary regimen as above, followed by EAE induction. VitD had no significant effect on EAE, whereby PWD mice remained highly resistant to EAE induction on either diet (**Figure 2D**; EAE incidence: VitD-high 0/8, VitD-low 2/15; $p = 0.53$). Taken together, our results demonstrate that high VitD provides female-specific protection from EAE in susceptible B6 mice, in agreement with previous reports (41, 42).

In Vivo Modulation of CD4 T Cell Transcriptome by VitD Is Genotype-, Sex-, and Cell Type Specific

CD4 T cells are thought to initiate the inflammatory cascade in MS. Studies in EAE suggest that these cells are also the most likely target of VitD, either by modification of function of CD4 effector T cells (Teff) or by induction of regulatory CD4 T cells (Tregs) (38). Hence, to understand the molecular mechanisms underlying immune modulation by VitD *in vivo*, we carried out transcriptional profiling of Teff and Tregs isolated from B6 and PWD mice exposed to VitD-low or VitD-high diets. Mice were subjected to the dietary paradigm as described in **Figure 1**, followed by isolation of splenic Teff and Tregs using fluorescence-activated cell sorting (FACS) and transcriptional profiling (see Materials and Methods) at 5 weeks post-dietary intervention (Figure S1 in Supplementary Material). When gene expression data were analyzed for effect of genotype, sex, and VitD, it was found that genotype accounted for the largest effect size, with modest effects of sex and VitD (**Figure 3A**). This is consistent with our published data showing strikingly divergent transcriptomes between B6 and PWD immune cells (50). Consistent with these observations, when both strains and sexes were pooled and analyzed together for effect of VitD, very few differentially expressed (DE) genes were detected in either cell type (**Figures 3B,C**). Considering the sex- and strain-specific effects of VitD on EAE (see **Figure 2**), and the profound effect of genotype, we analyzed the effect of VitD in each of the four sex/strain combinations (B6 females, B6 males, PWD females, and PWD males) separately. Two major findings were noted. First, in Teff cells, a prominent effect of VitD on gene expression was detected in B6 females, which was absent in B6 males or PWD mice of either sex (**Figure 3B**), in concordance with the effect of VitD on EAE outcome (see **Figure 2**). Second, in Tregs, VitD exhibited the strongest effect in PWD females (**Figure 3C**). In both cases, high VitD predominantly induced upregulation of gene expression compared with low VitD (**Figures 3B,C**).

Bioinformatic pathway analyses of DE genes (see Materials and Methods) revealed divergent and sometimes opposing effects of VitD on gene expression, depending on sex and strain

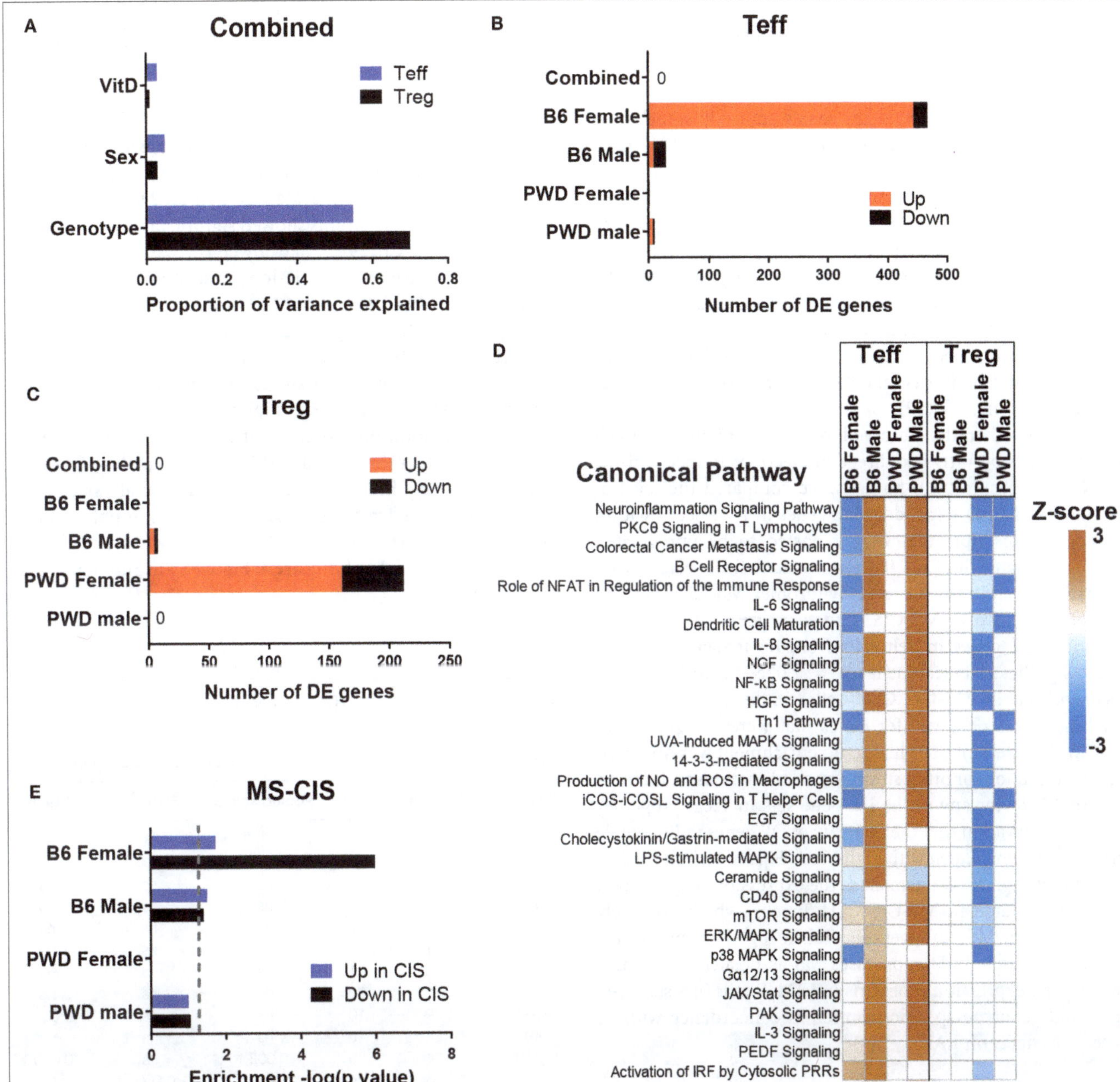

FIGURE 3 | *In vivo* transcriptional regulation by vitamin D3 (VitD). Female and male B6 and PWD mice ($N = 4$ for each sex/strain combination) were exposed to VitD-low and VitD-high diets as in **Figure 1**. At 5 weeks post-dietary intervention, transcriptional profiling was performed on Teff and regulatory T cells (Tregs) as described in Section "Materials and Methods." **(A)** The proportion of variance in gene expression explained by the indicated experimental variables is shown for Teff and Tregs. **(B,C)** The number of genes passing the differential expression threshold (|Fold Change| > 2, ANOVA $p < 0.001$) as a function of diet is shown for the indicated groups, in Teff **(B)** and Tregs **(C)**. Direction of change is depicted as expression level in VitD-high relative to VitD-low (e.g., "up" indicates higher expression in the VitD-high group). **(D)** Canonical pathway analysis was performed using IPA software (see Materials and Methods). *Z*-scores indicate predicted direction and relative strength of change (VitD-high relative to VitD-low). The top 30 pathways (ranked by *Z*-score) are shown. **(E)** Enrichment analysis of the indicated differentially expressed (DE) gene sets from Teff within transcripts DE (up or down) in CD4 cells from multiple sclerosis (MS)-CIS patients was performed using IPA (see Materials and Methods). *p*-Values for enrichment are shown as $-\log(p)$. Dotted line denotes $p = 0.05$.

(**Figure 3D**). Several canonical pathways relevant to EAE/MS pathogenesis (including neuroinflammation, Th1, and a number of other proinflammatory pathways) were downregulated by high VitD in Teff cells from B6 females, yet upregulated in B6 males or PWD males. The gene expression patterns in Teff cells were again concordant with EAE outcomes, whereby downregulation of proinflammatory activity by VitD was associated with EAE suppression in B6 females. Similarly, upstream regulator analysis in B6 female Teff cells predicted significant inhibition of several proinflammatory nodes by high VitD, including TNF,

NFκB, CSF2, and IFNγ as the top four nodes. Comparison of DE transcripts within the IFNγ node with two selected MS relevant canonical pathways, "Neuroinflammation Signaling Pathway" (ranked first) and "Th1 Pathway" (ranked 11th) revealed strong functional overlap and several key shared transcripts, including several MHC class II genes, and a central role for IFNγ itself (Figure S2 in Supplementary Material). The former is consistent with the documented regulation of the major MS risk MHC class II allele, HLA-DRB1*15:01, by VitD. The latter is consistent with the documented critical role of IFNγ in the regulation of EAE by VitD (36). Finally, this analysis implicated *Mapk14* (Figure S2 in Supplementary Material), encoding p38α MAP kinase, a gene that we have previously identified as a central regulator of differential sex-specific genetic effects on EAE in the B6.Chr^{PWD} model (51), a hypothesis that was validated in our targeted analysis of the role of p38α in EAE (52).

To test whether the observed regulation of immune cell transcriptomes by VitD had direct connections to mechanisms of CNS autoimmunity in humans, we compared the level of enrichment of VitD-dependent DE genes in PWD cells within the set of transcripts that were reported to be upregulated or downregulated in CD4 T cells isolated from early onset MS patients (clinically isolated syndrome; MS-CIS) relative to healthy controls (MS-CIS signature genes) (53). VitD-dependent DE genes in Teff cells from B6 females exhibited highly significant enrichment (p = 1.02e−6) within genes *downregulated* in MS-CIS CD4 cells, while marginal or no enrichment was observed for genes that were *upregulated* in MS-CIS (**Figure 3E**). Marginal to no enrichment was observed in either direction for other strain-sex combinations in Teff cells (**Figure 3E**) or for any of the DE gene sets in Tregs. Together with the observation that the majority of DE genes in B6 female Teff cells are *upregulated* with high VitD (**Figure 3B**), these data suggest that high VitD normalizes the expression of genes that are downregulated in MS-CIS CD4 T cells, which are likely associated with MS pathogenesis. Taken together, our results indicate that high VitD suppresses MS-associated proinflammatory gene expression programs in CD4 T cells in a sex-, cell type-, and genotype-specific manner, in concordance with its protective effects on EAE.

Sex and Genotype Dictate the Outcome of VitD Modulation in EAE

Since epidemiologic data (6, 26–29) and our findings above suggest the possibility that the outcome of VitD status in MS and EAE may be dependent on genotype, we deliberately introduced the segregation of natural genetic variation into our model. To achieve this, we utilized the B6.Chr^{PWD} consomic model, in which natural genetic variation exhibits a significant impact on EAE susceptibility (51). Twenty B6.Chr^{PWD} consomic strains, encompassing 17 autosomes, X and Y, and a conplastic strain with the PWD mitochondrial genome were included in the study. The mice were exposed to the VitD-high and VitD-low dietary paradigm, followed by EAE induction and evaluation, as in **Figure 2**. Surprisingly, in a combined analysis of all strains and sexes, no significant effect of dietary modulation of VitD on EAE course was detected (**Table 1**; **Figure 4A**). Similarly, when this combined analysis was stratified by sex, no significant effect of VitD in either sex was detected (**Table 1**; **Figure 4A**). Given the known variation in EAE susceptibility across the B6.Chr^{PWD} consomic/conplastic strains (51), and the sex- and strain-specific responses to VitD in EAE and gene expression (see above), each strain was analyzed individually for the effect of VitD on EAE, either combining both sexes or analyzing each sex separately. When analyzing males and females together, five strains showed significant effects of VitD. Chr11.1^{PWD} and Chr19^{PWD} had lower EAE severity on VitD-high diet compared with VitD-low, as seen in B6 females, but surprisingly, Chr10.2^{PWD}, Chr11.2^{PWD}, and Chr14^{PWD} exhibited the opposite effect (**Figure 4**; Figure S3 in Supplementary Material). Stratification by sex revealed that these effects were primarily driven by a single sex, either female or male, depending on the strain (e.g., **Figure 4**). Stratification by sex also revealed additional significant effects of VitD in females (Chr10.3^{PWD}, Chr15^{PWD}, and mt^{PWD}) and in males (Chr8^{PWD}, Chr12^{PWD}, and ChrY^{PWD}) (**Table 1**). Additional analyses of EAE quantitative trait variables (Table S1 in Supplementary Material) supported the conclusions drawn from disease course analyses (**Table 1**; **Figure 4**; Figure S4 in Supplementary Material).

TABLE 1 | Effects of vitamin D3 (VitD) on EAE disease course in B6.Chr^{PWD} consomic mice.

***N*/group**			**Effect of diet on EAE course**[a]		
Strain	**Female**	**Male**	**Pooled sexes**	**Females**	**Males**
All strains	449	448	ns	ns	ns
B6	52	36	ns	0.006 ↓	ns
PWD	10	13	ns	ns	ns
Chr1	21	18	ns	ns	ns
Chr2	6	6	ns	ns	ns
Chr5	21	24	ns	ns	ns
Chr6	30	21	ns	ns	ns
Chr7	11	22	ns	ns	ns
Chr8	9	10	ns	ns	0.006 ↑
Chr9	22	19	ns	ns	ns
Chr10.2	14	20	0.002 ↑	ns	0.006 ↑
Chr10.3	25	24	ns	<0.0001 ↑	ns
Chr11.1	19	21	0.01 ↓	ns	<0.0001 ↓
Chr11.2	16	13	0.002 ↑	ns	0.002 ↑
Chr12	29	29	ns	ns	0.0001 ↓
Chr14	18	22	<0.0001 ↓	ns	<0.0001 ↓
Chr15	20	23	ns	0.03 ↓	ns
Chr17	19	19	ns	ns	ns
Chr18	26	25	ns	ns	ns
Chr19	18	22	<0.0001 ↓	<0.0001 ↓	ns
ChrY	27	26	ns	ns	<0.0001 ↓
ChrX.3	11	12	ns	ns	ns
mt	25	23	ns	<0.0001 ↑	ns

[a]*The significance of the observed differences in the severity of the EAE clinical disease course for each of the B6.Chr^{PWD} consomic strains was analyzed for the effect of VitD diet, as described in Section "Materials and Methods." Data for females and males were analyzed together (pooled) and following stratification by sex. ANOVA p-values for the effect of diet on overall EAE course are shown where significant; ns, not significant; ND, not done. Direction of arrow indicates the direction of change for EAE severity in the VitD-high diet group relative to the VitD-low group (i.e., downward arrow indicates suppression of EAE by VitD-high diet).*

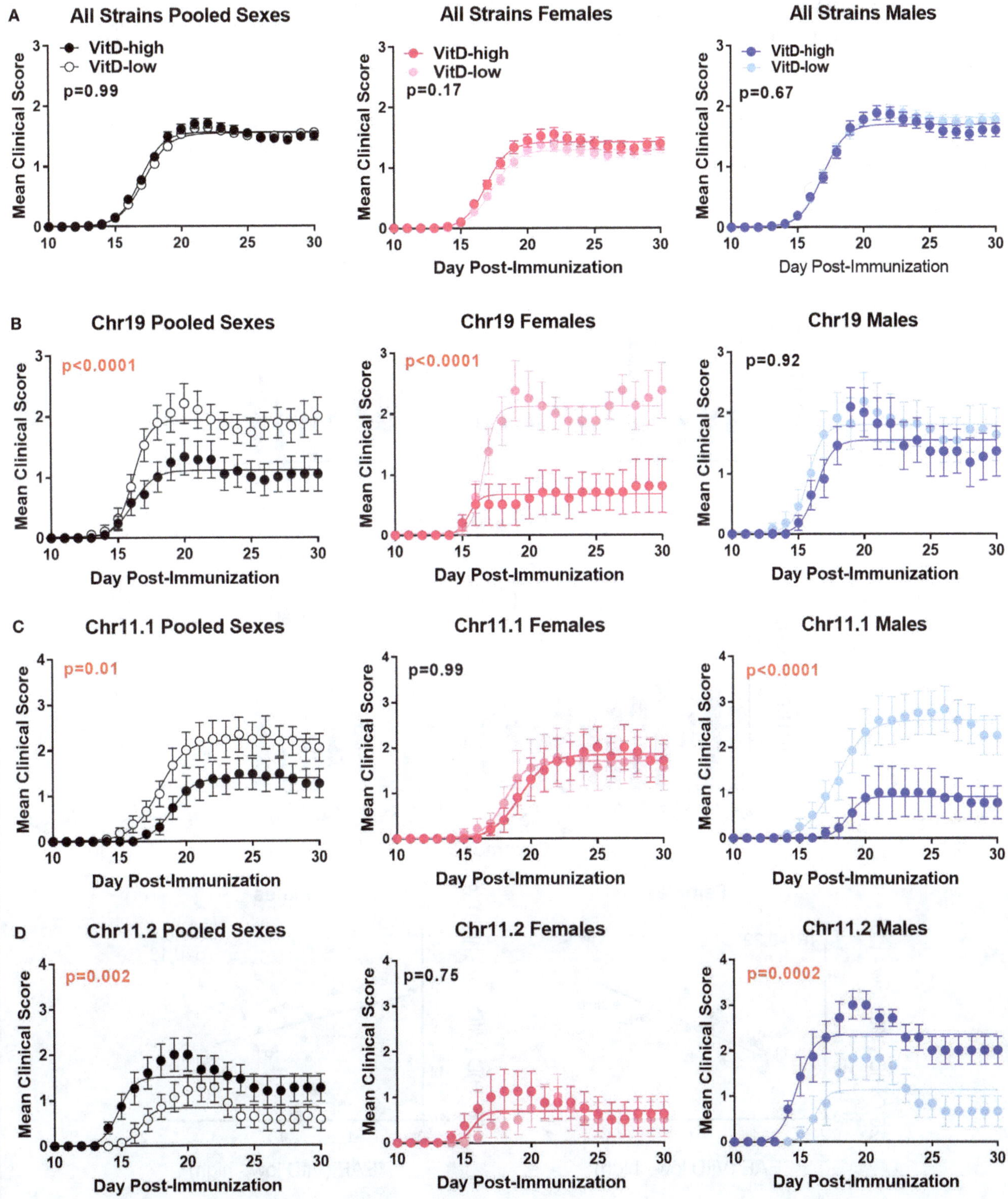

FIGURE 4 | Effects of vitamin D3 (VitD) on EAE disease course in B6.Chr^{PWD} consomic mice. B6.Chr^{PWD} consomic mice were exposed to VitD-high and VitD-low diets, as in **Figure 2**, followed by induction of EAE. Disease course in a pooled analysis of all consomic strains **(A)**, or in three representative consomic strains, Chr19^{PWD} **(B)**, Chr11.1^{PWD} **(C)**, and Chr11.2^{PWD} **(D)**, is shown for pooled sexes, or for each sex separately, as indicated. *p*-Values for the effect of diet on overall EAE course (representing the interaction term for treatment × time, repeated measures two-way ANOVA) are shown. Numbers of animals per group are shown in Table S1 in Supplementary Material.

Systemic 25(OH)D Levels Predict EAE Outcome in Female B6.Chr^{PWD} Consomic Mice

Since circulating VitD levels are genetically controlled in humans (54) and in B6 and PWD mice (**Figure 1**), we determined whether B6.Chr^{PWD} consomic/conplastic strains subjected to our dietary paradigm exhibited any differences in systemic VitD levels. Because the 25(OH)D levels reached on the VitD-high diet were dramatically different from those on the VitD-low diet (see **Figure 1**), the data were analyzed separately for each diet, to assess the effect of strain and sex. Significant differences in 25(OH)D levels were observed between several consomic strains and B6. On the VitD-high diet, a number of strains presented with significantly lower levels of 25(OH)D3 compared with B6, but no strains exhibited higher levels (**Figure 5A**). On the

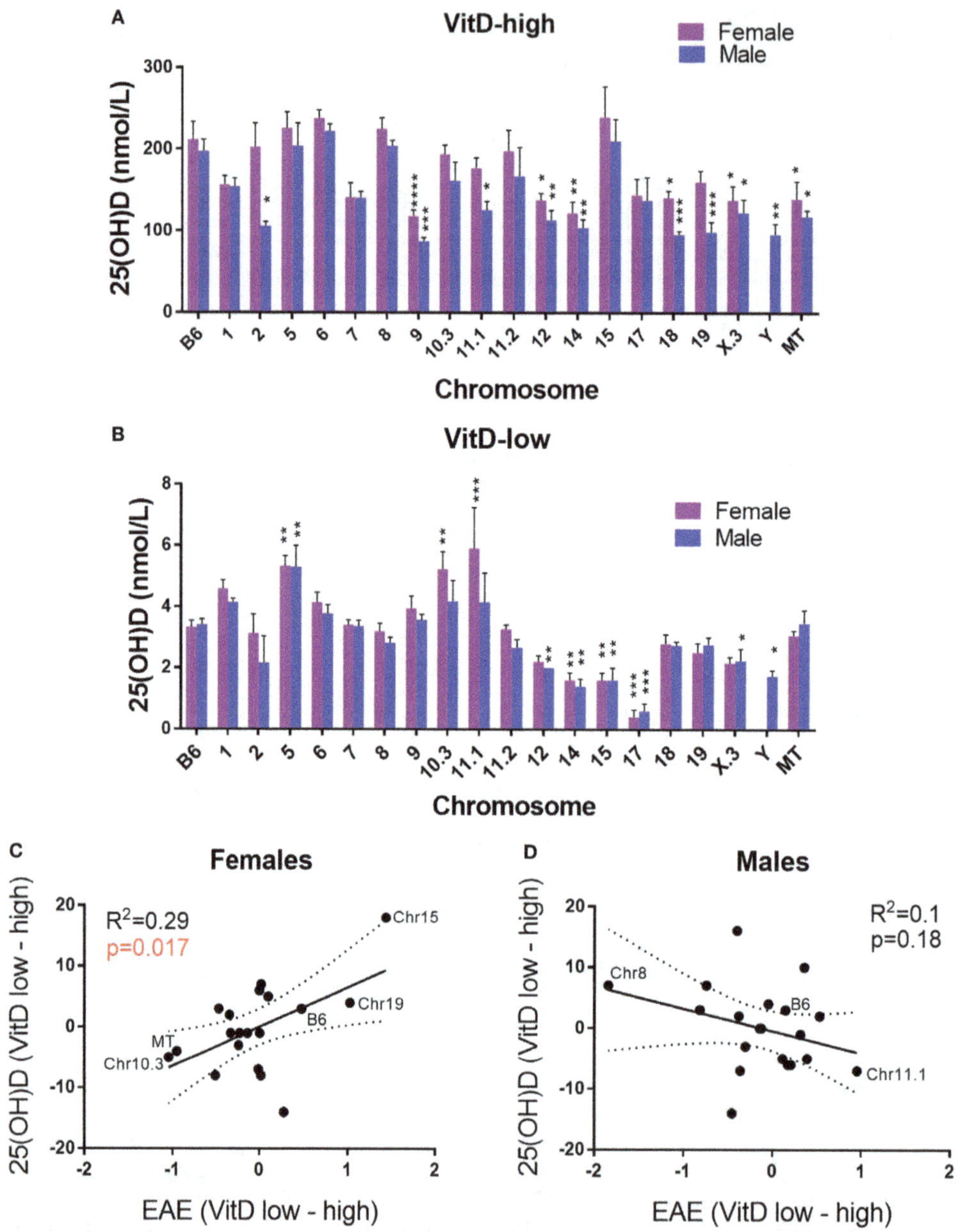

FIGURE 5 | Effects of genotype and sex on systemic vitamin D3 (VitD) levels as related to EAE outcomes. B6.Chr^{PWD} consomic mice were exposed to VitD-high **(A)** and VitD-low **(B)** diet, followed by EAE induction, as in **Figure 4**. Sera were collected at day 30 post-EAE induction. 25(OH)D levels were measured by enzyme-linked immunoassay in five males and five females of each strain for each diet type. The significance of the observed differences was assessed by two-way ANOVA, followed by Holm–Sidak's *post hoc* comparisons, comparing each consomic strain to B6. Symbols indicate a significant difference between B6 and the indicated groups, as follows: *$p < 0.05$; **$p < 0.01$; ***$p < 0.001$; ****$p < 0.0001$. **(C,D)** The relationship between serum 25(OH)D levels and EAE severity was examined, as described in Section "Materials and Methods." Linear regression was used to determine the significance of the correlation between the ranked 25(OH)D response [difference in 25(OH)D between VitD-low and -high diets] and normalized EAE response (difference in cumulative disease score between VitD-low and high diets). R^2 values and p-values for regression analysis are shown. Selected B6.Chr^{PWD} consomic strains are labeled as specific examples.

VitD-low diet, several strains exhibited significantly higher or lower levels of 25(OH)D compared with B6 (**Figure 5B**). Next, we tested whether any of these changes in 25(OH)D levels were correlated with EAE outcomes, e.g., whether a larger change in VitD levels corresponded to a higher degree of disease protection by VitD. EAE cumulative disease score (CDS), as the quantitative trait variable that most accurately reflects the overall severity of the EAE clinical disease course, was used to calculate a normalized difference in CDS between VitD-low and -high diets, for each strain. Similarly, a relative difference in serum 25(OH)D between VitD-low and -high diets was calculated for each strain. The relationship between these two parameters was examined using linear regression. For female consomic mice, a significant positive relationship was observed, suggesting that those strains that had higher serum 25(OH)D responses exhibited protective effects of VitD (e.g., B6, Chr15, and Chr19), while those with low responses had the opposite effects (e.g., Chr10.3), albeit the association was modest ($r^2 = 0.29$) (**Figure 5C**). Surprisingly, in males, the trend was reversed, although it did not reach significance (**Figure 5D**). Taken together, these results suggest that genotype controls systemic levels of VitD, which in turn may contribute to EAE susceptibility in a sex-specific manner.

Tissue-Specific Differential Expression of VitD Metabolic Pathway Genes in B6 and PWD Mice

Systemic 25(OH)D levels in humans are genetically regulated, and recent GWAS studies have identified common variants in four major genes in the VitD metabolism pathway: *GC*, *DHCR7*, *CYP2R1*, and *CYP24A1*, which together explain a large proportion of the variation in 25(OH)D (54). Subsequent Mendelian randomization studies showed that the genetic control of low 25(OH)D levels by alleles of the four genes is associated with increased susceptibility to MS (11–13). To begin to identify potential candidate genes underlying differential responses across different B6.Chr^{PWD} consomic strains, we examined the level of expression of mouse orthologs of these four key genes (*Gc*, *Dhcr7*, *Cyp2r1*, and *Cyp24a1*) in several relevant tissues (kidney, liver, and spleen) in male and female B6 and PWD mice, using publically available datasets (see Materials and Methods). We included three additional key VitD metabolism genes: *Cyp27a1*, *Cyp27b1*, and *Vdr* (55). A number of these genes were DE across different tissues. In all three tissues, vitamin D-25 hydroxylase, *Cyp27a1*, exhibited twofold to threefold lower expression in PWD compared with B6, with significantly lower expression in females compared with males in both strains in the kidney (**Figures 6A–C**). In the kidney, 1-α-hydroxylase, *Cyp27b1*, exhibited a modest significant increase in expression in PWD compared with B6 (**Figure 6D**), while 1,25(OH)$_2$D$_3$-inactivating 24-hydroxylase, *Cyp24a1*, exhibited a significant increase in expression in B6 (**Figure 6E**). *Vdr* also exhibited higher expression in PWD compared with B6 in the spleen (**Figure 6F**). These results demonstrate genetic control of tissue-specific differential expression of several components of the VitD metabolic pathway which may underlie some of the differences in serum 25(OH)D levels (**Figures 1** and **5**) and EAE responses (**Table 1**; **Figure 4**) in B6.Chr^{PWD} mice. Of these

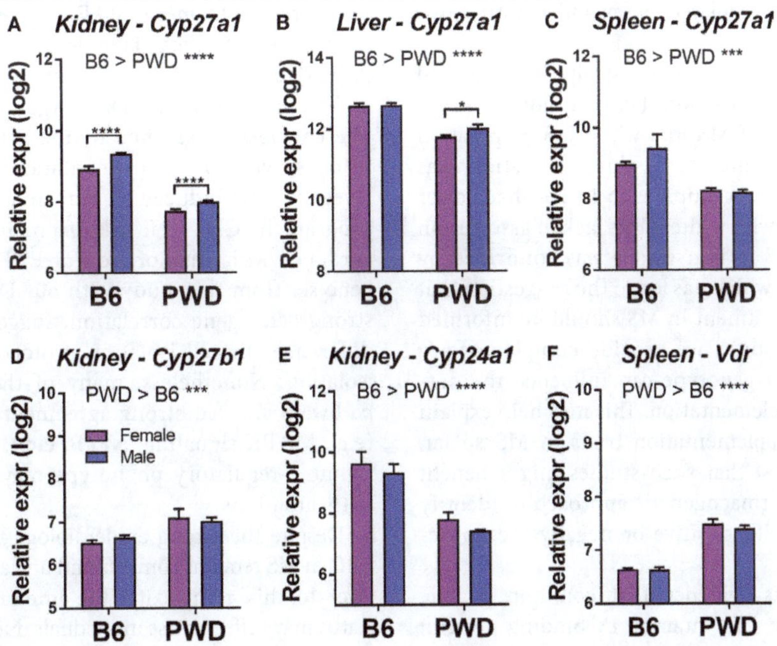

FIGURE 6 | Tissue-specific differential expression of vitamin D3 metabolic pathway genes in B6 and PWD mice. Gene expression data were obtained from the Gene Expression Miner database, as described in Section "Materials and Methods." Genes showing a significant differential expression (with a greater than 30% change in expression) as a function of strain or sex are shown in **(A–F)**. The significance of the observed differences was assessed by two-way ANOVA, with Holm–Sidak's *post hoc* comparisons: B6 vs. PWD (overall effect of strain; indicated above the graphs), and female vs. male (within strain; indicated with brackets). The data included 12 C57BL/6J mice (6 females and 6 males), and 11 PWD/PhJ mice (6 females and 5 males). Symbols indicate a significant difference between the indicated groups, as follows: *$p < 0.05$; **$p < 0.01$; ***$p < 0.001$; ****$p < 0.0001$.

genes, two lie within consomic intervals of interest (carried by consomic strains exhibiting significant effects in **Table 1**): *Cyp27b1* (Chr10.3) and *Vdr* (Chr15). As such, they represent candidate genes controlling differential responsiveness to VitD in EAE (see Discussion), and their relevance will be assessed in future studies.

DISCUSSION

Genetic and environmental influences on MS risk are well documented. However, gene–environment interactions have been more elusive, with the exception of HLA alleles and their putative interactions with smoking, EBV, and obesity (56). Part of the difficulty in identifying such interactions is the inability to clearly define over time the presence/absence/level of environmental variables/exposures and possible confounding variables (57). The other difficulty inherent to all epidemiologic studies is the inability to separate cause and effect from association/correlation. The association of low VitD with MS risk is an example of such an association, where cause and effect have been difficult to parse out, and therapeutic intervention has not yet provided a clear answer (58). Animal models provide an opportunity to bridge the gap between observation and causation, as putative genetic and environmental risk factors can be precisely controlled (45). As such, they also provide an opportunity to identify gene–environment interactions in a highly controlled experimental setting. In this study, we have applied a well-defined dietary paradigm to intentionally modulate systemic VitD levels, while at the same time introducing controlled genetic variation. This approach revealed that the effects of VitD in a mouse model of MS are regulated by sex and genotype in a cell type-specific fashion.

In a seminal prospective case–control study, Ascherio and colleagues identified an association between low 25(OH)D levels and increased risk of MS in a white U.S. population (6). Interestingly, in the same study, this association was absent in black and Hispanic groups, who in fact had lower 25(OH)D levels compared with whites. This lack of association between 25(OH)D and MS in non-whites was confirmed by several groups (22, 26–29), which has led to the suggestion that VitD-related testing and treatment in MS should be informed by ethnicity (59). In our study, we provide complementary experimental evidence that genotype can influence the outcome of VitD status or supplementation. This may help explain the variability in VitD supplementation trials in MS so far, and our results also suggest that such studies might benefit from a complementary pharmacogenetic approach to identify gene variants associated with positive or negative responses to VitD.

In this regard, there is evidence that common genetic variants in *GC* (encoding the vitamin D binding-protein; DBP) may lead to profound ethnic-specific variations in DBP levels, DBP binding avidity, and bioavailablity of VitD and its metabolites (31). However, a recent study by Barcellos and colleagues found that these variants in *GC* do not account for the lack of association between serum VitD levels and MS in blacks and Hispanics (30). This suggests that other unknown ethnic-specific genetic determinants can regulate VitD metabolism and/or subsequent physiologic responses, such as those underlying MS susceptibility.

In some B6.Chr^{PWD} consomic strains (e.g., male Chr11.2^{PWD}), an unexpected phenotype was observed, whereby higher EAE severity was seen on the VitD-high diet compared with VitD-low diet. However, several previous reports have documented similar unexpected EAE-suppressing effects of VitD insufficiency or deficiency, depending on length and timing of the exposure (60, 61). In addition, mice completely deficient in *Vdr* are unexpectedly resistant to EAE (62), suggesting that VitD signaling is needed to mount a robust T cell response. Thus, we hypothesize that VitD status can serve as a bi-directional rheostat regulating autoimmunity, and this balance can be further modified by genetic background and sex. Interestingly, Chr10.3^{PWD} female mice exhibited lower 25(OH)D responses associated with increased EAE on the VitD-high diet (**Figure 5C**; Figure S3 in Supplementary Material). It is possible that increased kidney *Cyp27b1* expression from the PWD allele in the Chr10.3 locus (**Figure 6D**) drives faster 25(OH)D to 1,25(OH)D metabolism, which could result in different levels or kinetics of VDR activation and divergent EAE outcomes. Conversely, female Chr15^{PWD} mice exhibit the opposite phenotype with regard to VitD status and EAE outcome (**Figure 5C**), while the PWD allele of *Vdr* (located on Chr15) shows higher expression (**Figure 6F**). Since for *Cyp27b1* and *Vdr* the expression differences were not sex specific (**Figures 6D,F**), we postulate that other sex-specific factors (e.g., lower expression of *Cyp27a1* in females; **Figures 6A,B**) interact with the genetically determined differential expression of these VitD pathway genes to give rise to different outcomes in EAE.

In a recent study, Jagodic and colleagues used a dietary paradigm highly similar to ours to examine genomic effects of VitD in the inbred Dark Agouti rat model of EAE (44). The conclusions reached by the authors were largely similar to ours, whereby supplementation of female rats with high levels of VitD induced an anti-inflammatory gene expression program in CD4 Teff cells from immunized mice, in concordance with amelioration of EAE. Comparison of the DE gene set from this study with our DE gene set did not reveal strong gene–gene correlation, suggesting species differences, differences in cell isolation protocols, and/or timing of cell isolation. Nonetheless, many of the differentially regulated pathways showed strong agreement between the two studies (e.g., MAPK signaling, NFκB, etc.), suggesting that a similar immune-regulatory phenotype may be achieved by VitD in both situations.

Despite the strong epidemiological associations, the role of VitD in MS remains complex and unclear. Our studies add another layer to this complexity: the immunologic response to VitD status may differ across individuals due to genetic and sex effects. The sex effects have been shown in mouse models to be likely due to the influence of estrogen (42). Our future studies will be aimed at identifying genetic modifiers of the VitD response in CNS autoimmunity. This information will help inform future VitD supplementation trials, as well as the use of VitD status as a prognostic.

MATERIALS AND METHODS

Animals and Dietary Treatments

C57BL/6J (B6), PWD/PhJ (PWD), and B6.Chr^{PWD} consomic mice were purchased from Jackson Laboratories (Bar Harbor, ME, USA), then bred and housed in a single room within the vivarium at the Larner College of Medicine at the University of Vermont for two to four generations prior to any experimentation. The experimental procedures used in this study were approved by the Animal Care and Use Committee of the University of Vermont.

To ensure their correct identity and to enhance rigor and reproducibility of these studies, B6.Chr^{PWD} consomic mice were subjected to genome-wide SNP genotyping using Dartmouse genotyping services (Dartmouth College, NH, USA). All mice used in this study were of the expected genotypes, with the following exceptions. B6.Chr4^{PWD} mice were excluded from the study, because they were found to be a mix of various genotypes, where much of the Chr4^{PWD} had been replaced with B6 genome. Chr17^{PWD} mice were found to carry a homozygous B6-derived interval between 30 and 45 Mb on Chr17, encompassing *H2*.

At weaning (3 weeks of age), littermate mice were randomly assigned to one of two diets: VitD-low (0 IU VitD/g; 0.87% Ca^{2+}, 0.3% phosphorus, alcohol extracted casein as protein source) or VitD-high [identical composition to VitD-low, supplemented with 5 IU VitD (cholecalciferol)/g]. The composition of the diets was based on the study those described by Spach and Hayes (41) and was prepared by Harlan-Teklad (WI, USA), designated by the following company product numbers: VitD-low, TD.10837; VitD-high, TD.140867.

Induction and Evaluation of EAE

EAE was induced in B6 and B6.Chr^{PWD} consomic mice using the 2× MOG35-55/CFA protocol, as previously described (63). Mice were injected subcutaneously with 0.1 ml of emulsion containing 0.1 mg of myelin oligodendrocyte glycoprotein peptide 35–55 (MOG_{35-55}) peptide (Anaspec Inc., MA, USA) in PBS and 50% complete Freund's adjuvant (CFA; Sigma, USA) on day 0 on the lower flanks (50 μl per flank), followed by an identical injection on upper flanks on day 7. CFA was supplemented with 4 mg/ml *Mycobacterium tuberculosis* H37Ra (Difco, USA). EAE was induced in PWD mice using the following modifications to the protocol above, as previously described (50). Mice were injected subcutaneously with 0.1 ml of emulsion containing 2.5 mg of MSCH in PBS and 50% CFA on day 0 and day 7. On day 0 and day 2, mice also received an i.p. injection of 200 ng pertussis toxin (List Laboratories, USA) as an ancillary adjuvant.

Starting on day 10, mice were scored visually, as follows: 1—partial loss of tail tone, 2—full loss of tail tone, 3—loss of tail tone and weakened hind limbs, 4—hind limb paralysis, 5—hind limb paralysis and incontinence, and 6—quadriplegia or death. EAE scoring was performed by a non-biased observer. EAE quantitative traits were calculated essentially as previously described (64), as follows. The incidence of EAE was recorded as positive for any mouse with clinical signs of EAE (clinical score ≥1) for two or more consecutive days. CDS was calculated as the sum of all daily scores over the course of 30 days. Days affected was calculated as the number of days an animal displayed a clinical score ≥1 for at least two consecutive days. Day of onset was the day a clinical score ≥1 was first observed (not calculated for animals without clinical signs for at least two consecutive days). Severity index was generated by averaging the clinical scores for each animal over the number of days that it exhibited clinical symptoms (unaffected animals were included as 0). Peak score represents the maximum daily score (unaffected animals were included as 0).

Cell Sorting and RNA Isolation

B6 and PWD mice were subjected to the dietary paradigms, as described in Section "Results." At 5 weeks post-dietary intervention, mice were euthanized, and spleens were collected. Spleens were digested using Spleen Dissociation Medium (STEMCELL Technologies, Inc., Canada). B cells were depleted using the EasySep B cell positive selection kit and EasySep magnet (STEMCELL Technologies, Inc., Canada). The remaining cells were purified by FACS using fluorophore-conjugated antibodies against cell surface markers as follows: CD4 (Tconv) cells ($CD19^-$ $TCR\beta^+$ $CD4^+$ $CD8^-$ $CD25^-$) and Tregs ($CD19^-$ $TCR\beta^+$ $CD4^+$ $CD8^-$ $CD25^+$). Dead cells were excluded using the Far Red Live-Dead staining kit (Thermo Fisher Scientific, USA). Antibodies were purchased from BioLegend, Inc. (San Diego, CA, USA); catalog numbers were as follows: CD19, CD4, CD25, CD8, CD11b, CD11c, and TCRβ; 115534, 100531, 102016, 101206, 117319, and 109222, respectively. RNA was isolated using the Qiagen RNeasy Mini or Micro Kits. RNA quality was assessed using the Agilent Bioanalyzer 2100, and samples were selected for downstream analysis based on RNA integrity number (typically 6–9). RNA quantity was determined using Qubit Fluorometric Quantification (Thermo Fisher Scientific, USA). Four biological replicates (individual mice) for each strain, sex, and diet combination were selected.

Transcriptional Profiling

For transcriptional profiling, microarray analysis was performed at the UVM Cancer Center Genomics Facility using the Mouse Affymetrix Clariom D Genechip and the GeneChip™ WT Pico Target Preparation reagent kit (Thermo Fisher Scientific 9026220) as described by the manufactures procedures. Briefly, 5 ng of RNA was used to synthesize cDNA through a First-Strand and Second-Strand reverse transcription reaction followed by conversion to cRNA through an overnight T7 InvitroTranscription reaction. The resulting cRNA was purified and 5.5 μg was converted to sense, single-strand cDNA using UDG (10 U/μL) and APE1 (1,000 U/μL), provided in the GeneChip® WT PLUS Reagent Kit. cDNA was end labeled with biotin using TdT (30 U/μL), and used as input for the hybridization mix for the GeneChip. Mouse Clariom D arrays were incubated in the Affymetrix® GeneChip® Hybridization Oven 645 at 45°C/60 RPM for 16–18 h. Arrays were stained using the Affymetrix® GeneChip® staining reagents and scanned with the 7 G Affymetrix® GeneChip® Scanner 3000.

Statistical Analyses of Microarray Data

Raw intensity CEL files were imported into Expression Console software (Affymetrix, USA), and CHP files were generated for gene level analysis. CHP files were imported into Transcriptome Analysis Console (TAC) software v4.0.0.25 (Affymetrix, USA), and gene level expression analysis was performed using the default ANOVA settings (e-Bayesian method), analyzing Tconv and Treg data separately. The following comparison variables were used: strain (B6, PWD), sex (male, female), diet (VitD-high, VitD-low), as well as a batch variable (cDNA samples were processed and scanned in batches over several different days). To detect DE genes as a function of VitD status, pairwise comparisons were done between VitD-high and VitD-low groups for the following sample groupings: (all mice together, B6 females only, B6 males only, PWD females only, and PWD males only). All raw microarray data have been deposited into the Gene Expression Omnibus database, accession number GSE116457.

Bioinformatic Analyses

Pathway analysis was performed using Ingenuity Pathway Analysis™ (IPA; Qiagen, Inc., USA) software. The gene expression datasets were exported from TAC software and uploaded into IPA. A relaxed cutoff filter of $|FC| > 1.5$ and ANOVA $p < 0.05$ was used to maximize the number of genes in the analysis (recommended by IPA to enhance the analysis power and accuracy). The IPA Core Analysis function, followed by the Comparison Analysis function was used to compare the effect of VitD across the four strain-sex combinations (B6 females, B6 males, PWD females, and PWD male), as follows. The Canonical Pathway function was used to identify the top canonical pathways ($p < 0.01$, Z-score $> |2|$) affected by the DE genes between VitD-high and VitD-low conditions. The sign and magnitude of the Z-scores are indicative of the predicted strength and direction of the VitD-high effect. The upstream regulator analysis function was similarly used to predict Z-scores and p-values for putative upstream regulators.

Enrichment analysis of VitD-regulated genes compared with genes DE in CD4 T cells in MS as performed as follows. The list of transcripts reported to be upregulated in CD4 T cells from MS-CIS subjects vs. controls (53) was imported into IPA. The Core Analysis function was used to determine the significance of enrichment of VitD DE genes within the MS-CIS list.

Serum 25(OH)D and Ca^{2+} Measurements

Whole blood was collected at the indicated time points, allowed to coagulate for 30 min at room temperature, followed by centrifugation and collection of serum. Sera were stored at −80°C prior to analysis. 25(OH)D levels were determined using a commercially available enzyme-linked immunoassay kit (ImmunoDiagnosticSystems, Inc., MD, USA), which detects $25(OH)D_3$ and $25(OH)D_2$. Sera from mice on the high VitD diet were diluted 1:10 with PBS + 1% BSA prior to analysis, to maintain readings within the range of the standard curve. Kit-supplied standards were used with 4-parameter logistic regression to determine concentrations in unknown samples.

Serum Ca^{2+} measurements were performed at the University of Vermont Medical Center Clinical Chemistry laboratory.

Statistical Analyses

Statistical analyses not pertaining to microarray data were carried out using GraphPad Prism software, version 6. Details of the analyses are provided in the figure legends and below. All statistical tests were two-sided, and adjustments for multiple comparisons were made as indicated. All center values represent the mean, and error bars represent the SEM. p-Values below 0.05 were considered significant. Sample sizes for animal experiments were chosen based on previous experience with similar analyses. Animals were randomly assigned to different treatment groups (diet), assigning littermates to both groups evenly, whenever possible. For some consomic strains, sample sizes studied were lower due to inadequate breeding performance.

Analyses of EAE clinical scores were performed as follows. Clinical disease time course was analyzed for the effect of diet (VitD) for each strain, using two-way repeated measures ANOVA. The effect of diet was considered significant when a significant strain and/or strain × time interaction term was observed. The latter term is shown in the figures and tables, to indicate overall significance of effect of diet on overall EAE course.

The relationship between serum 25(OH)D levels and EAE severity was determined as follows. First, a weighted difference in EAE severity was calculated, using CDS, as a single quantitative measure of overall disease severity and duration. For each strain, the diet-driven change in CDS was calculated by substracting the mean CDS for the VitD-high diet from the mean CDS for the VitD-low diet. Since the absolute CDS varied significantly across strains independent of VitD, this change was normalized by dividing by the overall mean CDS for that strain:

$$\text{Normalized change in EAE CDS} = \frac{CDS_{\text{VitD-low}} - CDS_{\text{VitD-high}}}{\text{mean } CDS_{\text{VitD-low+high}}}.$$

Because serum 25(OH)D levels varied by strain, to determine the relative serum 25(OH)D response to diet, a ranked change was calculated for each strain, as follows. 25(OH)D3 levels were ranked for across the consomic strains separately for VitD-high and VitD-low diets. For each strain, the ranked change in 25(OH)D as a function of diet was calculated by substracting the ranked 25(OH)D for the VitD-high diet from the ranked 25(OH)D for the VitD-low diet:

$$\text{Ranked change in 25(OH)D} = \text{ranked } 25(OH)D_{\text{VitD-low}} - \text{ranked } 25(OH)D_{\text{VitD-high}}.$$

Subsequently, linear regression was used to determine measure the association between the ranked 25(OH)D3 response and normalized EAE response. R^2 and the significance for the slope not being equal to zero were calculated as a measure of strength of association.

Differential Expression Analyses of VitD-Related Genes in B6 and PWD Mice

Differential expression data were obtained from the Gene Expression Miner database from Jackson Laboratories (http://cgd.jax.org/gem/strainsurvey26/v1), which contains microarray data from a gene expression survey across 26 inbred strains of mice, in 4 tissues: spleen, liver, and left and right kidneys. The data set included data on 12 C57BL/6J mice (6 females and 6 males), and 11 PWD/PhJ mice (6 females and 5 males). Log2-normalized gene expression data were downloaded for the following genes of interest: *Gc*, *Dhcr7*, *Cyp2r1*, *Cyp24a1*, *Cyp27a1*, *Cyp27b1*, and *Vdr*. *Gc* and *Cyp2r1* did not show appreciable levels of expression in any of the tissues, and thus were not analyzed further. The rest of the gene expression data were analyzed in Graphpad Prism, version 6, as detailed in the figure legends.

AUTHOR CONTRIBUTIONS

DK and CT designed experiments. DK, LA, and CT analyzed data and wrote manuscript. DK, QF, and MM performed experiments and analyzed data.

FUNDING

This work was supported by the following grants: RG-5170A6/1 from the National Multiple Sclerosis Society (NMSS) to CT, R21 NS095007 from NIH/NINDS to CT, and R01 NS097596 from NIH/NINDS to DK. Additionally, the research performed at the VGN microarray facility was partially supported by an Institutional Development Award (IDeA) from the National Institute of General Medical Sciences (NIGMS) of the National Institutes of Health under grant number P20GM103449, and research performed at the Flow Cytometry and Cell Sorting Facility was partially supported by NIGMS P20GM103496. The manuscript's contents are solely the responsibility of the authors and do not necessarily represent the official views of NIGMS or NIH.

REFERENCES

1. Hollenbach JA, Oksenberg JR. The immunogenetics of multiple sclerosis: a comprehensive review. *J Autoimmun* (2015) 64:13–25. doi:10.1016/j.jaut.2015.06.010
2. Baranzini SE, Oksenberg JR. The genetics of multiple sclerosis: from 0 to 200 in 50 years. *Trends Genet* (2017) 33(12):960–70. doi:10.1016/j.tig.2017.09.004
3. Ebers GC. Environmental factors and multiple sclerosis. *Lancet Neurol* (2008) 7(3):268–77. doi:10.1016/S1474-4422(08)70042-5
4. Disanto G, Morahan JM, Ramagopalan SV. Multiple sclerosis: risk factors and their interactions. *CNS Neurol Disord Drug Targets* (2012) 11(5):545–55. doi:10.2174/187152712801661266
5. Plum LA, DeLuca HF. Vitamin D, disease and therapeutic opportunities. *Nat Rev Drug Discov* (2010) 9(12):941–55. doi:10.1038/nrd3318
6. Munger KL, Levin LI, Hollis BW, Howard NS, Ascherio A. Serum 25-hydroxyvitamin D levels and risk of multiple sclerosis. *JAMA* (2006) 296(23):2832–8. doi:10.1001/jama.296.23.2832
7. Smolders J, Menheere P, Kessels A, Damoiseaux J, Hupperts R. Association of vitamin D metabolite levels with relapse rate and disability in multiple sclerosis. *Mult Scler* (2008) 14(9):1220–4. doi:10.1177/1352458508094399
8. Ascherio A, Munger KL, White R, Kochert K, Simon KC, Polman CH, et al. Vitamin D as an early predictor of multiple sclerosis activity and progression. *JAMA Neurol* (2014) 71(3):306–14. doi:10.1001/jamaneurol.2013.5993
9. Ramagopalan SV, Heger A, Berlanga AJ, Maugeri NJ, Lincoln MR, Burrell A, et al. A ChIP-seq defined genome-wide map of vitamin D receptor binding: associations with disease and evolution. *Genome Res* (2010) 20(10):1352–60. doi:10.1101/gr.107920.110
10. Berlanga-Taylor AJ, Disanto G, Ebers GC, Ramagopalan SV. Vitamin D-gene interactions in multiple sclerosis. *J Neurol Sci* (2011) 311(1–2):32–6. doi:10.1016/j.jns.2011.08.041
11. Mokry LE, Ross S, Ahmad OS, Forgetta V, Smith GD, Goltzman D, et al. Vitamin D and risk of multiple sclerosis: a Mendelian Randomization Study. *PLoS Med* (2015) 12(8):e1001866. doi:10.1371/journal.pmed.1001866
12. Rhead B, Baarnhielm M, Gianfrancesco M, Mok A, Shao X, Quach H, et al. Mendelian randomization shows a causal effect of low vitamin D on multiple sclerosis risk. *Neurol Genet* (2016) 2(5):e97. doi:10.1212/NXG.0000000000000097
13. Gianfrancesco MA, Stridh P, Rhead B, Shao X, Xu E, Graves JS, et al. Evidence for a causal relationship between low vitamin D, high BMI, and pediatric-onset MS. *Neurology* (2017) 88(17):1623–9. doi:10.1212/WNL.0000000000003849
14. Ozerlat I. Multiple sclerosis: multiple sclerosis therapy – vitamin D under spotlight. *Nat Rev Neurol* (2012) 8(4):177. doi:10.1038/nrneurol.2012.37
15. Stein MS, Liu Y, Gray OM, Baker JE, Kolbe SC, Ditchfield MR, et al. A randomized trial of high-dose vitamin D2 in relapsing-remitting multiple sclerosis. *Neurology* (2011) 77(17):1611–8. doi:10.1212/WNL.0b013e3182343274
16. Kampman MT, Steffensen LH, Mellgren SI, Jorgensen L. Effect of vitamin D3 supplementation on relapses, disease progression, and measures of function in persons with multiple sclerosis: exploratory outcomes from a double-blind randomised controlled trial. *Mult Scler* (2012) 18(8):1144–51. doi:10.1177/1352458511434607
17. James E, Dobson R, Kuhle J, Baker D, Giovannoni G, Ramagopalan SV. The effect of vitamin D-related interventions on multiple sclerosis relapses: a meta-analysis. *Mult Scler* (2013) 19(12):1571–9. doi:10.1177/1352458513489756
18. Hart PH, Gorman S, Finlay-Jones JJ. Modulation of the immune system by UV radiation: more than just the effects of vitamin D? *Nat Rev Immunol* (2011) 11(9):584–96. doi:10.1038/nri3045
19. Breuer J, Schwab N, Schneider-Hohendorf T, Marziniak M, Mohan H, Bhatia U, et al. Ultraviolet B light attenuates the systemic immune response in central nervous system autoimmunity. *Ann Neurol* (2014) 75(5):739–58. doi:10.1002/ana.24165
20. Lucas RM, Ponsonby AL, Dear K, Valery PC, Pender MP, Taylor BV, et al. Sun exposure and vitamin D are independent risk factors for CNS demyelination. *Neurology* (2011) 76(6):540–8. doi:10.1212/WNL.0b013e31820af93d
21. Baarnhielm M, Hedstrom AK, Kockum I, Sundqvist E, Gustafsson SA, Hillert J, et al. Sunlight is associated with decreased multiple sclerosis risk: no interaction with human leukocyte antigen-DRB1*15. *Eur J Neurol* (2012) 19(7):955–62. doi:10.1111/j.1468-1331.2011.03650.x
22. Langer-Gould A, Lucas R, Xiang AH, Chen LH, Wu J, Gonzalez E, et al. MS Sunshine Study: sun exposure but not vitamin D is associated with multiple sclerosis risk in blacks and Hispanics. *Nutrients* (2018) 10(3):E268. doi:10.3390/nu10030268
23. Hauser SL, Weiner HL, Che M, Shapiro ME, Gilles F, Letvin NL. Prevention of experimental allergic encephalomyelitis (EAE) in the SJL/J mouse by whole body ultraviolet irradiation. *J Immunol* (1984) 132(3):1276–81.
24. Becklund BR, Severson KS, Vang SV, DeLuca HF. UV radiation suppresses experimental autoimmune encephalomyelitis independent of vitamin D production. *Proc Natl Acad Sci U S A* (2010) 107(14):6418–23. doi:10.1073/pnas.1001119107
25. Wang Y, Marling SJ, McKnight SM, Danielson AL, Severson KS, Deluca HF. Suppression of experimental autoimmune encephalomyelitis by 300-315nm ultraviolet light. *Arch Biochem Biophys* (2013) 536(1):81–6. doi:10.1016/j.abb.2013.05.010
26. Gelfand JM, Cree BA, McElroy J, Oksenberg J, Green R, Mowry EM, et al. Vitamin D in African Americans with multiple sclerosis. *Neurology* (2011) 76(21):1824–30. doi:10.1212/WNL.0b013e31821cccf5
27. Amezcua L, Chung RH, Conti DV, Langer-Gould AM. Vitamin D levels in Hispanics with multiple sclerosis. *J Neurol* (2012) 259(12):2565–70. doi:10.1007/s00415-012-6537-z
28. Espinosa-Ramirez G, Ordonez G, Flores-Rivera J, Sotelo J. Sunlight exposure and multiple sclerosis in a tropical country. *Neurol Res* (2014) 36(7):647–50. doi:10.1179/1743132813Y.0000000307
29. Rito Y, Flores J, Fernandez-Aguilar A, Escalante-Membrillo C, Barboza MA,

Amezcua L, et al. Vitamin D and disability in relapsing-remitting multiple sclerosis in patients with a Mexican background. *Acta Neurol Belg* (2018) 118(1):47–52. doi:10.1007/s13760-017-0834-3

30. Langer-Gould A, Lucas RM, Xiang AH, Wu J, Chen LH, Gonzales E, et al. Vitamin D-binding protein polymorphisms, 25-hydroxyvitamin D, sunshine and multiple sclerosis. *Nutrients* (2018) 10(2):E184. doi:10.3390/nu10020184
31. Powe CE, Evans MK, Wenger J, Zonderman AB, Berg AH, Nalls M, et al. Vitamin D-binding protein and vitamin D status of black Americans and white Americans. *N Engl J Med* (2013) 369(21):1991–2000. doi:10.1056/NEJMoa1306357
32. Simmons SB, Pierson ER, Lee SY, Goverman JM. Modeling the heterogeneity of multiple sclerosis in animals. *Trends Immunol* (2013) 34(8):410–22. doi:10.1016/j.it.2013.04.006
33. Lemire JM, Archer DC. 1,25-Dihydroxyvitamin D3 prevents the in vivo induction of murine experimental autoimmune encephalomyelitis. *J Clin Invest* (1991) 87(3):1103–7. doi:10.1172/JCI115072
34. Cantorna MT, Hayes CE, DeLuca HF. 1,25-Dihydroxyvitamin D3 reversibly blocks the progression of relapsing encephalomyelitis, a model of multiple sclerosis. *Proc Natl Acad Sci U S A* (1996) 93(15):7861–4. doi:10.1073/pnas.93.15.7861
35. Mayne CG, Spanier JA, Relland LM, Williams CB, Hayes CE. 1,25-Dihydroxyvitamin D3 acts directly on the T lymphocyte vitamin D receptor to inhibit experimental autoimmune encephalomyelitis. *Eur J Immunol* (2011) 41(3):822–32. doi:10.1002/eji.201040632
36. Spanier JA, Nashold FE, Olson JK, Hayes CE. The IFNg gene is essential for VDR gene expression and vitamin D(3)-mediated reduction of the pathogenic T cell burden in the central nervous system in experimental autoimmune encephalomyelitis, a multiple sclerosis model. *J Immunol* (2012) 189(6):3188–97. doi:10.4049/jimmunol.1102925
37. Nashold FE, Nelson CD, Brown LM, Hayes CE. One calcitriol dose transiently increases Helios+ FoxP3+ T cells and ameliorates autoimmune demyelinating disease. *J Neuroimmunol* (2013) 263(1–2):64–74. doi:10.1016/j.jneuroim.2013.07.016
38. Hayes CE, Hubler SL, Moore JR, Barta LE, Praska CE, Nashold FE. Vitamin D Actions on CD4(+) T cells in autoimmune disease. *Front Immunol* (2015) 6:100. doi:10.3389/fimmu.2015.00100
39. Cantorna MT, Humpal-Winter J, DeLuca HF. Dietary calcium is a major factor in 1,25-dihydroxycholecalciferol suppression of experimental autoimmune encephalomyelitis in mice. *J Nutr* (1999) 129(11):1966–71. doi:10.1093/jn/129.11.1966
40. Meehan TF, Vanhooke J, Prahl J, Deluca HF. Hypercalcemia produced by parathyroid hormone suppresses experimental autoimmune encephalomyelitis in female but not male mice. *Arch Biochem Biophys* (2005) 442(2):214–21. doi:10.1016/j.abb.2005.08.011
41. Spach KM, Hayes CE. Vitamin D3 confers protection from autoimmune encephalomyelitis only in female mice. *J Immunol* (2005) 175(6):4119–26. doi:10.4049/jimmunol.175.6.4119
42. Nashold FE, Spach KM, Spanier JA, Hayes CE. Estrogen controls vitamin D3-mediated resistance to experimental autoimmune encephalomyelitis by controlling vitamin D3 metabolism and receptor expression. *J Immunol* (2009) 183(6):3672–81. doi:10.4049/jimmunol.0901351
43. Adzemovic MZ, Zeitelhofer M, Hochmeister S, Gustafsson SA, Jagodic M. Efficacy of vitamin D in treating multiple sclerosis-like neuroinflammation depends on developmental stage. *Exp Neurol* (2013) 249:39–48. doi:10.1016/j.expneurol.2013.08.002
44. Zeitelhofer M, Adzemovic MZ, Gomez-Cabrero D, Bergman P, Hochmeister S, N'Diaye M, et al. Functional genomics analysis of vitamin D effects on CD4+ T cells in vivo in experimental autoimmune encephalomyelitis. *Proc Natl Acad Sci U S A* (2017) 114(9):E1678–87. doi:10.1073/pnas.1615783114
45. Krementsov DN, Teuscher C. Environmental factors acting during development to influence MS risk: insights from animal studies. *Mult Scler* (2013) 19(13):1684–9. doi:10.1177/1352458513506954
46. Guenet JL, Bonhomme F. Wild mice: an ever-increasing contribution to a popular mammalian model. *Trends Genet* (2003) 19(1):24–31. doi:10.1016/S0168-9525(02)00007-0
47. Chang PL, Kopania E, Keeble S, Sarver BAJ, Larson E, Orth A, et al. Whole exome sequencing of wild-derived inbred strains of mice improves power to link phenotype and genotype. *Mamm Genome* (2017) 28(9–10):416–25. doi:10.1007/s00335-017-9704-9
48. Gregorova S, Divina P, Storchova R, Trachtulec Z, Fotopulosova V, Svenson KL, et al. Mouse consomic strains: exploiting genetic divergence between *Mus m. musculus* and *Mus m domesticus* subspecies. *Genome Res* (2008) 18(3):509–15. doi:10.1101/gr.7160508
49. Gregorova S, Forejt J. PWD/Ph and PWK/Ph inbred mouse strains of *Mus m. musculus* subspecies – a valuable resource of phenotypic variations and genomic polymorphisms. *Folia Biol* (2000) 46(1):31–41.
50. Bearoff F, Del Rio R, Case LK, Dragon JA, Nguyen-Vu T, Lin CY, et al. Natural genetic variation profoundly regulates gene expression in immune cells and dictates susceptibility to CNS autoimmunity. *Genes Immun* (2016) 17(7):386–95. doi:10.1038/gene.2016.37
51. Bearoff F, Case LK, Krementsov DN, Wall EH, Saligrama N, Blankenhorn EP, et al. Identification of genetic determinants of the sexual dimorphism in CNS autoimmunity. *PLoS One* (2015) 10(2):e0117993. doi:10.1371/journal.pone.0117993
52. Krementsov DN, Noubade R, Dragon JA, Otsu K, Rincon M, Teuscher C. Sex-specific control of central nervous system autoimmunity by p38 mitogen-activated protein kinase signaling in myeloid cells. *Ann Neurol* (2014) 75(1):50–66. doi:10.1002/ana.24020
53. Corvol JC, Pelletier D, Henry RG, Caillier SJ, Wang J, Pappas D, et al. Abrogation of T cell quiescence characterizes patients at high risk for multiple sclerosis after the initial neurological event. *Proc Natl Acad Sci U S A* (2008) 105(33):11839–44. doi:10.1073/pnas.0805065105
54. Wang TJ, Zhang F, Richards JB, Kestenbaum B, van Meurs JB, Berry D, et al. Common genetic determinants of vitamin D insufficiency: a genome-wide association study. *Lancet* (2010) 376(9736):180–8. doi:10.1016/S0140-6736(10)60588-0
55. Zhu J, DeLuca HF. Vitamin D 25-hydroxylase – four decades of searching, are we there yet? *Arch Biochem Biophys* (2012) 523(1):30–6. doi:10.1016/j.abb.2012.01.013
56. Olsson T, Barcellos LF, Alfredsson L. Interactions between genetic, lifestyle and environmental risk factors for multiple sclerosis. *Nat Rev Neurol* (2017) 13(1):25–36. doi:10.1038/nrneurol.2016.187
57. Clayton DG. Prediction and interaction in complex disease genetics: experience in type 1 diabetes. *PLoS Genet* (2009) 5(7):e1000540. doi:10.1371/journal.pgen.1000540
58. Sintzel MB, Rametta M, Reder AT. Vitamin D and multiple sclerosis: a comprehensive review. *Neurol Ther* (2018) 7(1):59–85. doi:10.1007/s40120-017-0086-4
59. Avasarala J, Zachariah P. Vitamin D deficiency in multiple sclerosis: should testing and treatment be based on racial background? *J Neurol Sci* (2015) 358(1–2):417–8. doi:10.1016/j.jns.2015.08.018
60. DeLuca HF, Plum LA. Vitamin D deficiency diminishes the severity and delays onset of experimental autoimmune encephalomyelitis. *Arch Biochem Biophys* (2011) 513(2):140–3. doi:10.1016/j.abb.2011.07.005
61. Fernandes de Abreu DA, Ibrahim EC, Boucraut J, Khrestchatisky M, Feron F. Severity of experimental autoimmune encephalomyelitis is unexpectedly reduced in mice born to vitamin D-deficient mothers. *J Steroid Biochem Mol Biol* (2010) 121(1–2):250–3. doi:10.1016/j.jsbmb.2010.03.006
62. Wang Y, Marling SJ, Zhu JG, Severson KS, DeLuca HF. Development of experimental autoimmune encephalomyelitis (EAE) in mice requires vitamin D and the vitamin D receptor. *Proc Natl Acad Sci U S A* (2012) 109(22):8501–4. doi:10.1073/pnas.1206054109
63. Krementsov DN, Case LK, Hickey WF, Teuscher C. Exacerbation of autoimmune neuroinflammation by dietary sodium is genetically controlled and sex specific. *FASEB J* (2015) 29(8):3446–57. doi:10.1096/fj.15-272542

17

Pregnancy Outcomes in Men and Women Treated With Teriflunomide: A Population-Based Nationwide Danish Register Study

Johanna Balslev Andersen [1]*, *Julie Yoon Moberg* [1], *Tim Spelman* [1] *and Melinda Magyari* [1,2]

[1] *Danish Multiple Sclerosis Registry, Department of Neurology, Copenhagen University Hospital, Rigshospitalet, Denmark,*
[2] *Department of Neurology, Danish Multiple Sclerosis Center, Copenhagen University Hospital, Rigshospitalet, Denmark*

***Correspondence:**
Johanna Balslev Andersen
johanna.balslev.andersen@regionh.dk

Background: The majority of persons diagnosed with multiple sclerosis (MS) experience their first MS symptoms in the reproductive age. Teriflunomide (TFL, Aubagio), was first released in Denmark for relapsing-remitting MS in December 2013. TFL treatment is contraindicated in women of childbearing potential who are not using reliable contraception. TFL can be transmitted via semen and a low risk of male-mediated embryo-fetal toxicity is described.

Objective: To report pregnancy outcomes of TFL-treated women and partners to TFL-treated men: gestation week.

Methods: Prospective cohort study comparing pregnancy outcomes of TFL-treated men and women, matched on age at conception, 1:4 with controls from the general population. Data on TFL-treated patients treated 1st of January 2014–31st of December 2016 for at least 30 consecutive days prior to conception, and with conception occurring latest 2 years after treatment discontinuation were extracted from The Danish Multiple Sclerosis Registry and merged with several national reproductive registries. Logistic regression was used to analyse the association between TFL exposure and any adverse event.

Results: A total of 31 pregnancies were recorded, 13 women and 18 of partners to a TFL-treated man. All 18 partners of TFL-treated men completed their pregnancies: livebirth (18), gestation time >37 weeks (17), gestation time 33–36 weeks (1), normal birth weight (18), spontaneous and elective abortion (0), congenital malformation (plagiocephali) (1), normal delivery (14), induced delivery (2), cesarean section (2), Apgar score ≥7 (18). Among the 13 pregnancies in women exposed to TFL: elective abortion (11), spontaneous abortion (0), livebirth (2), gestation time >37 weeks (2), normal birth weight (2), congenital malformations (0), normal delivery (1), induced delivery (1), Apgar score ≥7 (2). The TFL group was associated with a 22% reduction in the odds of any adverse event relative to controls, although this association was not significant (OR 0.78; 95% CI 0.16–3.72, $p = 0.753$).

Conclusion: Pregnancy outcomes were consistent with those of the general population. The malformation reported of the partner to a TFL-treated man is comparable to the rate of plagiocephaly reported in Denmark.

Keywords: teriflunomide, pregnancy-related outcomes, nationwide Danish register study, teriflunomide treated men and women, pregnancy-related outcomes for mother and child

INTRODUCTION

Multiple sclerosis (MS) is a progressive chronic neurological disease manifesting in two main phenotypes, relapse-remitting (RR) and primary progressive course. Approximately 85% of MS patients have a RR onset with recurring acute relapses over a period of decades, transitioning at some point to a progressive, secondary phase with or without relapses (1). MS occurs more frequently in women than men, and the mean age in recent years at onset according to the Danish Multiple Sclerosis Registry (DMSR) is 35.5 years [standard deviation (SD) 10.5] for men and 34.6 (SD 10.7) for women, which means the majority of the patients is in their reproductive years at disease onset.

Teriflunomide (TFL) is a once-daily oral immunomodulator, which was approved for the treatment of RRMS in the European Union in 2013. TFL is a first-line disease-modifying therapy (DMT) with prolonged half-life. Over 21 days, 60.1% of the administered dose is excreted but it may be detectable up to 2 years after discontinuation. The elimination of TFL from the circulation can be expedited using an accelerated elimination procedure (AEP) (2). Based on animal studies, TFL is contraindicated in women who are planning pregnancy due to the occurrence of teratogenicity and embryo lethality in rats and rabbits (3, 4). TFL can be detected in human semen, but the risk of male-mediated embryo fetal toxicity through TFL-treatment is considered low (5). In the United States, the Food and Drug Administration (FDA) advises men to use barrier contraception to prevent the active substance from transferring to their female partner and potentially her fetus. This has not been a requirement in Europe. A recent report (6) presenting post-marketing and clinical study data on 231 female MS patients with TFL-exposed pregnancies (with known outcomes in 129) found no evidence of a teratogenic signal, although three structural abnormalities were reported. Exposure to TFL among the majority of these women had been limited to the first trimester since patients were recommended to undergo an AEP in case of conception.

After discovering the teratogenic link between thalidomide and malformations in more than 10,000 children worldwide, registries were founded to facilitate epidemiological research and surveillance concerning causes of congenital malformation due to genetic, environmental, or medical exposures. Congenital malformations, such as spontaneous abortions, pre-mature birth, physical anomalies, or neurobehavioral outcomes can indicate adverse pregnancy outcomes linked to teratogenic exposure.

The objective of our study was to investigate pregnancy-related outcomes in in TFL-treated female MS patients, in women whose sexual male partners are MS patients treated with TFL registered in the DMSR, and in the new-born of such. Furthermore, we want to investigate any association between TFL exposure during pregnancy and adverse pregnancy-related events.

MATERIALS AND METHODS

Registries

All Danish citizens have access to universal health care, which is government-funded through taxation. Most Danish registries have existed for decades, and they are nationwide and population-based, and which provide an excellent foundation for epidemiological research. Persons residing in Denmark have a unique 10 digit ID-number (Civil Registration Number CPR) which can be used to identify and merge data from all Danish registries (7).

The Danish Multiple Sclerosis Registry (DMSR)

The DMSR was established in 1956 and contains data on all Danes who have been diagnosed by a neurologist as having MS. Data are collected continuously and provide information on a number of baseline and clinical variables (8). Since 1996, a mandatory notification of all MS patients treated with a DMT has been carried out, thus ensuring a high level of data completeness. The registry contains baseline and clinical information on all Danish MS patients with year of onset and diagnosis, disease course, information on DMT, treatment start, treatment stop, previous DMTs and current DMT in addition to first clinical symptom, diagnosis (phenotype), relapses, and Expanded Disability Status Scale (EDSS) (8).

The Danish Medical Birth Register (DMBR)

The DMBR was established in 1973 and was reconstructed and updated in 1997. The register monitors the health of pregnant women and contains data on all births in Denmark. Several sources feed data into DMBR, such as the Danish National Patient Registry, the Danish Civil Registration System, and data on stillbirths and home deliveries. Data on the mother include height, weight, age, smoking status, and several variables related to the birth, such as pregnancy and birth complications, parity, infection, pain relief during labor, cesarean section, induction of labor etc. In relation to the new-born, it contains a variety of information including sex, gestational age, congenital malformations, Apgar score after 5 min, height, weight, head circumference, and birth status (live birth/stillborn) (9).

The Danish National Patient Registry (DNPR)

The DNPR registers every individual episode of a person's contact with hospitals and outpatient clinics in Denmark. It contains multiple information including date of visit, type of contact, examinations, admission type, tests, surgery, treatment, diagnosis, residence, and hospital visited. Diagnoses, surgery, other treatment, anesthesia, and examinations are provided with a code that translates to the standard coding system of the International Coding of Diseases (ICD) (10). The DNPR provides data for several other registries in Denmark including the DMBR and The Register of Legally Induced Abortions. All Danish regions report data to the DNPR, and data are updated at least monthly.

The Register of Legally-Induced Abortions (RLIA)

The RLIA was established in 1973 when abortion before the end of gestation week 12 became legal in Denmark. The data are mainly from the DNPR, but also includes data from specialized clinicians who carry out legal abortions. Data from the RLIA contain a variety of information including age of the woman, gestational week, prior abortion, type of procedure, legal reason for abortion, complications and admission date (11).

Data Collection

This study was a cohort study comparing outcomes of TFL-treated female MS patients and partners to TFL-treated male patients using prospectively collected nationwide data from the DMSR. The TFL-treated men and women were matched at age of conception 1:4 with controls from the general population. Patients were included from 1st of January 2014 until 31st of December 2016. Included patients should have a confirmed MS diagnosis according to the McDonald criteria, treatment start date with TFL at least 30 consecutive days prior to conception, and conception occurring at the latest 2 years after discontinuation of TFL. The data were merged with the Danish Medical Birth Register, Danish National Patient Registry, and the Register of Legally-Induced Abortions by a unique personal identification number.

In Denmark, pre-term birth is defined as birth before gestation week 37 as described in the literature (12–14). Low birth weight in relation to gestational age was based on the Danish guidelines from the Department of Neonatology, Copenhagen University Hospital (15). Low birthweight for children born after week 37 is defined as a birthweight <2,500 g, and low birthweight for children born week 33–36 is defined as a birthweight <2,300 g.

Registration of congenital malformations in Denmark is reported and registered at birth and up to 1 year after birth to allow for delayed identification, as some anomalies are undiagnosed until sometimes after birth e.g., congenital heart disease.

The Apgar score has been used since 1952 and is a quick way to assess the postnatal condition of the new-born. The perspective is to assess for asphyxia, as well as, determine the risk of neurological deficits (16). The assessment is comprised of five components with a maximum of total 10 points, where 7–10 points is considered "reassuring" of normality.

Controls

The reference cohort was selected randomly from the general population using the Danish Civil Registration System (7), and pregnant women were chosen as controls. We sampled four controls per one TFL-treated man or woman matched by age at conception. Matching of the control population for the female partners of TFL-treated men was done by the age of the man at conception, due to lack of availability of information on the female partners of TFL-treated men.

Statistical Analysis

Categorical variables were summarized using frequency and percentage. Continuous variables were summarized using mean and standard deviation (SD) or median and interquartile range (IQR) as appropriate. Logistic regression was used to analyse the association between TFL-treated patients and any adverse event (defined as congenital malformation, spontaneous abortion, pre-term birth, or Apgar score <7), relative to the control group. A Hosmer & Lemeshow test was used to assess the logistic regression for goodness-of-fit. For all statistical comparisons, $p < 0.05$ was considered significant. All analysis was conducted using SAS version 9.4 (SAS Institute Inc., Cary, NC, USA).

RESULTS

A total of 2,450 TFL-treated patients with MS were identified through the DMSR, of which 31 (18 men and 13 women) met all inclusion criteria. The women had a mean age of 26.6 years (SD 4.9) when diagnosed with MS and 28.5 years (SD 4.7) at conception, while the men had a mean age of 30.7 years (SD 6.7) at diagnosis and 34.1 years (SD 3.9) at conception (**Tables 1, 2**). In the female study group, 7 of 13 (53.8%) were being treated with

TABLE 1 | Baseline characteristics of patients in the study group $n = 31$ (MS* patients exposed to TFL** >30 consecutive days when becoming/partner becoming pregnant and up to 2 years after discontinuation of TFL treatment), and the reference group ($n = 124$).

	Study group $n = 31$		Reference group $n = 124$	
	Male	**Female**	**Male**	**Female**
N (%)	18 (59%)	13 (41%)	72 (59%)	52 (41%)
YEAR OF BIRTH, *n*				
1965–1984	16	3	64	23
1985–2002	2	10	8	29
AGE AT ONSET IN YEARS, *n*				
0–24	4	6	N/A***	N/A
25–34	11	6	N/A	N/A
35–44	3	1	N/A	N/A
Mean (min;max)sd***	29.16 (12;38)6.76	25.23 (16;36)5.18	N/A	N/A
AGE AT DIAGNOSIS IN YEARS, *n*				
0–24	2	5	N/A	N/A
25–34	9	7	N/A	N/A
35–44	7	1	N/A	N/A
Mean (min;max)sd****	30.72 (13;39)6.79	26.61 (19;37)4.91	N/A	N/A

*Multiple sclerosis.
**Teriflunomide.
***Not applicable.
****Standard deviation.

TABLE 2 | Data regarding conception within the study group $n = 31$ (MS* patients exposed to TFL** >30 consecutive days when becoming/partner becoming pregnant and up to 2 years after discontinuation of TFL treatment), and the reference group ($n = 124$).

	Study group $n = 31$		Reference group $n = 124$	
	Male ($n = 18$)	Female ($n = 13$)	Male ($n = 72$)	Female ($n = 52$)
AGE AT CONCEPTION				
19–24	0	3	0	12
25–30	3	6	13	24
31–35	10	3	40	12
36–40	3	1	12	4
>40	2	0	8	0
Mean (min;max)sd***	34.1 (27;42)3.9	28.5 (19;38)4.8	34.1 (27;42)3.9	28.5 (19;38)4.6
DURATION ON TFL AT CONCEPTION IN DAYS				
31–90	5	2	N/A****	N/A
91–180	4	3	N/A	N/A
181–365	5	1	N/A	N/A
>365	3	1	N/A	N/A
Mean (min;max)sd	198 (34;463)148.1	154 (47;380)111.3	N/A	N/A
CONCEPTION AFTER TREATMENT STOP IN DAYS				
31–90	0	1	N/A	N/A
91–180	0	1	N/A	N/A
181–365	1	2	N/A	N/A
366–730	0	2	N/A	N/A
Mean (min;max)sd***	343	316.5 (35;688)234.8	N/A	N/A

*Mulitple sclerosis.
**Teriflunomide.
***Standard deviation.
****Not applicable.

TABLE 3 | Characteristics of delivery outcomes; namely still or live birth, abortions and delivery mode in the study group $n = 31$ (MS* patients exposed to TFL** >30 consecutive days when becoming/partner becoming pregnant and up to 2 years after discontinuation of TFL treatment), and the reference group ($n = 124$).

	Study group ($n = 31$)		Reference group ($n = 124$)	
	Male ($n = 18$)	Female ($n = 13$)	Male ($n = 72$)	Female ($n = 52$)
BIRTHS				
Still births	0	0	0	0
Live births	18	2	72	37
ABORTIONS				
Elective	0	11	0	12
Spontaneous	0	0	0	3
DELIVERY				
Normal birth singleton	14	1	42	24
Normal birth multiples	0	0	1	0
Induced	2	1	19 (1 missing)	5
CESAREAN				
Acute	2	0	5	6
Elective	0	0	4	2

*Multiple sclerosis.
**Teriflunomide.

TFL at conception, with an average treatment period of 154 days (SD 111.3). The remaining six conceived on average 316 days (SD 234.8) after discontinuation. Two TFL treated women decided to continue their pregnancy to term, one conceived 35 days after discontinuation of TFL (352 total days on TFL), and the other 95 days after discontinuation of TFL (179 total days on TFL). Only one man fathered a child after discontinuing TFL (343 days later), while the remaining 17 men had been treated with TFL an average of 198 days (SD 148.2 days) at child conception (**Table 2**).

A total of 31 pregnancies were included in the analysis, matched to 124 controls. Of the 31 pregnancies comprising the study group, 13 were women treated with TFL whilst the remaining 18 were female partners of TFL-treated men. All 18 female partners of TFL-treated men completed their pregnancies resulting in live births. Of these, 17 had a normal gestation time (>37 weeks) and one gave birth in week 36. All new-borns recorded a normal birth weight relative to gestation week, and no spontaneous or elective abortions were reported. 88.89% (16 out of 18) of the female partners to a TFL-treated man had vaginal delivery, of which two were induced, and the remaining two had cesarean section (**Table 3**). All 18 new-borns had Apgar score ≥7, and one new-born had a congenital malformation (plagiocephaly) (**Table 4**).

Among the 13 pregnant women treated with TFL, 11 (85%) chose an elective abortion. There were no reports of spontaneous abortions. Two women chose to continue the pregnancy to term, both of which resulted in live births. Both pregnancies were carried to term with normal gestation time >37 weeks, normal birth weight, one vaginal delivery, and one induced. Both new-borns had an Apgar score ≥7 with no reports of congenital malformations (**Tables 3, 4**).

The study group had two adverse events, namely one congenital malformation and one pre-term birth (week 36). The comparison group presented 14 adverse events, namely three spontaneous abortions, eight pre-term deliveries, and three congenital malformation (**Table 4**). Stillbirth has not been included as an adverse event, as no such event occurred in either of the groups. The study group was associated with a 22% reduction in the odds of any adverse event relative to controls, although this association was not significant (OR 0.78; 95% CI 0.16–3.72, $p = 0.753$).

DISCUSSION

In this nationwide population-based study, we did not find any deviations in either women or new-borns among female patients treated with TFL or in women of male partners treated with TFL in terms of spontaneous abortions, pre-term delivery (<week 37), low Apgar score (<7), or congenital malformations when compared to the general population. Elective abortions among

TABLE 4 | Characteristics of birth-related outcome; namely gestation time, birth weight in relation to gestation time, Apgar score, and congenital malformations in the study group $n = 31$ (MS* patients exposed to TFL** >30 consecutive days when becoming/partner becoming pregnant and up to 2 years after discontinuation of TFL treatment), and the reference group ($n = 124$).

	Study group ($n = 31$)		Reference group ($n = 124$)	
	Male ($n = 18$)	Female ($n = 13$)	Male ($n = 72$)	Female ($n = 52$)
GESTATION TIME				
Normal >37 weeks	17	2	67	34
Pre-term birth <37 weeks	1	0	5	3
BIRTH WEIGHT IN RELATION TO GESTATIONAL WEEK				
Normal	18	2	68	37
Low	0	0	3	0
APGAR SCORE				
Low <7	0	0	0	0
Normal ≥7	18	2	71 (1 missing)	37
CONGENITAL MALFORMATIONS				
Plagiocephaly	1	0	1	0
Cardiac septum	0	0	1	0
Respiratory system	0	0	0	1

*Multiple sclerosis.
**Teriflunomide.

women treated with TFL were unsurprisingly higher, although the two women who continued the pregnancy had healthy live births. None of the female partners of the TFL-treated men chose an elective abortion.

Overall, studies investigating the perinatal characteristics and obstetric complications in mothers with MS compared to the background population have not found any differences in either neonatal or obstetric complications (17, 18), although one study found a slightly higher rate of induced labor and cesarean delivery among women with MS than in the reference group (19).

In general, female MS patients who intend to get pregnant are advised to discontinue their DMT based on the potential risk of adverse events in relation to DMT exposure during pregnancy. However, this might result in a worsening of the disease (20).

Teriflunomide is contraindicated in women who are pregnant and women of childbearing potential who are not using effective contraception during treatment based on preclinical findings of embryotoxicty and teratogenicity in rats and rabbits when treated with clinically relevant doses of TFL. Later research showed a difference in the affinity of dihydroorotate dehydrogenase for TFL between rats and humans. Thus, TFL is a more potent inhibitor of the rat enzyme than the human enzyme, which may reflect the observed embryotoxicity and teratogenicity in rats (21–23). In Europe, it is not advised against fathering children during TFL treatment. Also, although women are required to use reliable contraception when treated with TFL, pregnancies in women treated with TFL have been reported.

In Denmark, the estimated incidence of spontaneous abortions in the general population is 13.5% (24), and the incidence of pre-mature new-born (<37 weeks) has been stable at 6% during the last 5 years based on numbers from the Danish National Birth Register (25). In this study, there were no cases of registered spontaneous abortions among the TFL study group, and one pre-term birth in the TFL-exposed group equivalent to an incidence rate of 5.5%; corresponding to that of the general population.

Previous research investigating pregnancy-related outcomes of mother and new-born in relation to TFL exposure (6, 26) reported a higher incidence rate for spontaneous abortions in the TFL-treated patients, respectively, 18.6 and 21%, respectively, than that reported for the general population in Denmark. Kieseier et al. reported a mean of gestation week 39 (range 36–44 weeks) among women treated with TFL equivalent to what is reported in this study (both >week 37).

Plagiocephaly, the congenital malformation reported in the TFL-exposed group in this study, is also known as "flat head syndrome." It is a condition characterized by an asymmetrical distortion of the infant's skull. It is important to differentiate between craniosynostosis and positional skull deformities, also known as synostotic and non-synostotic plagiocephaly (27). In case of skull deformity at birth, a pediatrician should differentiate whether the cause is synostotic, as synostotic plagiocephaly worsens over time, causes severe complications, and often requires surgery. Deformational plagiocephaly (DP), or non-synostotic plagiocephaly, is normally benign and the most common cause of plagiocephaly with prevalence of 5–48% in healthy new-borns (27, 28). It can be caused when the child passes through the birth canal, or due to gravitational forces, such as the dramatic increase in DP that was seen in the 1990's after implementing the recommendation for infants to sleep in a supine position to decrease the risk of sudden infant death syndrome.

Kieser et al. found no structural or functional abnormalities at birth among new-borns of either TFL treated women or in women whose male partners were treated with TFL. It is not mentioned if abnormalities appearing after birth were considered. Vukusic et al. reported one fetal death ≥20 weeks of gestation, and three structural abnormalities, but without comparison of the results to any reference group or general population. Both previous studies conclude no evidence of teratogenic signals in TFL-treated women or in females whose male partners were treated with TFL.

A strength of this study is the use of nationwide population-based data, although the small sample size is a limitation in terms of generalizations or absolute recommendations. The incidence of spontaneous abortion, pre-term delivery, or congenital malformation in female partners of TFL-treated men and TFL-treated women is no different than that of the general Danish population. A possible limitation of this study is the unknown age of the female partners of the men treated with TFL.

CONCLUSION

The post-marketing analyses of this report, based on nationwide register-based data from the availability of TFL in Denmark until 1st of January 2017 do not indicate teratogenicity due to TFL in pregnancy or pregnancy-related outcomes. This is in line with the known outcomes from both clinical trials and post-marketing studies.

Further analyses of available pregnancy data with TFL are warranted to better quantify the risk associated with TFL exposure in pregnancy before concluding against teratogenicity.

AUTHOR CONTRIBUTIONS

JA study concept and design, data acquisition, statistical analyses, interpretation of the results, drafting, and revision of the manuscript. JM study concept and critical revision of the manuscript. TS revision of the manuscript and statistical analyses. MM study concept and design, data acquisition, interpretation of results, revision of the manuscript.

REFERENCES

1. Lublin FD. New multiple sclerosis phenotypic classification. *Eur Neurol.* (2014) 72:1–5. doi: 10.1159/000367614
2. Freedman MS. Teriflunomide in relapsing multiple sclerosis: therapeutic utility. *Ther Adv Chronic Dis.* (2013) 4:192–205. doi: 10.1177/2040622313492810
3. Cada DJ, Demaris K, Levien TL, Baker DE. Teriflunomide. *Hosp Pharm.* (2013) 48:231–40. doi: 10.1310/hpj4803-231
4. FDA. *Aubagio [Package Insert].* Cambridge, MA: Genzyme Corporation (2012). Available online at: https://www.accessdata.fda.gov/drugsatfda_docs/label/2012/202992s000lbl.pdf
5. Kieseier BC, Benamor M. Pregnancy outcomes following maternal and paternal exposure to teriflunomide during treatment for relapsing-remitting multiple sclerosis. *Neurol Ther.* (2014) 3:133–8. doi: 10.1007/s40120-014-0020-y
6. Vukusic S, Coyle PK, Jurgensen S, Truffinet P, Benamor M, Poole E, et al. Pregnancy outcomes in patients with MS treated with teriflunomide: clinical study and postmarketing data (P.4.361). *Neurol. Adv. Commun.* (2018) 90:202563. Available online at: http://onlinelibrary.ectrims-congress.eu/ectrims/2017/ACTRIMS-ECTRIMS2017/202563/sandra.vukusic.pregnancy.outcomes.in.patients.with.ms.treated.with.html
7. Schmidt M, Pedersen L, Sørensen HT. The Danish civil registration system as a tool in epidemiology. *Eur J Epidemiol.* (2014) 29:541–9. doi: 10.1007/s10654-014-9930-3
8. Magyari M, Koch-Henriksen N, Sørensen PS. The danish multiple sclerosis treatment register. *Clin Epidemiol.* (2016) 8:549–52. doi: 10.2147/CLEP.S99500
9. Bliddal M, Broe A, Pottegård A, Olsen J, Langhoff-Roos J. The Danish medical birth register. *Eur J Epidemiol.* (2018) 33:27–36. doi: 10.1007/s10654-018-0356-1
10. Schmidt M, Schmidt SAJ, Sandegaard JL, Ehrenstein V, Pedersen L, Sørensen HT. The Danish national patient registry: a review of content, data quality, and research potential. *Clin Epidemiol.* (2015) 7:449–90. doi: 10.2147/CLEP.S91125
11. Tølbøll Blenstrup L, Knudsen LB. Danish registers on aspects of reproduction. *Scand J Public Health* (2011) 39:79–82. doi: 10.1177/1403494811399957
12. Tsimis ME, Abu Al-Hamayel N, Germaine H, Burd I. Prematurity: present and future. *Minerva Ginecol.* (2015) 67:35–46.
13. Quinn JA, Munoz FM, Gonik B, Frau L, Cutland C, Mallett-Moore T, et al. Preterm birth: case definition & guidelines for data collection, analysis, and presentation of immunisation safety data. *Vaccine* (2016) 34:6047–56. doi: 10.1016/j.vaccine.2016.03.045
14. Mazaki-Tovi S, Romero R, Kusanovic JP, Erez O, Pineles BL, Gotsch F, et al. Recurrent preterm birth. *Semin Perinatol.* (2007) 31:142–58. doi: 10.1053/j.semperi.2007.04.001
15. Videnscenter R. *Definitioner for Tidligt Født – Riget.* Available online at: https://www.rigshospitalet.dk/afdelinger-og-klinikker/julianemarie/videnscenter-for-tidligt-foedte-boern/om-tidligt-foedte/Sider/Definitioner.aspx
16. American Academy of Pediatrics Committee on Fetus and Newborn. Use and abuse of the apgar score. *Pediatrics.* (1996) 98:141–2.
17. Goldacre A, Pakpoor J, Goldacre M. Perinatal characteristics and obstetric complications in mothers with multiple sclerosis: record-linkage study. *Mult Scler Relat Disord.* (2017) 12:4–8. doi: 10.1016/j.msard.2016.11.011
18. Yalcin SE, Yalcin Y, Yavuz A, Akkurt MO, Sezik M. Maternal and perinatal outcomes in pregnancies with multiple sclerosis: a case-control study. *J Perinat Med.* (2017) 45:455–60. doi: 10.1515/jpm-2016-0060
19. Fong A, Chau CT, Quant C, Duffy J, Pan D, Ogunyemi DA. Multiple sclerosis in pregnancy: prevalence, sociodemographic features, and obstetrical outcomes. *J Matern Neonatal Med.* (2018) 31:382–7. doi: 10.1080/14767058.2017.1286314
20. Fragoso YD, Boggild M, MacIas-Islas MA, Carra A, Schaerer KD, Aguayo A, et al. The effects of long-term exposure to disease-modifying drugs during pregnancy in multiple sclerosis. *Clin Neurol Neurosurg.* (2013) 115:154–9. doi: 10.1016/j.clineuro.2012.04.024
21. Davenport L, Edling A, Finn P, Truffinet P. *Teriflunomide Mechanism of Action: Linking Species' Sensitivities to Pregnancy Outcomes.* Vol. 23. Copenhagen: 29th Congress of the European Commitee for Treatment and Research in Multiple Sclerosis, 2013 (2015). Available online at: http://ovidsp.ovid.com/ovidweb.cgi?T=JS&PAGE=reference&D=emed17&NEWS=N&AN=72058744
22. Cassina M, Johnson DL, Robinson LK, Xu R, Jimenez JL, Mirrasoul N, et al. Pregnancy outcome in women exposed to leflunomide before or during pregnancy. *Arthritis Rheum.* (2012) 64:2085–94. doi: 10.1002/art.34419
23. Alwan S, Chambers CD, Armenti VT, Sadovnick AD. The need for a disease-specific prospective pregnancy registry for multiple sclerosis (MS). *Mult Scler Relat Disord.* (2015) 4:6–17. doi: 10.1016/j.msard.2014.10.001
24. Andersen A-MN. Maternal age and fetal loss: population based register linkage study. *BMJ.* (2000) 320:1708–12. doi: 10.1136/bmj.320.7251.1708
25. *The Danish National Birth Register.* Available online at: http://www.esundhed.dk/sundhedsregistre/MFR/Sider/MFR06A.aspx
26. Kieseier B, Truffinet P, Jung Henson LBM. Pregnancy outcomes for female patients and partners of male patients in the teriflunomide clinical development program. *Mult Scler.* (2014) 20(1 Suppl. 1):438. doi: 10.1016/j.msard.2014.09.192
27. Ghizoni E, Denadai R, Raposo-Amaral CA, Joaquim AF, Tedeschi H, Raposo-Amaral CE. Diagnosis of infant synostotic and nonsynostotic cranial deformities: a review for pediatricians. *Rev Paul Pediatr.* (2016) 34:495–502. doi: 10.1016/j.rppede.2016.02.005
28. Losee JE, Mason AC. Deformational plagiocephaly: diagnosis, prevention, and treatment. *Clin Plast Surg.* (2005) 32:53–64. doi: 10.1016/j.cps.2004.08.003

18

Serum Lipoprotein Profile Is Associated With Protective Effects of Oral Contraceptive Use on Multiple Sclerosis Severity

Armando Sena[1,2,3]*, *Ana Macedo*[4,5], *Véronique Ferret-Sena*[1], *Carlos Capela*[3] *and Rui Pedrosa*[3]

[1] *Centro de Investigação Multidisciplinar Egas Moniz (CiiEM), Instituto Universitário Egas Moniz, Caparica, Portugal,* [2] *Faculdade de Ciências Médicas, Universidade Nova de Lisboa, Lisbon, Portugal,* [3] *Departamento de Neurociências, Serviço de Neurologia, Centro Hospitalar de Lisboa-Central, Lisbon, Portugal,* [4] *Keypoint, Consultora Científica, Algés, Portugal,* [5] *Departamento de Ciências Biomédicas e Medicina (DCBM), Universidade do Algarve, Faro, Portugal*

***Correspondence:**
Armando Sena
asena@egasmoniz.edu.pt

Background: The mechanisms underlying the influence of sex hormones in multiple sclerosis (MS) are uncertain. Sex steroids interact with cholesterol metabolism and the serum lipid profile has been associated with the severity of the disease. We hypothesized that the putative associations between lipoprotein metabolism and MS could be modulated by sex steroids exposure. The aim of this study was to investigate whether oral contraceptives (OC) use changes the lipoprotein profile associated with disability in patients with multiple sclerosis.

Methods: Clinical data was collected from 133 relapsing-remitting multiple sclerosis (RRMS) women with a mean of 6.5 years of disease duration and prior to the start of disease-modifying therapies. Patients who were using OC after disease onset (DO) (OC+, $n = 57$) were compared to those who never used OC or discontinued its intake before DO (OC–, $n = 76$). In both cohorts of subjects, the associations between the apolipoprotein E (ApoE) polymorphism, and plasma lipid levels, and the annualized relapse rate (RR), the Expanded Disability Status Score (EDSS), and the Multiple Sclerosis Severity Score (MSSS) were evaluated using a hierarchic multiple regression analysis after adjustment for confounders.

Results: Low density lipoprotein (LDL) levels were associated with higher EDSS ($p = 0.010$) and MSSS ($p = 0.024$) in the whole studied cohort. In E3/E3 phenotype carriers (73.7%), EDSS and MSSS were lower in OC+ in comparison with OC– subgroup of patients ($p < 0.01$). LDL and total cholesterol were associated with EDSS ($p = 0.005$ and $p = 0.043$, respectively), and LDL and the triglyceride/high density lipoprotein ratio with MSSS ($p = 0.011$ and $p = 0.048$, respectively) in OC+ patients. In OC– subgroup of patients, ApoE levels were associated with EDSS ($p = 0.012$) and MSSS ($p = 0.031$). No significant interactions between the lipid variables or OC use and RR were observed.

Conclusions: Serum lipid profile is associated with protective effects of OC use on disability of RRMS patients. Lipoprotein metabolism may be involved in the modulatory effects of sex steroids on the severity of the disease.

Keywords: multiple sclerosis, lipoproteins, cholesterol, apolipoprotein E, oral contraceptives, sex steroids

INTRODUCTION

Multiple sclerosis (MS) is an inflammatory demyelinating and neurodegenerative disease in which onset and course may be modulated by gender and sex hormones (1). The mechanisms underlying sex differences and effects of sex steroids in the disease are poorly understood. Recent studies have implicated serum cholesterol metabolism and lipoprotein profile in the pathophysiology and severity of the disease (2). Nevertheless, results are mixed, and whether these relations are causal or secondary to the disease process, treatment regimens or other confounding factors remain uncertain. Complex interactions between cholesterol metabolism and sex steroids are well-known (3) and may modulate the clinical activity of experimental autoimmune encephalomyelitis (EAE), the animal model for MS (4, 5). Therefore, we hypothesized that the putative associations between lipoprotein metabolism and the severity of MS could be modulated by sex hormone exposure.

Oral contraceptives (OC) use has provided an opportunity to assess the influence of sex hormones on the risk and course of MS. Recent data suggested a less severe clinical course (6, 7) and decreased inflammatory brain lesions (8) in relapsing-remitting (RRMS) women taking OC. Protective effects of estriol, the estrogen unique to parity (9), and of hormone therapy in postmenopausal MS women were also reported (10). In healthy women, OC use induces variable alterations in serum lipids and apolipoproteins levels modulated by ApoE polymorphism (11, 12). Although ApoE polymorphism is not generally considered to affect the risk of MS, its association with the neurodegenerative process and severity of the disease is still controversial (4, 5). ApoE is implicated in the immune dysfunction and clinical activity of EAE (5) and recent studies have suggested that EAE disease severity is differently modulated by cholesterol and ApoE metabolism in female and male mice (4, 13). Oestrogens may regulate the expression of ApoE gene (2) and estrogen treatment has protective effects in EAE (14). Oestrogens-ApoE interactions are suggested to be involved in other neurological conditions with a sex bias and abnormal cholesterol metabolism, such as Alzheimer disease (15). Based on these data, the aim of the present study was to investigate whether OC intake in RRMS patients influence the associations between the serum lipoprotein profile and the clinical severity of the disease.

MATERIALS AND METHODS

Study Population

The studied population include 133 women with the diagnosis of RRMS according to the revised McDonald criteria (16) followed at the MS outpatient clinic of a University Hospital in Lisbon (Portugal). Most women enrolled in this study belong to a population of Caucasian origin included in a previous work published by our group (7). The present study includes all patients followed in our clinic since 1995 diagnosed with RRMS with at least 2 years of disease duration and whose lipid data were available prior to the start of disease-modifying therapies. No woman was taking lipid-lowering agents. Disease onset (DO) was defined as the age of appearance of the first symptoms suggestive of MS. The annualized relapse rate (RR) and the Expanded Disability Status Scale (EDSS) and Multiple Sclerosis Severity (MSSS) values were determined at a stable phase of the disease. MSSS scores were obtained from Figure 3 of the paper of Roxburg et al. (17). The MSSS is based on EDSS scores adjusted for disease duration and it is a method to compare disability progression in groups of patients (7, 17). Women in menopause or history of gynecological surgical interventions or a delivery the last 6 months were excluded. Clinical indexed information included the body mass index (BMI) (Kg/m^2), age of first menstruation (menarche) and history of childbirths (parity), smoking habit, and OC intake. Patients labeled smokers reported to smoke regularly at least five cigarettes per day since DO. Women were classified as OC non-users if they never used OC or discontinued its intake for at least 1 year before DO (OC−); and OC users if they maintained pill intake after DO for at least a continuous period of 1 year (OC+). We were unable to take the composition of the prescribed pill into account because this information was lacking for some patients and many changed the brand of the drug. However, all women who remembered the formulation of OC used took formulations of 20 or 30 μg of ethinyl estradiol combined with progestin. No woman reported to use progestin-only formulations. This study was approved by the Ethics Committee of the Centro Hospitalar, Lisboa Central (Lisbon, Portugal). All patients gave written informed consent, including for publication of results, in accordance with the Declaration of Helsinki.

Biochemical Analysis

Blood samples were collected in fasting conditions shortly after clinical data collection and neurological examination. Plasma or serum samples were stored at −80°C and biochemical measurements performed in blind conditions regarding subject participants. At sampling, patients were in a remission phase of RRMS and none of them had initiated disease-modifying therapies, suffered from a relapse or were treated with steroids for at least 1 month. Serum triglycerides (TG), total cholesterol (TC), high density lipoprotein (HDL)-cholesterol, apolipoprotein A-1 (ApoA1), and apolipoprotein B (ApoB) were determined with enzymatic methods and lipoprotein (a) [Lp(a)] by turbidimetric immunoassay by using a Hitachi 911 autoanalyzer and commercial kits (Roche Diagnostic, Mannheim, Germany). Non-HDL cholesterol levels were calculated by subtracting HDL from TC. Low density lipoprotein (LDL)-cholesterol was determined by using the Friedewald equation (18) and oxidized LDL (oxLDL) by Enzyme-Linked Immunosorbent Assay (Mercodia, eBioscience). Apolipoprotein E (ApoE) protein levels were determined by electroimmunodiffusion (Sebia, Emery, France) and ApoE polymorphism examined by using an isoelectric focusing (IEF) method as described previously (19). Briefly, 15 μl of delipidated plasma samples was run on agarose with sorbitol, urea, ampholine (pH 5–7) and pharmalyte (pH 4–6.5) (Amersham Pharmacia Biotech, Little Chalfont, UK). After IEF, the proteins were transferred to nitrocellulose membranes (Immobilon, pore size 0.2 μm; Millipore Corporate Headquarters, Billerica, USA). The membranes were incubated with polyclonal-goat anti-human ApoE antibody (Daichi Pure Chemicals, Tokyo, Japan) and IgG peroxidase-conjugate anti-goat antibody (Sigma-Aldrich Biotechnology, St Louis, USA). The ApoE isoforms were visualized in a solution containing 3,3' diaminobenzidine tetrahydrochloride reagent (Sigma). For common ApoE polymorphism, protein phenotyping is in good agreement with DNA-based genotyping (20).

Statistical Analysis

Patient demographic and clinical characteristics were described using mean, median, standard deviation, and interquartile range for continuous variables. In the text, standard deviation is presented as mean (standard deviation). For categorical variables absolute and relative frequencies were calculated. The relation between severity parameters of clinical disease activity (RR, MSSS, and EDSS) and ApoE phenotypes was evaluated using Kruskal-Wallis ranking test. Comparisons of disease severity between OC+ and OC− subgroups of patients were performed using a Mann Whitney test. The associations between disease severity parameters such as MSSS, EDSS, and RR and the lipid profile were evaluated using a two tailed Spearman Correlation analysis. The correlation analysis was performed for the total subset of patients carrying the E3/E3 phenotype and also split for those in OC+ and OC− subgroups. A hierarchical multiple linear regression was used assuming the EDSS and MSSS as dependent variables and characterization variables such as age, disease onset, oral contraception, disease duration and parity (block 1), and lipid profile parameters that had significant correlation with EDSS and MSSS in the correlation analysis (block 2), as independent variables. A enter model was used for the variables in the block 1 and a stepwise model was used for variables in block 2.A significance level of 0.05 was considered in all analysis.

RESULTS

The main demographic and clinical characteristics of the studied population are summarized in **Table 1**. Twenty-nine patients (21.8%) were classified as overweight ($25 \geq$ BMI < 30) or obese (BMI ≥ 30). In the OC+ subgroup ($n = 57$), the mean duration of OC use was 10 years (6.6) and all but nine women started intake before DO. In the OC− subgroup, fifty patients were never prescribed with OC and 26 discontinued the intake before DO. OC+ patients were younger and had the onset of the disease at an earlier age than OC− subgroup of patients. Significant associations were found between EDSS and MSSS and age ($p < 0.001$ and $p = 0.013$), DO ($p = 0.004$ and $p < 0.001$), disease duration ($p = 0.004$ and $p < 0.001$), OC use ($p = 0.001$ and $p = 0.002$), and parity after DO ($p < 0.001$ and $p = 0.006$). RR was only associated with disease duration ($p = 0.006$). Menarche age, duration of OC intake, BMI, and smoker habit were not associated with RR or disability scores (data not shown). Concerning the lipid data, HDL and Apo A1 levels were higher in OC+ patients. In a hierarchic multiple regression analysis adjusted for age, DO, disease duration, and OC use, LDL was the only lipid variable associated with EDSS and MSSS (β = 0.008, 95% CI (0.002 to 0.015) $p = 0.010$ and β = 0.013, 95% CI (0.002 to 0.025) $p = 0.024$, respectively). ApoE phenotypes found in the studied cohort were E3/E3 ($n = 98$, 73.7%), E4/E3 ($n = 20$, 15%), E2/E3 ($n = 12$, 9%). Analysis of ApoE polymorphism was missing from one patient and two additional patients carried the E4/E2 phenotype. No homozygotes for the E4 and E2 alleles were detected. The observed frequencies of ApoE alleles were comparable with those reported for the general populations in Portugal and other countries in South Europe (21).

No associations between the three common ApoE phenotypes and EDSS, MSSS, or RR were found. However, in the E3/E3 subset of subjects, EDSS, and MSSS values were lower in OC+ in comparison to OC− subgroup of patients ($p < 0.01$) (**Figure 1**). These results remain significant after hierarchical multiple linear regression analysis adjusting for demographic features among the ApoE genetic groups. RR was not significantly changed by OC intake ($p = 0.457$). In consequence, serum lipid and apolipoprotein levels were investigated in this subset of patients according to OC use. Overall, there was no statistical difference in the lipid profile with the exception of higher ApoA1 and lower ApoE levels in OC+ in comparison to OC− patients [171.3 mg/dl (40.6) vs. 151.5 mg/dl, (27.5); $p < 0.01$ and 67.3 mg/dl (29.6) vs. 80.1 mg/dl (28.7); $p < 0.05$, respectively]. Correlation between lipoprotein levels and disability scores were analyzed in E3/E3 subset of patients stratified according to OC use. In OC+ subgroup of patients, LDL was associated with EDSS ($p = 0.018$) and ApoB was associated with MSSS ($p = 0.043$). In contrast, in the OC− subgroup of patients, ApoE was associated with MSSS values ($p = 0.008$); TC and non-HDL were associated with EDSS ($p = 0.025$ and $p = 0.035$, respectively); and TC ($p = 0.035$), LDL ($p = 0.028$), non-HDL ($p = 0.005$), and ApoB ($p = 0.008$) with RR (**Table 2**).

A hierarchic multiple regression analysis in E3/E3 subjects split for OC+ and OC− patients and adjusted for age, DO and disease duration was then performed (**Table 3**). EDSS was related to LDL [β = 0.026, 95% CI (0.009 to 0.044); $p = 0.005$] and TC [β = −0.018, 95% CI (−0.034 to −0.001); $p = 0.043$]; model R square = 0.328 ($p = 0.015$) in OC+ population; and to ApoE [β = 0.015, 95% CI (0.004 to 0.028); $p = 0.012$]; model R square = 0.312 ($p = 0.001$) in the OC− subgroup of patients. In a similar model, MSSS was related to LDL, [β = 0.022, 95% CI (0.002 to 0.033); $p = 0.011$] and to TG/HDL ratio, [β = 0.389, 95% CI (0.088 to 0.800); $p = 0.048$];

TABLE 1 | Patient demographic and clinical characteristics.

Characteristics	Total (n = 133)	OC+ (n = 57)	OC– (n = 76)	*p-value*
Age (years)	35.2 ± 8.4	32.4 ± 6.9	37.3 ± 8.8	**0.001**
Disease onset (age)	28.6 ± 8.2	25.7 ± 6.7	30.8 ± 8.5	**<0.001**
Disease duration (years)	6.5 ± 5.3	6.6 ± 5.0	6.4 ± 5.5	0.836
EDSS	2.1 ± 1.3 2.0 [1.0;3.0]$	1.7 ± 1.1 1.5 [1.0;2.0]$	2.4 ± 1.4 2.5 [1.6;3.5]$	**<0.001**
MSSS	3.5 ± 2.4 3.4 [1.5;5.2]$	2.8 ± 2.0 2.3 [1.3;4.5]$	4.1 ± 2.6 3.9 [2.0;6.0]$	**0.003**
Relapse rate	0.9 ± 0.6 1.0 [0.5;1.0]$	0.9 ± 0.5 1.0 [0.5;1.0]$	± 0.6 1.0 [0.5;1.0]$	0.317
TC (mg/dl)	201.5 ± 36.5	202.9 ± 34.7	200.5 ± 37.9	0.708
LDL (mg/dl)	126.0 ± 34.1	123.2 ± 33.1	128.1 ± 34.9	0.418
HDL (mg/dl)	57.9 ± 15.2	60.9 ± 17.8	55.7 ± 12.5	**0.049**
Non HDL (mg/dl)	143.6 ± 37.4	142.0 ± 35.8	144.8 ± 38.9	0.670
Oxidized LDL (u/L)	60.3 ± 24.3	61.0 ± 25.3	59.4 ± 23.9	0.863
TG (mg/dl)	95.3 ± 47.6	102.2 ± 49.5	90.1 ± 45.8	0.149
ApoA1 (mg/dl)	159.1 ± 33.7	173.0 ± 37.6	148.5 ± 26.1	**<0.001**
ApoB (mg/dl)	90.2 ± 24.7	91.2 ± 22.9	89.5 ± 26.1	0.698
Lp(a) (mg/dl)	29.4 ± 29.5	32.4 ± 29.5	27.5 ± 29.6	0.377
ApoE (mg/l)	77.2 ± 31.8	70.4 ± 29.1	81.9 ± 32.9	0.052
ApoE 3/3 n (%)	98 (73.7)	42 (73.7)	56 (73.7)	0.184
ApoE 4/3 n (%)	20 (15.0)	12 (21.1)	8 (10.5)	
ApoE 2/3 n (%)	12 (9.0)	3 (5.3)	9 (11.8)	

The continues variables are expressed as mean ± SD; $ median and IQR [].
Categorical variables are expressed as frequency n (%). p represents the significance of the comparison between OC user (OC+) and non-user (OC–) patients (Mann–Whitney test). EDSS, Expanded Disability Status Scale; MSSS, Multiple Sclerosis Severity Score; TC, total cholesterol; LDL, low density lipoprotein; HDL, high density lipoprotein TG, triglyceride; Apo A1, apolipoprotein A1; ApoB, apolipoprotein B; Lp(a), lipoprotein (a) ApoE, apolipoprotein E; ApoE phenotypes (3/3, 4/3,2/3). Analysis of ApoE polymorphism was missing from one patient and two additional patients carried the E4/E2 phenotype (not shown). Bold values mean significant differences.

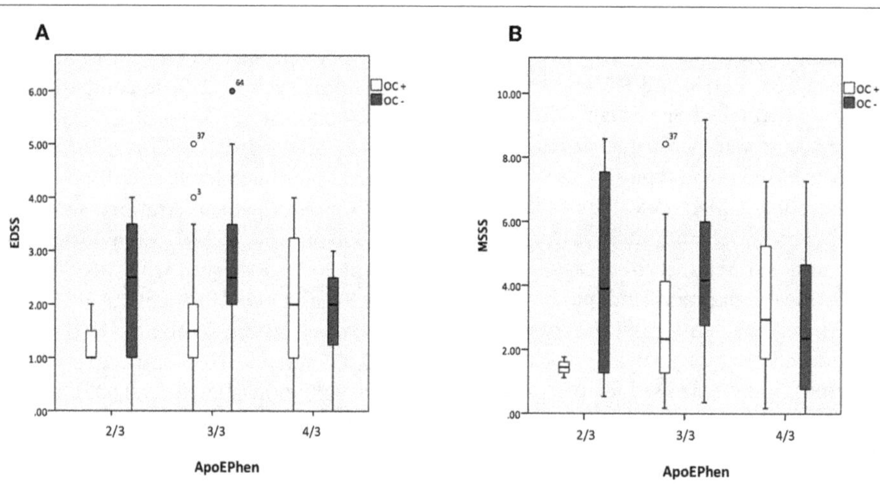

FIGURE 1 | Association between Apolipoprotein E phenotypes and disability changes stratified according to oral contraceptive use. Dependence of the Expanded Disability Status Scale (EDSS) **(A)** and of the Multiple Sclerosis Severity Score (MSSS) **(B)** with Apo E phenotypes (ApoEPhen) (2/3, 3/3, 4/3) in oral contraceptive users (n = 57 in white) and non-users (n = 73 in gray) subgroups of patients. The bars represent inter-quartile range (percentiles 25 and 75); OC+, ApoEPhen 2/3- only 3 patients analyzed. EDSS and MSSS values are lower in OC users in comparison to non-user patients carrying the E3/E3 phenotype (Mann-Whitney test, $p < 0.001$ and $p = 0.001$, respectively).

model R square = 0.333 (p = 0.016) in OC+ patients; and to ApoE, [β = 0.024, 95% CI (0.003 to 0.046); p = 0.031]; model R square = 0.299 (p = 0.002) in OC− population (see **Supplementary Material**). No significant associations between the lipids variables and RR were observed using this model (not shown).

TABLE 2 | Associations between the lipid profile and clinical variables in patients carrying the E3/E3 phenotype stratified according to oral contraceptive use.

Lipid variables	OC+			OC–		
	RR	EDSS	MSSS	RR	EDSS	MSSS
TC (mg/dl)	−0.034 (0.833)	0.211 (0.180)	0.186 (0.239)	**0.283 (0.035)**	**0.299 (0.025)**	0.203 (0.134)
LDL (mg/dl)	−0.017 (0.917)	**0.363 (0.018)**	0.255 (0.103)	**0.294 (0.028)**	0.246 (0.067)	0.128 (0.346)
Non-HDL (mg/dl)	−0.045 (0.778)	0.268 (0.086)	0.152 (0.338)	**0.366 (0.005)**	**0.283 (0.035)**	0.221 (0.101)
Apo B (mg/dl)	0.103 (0.517)	0.270 (0.084)	**0.313 (0.043)**	**0.357 (0.008)**	0.230 (0.094)	0.199 (0.150)
Apo E (mg/l)	−0.001 (0.995)	−0.002 (0.993)	0.030 (0.863)	0.154 (0.266)	0.206 (0.136)	**0.356 (0.008)**

The results show Spearman Correlation significance between subgroups of patients carrying the E3/E3 phenotype. OC+: oral contraceptives user (n = 36); OC– oral contraceptives non-user (n = 51); RR, annualized relapse Rate; EDSS, Expanded Disability Status Scale; MSSS, Multiple Sclerosis Severity Score; TC, total cholesterol; LDL, low density lipoprotein; HDL, high density lipoprotein; ApoB, apolipoprotein B; ApoE, apolipoprotein E. No significant associations were found for other lipid variables (not shown). Bold values mean significant differences.

TABLE 3 | Hierarchical multiple linear regression model to determine the association between lipid variables and disability changes in patients carrying the E3/E3 phenotype stratified according to oral contraceptive use.

Factors	β coefficient*	CI 95%*	*p-value*	*R* square	Sig (ANOVA)
DEPENDENT VARIABLE: EDSS					
OC+					
TC (mg/dl)	**−0.018**	−0.034 to −0.001	**0.043**	0.328	**0.015**
LDL (mg/dl)	**0.026**	0.009 to 0.044	**0.005**		
OC–					
ApoE (mg/l)	**0.015**	0.004 to 0.028	**0.012**	0.312	**0.001**
DEPENDENT VARIABLE: MSSS					
OC+					
LDL (mg/dl)	**0.022**	0.002 to 0.033	**0.011**	0.333	**0.016**
TG/HDL ratio	**0.389**	0.088 to 0.800	**0.048**		
OC–					
ApoE (mg/l)	**0.024**	0.003 to 0.46	**0.031**	0.299	**0.002**

**Adjusted for age, disease onset, disease duration, and oral contraception (OC) intake. EDSS, Expanded Disability Status Scale; MSSS, Multiple Sclerosis Severity Score; Oral contraceptive users (OC+, n = 34) and non-users (OC–, n = 51) subgroups of patients carrying the E3/E3 phenotype; TC, total cholesterol; LDL, low-density lipoprotein; ApoE, apolipoprotein E; TG, triglycerides; HDL, high-density lipoprotein. No significant associations were found for other lipid variables (not shown). Bold values mean significant differences.*

DISCUSSION

The results reported in this study suggest that oral OC use modifies the serum lipoprotein profile associated with disability in patients with MS. Recent prospective studies have shown variably associations between serum lipid and apolipoprotein levels and the risk of new lesions accumulation and disability progression in patients with RRMS and/or the first symptoms suggestive of the disease (clinical isolated syndrome, CIS) (2). However, most research has included patients under immunomodulatory therapies and have not assessed possible influences of OC use. In consequence, in this cohort, lipid data was analyzed before the introduction of disease-modifying therapies and comparing women who never used OC or stopped its intake before disease onset (OC–) to those who were OC users after disease onset (OC+).

The serum lipoprotein profile is in part genetically regulated by the common human isoforms of ApoE designated E2, E3, and E4, which display different modulatory roles in cholesterol metabolism, immune function, and neuronal homeostasis (3, 5, 11). In agreement with most studies (4, 5), no association between the ApoE polymorphism and the clinical activity and severity of MS was found. However, in individuals carrying the major E3/E3 phenotype, EDSS and MSSS were significant lower in the OC+ group, when compared to OC– patients. In line with previous retrospective work (6, 7) and a recent longitudinal study (22) no influence of OC use on relapse risk was observed. Future research in a larger population of carriers of the ε2 and ε4 alleles is needed. In particular, the apparent lack of effect on disability in E4/E3 patients is of considerable interest. In fact, experimental and clinical studies have shown that the neuroprotective and anti-inflammatory effects of estrogen are attenuated by the ApoE4 isoform (3) and the risk conferred by this allele for Alzheimer disease is amplified in women (15). These results lead us to perform an analyse of serum lipid variables and their associations with clinical parameters restricted to carriers of the E3/E3 phenotype.

In healthy women, the use of OC formulations containing combinations of ethinyl estradiol and a progestin induce in general an increase of serum TG, ApoA1, and ApoB(11, 12). Higher levels of HDL and/or of its major apolipoprotein, ApoA1, were suggested to be protective for the genesis of new lesions in the MS (23, 24). Although ApoA1 levels were higher in OC+ than in OC– patients, no evidence for a protective effect was observed in agreement with other studies (25–27). In accordance with most studies (27), no independent association between lipid parameters and RR were observed after adjustments in multivariable analysis. In contrast, when all the variables were analyzed in a hierarchic model, significant associations were found between disability and TC, LDL, and the TG/HDL ratio only in the OC+ population. The TG/HDL ratio is a parameter recently associated with insulin resistance, obesity, metabolic syndrome, and clinical outcome in stroke (28). Our finding is consistent with some studies reporting worsening disability in patients with high TG levels (24, 26).

In healthy women, OC intake consistently decreases ApoE levels and changes the distribution of this protein between lipoprotein fractions containing ApoB (LDL and triglyceride-rich lipoproteins) and those devoid of ApoB and rich in ApoA1 (HDL). Interestingly, these alterations are not induced in E4 carriers (12). Recently, differences in LDL particle size were observed between male and female RRMS patients, supporting gender differences in lipid metabolism (29). These data indicate that further work is needed to analyse whether OC intake in these patients modify ApoE distribution among lipid fractions. Nevertheless, ApoE levels were lower in OC+ than in OC− patients, and were correlated in these latter subjects with disability. Previous studies have linked higher plasma ApoE levels with severity of EAE (5), higher disability in RRMS (26) and deep gray matter atrophy in CIS patients (25). Several experimental studies have shown that oestrogens may modulate the interactions between Apo E gene expression and LDL metabolism (3, 13). In this context, it is of great interest that an altered gene expression for ApoE and other proteins implicated in cholesterol synthesis and transport occurs during the development and resolution of CNS lesions in EAE and MS patients (30, 31). In addition, Mailleux et al. (13) have shown that LDL receptor deficiency reduces EAE disease severity in female, but not in male rats, through the induction of ApoE release by macrophages. In line with the reviewed data, the present results strongly support a role of sex steroids in modulating ApoE and related cholesterol metabolism in MS patients.

Beyond the relative small dimension of the cohort, absence of a healthy control population and its cross-sectional design, this study has several other limitations. Considering the models statistical assumptions and the nature of the included clinical variables, the results should be interpreted carefully. Prospective studies are necessary to substantiate a causal role of the lipid profile associated with OC behavior in disability progression. It should be noted that many patients are at present medicated following a first clinical episode and paraclinical evidence suggestive of MS (CIS). Therefore, it is increasingly impractical or unethical to carry out a study on a larger population of patients with the diagnosis of RRMS without taking disease-modifying therapies, which may variably interfere with lipid metabolism (32, 33). Although a healthy control population has not be analyzed, as discussed above, our results suggest that OC intake in these patients and healthy women might interact with similar pathways of lipid metabolism. Further work is warranted to investigate this interesting issue. We were unable to include neuroimaging information, analysis of vitamin D, and inflammatory markers. In particular, vitamin D levels could affect the serum lipid profile in MS patients (34) and the mutual metabolic relationships between oestrogens and vitamin D may be relevant for the pathogenesis of the disease (1). However, in a previous work, we have found no evidence for significant alterations of serum 25-hydroxyvitamin D levels associated with OC use in these patients (7). Information concerning the intake of vitamin D supplements was not available. Nonetheless, the population included in this study was analyzed before the intake of these supplements became a common practice by these patients. Dietary and physical activities were not controlled and the impact of different contraceptive formulations could not be evaluated. Gava et al. (6) did not find any differences in the protective effects of OC use in the clinical course of MS depending on the dose of ethinyl estradiol or the type of progestin. However, the anti-inflammatory effects of oestrogens are dose-dependent (8) and future randomized, double-blind, controlled studies are needed to investigate this issue. The progestin content of these formulations could change the lipid profile (11, 12) and were suggested to affect the risk for MS (35). In conclusion, despite these limitations, our results report new findings, supporting a role of the serum lipid profile in mediating modulatory effects of sex steroids in the severity of MS. In addition, they indicate that further work assessing the effects of specific OC doses and formulations in lipoprotein metabolism of these patients may provide new therapeutic strategies for the disease.

AUTHOR CONTRIBUTIONS

AS, CC, and RP contributed to the study design and data collection. AM performed the data analysis. AS wrote the manuscript, which was critically reviewed, and drafted by VF-S. All authors contributed to data interpretation and approved the final version of the manuscript.

FUNDING

This work was supported by Merck, Bayer Health Care and Teva (Projects PPAR/2006, LIPESBETA/2005, LILERICOP/2004) and by national funds through the FCT-Foundation of Science and Technology, I.P. (Portugal) under the project UID/BIM/04585/2019.

ACKNOWLEDGMENTS

The authors are grateful to all patients who participated in this study, to nurse Cristina Araújo for help in research and to Maria de Lurdes Andrade, Maria Adalgisa Tavares, and Firmina Lebre for technical assistance.

REFERENCES

1. Bove R, Chitnis T. The role of gender and sex hormones in determining the onset and outcome of multiple sclerosis. *Multiple Sclerosis J.* (2014) 20:520–6. doi: 10.1177/1352458513519181
2. Zhornitsky S, McKay KA, Metz LM, Teunissen CE, Rangachari M. Cholesterol and markers of cholesterol turnover in multiple sclerosis: relationship with disease outcomes. *Multiple Sclerosis Relat Disord.* (2016) 5:53–65. doi: 10.1016/j.msard.2015.10.005
3. Xing Y, Jia JP, Ji XJ, Tian T. Estrogen associated gene polymorphisms and their interactions in the progress of Alzheimer's disease. *Prog Neurobiol.* (2013) 111:53–74. doi: 10.1016/j.pneurobio.2013.09.006
4. Schrewe L, Lill CM, Liu T, Salmen A, Gerdes LA, Guillot-Noel L, et al. Investigation of sex-specific effects of apolipoprotein E on severity of EAE and MS. *J Neuroinflamm.* (2015) 12:234. doi: 10.1186/s12974-015-0429-y

5. Zhang H-L, Wu J, Zhu J. The immune-modulatory role of apolipoprotein E with emphasis on multiple sclerosis and experimental autoimmune encephalomyelitis. *Clin Dev Immunol.* (2010) 2010:186813. doi: 10.1155/2010/186813
6. Gava G, Bartolomei I, Costantino A, Berra M, Venturoli S, Salvi F, et al. Long-term influence of combined oral contraceptive use on the clinical course of relapsing-remitting multiple sclerosis. *Fertility Sterility* (2014) 102:116–22. doi: 10.1016/j.fertnstert.2014.03.054
7. Sena A, Couderc R, Vasconcelos JC, Ferret-Sena V, Pedrosa R. Oral contraceptive use and clinical outcomes in patients with multiple sclerosis. *J Neurol Sci.* (2012) 317:47–51. doi: 10.1016/j.jns.2012.02.033
8. Pozzilli, C., De Giglio, L., Barletta, V. T., Marinelli, F., Angelis, F., De, G.allo, V., et al. (2015). Oral contraceptives combined with interferon β in multiple sclerosis. *Neurol Neuroimmunol Neuroinflamm.* 2:e120. doi: 10.1212/NXI.0000000000000120
9. Voskuhl RR, Wang H, Wu TCJ, Sicotte NL, Nakamura K, Kurth F, et al. Estriol combined with glatiramer acetate for women with relapsing-remitting multiple sclerosis: a randomised, placebo-controlled, phase 2 trial. *Lancet Neurol.* (2016) 15:35–46. doi: 10.1016/S1474-4422(15)00322-1
10. Bove R, White CC, Fitzgerald KC, Chitnis T, Chibnik L, Ascherio A, et al. Hormone therapy use and physical quality of life in postmenopausal women with multiple sclerosis. *Neurology* (2016) 87:1457–63. doi: 10.1212/WNL.0000000000003176
11. Scharnagl H, Petersen G, Nauck M, Teichmann AT, Wieland H, März W. Double-blind, randomized study comparing the effects of two monophasic oral contraceptives containing ethinylestradiol (20 microg or 30 microg) and levonorgestrel (100 microg or 150 microg) on lipoprotein metabolism. *Contraception* (2004) 69:105–13. doi: 10.1016/j.contraception.2003.10.004
12. Starck M, Schiele F, Herbeth B, Vincent-Viry M, Beaud B, Siest G, et al. Apolipoproteins E and C-III in apo B- and non-apo B-containing lipoproteins in middle-aged women from the Stanislas cohort. effect of oral contraceptive use and common apolipoprotein E polymorphism. *Atherosclerosis* (2001) 155:509–16.
13. Mailleux J, Timmermans S, Nelissen K, Vanmol J, Vanmierlo T, van Horssen J, et al. Low-density lipoprotein receptor deficiency attenuates neuroinflammation through the induction of apolipoprotein E. *Front Immunol.* (2017) 8:1701. doi: 10.3389/fimmu.2017.01701
14. Seifert HA, Benedek G, Nguyen H, Kent G, Vandenbark AA, Offner H. Estrogen protects both sexes against EAE by promoting common regulatory cell subtypes independent of endogenous estrogen. *Metabol Brain Dis.* (2017) 32:1747–54. doi: 10.1007/s11011-017-0063-8
15. Altmann A, Tian L, Henderson VW, Greicius MD, Alzheimer's Disease Neuroimaging Initiative Investigators. Sex modifies the APOE-related risk of developing Alzheimer disease. *Ann Neurol.* (2014) 75:563–73. doi: 10.1002/ana.24135
16. Polman CH, Reingold SC, Edan G, Filippi M, Hartung HP, Kappos L, et al. Diagnostic criteria for multiple sclerosis: 2005 revisions to the "McDonald Criteria." *Ann Neurol.* (2005) 58:840–6. doi: 10.1002/ana.20703
17. Roxburgh RHSR, Seaman SR, Masterman T, Hensiek AE, Sawcer SJ, Vukusic S, et al. Multiple Sclerosis Severity Score: using disability and disease duration to rate disease severity. *Neurology* (2005) 64:1144–51. doi: 10.1212/01.WNL.0000156155.19270.F8
18. Friedewald WT, Levy RI, Fredrickson DS. Estimation of the concentration of low-density lipoprotein cholesterol in plasma, without use of the preparative ultracentrifuge. *Clin Chem.* (1972) 18:499–502.
19. Bailleul S, Couderc R, Landais V, Lefandegravevre G, Raichvarg D, Etienne J. Direct phenotyping of human apolipoprotein E in plasma: application to population frequency distribution in Paris (France). *Human Hered.* (1993) 43:159–65. doi: 10.1159/000154172
20. Hansen PS, Gerdes LU, Klausen IC, Gregersen N, Faergeman O. Genotyping compared with protein phenotyping of the common apolipoprotein E polymorphism. *Clin Chim Acta* (1994) 224:131–7.
21. Sena A, Couderc R, Ferret-Sena V, Pedrosa R, Andrade ML, Araujo C, et al. Apolipoprotein E polymorphism interacts with cigarette smoking in progression of multiple sclerosis. *Eur J Neurol.* (2009) 16:832–7. doi: 10.1111/j.1468-1331.2009.02603.x
22. Bove R, Rankin K, Chua AS, Saraceno T, Sattarnezhad N, Greeke E, et al. Oral contraceptives and MS disease activity in a contemporary real-world cohort. *Multiple Sclerosis J.* (2018) 24:227–30. doi: 10.1177/1352458517692420
23. Fellows K, Uher T, Browne RW, Weinstock-Guttman B, Horakova D, Posova H, et al. Protective associations of HDL with blood-brain barrier injury in multiple sclerosis patients. *J Lipid Res.* (2015) 56:2010–8. doi: 10.1194/jlr.M060970
24. Weinstock-Guttman B, Zivadinov R, Mahfooz N, Carl E, Drake A, Schneider J, et al. Serum lipid profiles are associated with disability and MRI outcomes in multiple sclerosis. *J Neuroinflamm.* (2011) 8:127. doi: 10.1186/1742-2094-8-127
25. Browne RW, Weinstock-Guttman B, Horakova D, Zivadinov R, Bodziak M, Lou Tamaño-Blanco M, et al. Apolipoproteins are associated with new MRI lesions and deep grey matter atrophy in clinically isolated syndromes. *J Neurol Neurosurg Psychiatry* (2014) 85:859–64. doi: 10.1136/jnnp-2013-307106
26. Tettey P, Simpson S, Taylor B, Blizzard L, Ponsonby A-L, Dwyer T, et al. An adverse lipid profile is associated with disability and progression in disability, in people with MS. *Multiple Sclerosis J.* (2014) 20:1737–44. doi: 10.1177/1352458514533162
27. Tettey P, Simpson S, Taylor B, Ponsonby A-L, Lucas RM, Dwyer T, et al. An adverse lipid profile and increased levels of adiposity significantly predict clinical course after a first demyelinating event. *J Neurol Neurosurg Psychiatry* (2017) 88:395–401. doi: 10.1136/jnnp-2016-315037
28. Deng Q-W, Wang H, Sun C-Z, Xing F-L, Zhang H-Q, Zuo L, et al. Triglyceride to high-density lipoprotein cholesterol ratio predicts worse outcomes after acute ischaemic stroke. *Eur J Neurol.* (2017) 24:283–91. doi: 10.1111/ene.13198
29. Jorissen W, Wouters E, Bogie JF, Vanmierlo T, Noben J-P, Sviridov D, et al. Relapsing-remitting multiple sclerosis patients display an altered lipoprotein profile with dysfunctional HDL. *Sci Rep.* (2017) 7:43410. doi: 10.1038/srep43410
30. Lavrnja I, Smiljanic K, Savic D, Mladenovic-Djordjevic A, Tesovic K, Kanazir S, et al. Expression profiles of cholesterol metabolism-related genes are altered during development of experimental autoimmune encephalomyelitis in the rat spinal cord. *Sci Rep.* (2017) 7:2702. doi: 10.1038/s41598-017-02638-8
31. Mailleux J, Vanmierlo T, Bogie JF, Wouters E, Lütjohann D, Hendriks JJ, et al. Active liver X receptor signaling in phagocytes in multiple sclerosis lesions. *Multiple Sclerosis J.* (2018) 24:279–89. doi: 10.1177/1352458517696595
32. Sena A, Pedrosa R, Ferret-Sena V, Almeida R, Andrade ML, Morais MG, et al. Interferon β1a therapy changes lipoprotein metabolism in patients with multiple sclerosis. *Clin Chem Lab Med.* (2000) 38:209–13. doi: 10.1515/CCLM.2000.030
33. Uher T, Fellows K, Horakova D, Zivadinov R, Vaneckova M, Sobisek L, et al. Serum lipid profile changes predict neurodegeneration in interferon-β1a-treated multiple sclerosis patients. *J Lipid Res.* (2017) 58:403–11. doi: 10.1194/jlr.M072751
34. Weinstock-Guttman B, Zivadinov R, Ramanathan M. Inter-dependence of vitamin D levels with serum lipid profiles in multiple sclerosis. *J Neurol Sci.* (2011) 311:86–91. doi: 10.1016/j.jns.2011.07.024
35. Hellwig K, Chen LH, Stancyzk FZ, Langer-Gould AM. Oral contraceptives and multiple sclerosis/clinically isolated syndrome susceptibility. *PLoS ONE* (2016) 11:e0149094. doi: 10.1371/journal.pone.0149094

19

Latitude, Vitamin D, Melatonin, and Gut Microbiota Act in Concert to Initiate Multiple Sclerosis: A New Mechanistic Pathway

Majid Ghareghani[1,2], *Russel J. Reiter*[3], *Kazem Zibara*[4*] *and Naser Farhadi*[5*]

[1] *CERVO Brain Research Center, Quebec City, QC, Canada,* [2] *Medicinal Plants Research Center, Yasuj University of Medical Sciences, Yasuj, Iran,* [3] *Department of Cell Systems and Anatomy, The University of Texas Health Science Center, San Antonio, TX, United States,* [4] *PRASE, Biology Department, Faculty of Sciences-I, Lebanese University, Beirut, Lebanon,* [5] *Cellular and Molecular Research Center, Yasuj University of Medical Sciences, Yasuj, Iran*

Correspondence:
Kazem Zibara
kzibara@ul.edu.lb
Naser Farhadi
naserfarhadi42@yahoo.com

Multiple sclerosis (MS) is an inflammatory demyelinating disease of the central nervous system (CNS). While the etiology of MS is still largely unknown, scientists believe that the interaction of several endogenous and exogenous factors may be involved in this disease. Epidemiologists have seen an increased prevalence of MS in countries at high latitudes, where the sunlight is limited and where the populations have vitamin D deficiency and high melatonin levels. Although the functions and synthesis of vitamin D and melatonin are contrary to each other, both are involved in the immune system. While melatonin synthesis is affected by light, vitamin D deficiency may be involved in melatonin secretion. On the other hand, vitamin D deficiency reduces intestinal calcium absorption leading to gut stasis and subsequently increasing gut permeability. The latter allows gut microbiota to transfer more endotoxins such as lipopolysaccharides (LPS) into the blood. LPS stimulates the production of inflammatory cytokines within the CNS, especially the pineal gland. This review summarizes the current findings on the correlation between latitude, sunlight and vitamin D, and details their effects on intestinal calcium absorption, gut microbiota and neuroinflammatory mediators in MS. We also propose a new mechanistic pathway for the initiation of MS.

Keywords: multiple sclerosis, latitude, sunlight, vitamin D, melatonin, gut microbiota

INTRODUCTION

Multiple sclerosis (MS) is an inflammatory demyelinating disease of the central nervous system (CNS) affecting over 2.5 million young adults worldwide; this condition develops when activated immune cells attack the CNS (1). Previous studies using advanced neuroimaging, neuroimmunological, and neuropathological technologies demonstrated that MS is not a single disease but rather a spectrum at disease (2). Symptoms of MS may differ greatly between patients and its progression depends on various factors affecting mainly the nerve processes. The exact mechanism responsible for this destructive disease is still unknown. Several immunological pathways have been suggested to be involved in MS owing to the use of the experimental autoimmune encephalomyelitis (EAE) animal model, the most widely used and best model for clinical MS (3). In the absence of a firm understanding of the mechanisms underlying MS, researchers have suggested a combination of risk factors that are involved in this disease; however, their specific contribution to MS pathogenesis is largely unknown. Among others, these risk factors include age, sex, family history, infections, race, climate, environment, and smoking (4).

Environmental factors, such as exposure to infectious agents, sunlight and vitamin D levels have long been considered as potent risk factors in people under 15 years of age (5). Both epidemiological and immunological data support the idea that some chronic bacterial infections may reside within the CNS and initiate pathological states (6, 7). On the other hand, high prevalence of MS has been reported in areas with short days and long night periods that may last 6–8 months per year (8). Moreover, vitamin D deficiency is commonplace in these regions of limited sunshine durations.

This survey critically reviews the literature in an attempt to clarify whether any connection exists between sunlight, vitamin D, and bacterial infection toward causing MS and suggests a new mechanism by which MS may be triggered.

LATITUDE, SUNLIGHT, AND VITAMIN D IN MULTIPLE SCLEROSIS

About 85% of the world population lives at latitudes between the 40th parallels North and South, as a result, these individual are routinely exposed to sunlight (8). However, the remainder of the population (15%) lives at higher latitudes in the northern half of the USA, Europe, Canada, and Russia or in the southern hemisphere in New Zealand, Tasmania and Patagonia. The individuals at these high latitudes receive relatively lower amounts of sunshine while they have the highest rate of MS. Indeed, the incidence of MS in these individuals ranges from 110 to 140 cases per 100,000 people, which is two-fold greater than the rate between the 40th parallels which has about 57 to 78 cases per 100,000 (9). The incidence of MS is also higher in colder climates (10).

Inadequate exposure to sunlight has been introduced as the main risk factor for vitamin D deficiency (11). It is well documented that short days and weak sunlight do not trigger vitamin D synthesis in the skin at latitudes above 40 degrees North (10, 12) where the population relies on dietary rather than light-synthetized vitamin D (13). Two forms of vitamin D are present: D2 and D3, ergocalciferol, and cholecalciferol, respectively. Vitamin D2 is produced by some plants in response to UV radiation whereas vitamin D3 is synthesized in the skin of humans and animals via the UV irradiation of 7-dehydrocholesterol to provitamin D3, the most biologically active form (14–16). Importantly, vitamin D is a major regulator of the immune system (17) and various immunological diseases, especially MS (18).

We have reviewed the literature related to MS prevalence and vitamin D levels in Sweden, a country that is mostly present above 60° North latitude (12), where people experience long nights, especially during the winter. The prevalence of MS in 2011 was 189/100,000 individuals (19). Ultraviolet radiation in Sweden, particularly at northern latitudes, is too low to allow the synthesis of vitamin D during the winter months where the sun is above the horizon (20, 21). Concerning vitamin D levels in the Swedish population, several studies clearly reported vitamin D deficiency (22, 23). These observations are similar to those for New Zealand in the south hemisphere (24). Geographically, the prevalence of MS decreases by moving toward the equator (25), which further implicates sunlight and vitamin D as contributors to this serious disease (26).

MELATONIN, VITAMIN D, AND MULTIPLE SCLEROSIS

Melatonin, known as the chemical expression of darkness, is a sunlight dependent molecule released from pineal gland in response to darkness (27). Melatonin levels correlate with neuroimmunological diseases and are inversely related to the severity of MS and its relapse (28–32). These observations prompted researchers to investigate melatonin's effect on MS using experimental autoimmune encephalomyelitis (EAE) animal models. When tested, the severity of this condition was ameliorated using melatonin (33–35). We previously reported, however, that the action of melatonin in EAE rats may be age related (36). At the clinical level, MS patients administered melatonin as a sole treatment for 4 years recovered to 6.0 at the Expanded Disability Status Scale (EDSS), from an initial 8.0 level (32).

While several clinical studies investigated vitamin D-mediated functions in MS, the mechanisms by which vitamin D or melatonin functions relate to MS are not known. Previous studies clearly noted a reduction of vitamin D levels in MS patients, compared to healthy subjects; hence, hypovitaminosis D has been suggested to be a risk factor for MS (37). However, the evidence for a role of vitamin D as a treatment for MS is inconclusive and larger studies are needed (38). As a strategy to ameliorate the severity of MS, low-dose vitamin D supplementation did not show a significant effect on the EDSS score or relapse rate of MS patients (39). Conversely, some studies reported that increased vitamin D levels reduce the incidence and disease course of MS (40–42). A recent study showed an inverse correlation between changes in serum levels of vitamin D and melatonin. Indeed, the night secretion of melatonin was shown to be reduced after 3 months' administration of high dose vitamin D in IFN-β treated MS patients. Moreover, there was a reduction in serum vitamin D levels when melatonin levels rose at night (43).

VITAMIN D, MELATONIN, AND THE EYE

Both vitamin D and melatonin are individually essential for cellular physiology; their rhythms are contrary to each other. Vitamin D is synthesized in the skin when it is exposed to ultra

---

Abbreviations: CNS, central nervous system; MS, multiple sclerosis; LPS, lipopolysaccharides; EAE, experimental autoimmune encephalomyelitis; ipRGCs, intrinsically photosensitive retinal ganglion cells; RGCs, retinal ganglion cells; SCN, suprachiasmatic nucleus; BBB, blood brain barrier; SMCs, smooth muscle cells; TLR4, Toll like receptor 4; LBP, LPS-binding protein.

violet radiation from the sun whereas melatonin synthesis by the pineal gland occurs primarily at night. While vitamin D is present in certain foods, the bulk of it is obtained through exposure to sunlight. Conversely, the pineal gland produces melatonin primarily at night (44, 45), but it is also, like vitamin D, consumed in the diet (46). It is well established that melatonin secretion from the pineal gland peaks near the middle of the dark phase and then declines slowly and gradually (47, 48). It is possible that increasing vitamin D levels during the day may act, in part, as a signal that suppresses melatonin generation (43).

In the mammalian retina, rod and cone photoreceptors, whose photopigments are rhodopsin and photopsin, are responsible for the image-forming vision. Newly identified photoreceptors in the inner retina named "intrinsically photosensitive retinal ganglion cells (ipRGCs)" are responsible for non-image-forming vision such as regulation of circadian rhythms and pupil size (49–52). These retinal ganglion cells (RGCs) are also involved in melatonin regulation where ipRGCs selectively express melanopsin, a novel opsin-like protein and a photopigment whose expression is restricted to <2% of RGCs (53). Melanopsin regeneration is different from that of rhodopsin (54, 55). Melanopsin exists in equilibrium in two stable states under broadband light conditions and exhibits a peak spectral sensitivity in the blue wavelengths at ~482 nm. It is important to note that ipRGSc are involved in non-visual responses to light, especially blue light (56). The circadian rhythm of pineal melatonin is regulated by signals coming from suprachiasmatic nucleus (SCN) of the hypothalamus (57). ipRGC axons project to the SCN and it is this pathway that ultimately controls pineal melatonin production (58).

It is now known that exposure to blue light activates melanopsin and inhibits the SCN to synthesize and release melatonin (59–61). A recent study indicated that loss of visual axons and RGCs could be associated with vitamin D deficiency, consistent with the neuro-steroid effects of vitamin D in the CNS (62). While RGCs play a critical role in regulating melatonin production/release, the effect of vitamin D deficiency on RGCs could relate vitamin D deficiency with melatonin. This is a subject worthy of investigation. Immunologically, both hormones play a critical role in the blood brain barrier (BBB) integrity (63, 64).

VITAMIN D AND INTESTINAL CALCIUM ABSORPTION

Calcium is an abundant element in the human body and exhibits key roles in many physiological processes including blood clotting, hormone secretion, bone mineralization, nerve impulse transmission, and muscle contraction (65). While melatonin influences calcium absorption (66), vitamin D3 is the main hormone controlling intestinal calcium uptake (67). The importance of vitamin D deficiency in impairing calcium absorption from the intestine has been known for decades (68, 69). Several studies have shown, using vitamin D receptor (VDR) knockout mice, that vitamin D directly enhances intestinal calcium absorption (70, 71). In addition, it has been clearly documented that intestinal calcium absorption is reduced in vitamin D deficient animals and patients with low circulating vitamin D levels (72, 73).

Gastrointestinal motility involves a complex tightly coordinated series of contractions and relaxations of gastrointestinal smooth muscles, which are essential to maintain the orderly process of digestion. While most muscle cells use free calcium present in the cytosol for this process, gastrointestinal smooth muscle cells (SMCs) use calcium that has been imported from the extracellular fluid through special channels (74). Intestinal muscle cells need to increase and then reduce the concentration of calcium to initiate the contraction and relaxation of the intestinal muscles, respectively (75). This calcium variation is one of the main regulatory factors that affects intestinal motility. This observation led for simultaneous administration of vitamin D and calcium as a therapeutic strategy to stimulate normal intestinal motility in humans (76). In addition to the critical role of vitamin D3 in intestinal calcium absorption and intestinal motility, it may be involved in maintaining the integrity of the intestinal barrier and protecting it against mucosal injury (77).

INTESTINAL CALCIUM ABSORPTION, GUT MICROBIOTA, AND MULTIPLE SCLEROSIS

The reduction in intestinal calcium absorption leads to disruptions in intestinal motility and subsequently causes stasis of aboral movement (gut stasis) and gastroparesis in the long term (78). Gut stasis is a potentially deadly condition in which the digestive system slows down or stops completely whereas gastroparesis is a chronic disorder of delayed gastric emptying characterized by food remaining in the stomach for a longer time than normal (79). Gill etal. (80) reported for the first time a role of intestinal aboral movement in MS patients with intractable constipation. Two other studies in MS patients complaining of constipation or fecal incontinence reported that an efficient therapy for MS patients is gut focused behavioral treatment (biofeedback), especially for those with non-progressive limited disability (81, 82). In addition, a similar study in MS patients with constipation symptoms suggested a positive effect of abdominal massage on constipation symptoms and alleviation of MS severity (83).

Abnormalities of slow intestinal movement such as gut stasis, gastroparesis, and constipation seems to cause a rise in intestinal absorption including bacterial toxins. In support of this hypothesis, several previous studies clearly showed that gut stasis leads to elevated gut permeability and bacterial translocation (75, 84–87). This ultimately releases toxic mediators which further increases gut permeability (88–91). Conversely, alterations in the gut microbiota may to be involved in some neurological and autoimmune conditions (92), especially MS (93). For instance, it has been reported that patients in the active or remission phases of relapsing-remitting MS (RRMS) have gut microbial dysbiosis (94). Another similar study in children (≤18 years old within 2 years of MS) showed increased levels of gut gram-negative bacteria that could be associated with neurodegeneration (95). Moreover, gut bacteria can also affect the integrity of BBB, which is critical in MS (96).

TABLE 1 | Clinical and review studies.

Study	Main results	References
Systematic review	Overall incidence rate of MS was 3.6/100,000 person-years	(116)
	Higher latitude was associated with higher MS incidence	
	Latitude gradient was attenuated after 1980, increase in ratio of female-to-male in MS incidence in lower latitudes	
Review and meta-regression analysis	Universal increase in prevalence and incidence of MS over time	(115)
	A general increase in incidence of MS in females	
	Latitude gradient of incidence of MS is apparent for Australia and New Zealand	
Medical hypothesis	Low incidence of MS near the equator may be due to UV light induced suppressor cells to melanocyte antigens	(25)
Ecological study	Strong association between MS prevalence and annual UVB	(114)
	Female and male prevalence rates were correlated with annual UVB	
	The effect of UVB on prevalence rates differed by sex	
Review and meta-regression analyses	Statistically significant positive association between MS prevalence and latitude globally	(10)
	The latitude-dependent incidence of MS, possibly due to UV radiation/vitamin D	
Case-control study	Lower nocturnal serum melatonin levels in MS patients with major depression (MD) compared to patients without MD	(28)
	Negative correlation between Beck Depression Scale (BDS) scores and serum melatonin levels	
Case-control study	No significant difference between saliva melatonin levels of MS patients vs. healthy subjects; however, when taking the effect of age, a significant difference was found	(29)
Case-control study	Decreased levels of 6-sulphatoxy-melatonin (6-SMT) in MS patients	(30)
	IFN-β treatment increased 6-SMT in patients with improved fatigue	
Case report	4-years of melatonin therapy improved primary progressive MS	(32)
Systematic review	The evidence for vitamin D as a treatment for MS is inconclusive	(38)
	Larger studies are warranted to assess the effect of vitamin D on clinical outcomes in patients with MS	
Randomized placebo-controlled trial	Low-dose vitamin D therapy had no significant effect on the EDSS score or relapse rate of MS patient.	(39)
	A larger multicenter study of vitamin D in RRMS is warranted to assess the efficacy of this intervention	
Prospective cohort study	Higher vitamin D levels associated with a reduced hazard of relapse	(40)
	Each 10 nmol/l increase in vitamin D resulting in up to a 12% reduction in risk of relapse	
	Raising 25-OH-D levels by 50 nmol/l could cause relapse	
Randomized, double blind study	Melatonin secretion is negatively correlated with alterations in serum vitamin D in IFN-β treated MS patients	(43)
	Melatonin should be considered as a potential mediator of vitamin D neuro-immunomodulatory effects in MS patients	

TABLE 2 | Experimental studies on EAE.

Main result	References
Melatonin therapy reduced the clinical severity of EAE	(33)
Melatonin reduced immune cell infiltration into the spinal cord of EAE	
Melatonin protects against EAE by controlling peripheral and central T effector/regulatory responses	(34)
Melatonin modulates adaptive immunity centrally and peripherally in EAE mice	(35)
Melatonin suppresses the expression of IFN-γ, IL-17, IL-6, and CCL20 in the CNS of EAE and inhibits antigen-specific T cell proliferation	
A relationship exists between age and the development of EAE	(36)
Melatonin in young EAE rats exacerbated disease severity	
Vitamin D therapy suppresses the severity of clinical scores and reduces IL-6 and IL-17	(126)
Dietary calcium and vitamin D are both involved in the prevention of symptomatic EAE	(121)
Vitamin D could reduce the severity of disease only when accompanied by elevated serum calcium	
Exposure to UVB reduced EAE incidence by 74%	(122)
Exposure to UVB increased the conversation of skin trans-urocanic acid to cis-urocanic acid	
Enhanced skin cis-urocanic acid levels independent of UVB was unable to reduce EAE	
Vitamin D therapy prevents blood brain barrier disruption caused by relapse–remitting MS and secondary progressive MS	(18)
Women are more susceptible to gastroparesis than men	(125)

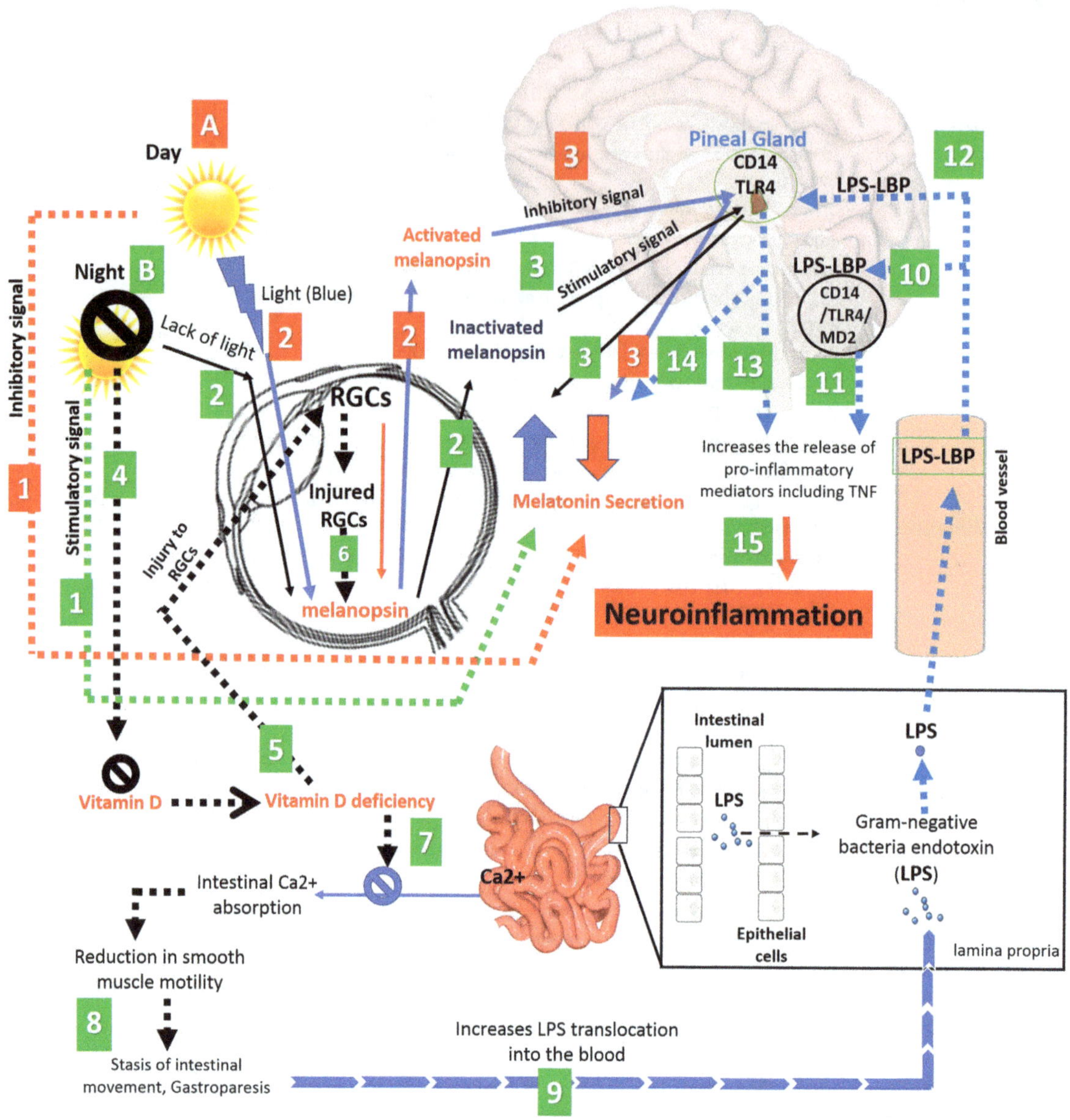

FIGURE 1 | Schematic representation correlating various factors such as light, eye, melanopsin, pineal gland, vitamin D, intestinal calcium, and gut microbiota to neuroinflammation and MS. **(A)** Adequate exposure to sunlight; (1) Long days and adequate exposure to sunlight suppresses the melatonin secretion and (2) leads to activation of melanopsin, generated by RGCs. (3) Activated melanopsin by sunlight sends an inhibitory signal to pineal gland to decreases the melatonin secretion. (Red numbered rectangle). **(B)** Inadequate exposure to sunlight; (1) Long nights and/or inadequate exposure to sunlight increase the level of melatonin (black arrow), (2) causes melanopsin inactivation and. (3) Promotion in level of inactivated melanopsin by darkness leads to sending a stimulatory signal to pineal gland to cause a further increase in melatonin levels. (4) On the other hand, darkness leads to Vitamin D deficiency. (5) Vitamin D deficiency causes injury to RGCs, (6) reducing melanopsin secretion (dashed black arrow). (7) Vitamin D deficiency also causes disruption in intestinal calcium absorption, which (8) leads to a reduction in smooth muscles of the intestine and subsequently gut stasis. (9) The latter increases gut permeability and LPS translocation toward the CNS. (10) LPS activates CD14/TLR4/MD2 complex which (11) increases the proinflammatory mediators in the brain such as TNF-α. (12) CD14 and TLR4 receptors in the pineal gland respond to LPS by (13) TNF secretion and (14) suppression of melatonin synthesis. (15) Eventually, secreted proinflammatory mediators and activated NF-kB pathway leads to neuroinflammation and possible demyelination at the long term. (Green numbered rectangle).

GUT MICROBIOTA, CD14, TOLL LIKE RECEPTOR 4 (TLR4), AND MELATONIN

The intestine of animals and humans contain gut microbiota which produce endotoxic compounds including lipopolysaccharides (LPS), a component of gram-negative bacterial outer membrane (97, 98). The rise in LPS levels in gut microbiota increases the blood LPS through gut inflammation (99). LPS is recognized by LPS-binding protein (LBP) in the serum which brings the LPS to the surface of various cells such as macrophages and endothelial cells to form a complex with CD14, a receptor molecule for LPS. CD14 splits LPS aggregates into monomeric molecules and facilitates the transfer of LPS to TLR4/MD2 complex. MD2 is a secreted glycoprotein that functions as an indispensable extracellular adaptor molecule for LPS-signaling events. Activation of TLR4/MD2 complex upon binding to LPS leads to LPS-mediated NF*k*B activation and production of pro-inflammatory cytokines such as tumor necrosis factor-alpha (TNF-α) (100–107).

The role of the pineal gland/melatonin in response to LPS is controversial. Melatonin was shown to inhibit the LPS-CD14-TLR4 signaling pathway in bovine mammary epithelial cells and decreased LPS-induced expression of pro-inflammatory cytokines such as TNF-α, IL-1β, and IL-6 (108). In contrast, pineal cells possess both TLR4 and CD14 that bind to LPS and activate NF-*k*B pathway by increasing the level of TNF, which subsequently suppresses melatonin synthesis (109). Since CD14 is the major cell surface receptor for LPS on monocytes/macrophages (110), the authors established that melatonin increased the secretion of IL-1 *in vitro* and *in vivo* (111, 112) and TNF-α and IL-6 *in vivo* (112, 113). These data support the hypothesis that LPS produced by gut microbiota causes neuroinflammation that in turn induces higher levels of LPS stimulating the pineal gland to activate the NF-kB pathway and to produce TNF-α while suppressing melatonin synthesis.

UV IRRITATION, VITAMIN D, GASTROPARESIS

Higher latitude has been associated with higher MS incidence and lower UV exposure. In support of the role of latitude in MS susceptibility, a recent study suggested that regional UVB radiation affects MS prevalence which supports the hypothesis that exposure to sunlight can influence MS risk (114). The latter study highlighted the potential role of gender-specific effects of UVB, a suggestion that is also proposed by meta-regression analyses (115) and by incidence studies of MS (116). In fact, an experimental study demonstrated that UVB therapy can suppress EAE; however, its effect does not proceed via the production of vitamin D (117). On the other hand, although vitamin D levels are low in MS patients, evidence that vitamin D prescription can reduce the incidence of MS has not been obtained yet (118–120). Importantly, vitamin D could reduce the severity of disease only when it was accompanied by elevated serum calcium (121).

To investigate the involvement of UV in MS progression, Irving and colleagues demonstrated that EAE incidence was reduced by 74% following UVB radiation (122). Since UVB photons enter the skin to produce vitamin D3 during exposure to sunlight (123), Irving and colleagues showed that UVB therapy in EAE caused an increase in the levels of skin cis-urocanic acid levels, an intermediate in the catabolism of l-histidine. Moreover, they also observed that enhancement of skin cis-urocanic acid levels independent of UVB cannot affect the disease onset or progression (122). On the other hand, it has been demonstrated that cis-urocanic acid causes a reduction in the severity of colitis, a chronic inflammatory condition of the gut (124). In addition, colitis was shown to delay gastric emptying and leads to colitis-induced gastroparesis in animal models (124). In accordance, it has been reported that women are more susceptible to gastroparesis than men (125), while the incidence of MS is about 3-fold higher in women than in men. We therefore suggest that gastroparesis could be one of the main factors involved in triggering MS.

The summarized results and highlights about the clinical and experimental studies on MS patients and EAE model have been demonstrated in **Table 1** and **Table 2**, respectively.

CONCLUSION

We suggest a new pathway that lead to neuroinflammation and MS by including different factors such as latitude, sunlight, vitamin D, melanopsin, intestinal calcium, pineal gland, gut stasis, gut endotoxins (LPS), and CD14/TLR4 (**Figure 1**). While the prevalence of MS is dramatically higher at latitudes above 40 degrees North and South, populations in these areas receive limited sunlight that may lead to a longer increase in melatonin synthesis and release. Since the functions and synthesis of melatonin and vitamin D are contrary to each other, we believe that therapy using these hormones would not be an effective strategy for the treatment of MS patients with low melatonin levels or vitamin D deficiency. We suggest that a balance should exist between these two hormones. In dark periods, melanopsin in the RGCs is inactivate allowing the pineal gland to synthesize melatonin; however, vitamin D levels decrease dramatically and patients face vitamin D deficiency with long term sunlight deprivation. This low level of vitamin D causes RGC injury which contain melanopsin and also reduces intestinal calcium absorption, essential for intestinal smooth muscle contraction. Vitamin D deficiency and reduction of calcium absorption leads to gut stasis and subsequently increases the gut permeability allowing gut microbiota to transfer more endotoxins such as LPS into the blood. Translocated LPS migrates to the brain and triggers the production of pro-inflammatory mediators through CD14/TLR4/MD2 complex. CD14 and TLR4 receptors within the pineal gland respond to LPS with induced TNF secretion while melatonin synthesis is suppressed causing neuroinflammation and contributing to the development of MS in the long term. Further experimental and clinical studies are needed to unravel the mechanisms of MS induction.

AUTHOR CONTRIBUTIONS

MG, RR, KZ, and NF: concept and design of the review, drafting the manuscript and figures. All authors have read, critically revised, and approved the final manuscript before submission. KZ and NF have equal contribution and are co-last and corresponding authors.

REFERENCES

1. Haase CG, Tinnefeld M, Faustmann PM. The influence of immunomodulation on psycho-neuroimmunological functions in benign multiple sclerosis. *Neuroimmunomodulation* (2004) 11:365–72. doi: 10.1159/000080146
2. Golan D, Staun-Ram E, Miller A. Shifting paradigms in multiple sclerosis: from disease-specific, through population-specific toward patient-specific. *Curr Opin Neurol.* (2016) 29:354–61. doi: 10.1097/WCO.0000000000000324
3. Loma I, Heyman R. Multiple sclerosis: pathogenesis and treatment. *Curr Neuropharmacol.* (2011) 9:409–16. doi: 10.2174/157015911796557911
4. Giulio D, Julia MM, Sreeram VR. Multiple sclerosis: risk factors and their interactions. *CNS Neurol Disord Drug Targets* (2012) 11:545–55. doi: 10.2174/187152712801661266
5. Milo R, Kahana E. Multiple sclerosis: geoepidemiology, genetics and the environment. *Autoimmun Rev.* (2010) 9:A387–94. doi: 10.1016/j.autrev.2009.11.010
6. Estanislao LB, Pachner AR. Spirochetal infection of the nervous system. *Neurol Clin.* (1999) 17:783–800. doi: 10.1016/S0733-8619(05)70166-3
7. Pawate S, Sriram S. The role of infections in the pathogenesis and course of multiple sclerosis. *Ann Indian Acad Neurol.* (2010) 13:80–6. doi: 10.4103/0972-2327.64622
8. Pierrot-Deseilligny C, Souberbielle JC. Is hypovitaminosis D one of the environmental risk factors for multiple sclerosis? *Brain* (2010) 133:1869–88. doi: 10.1093/brain/awq147
9. Goodin DS. The causal cascade to multiple sclerosis: a model for Ms pathogenesis. *PLoS ONE* (2009) 4:E4565. doi: 10.1371/journal.pone.0004565
10. Simpson S, Blizzard L, Otahal P, Van Der Mei I, Taylor B. Latitude is significantly associated with the prevalence of multiple sclerosis: a meta-analysis. *J Neurol Neurosurg Psychiatry* (2011) 82:1132. doi: 10.1136/jnnp.2011.240432
11. Holick MF, Binkley NC, Bischoff-Ferrari HA, Gordon CM, Hanley DA, Heaney RP, et al. Evaluation, treatment, and prevention of vitamin D deficiency: an endocrine society clinical practice guideline. *J Clin Endocrinol Metab.* (2011) 96:1911–30. doi: 10.1210/jc.2011-0385
12. Spiro A, Buttriss JL. Vitamin D: an overview of vitamin D status and intake in Europe. *Nutr Bull/BNF* (2014) 39:322–50. doi: 10.1111/nbu.12108
13. O'connor A, Benelam B. An update on UK vitamin D intakes and status, and issues for food fortification and supplementation. *Nutr Bull.* (2011) 36:390–6. doi: 10.1111/j.1467-3010.2011.01918.x
14. Plum LA, Deluca HF. Vitamin D, disease and therapeutic opportunities. *Nat Rev Drug Discov.* (2010) 9:941–55. doi: 10.1038/nrd3318
15. Tripkovic L, Lambert H, Hart K, Smith CP, Bucca G, Penson S, et al. Comparison Of vitamin D(2) and vitamin D(3) supplementation in raising serum 25-hydroxyvitamin D status: a systematic review and meta-analysis. *Am J Clin Nutr.* (2012) 95:1357–64. doi: 10.3945/ajcn.111.031070
16. Veldurthy V, Wei R, Oz L, Dhawan P, Jeon YH, Christakos S. Vitamin D, calcium homeostasis and aging. *Bone Res.* (2016) 4:16041. doi: 10.1038/boneres.2016.41
17. Aranow C. Vitamin D and the immune system. *J Invest Med.* (2011) 59:881–6. doi: 10.2310/JIM.0b013e31821b8755
18. Takahashi S, Maeda T, Sano Y, Nishihara H, Takeshita Y, Shimizu F, et al. Active form of vitamin D directly protects the blood–brain barrier in multiple sclerosis. *Clin Exp Neuroimmunol.* (2017) 8:244–54. doi: 10.1111/cen3.12398
19. Ahlgren C, Odén A, Lycke J. High nationwide prevalence of multiple sclerosis in Sweden. *Multiple Scler J.* (2011) 17:901–8. doi: 10.1177/1352458511403794
20. Klingberg E, Oleröd G, Konar J, Petzold M, Hammarsten O. Seasonal variations in serum 25-hydroxy vitamin D levels in a Swedish cohort. *Endocrine* (2015) 49:800–8. doi: 10.1007/s12020-015-0548-3
21. Engelsen O, Brustad M, Aksnes L, Lund E. Daily duration of vitamin D synthesis in human skin with relation to latitude, total ozone, altitude, ground cover, aerosols and cloud thickness. *Photochem Photobiol.* (2005) 81:1287–90. doi: 10.1562/2004-11-19-RN-375
22. Samefors M, Ostgren CJ, Molstad S, Lannering C, Midlov P, Tengblad A. Vitamin D deficiency in elderly people in Swedish nursing homes is associated with increased mortality. *Eur J Endocrinol.* (2014) 170:667–75. doi: 10.1530/EJE-13-0855
23. Andersson Å, Björk A, Kristiansson P, Johansson G. Vitamin D intake and status in immigrant and native Swedish women: a study at a primary health care centre located at 60°N in Sweden. *Food Nutr Res.* (2013) 57: 20089. doi: 10.3402/Fnr.V57i0.20089
24. Alla S, Pearson J, Debernard L, Miller D, Mason D. The increasing prevalence of multiple sclerosis in New Zealand. *Neuroepidemiology* (2014) 42:154–60. doi: 10.1159/000358174
25. Sharpe RJ. The low incidence of multiple sclerosis in areas near the equator may be due to ultraviolet light induced suppressor cells to melanocyte antigens. *Med Hypotheses* (1986) 19:319–23. doi: 10.1016/0306-9877(86)90104-0
26. Harandi AA, Harandi AA, Pakdaman H, Sahraian MA. Vitamin D and multiple sclerosis. *Iran J Neurol.* (2014) 13:1–6.
27. Reiter RJ. Melatonin: the chemical expression of darkness. *Mol Cell Endocrinol.* (1991) 79:C153–8. doi: 10.1016/0303-7207(91)90087-9
28. Akpinar Z, Tokgoz S, Gokbel H, Okudan N, Uguz F, Yilmaz G. The association of nocturnal serum melatonin levels with major depression in patients with acute multiple sclerosis. *Psychiatry Res.* (2008) 161:253–7. doi: 10.1016/j.psychres.2007.11.022
29. Ghorbani A, Salari M, Shaygannejad V, Norouzi R. The role of melatonin in the pathogenesis of multiple sclerosis: a case-control study. *Int J Prevent Med.* (2013) 4:S180–4.
30. Melamud L, Golan D, Luboshitzky R, Lavi I, Miller A. Melatonin dysregulation, sleep disturbances and fatigue in multiple sclerosis. *J Neurol Sci.* (2012) 314:37–40. doi: 10.1016/j.jns.2011.11.003
31. Sandyk R. Multiple sclerosis: the role of puberty and the pineal gland in its pathogenesis. *Int J Neurosci.* (1993) 68:209–25. doi: 10.3109/00207459308994277
32. Lopez-Gonzalez A, Alvarez-Sanchez N, Lardone PJ, Cruz-Chamorro I, Martinez-Lopez A, Guerrero JM, et al. Melatonin treatment improves primary progressive multiple sclerosis: a case report. *J Pineal Res.* (2015) 58:173–7. doi: 10.1111/jpi.12203
33. Kang JC, Ahn M, Kim YS, Moon C, Lee Y, Wie MB, et al. Melatonin ameliorates autoimmune encephalomyelitis through suppression of intercellular adhesion molecule-1. *J Vet Sci.* (2001) 2:85–9.
34. Alvarez-Sanchez N, Cruz-Chamorro I, Lopez-Gonzalez A, Utrilla JC, Fernandez-Santos JM, Martinez-Lopez A, et al. Melatonin controls experimental autoimmune encephalomyelitis by altering the T effector/regulatory balance. *Brain Behav Immun.* (2015) 50:101–14. doi: 10.1016/j.bbi.2015.06.021
35. Chen SJ, Huang SH, Chen JW, Wang KC, Yang YR, Liu PF, et al. Melatonin enhances interleukin-10 expression and suppresses chemotaxis to inhibit inflammation *in situ* and reduce the severity of experimental autoimmune encephalomyelitis. *Int Immunopharmacol.* (2016) 31:169–77. doi: 10.1016/j.intimp.2015.12.020
36. Ghareghani M, Dokoohaki S, Ghanbari A, Farhadi N, Zibara K, Khodadoust S, et al. Melatonin exacerbates acute experimental autoimmune encephalomyelitis by enhancing the serum levels of lactate: a potential biomarker of multiple sclerosis progression. *Clin Exp Pharmacol Physiol.* (2017) 44:52–61. doi: 10.1111/1440-1681.12678
37. Dudani SJ, Kalhan S, Sharma SP. Vitamin D and multiple sclerosis: potential pathophysiological role and clinical implications. *Int J Appl Basic Med Res.* (2011) 1:71–4. doi: 10.4103/2229-516X.91146
38. Pozuelo-Moyano B, Benito-Leon J, Mitchell AJ, Hernandez-Gallego J. A systematic review of randomized, double-blind, placebo-controlled trials examining the clinical efficacy of vitamin D in multiple sclerosis. *Neuroepidemiology* (2013) 40:147–53. doi: 10.1159/000345122
39. Shaygannejad V, Janghorbani M, Ashtari F, Dehghan H. Effects of adjunct low-dose vitamin D on relapsing-remitting multiple sclerosis progression: preliminary findings of a randomized placebo-controlled trial. *Multiple Scler Int.* (2012) 2012:452541. doi: 10.1155/2012/452541
40. Simpson S Jr, Taylor B, Blizzard L, Ponsonby AL, Pittas F, Tremlett H, et al. Higher 25-hydroxyvitamin D is associated with lower relapse risk in multiple sclerosis. *Ann Neurol.* (2010) 68:193–203. doi: 10.1002/ana.22043

41. Munger KL, Ascherio A. Prevention and treatment of MS: studying the effects of vitamin D. *Multiple Scler.* (2011) 17:1405–11. doi: 10.1177/1352458511425366
42. Holmøy T, Torkildsen Ø, Myhr KM, Løken-Amsrud KI. Vitamin D supplementation and monitoring in multiple sclerosis: who, when and wherefore. *Acta Neurol Scand.* (2012) 126:63–9. doi: 10.1111/ane.12028
43. Golan D, Staun-Ram E, Glass-Marmor L, Lavi I, Rozenberg O, Dishon S, et al. The influence of vitamin D supplementation on melatonin status in patients with multiple sclerosis. *Brain Behav Immun.* (2013) 32:180–5. doi: 10.1016/j.bbi.2013.04.010
44. Champney Thomas H, Holtorf AP, Steger RW, Reiter RJ. Concurrent determination of enzymatic activities and substrate concentrations in the melatonin synthetic pathway within the same rat pineal gland. *J Neurosci Res.* (1984) 11:59–66. doi: 10.1002/jnr.490110107
45. Brzezinski A. Melatonin in humans. *N Engl J Med.* (1997) 336:186–95. doi: 10.1056/NEJM199701163360306
46. Reiter RJ, Tan DX, Burkhardt S, Manchester LC. Melatonin in plants. *Nutr Rev.* (2001) 59:286–90. doi: 10.1111/j.1753-4887.2001.tb07018.x
47. Reiter RJ. The melatonin rhythm: both a clock and a calendar. *Experientia* (1993) 49:654–64. doi: 10.1007/BF01923947
48. Malpaux B, Migaud M, Tricoire H, Chemineau P. Biology of mammalian photoperiodism and the critical role of the pineal gland and melatonin. *J Biol Rhythms* (2001) 16:336–47. doi: 10.1177/074873001129002051
49. Yamazaki S, Goto M, Menaker M. No evidence for extraocular photoreceptors in the circadian system of the Syrian hamster. *J Biol Rhythms* (1999) 14:197–201. doi: 10.1177/074873099129000605
50. Ruby NF, Brennan TJ, Xie X, Cao V, Franken P, Heller HC, et al. Role of melanopsin in circadian responses to light. *Science* (2002) 298:2211–3. doi: 10.1126/science.1076701
51. Gamlin PD, Mcdougal DH, Pokorny J, Smith VC, Yau KW, Dacey DM. Human and macaque pupil responses driven by melanopsin-containing retinal ganglion cells. *Vision Res.* (2007) 47:946–54. doi: 10.1016/j.visres.2006.12.015
52. Paul KN, Saafir TB, Tosini G. The role of retinal photoreceptors in the regulation of circadian rhythms. *Rev Endocr Metab Disord.* (2009) 10:271–8. doi: 10.1007/s11154-009-9120-x
53. Hattar S, Liao HW, Takao M, Berson DM, Yau KW. Melanopsin-containing retinal ganglion cells: architecture, projections, and intrinsic photosensitivity. *Science* (2002) 295:1065–70. doi: 10.1126/science.1069609
54. Melyan Z, Tarttelin EE, Bellingham J, Lucas RJ, Hankins MW. Addition of human melanopsin renders mammalian cells photoresponsive. *Nature* (2005) 433:741–5. doi: 10.1038/nature03344
55. Mure LS, Rieux C, Hattar S, Cooper HM. Melanopsin-dependent nonvisual responses: evidence for photopigment bistability *in vivo*. *J Biol Rhythms* (2007) 22:411–24. doi: 10.1177/0748730407306043
56. Provencio I. *Circadian Photoreception A2 - Dartt, Darlene A. Encyclopedia of the Eye.* Oxford: Academic Press (2010).
57. Reppert SM, Weaver DR, Rivkees SA, Stopa EG. Putative melatonin receptors in a human biological clock. *Science* (1988) 242:78–81. doi: 10.1126/science.2845576
58. Gooley JJ, Lu J, Fischer D, Saper CB. A broad role for melanopsin in nonvisual photoreception. *J Neurosci.* (2003) 23:7093–106. doi: 10.1523/JNEUROSCI.23-18-07093.2003
59. Brainard GC, Hanifin JP, Greeson JM, Byrne B, Glickman G, Gerner E, et al. Action spectrum for melatonin regulation in humans: evidence for a novel circadian photoreceptor. *J Neurosci.* (2001) 21:6405–12. doi: 10.1523/JNEUROSCI.21-16-06405.2001
60. Mcdougal DH, Gamlin PD. The influence of intrinsically-photosensitive retinal ganglion cells on the spectral sensitivity and response dynamics of the human pupillary light reflex. *Vision Res.* (2010) 50:72–87. doi: 10.1016/j.visres.2009.10.012
61. Maynard ML, Zele AJ, Feigl B. Melanopsin-mediated post-illumination pupil response in early age-related macular degeneration. *Invest Ophthalmol Visual Sci.* (2015) 56:6906–13. doi: 10.1167/iovs.15-17357
62. Annweiler C, Beauchet O, Bartha R, Graffe A, Milea D, Montero-Odasso M. Association between serum 25-hydroxyvitamin D concentration and optic chiasm volume. *J Am Geriatr Soc.* (2013) 61:1026–8. doi: 10.1111/jgs.12249
63. Suzumura A. Effect of vitamin D on blood–brain barrier function in multiple sclerosis. *Clin Exp Neuroimmunol.* (2017) 8:180. doi: 10.1111/cen3.12410
64. Alluri H, Wilson RL, Anasooya Shaji C, Wiggins-Dohlvik K, Patel S, Liu Y, et al. Melatonin preserves blood-brain barrier integrity and permeability via matrix metalloproteinase-9 inhibition. *PLoS ONE* (2016) 11:E0154427. doi: 10.1371/journal.pone.0154427
65. Peacock M. Calcium metabolism in health and disease. *Clin J Am Soc Nephrol.* (2010) 5(Suppl. 1):S23–30. doi: 10.2215/CJN.05910809
66. Sjoblom M, Safsten B, Flemstrom G. Melatonin-induced calcium signaling in clusters of human and rat duodenal enterocytes. *Am J Physiol Gastrointest Liver Physiol.* (2003) 284:G1034–44. doi: 10.1152/ajpgi.00500.2002
67. Christakos S. Recent advances in our understanding of 1,25-dihydroxyvitamin D(3) regulation of intestinal calcium absorption. *Arch Biochem Biophys.* (2012) 523:73–6. doi: 10.1016/j.abb.2011.12.020
68. Devine A, Wilson SG, Dick IM, Prince RL. Effects of vitamin D metabolites on intestinal calcium absorption and bone turnover in elderly women. *Am J Clin Nutr.* (2002) 75:283–8. doi: 10.1093/ajcn/75.2.283
69. Fraser DR. Regulation of the metabolism of vitamin D. *Physiol Rev.* (1980) 60:551–613. doi: 10.1152/physrev.1980.60.2.551
70. Li YC, Pirro AE, Amling M, Delling G, Baron R, Bronson R, et al. Targeted ablation of the vitamin D receptor: an animal model of vitamin D-dependent rickets type II with alopecia. *Proc Natl Acad Sci USA.* (1997) 94:9831–5. doi: 10.1073/pnas.94.18.9831
71. Yoshizawa T, Handa Y, Uematsu Y, Takeda S, Sekine K, Yoshihara Y, et al. Mice lacking the vitamin D receptor exhibit impaired bone formation, uterine hypoplasia and growth retardation after weaning. *Nat Genet.* (1997) 16:391–6. doi: 10.1038/ng0897-391
72. Pansu D, Bellaton C, Roche C, Bronner F. Duodenal and ileal calcium absorption in the rat and effects of vitamin D. *Am J Physiol.* (1983) 244:G695–700.
73. Sheikh MS, Ramirez A, Emmett M, Santa Ana C, Schiller LR, Fordtran JS. Role of vitamin D-dependent and vitamin D-independent mechanisms in absorption of food calcium. *J Clin Invest.* (1988) 81:126–32. doi: 10.1172/JCI113283
74. Karaki H, Weiss GB. Calcium channels in smooth muscle. *Gastroenterology* (1984) 87:960–70.
75. Somlyo AP, Somlyo AV. Signal transduction and regulation in smooth muscle. *Nature* (1994) 372:231. doi: 10.1038/372231a0
76. Giraldi G, Fioravanti A, De Luca D'alessandro E, Palmery M, Martinoli L. Investigation of the effects of vitamin D and calcium on intestinal motility: *in vitro* tests and implications for clinical treatment. *Acta Pharm* (2015) 65:343–9. doi: 10.1515/acph-2015-0023
77. Kong J, Zhang Z, Musch MW, Ning G, Sun J, Hart J, et al. Novel role of the vitamin D receptor in maintaining the integrity of the intestinal mucosal barrier. *Am J Physiol Gastrointest Liver Physiol.* (2008) 294:G208–16. doi: 10.1152/ajpgi.00398.2007
78. Koenig J, Cote N. Equine gastrointestinal motility—ileus and pharmacological modification. *Can Veter J.* (2006) 47:551–9.
79. Parkman HP, Hasler WL, Fisher RS. American gastroenterological association technical review on the diagnosis and treatment of gastroparesis. *Gastroenterology* (2004) 127:1592–622. doi: 10.1053/j.gastro.2004.09.055
80. Gill KP, Chia YW, Henry MM, Shorvon PJ. Defecography in multiple sclerosis patients with severe constipation. *Radiology* (1994) 191:553–6. doi: 10.1148/radiology.191.2.8153339
81. Wiesel PH, Norton C, Roy AJ, Storrie JB, Bowers J, Kamm MA. Gut focused behavioural treatment (Biofeedback) for constipation and faecal incontinence in multiple sclerosis. *J Neurol Neurosurg Psychiatry* (2000) 69:240–3. doi: 10.1136/jnnp.69.2.240
82. Enck P, Van Der Voort I, Klosterhalfen S. Biofeedback therapy in fecal incontinence and constipation. *Neurogastroenterol Motility* (2009) 21:1133–41. doi: 10.1111/j.1365-2982.2009.01345.x
83. Mcclurg D, Hagen S, Hawkins S, Lowe-Strong A. Abdominal massage for the alleviation of constipation symptoms in people with multiple sclerosis: a randomized controlled feasibility study. *Multiple Scler J.* (2010) 17:223–33. doi: 10.1177/1352458510384899
84. Yacyshyn B, Meddings J, Sadowski D, Bowen-Yacyshyn MB. Multiple sclerosis patients have peripheral blood Cd45ro+ B cells and

increased intestinal permeability. *Dig Dis Sci.* (1996) 41:2493–8. doi: 10.1007/BF02100148

85. Nathens AB, Marshall JC. Sepsis, sirs, and mods: what's in a name? *World J Surg* (1996) 20:386–91.
86. Nieuwenhuijzen GA, Goris RJA. The gut: the "motor" of multiple organ dysfunction syndrome? *Curr Opin Critic Care* (1999) 5:126.
87. Hierholzer C, Kalff JC, Chakraborty A, Watkins SC, Billiar TR, Bauer AJ, et al. Impaired gut contractility following hemorrhagic shock is accompanied by Il-6 and G-Csf production and neutrophil infiltration. *Digest Dis Sci* (2001) 46:230–41. doi: 10.1023/A:1005524021552
88. Chieveley-Williams S, Hamilton-Davies C. The role of the gut in major surgical postoperative morbidity. *Int Anesthesiol Clin.* (1998) 37:81–110. doi: 10.1097/00004311-199903720-00006
89. Overhaus M, Tögel S, Pezzone MA, Bauer AJ. Mechanisms of polymicrobial sepsis-induced ileus. *Am J Physiol-Gastrointestinal Liver Physiol.* (2004) 287:G685–94. doi: 10.1152/ajpgi.00359.2003
90. Swank GM, Deitch EA. Role of the gut in multiple organ failure: bacterial translocation and permeability changes. *World J Surg.* (1996) 20:411–7. doi: 10.1007/s002689900065
91. Zheyu C, Qinghui Q, Lunan Y. Roles of calcium and Ip3 in impaired colon contractility of rats following multiple organ dysfunction syndrome. *Braz J Med Biol Res.* (2007) 40:1389–97. doi: 10.1590/S0100-879X2006005000147
92. Wang Y, Kasper LH. The role of microbiome in central nervous system disorders. *Brain Behav Immun.* (2014) 38:1–12. doi: 10.1016/j.bbi.2013.12.015
93. Wolfson C, Talbot P. Bacterial infection as a cause of multiple sclerosis. *Lancet* (2002) 360:352–3. doi: 10.1016/S0140-6736(02)09 603-4
94. Chen J, Chia N, Kalari KR, Yao JZ, Novotna M, Soldan MMP, et al. Multiple sclerosis patients have a distinct gut microbiota compared to healthy controls. *Sci Rep.* (2016a) 6:28484. doi: 10.1038/srep 28484
95. Tremlett H, Fadrosh DW, Faruqi AA, Zhu F, Hart J, Roalstad S, et al. Gut microbiota in early pediatric multiple sclerosis: a case-control study. *Eur J Neurol.* (2016) 23:1308–21. doi: 10.1111/ene.13026
96. Braniste V, Al-Asmakh M, Kowal C, Anuar F, Abbaspour A, Tóth M, et al. The gut microbiota influences blood-brain barrier permeability in mice. *Sci Trans Med.* (2014) 6:263ra158. doi: 10.1126/scitranslmed.30 09759
97. Poltorak A, He X, Smirnova I, Liu MY, Van Huffel C, Du X, et al. Defective LPS signaling in C3H/HEJ and C57bl/10sccr mice: mutations in Tlr4 gene. *Science* (1998) 282:2085–8. doi: 10.1126/science.282.5396.2085
98. Harmsen HJ, De Goffau MC. The human gut microbiota. *Adv Exp Med Biol.* (2016) 902:95–108. doi: 10.1007/978-3-319-31248-4_7
99. Jiang T, Gao X, Wu C, Tian F, Lei Q, Bi J, et al. Apple-derived pectin modulates gut microbiota, improves gut barrier function, and attenuates metabolic endotoxemia in rats with diet-induced obesity. *Nutrients* (2016) 8:126. doi: 10.3390/nu8030126
100. Schumann RR, Leong SR, Flaggs GW, Gray PW, Wright SD, Mathison JC, et al. Structure and function of lipopolysaccharide binding protein. *Science* (1990) 249:1429–31. doi: 10.1126/science.2402637
101. Dunzendorfer S, Lee HK, Soldau K, Tobias PS. Tlr4 is the signaling but not the lipopolysaccharide uptake receptor. *J Immunol.* (2004) 173:1166–70. doi: 10.4049/jimmunol.173.2.1166
102. Da Silva Correia J, Soldau K, Christen U, Tobias PS, Ulevitch RJ. Lipopolysaccharide is in close proximity to each of the proteins in its membrane receptor complex. Transfer from Cd14 to Tlr4 and Md-2. *J Biol Chem.* (2001) 276:21129–35. doi: 10.1074/jbc.M009164200
103. Akira S, Takeda K. Toll-like receptor signalling. *Nat Rev Immunol.* (2004) 4:499–511. doi: 10.1038/nri1391
104. Chow JC, Young DW, Golenbock DT, Christ WJ, Gusovsky F. Toll-like receptor-4 mediates lipopolysaccharide-induced signal transduction. *J Biol Chem.* (1999) 274:10689–92. doi: 10.1074/jbc.274.16. 10689
105. Buchholz BM, Bauer AJ. Membrane Tlr signaling mechanisms in the gastrointestinal tract during sepsis. *Neurogastroenterol Motil.* (2010) 22:232–45. doi: 10.1111/j.1365-2982.2009.01464.x
106. Zhang G, Ghosh S. Molecular mechanisms of Nf-Kappab activation induced by bacterial lipopolysaccharide through toll-like receptors. *J Endotoxin Res.* (2000) 6:453–7. doi: 10.1179/0968051001015 32414
107. Kawai T, Akira S. The role of pattern-recognition receptors in innate immunity: update on toll-like receptors. *Nat Immunol.* (2010) 11:373–84. doi: 10.1038/ni.1863
108. Yu G-M, Kubota H, Okita M, Maeda T. The anti-inflammatory and antioxidant effects of melatonin on Lps-stimulated bovine mammary epithelial cells. *PLoS ONE* (2017) 12:E0178525. doi: 10.1371/journal.pone.0178525
109. Da Silveira Cruz-Machado S, Carvalho-Sousa CE, Tamura EK, Pinato L, Cecon E, Fernandes PA, et al. Tlr4 and Cd14 receptors expressed in rat pineal gland trigger Nfkb pathway. *J Pineal Res.* (2010) 49:183–92. doi: 10.1111/j.1600-079X.2010.0 0785.x
110. Wright SD, Ramos RA, Tobias PS, Ulevitch RJ, Mathison JC. Cd14, a receptor for complexes of lipopolysaccharide (Lps) and Lps binding protein. *Science* (1990) 249:1431–3. doi: 10.1126/science.16 98311
111. Morrey KM, Mclachlan JA, Serkin CD, Bakouche O. Activation of human monocytes by the pineal hormone melatonin. *J Immunol.* (1994) 153:2671–80.
112. Pioli C, Caroleo MC, Nistico G, Doria G. Melatonin increases antigen presentation and amplifies specific and non specific signals for T-cell proliferation. *Int J Immunopharmacol.* (1993) 15:463–8. doi: 10.1016/0192-0561(93)90060-C
113. Barjavel MJ, Mamdouh Z, Raghbate N, Bakouche O. Differential expression of the melatonin receptor in human monocytes. *J Immunol.* (1998) 160:1191.
114. Orton SM, Wald L, Confavreux C, Vukusic S, Krohn JP, Ramagopalan SV, et al. Association of UV radiation with multiple sclerosis prevalence and sex ratio in France. *Neurology* (2011) 76:425–31. doi: 10.1212/WNL.0b013e31820a0a9f
115. Koch-Henriksen N, Sørensen PS. The changing demographic pattern of multiple sclerosis epidemiology. *Lancet Neurol.* (2010) 9:520–32. doi: 10.1016/S1474-4422(10)70064-8
116. Alonso A, Hernán MA. Temporal trends in the incidence of multiple sclerosis: a systematic review. *Neurology* (2008) 71:129–35. doi: 10.1212/01.wnl.0000316802.359 74.34
117. Wang Y, Marling SJ, Mcknight SM, Danielson AL, Severson KS, Deluca HF. Suppression of experimental autoimmune encephalomyelitis by 300–315nm ultraviolet light. *Arch Biochem Biophys.* (2013) 536:81–6. doi: 10.1016/j.abb.2013.05.010
118. Hart PH, Gorman S, Finlay-Jones JJ. Modulation of the immune system by UV radiation: more than just the effects of vitamin D? *Nat Rev Immunol.* (2011) 11:584–96. doi: 10.1038/nri3045
119. Kampman MT, Steffensen LH, Mellgren SI, Jørgensen L. Effect of vitamin D3 supplementation on relapses, disease progression, and measures of function in persons with multiple sclerosis: exploratory outcomes from a double-blind randomised controlled trial. *Multiple Scler J.* (2012) 18:1144–51. doi: 10.1177/1352458511434607
120. Rosjo E, Steffensen LH, Jorgensen L, Lindstrom JC, Saltyte Benth J, Michelsen AE, et al. Vitamin D supplementation and systemic inflammation in relapsing-remitting multiple sclerosis. *J Neurol.* (2015) 262:2713–21. doi: 10.1007/s00415-015-7902-5
121. Cantorna MT, Humpal-Winter J, Deluca HF. Dietary calcium is a major factor in 1,25-dihydroxycholecalciferol suppression of experimental autoimmune encephalomyelitis in mice. *J Nutr.* (1999) 129:1966–71. doi: 10.1093/jn/129.11.1966
122. Irving AA, Marling SJ, Plum LA, Deluca HF. Suppression of experimental autoimmune encephalomyelitis by ultraviolet light is not mediated by isomerization of urocanic acid. *BMC Neurosci.* (2017) 18:8. doi: 10.1186/s12868-016-0323-2
123. Holick MF. Sunlight, UV-radiation, vitamin D and skin cancer: how much sunlight do we need? *Adv Exp Med Biol.* (2008) 624:1–15. doi: 10.1007/978-0-387-77574-6_1

124. De Schepper HU, De Man JG, Van Nassauw L, Timmermans JP, Herman AG, Pelckmans PA, et al. Acute distal colitis impairs gastric emptying in rats via an extrinsic neuronal reflex pathway involving the pelvic nerve. *Gut* (2007) 56:195–202. doi: 10.1136/gut.2006.104745

125. Gangula PRR, Sekhar KR, Mukhopadhyay S. Gender bias in gastroparesis: is nitric oxide the answer? *Digest Dis Sci.* (2011) 56:2520–7. doi: 10.1007/s10620-011-1735-6

126. Chiuso-Minicucci F, Ishikawa LL, Mimura LA, Fraga-Silva TF, Franca TG, Zorzella-Pezavento SF, et al. Treatment with vitamin D/Mog association suppresses experimental autoimmune encephalomyelitis. *PLoS ONE* (2015) 10:E0125836. doi: 10.1371/journal.pone.0125836

20

Immunological Aspects of Approved MS Therapeutics

Paulus S. Rommer[1], Ron Milo[2,3], May H. Han[4], Sammita Satyanarayan[4], Johann Sellner[5,6], Larissa Hauer[7], Zsolt Illes[8,9], Clemens Warnke[10], Sarah Laurent[10], Martin S. Weber[11,12], Yinan Zhang[13] and Olaf Stuve[6,13,14]**

[1] Department of Neurology, Medical University of Vienna, Vienna, Austria, [2] Department of Neurology, Barzilai University Medical Center, Ashkelon, Israel, [3] Faculty of Health Sciences, Ben-Gurion University of the Negev, Beer-Sheva, Israel, [4] Neuroimmunology Division, Department of Neurology and Neurological Sciences, Stanford University, Stanford, CA, United States, [5] Department of Neurology, Christian Doppler Medical Center, Paracelsus Medical University, Salzburg, Austria, [6] Department of Neurology, Klinikum Rechts der Isar, Technische Universität, Munich, Germany, [7] Department of Psychiatry, Psychotherapy, and Psychosomatics, Christian Doppler Medical Center, Paracelsus Medical University, Salzburg, Austria, [8] Department of Neurology, Odense University Hospital, Odense, Denmark, [9] Institute of Clinical Research, University of Southern Denmark, Odense, Denmark, [10] Department of Neurology, Medical Faculty, University of Köln, Cologne, Germany, [11] Institute of Neuropathology, University Medical Center, Göttingen, Germany, [12] Department of Neurology, University Medical Center, Göttingen, Germany, [13] Department of Neurology and Neurotherapeutics, University of Texas Southwestern Medical Center, Dallas, TX, United States, [14] Neurology Section, VA North Texas Health Care System, Medical Service Dallas, VA Medical Center, Dallas, TX, United States

Correspondence:
Paulus S. Rommer
paulus.rommer@meduniwien.ac.at
Olaf Stuve
olaf.stuve@utsouthwestern.edu

Multiple sclerosis (MS) is the most common neurological immune-mediated disease leading to disability in young adults. The outcome of the disease is unpredictable, and over time, neurological disabilities accumulate. Interferon beta-1b was the first drug to be approved in the 1990s for relapsing-remitting MS to modulate the course of the disease. Over the past two decades, the treatment landscape has changed tremendously. Currently, more than a dozen drugs representing 1 substances with different mechanisms of action have been approved (interferon beta preparations, glatiramer acetate, fingolimod, siponimod, mitoxantrone, teriflunomide, dimethyl fumarate, cladribine, alemtuzumab, ocrelizumab, and natalizumab). Ocrelizumab was the first medication to be approved for primary progressive MS. The objective of this review is to present the modes of action of these drugs and their effects on the immunopathogenesis of MS. Each agent's clinical development and potential side effects are discussed.

Keywords: multiple sclerosis, immunotherapeutics, immunomodulation, immunosuppression, monoclonal antibodies

INTRODUCTION

Multiple sclerosis (MS) is the most common neuroinflammatory and neurodegenerative disease in young adults, with more than 2 million patients worldwide (1). Since the first insights into its pathogenesis were gained from anatomical studies on MS patients in the 19th century by Robert Carswell (2), Jean-Martin Charcot, and others (3), the understanding of pathophysiological concepts concerning MS has been broadened exceedingly. However, modification of the disease course was elusive until the approval of interferon beta-1b (IFN-ß) in 1993 (4). Over the past two decades, the treatment landscape has changed tremendously. Currently, more than a dozen drugs are approved for relapsing-remitting multiple sclerosis (RRMS), and one agent for primary progressive multiple sclerosis (PPMS) (5). These agents represent 10 different substance classes with different modes of action. Whereas, some drugs, including IFN-ß preparations and glatiramer acetate, have no clearly defined mechanisms of action, many of the other agents are target specific and the result of rational drug design. Consequently, much has been learnt about the pathogenesis of MS from the administration of these agents. Although T cells were thought to be the principal lymphocyte subset to initiate and perpetuate disease activity in MS (6), the efficacy of anti-CD20 agents, demonstrated in clinical trials, challenged that concept and pushed B cells together with T cells to the front stage of MS pathogenesis (7, 8).

The initial step in the immune cascade of MS seems to be the activation of T helper (Th) cells in lymph nodes through contact with antigens (either myelin antigens or non-self-antigens sharing similar epitopes to myelin antigens) presented by antigen-presenting cells (APC), including macrophages or dendritic cells (9). This results in the activation and differentiation of myelin-reactive T cells. Activated T cells exit the lymph nodes and circulate in peripheral blood (10), from where they can readily migrate into other tissues, including the central nervous system (CNS). There, these cells can proliferate and clonally expand if they encounter their cognate antigen. The level of chemokines and cytokines increases (e.g., interleukin [IL]-2, IL-1, interferon [IFN]-y, tumor necrosis factor [TNF]-α). As a consequence, additional T and B cells, as well as monocytes are recruited into the CNS and enhance the inflammatory cascade (11).

The monitoring of patients taking new and highly effective drugs that are associated with severe adverse events (AEs) or risks becomes increasingly important. Therefore, it is essential to understand the mode of action of MS drugs and their effects on the immune system. It supports remaining vigilant for unexpected novel AEs that in turn help to understand the mode of action more precisely, and explore the pathophysiology of MS.

This review aims to provide an overview of the approved MS drugs. The history of these drugs and their mode of action are presented considering the current understanding of the pathogenesis of MS.

The review starts with drugs for which the mechanisms of action are not entirely understood, followed by drugs with well-defined molecular and cellular targets.

INTERFERON BETA (IFN-ß)

Interferons are part of the cytokine family and are signaling proteins. They can be divided into three classes: type I (interferon alpha and beta), type II (interferon gamma), and type III (interferon delta), with different biological effects (12). IFN-ß belongs to the class of type I interferons and is produced by lymphocytes, fibroblasts, macrophages, and endothelial cells (12). Interferons play an important role in the regulation of the immune system. The effects modulated by IFN-ß are complex and have not been elucidated in detail. IFN-ß binds to the type I IFN receptors INFAR-1 and INFAR-2. Its affinity to INFAR-2 is higher than to INFAR-1. This binding activates the JAK/STAT (janus kinases/signal transducer and activator of transcription proteins) signaling pathway leading to the expression of cellular genes (e.g., Mx protein, ß2-microglobulin, 2′/5′-olygoadenylate synthetase, and neopterin) (13). Overall, the activation of signal-transduction pathways by IFN-ß leads to antiviral, immunomodulatory, and antiproliferative effects (14).

IFN-ß has a wide range of immunomodulatory effects. It reduces the number of dendritic cells and downregulates antigen presentation by APCs in the peripheral blood and also within the CNS (microglial cells and monocytes). The expression of Toll-like receptors (TLR) 3 and 7, as well as MyD88, on dendritic cells is upregulated, leading to altered immune responses. It induces $CD4^+$, $CD8^+$, $CD25^+$, $FOXP3^+$, and $FoxA1^+$ T cells (Treg cells). IFN-ß decreases inflammatory T cell responses by inhibiting the stimulation and activation of T cells (e.g., by modulating costimulatory molecules on dendritic cells and inhibiting the expression of MHC class II molecules and co-stimulatory factors such as CD80 and CD28 on APCs) (15, 16). The secretion of cytokines and chemokines is altered (e.g., increased levels of IL-10 and IL-4, and decreased levels of IL-12 and TNF α), and the differentiation of CD4+ T cells shifts from a T helper-1 (Th1) to Th2 phenotype, resulting in a less pro-inflammatory and more anti-inflammatory cytokine milieu (17). The number of Th17 cells decreases, leading to a reduction in the release of Il-17 (12), and the apoptosis of auto-reactive T cells is induced (5). Effects on cytokines and chemokines, matrix metalloproteinases (MMP), and adhesion molecules (e.g., VLA-4 on T cells) have been suggested (15, 18–20), thus the migration of leukocytes into the CNS via the blood-brain-barrier (BBB) is reduced.

Currently, IFN-ß is available as IFN-ß-1a (Avonex®, Rebif®, and Plegridy®) and IFN-ß-1b (Betaferon® or Extavia®). IFN-ß-1-a differs from IFN-ß-1b in its amino-acid sequence, tertiary structure, and glycosylation status (21). IFN-ß-1b was the first drug approved by the US Food and Drug Administration (FDA) for the treatment of MS in 1993 (22) and was granted market authorization in 1995 in Europe (23). The preparations differ with respect to their frequency and route of administration. The frequency of administration ranges from every other day/thrice a week (tiw) (Betaferon® or Extavia®/Rebif® subcutaneously [SC]), to once a week (Avonex®, intramuscular [IM]), to biweekly (Plegridy®, SC). PEGylation led to more stable preparations and a longer half-life (24).

When tested in patients with MS, IFN-ß-1b significantly lowered relapse rates in RRMS by approximately one third (25), with more patients free of relapses after 2 years in the IFN-ß-1b cohort (26). No significant differences in disease progression or the relapse rate were confirmed at 6 months in patients with mild (Expanded Disability Status Scale [EDSS] $\leq$3.5) or moderate (EDSS $>$3.5) disability (27). In patients with clinically isolated syndrome (CIS) treated with IFN-ß, the conversion rate to MS was lower during the study period compared to the control group (28–30). However, in secondary progressive MS (SPMS), conflicting results were reported between a European (31) and a North American study (32), with positive effects on progression confirmed at 3 months in the European study, which were explained partly by the younger and clinically more active patient population in the European study than the North American study (33). A prospective study of 2,570 IFN-ß-treated MS patients revealed that an early start within the first years after diagnosis significantly lowered the risk of EDSS progression and long term disability (milestone: EDSS 4) (34). A 16-year follow up study of pivotal trials of IFN-ß-1b revealed different mortality rates for the study groups in the pivotal studies, with the highest mortality rate for the cohort initially treated with a placebo (18.3%), followed by the study group given 50 μg every other day (8.3%), and was lowest mortality rate was found in the group given the high and subsequently approved dose of 250 μg (5.4%). Standard long-term assessments did not show differences between the study groups except for mortality (35).

Since IFN-ß is immunogenic, allergic reactions might occur, and importantly, neutralizing antibodies (NAbs) can be formed in response to treatment. NAbs can lead to the decreased efficacy of IFN-ß preparations and a worsening disease outcome might be observed (36). NAbs were more frequently reported during treatment with IFN-ß-1b than with IFN-ß-1a. Based on the data from various trials, IFN-ß-1b seems to be more immunogenic than IFN-ß-1a (4, 37). This was confirmed by samples from 20,695 MS patients from 6 European Countries. IM administered IFN-ß-1a is the least immunogenic IFN-ß preparation followed by SC administered IFN-ß-1a preparations, with SC IFN-ß-1b preparations being the most immunogenic ones (37). The reason for this has not been elucidated.

The most common AEs include influenza-like symptoms, injection-site reactions, headache, thyroid disorders including autoimmunity, depression, allergic reactions, and elevated liver enzymes with the possibility of severe hepatic injury, which are all frequently reported. Hematological abnormalities (leukopenia, lymphopenia) can also be found (4, 5, 23, 26, 27).

Monitoring requirements include blood counts, liver-enzyme assessments and thyroid testing at regular intervals. NAbs should be tested when treatment failure is suspected (5). According to preclinical studies, harm to the fetus cannot be excluded. The data on IFN-ß during pregnancy in MS patients has so far revealed no association between treatment and an increased teratogenic or abortive potential. The data on treatment during the second and third trimester is limited (38). **Table 1** shows data on all approved injectables.

GLATIRAMER ACETATE

Glatiramer acetate (GA, Copaxone®, formerly known as copolymer-1 or Cop-1, and Glatopa®, a biosimilar) is a mixture of random synthetic polypeptides composed of 4 amino acids (glutamate, lysine, alanine, and tyrosine) in a pre-defined molar ratio. GA initially was developed at the Weizmann Institute in Israel as a chemical and immunological analog of the major myelin antigen, myelin basic protein (MBP), to induce experimental autoimmune encephalomyelitis (EAE). Surprisingly, GA did not prove to be encephalitogenic, nor did it induce EAE in susceptible animals, but rather showed high efficacy in suppressing, and even preventing EAE induced by MBP and other myelin antigens in a variety of species and models of EAE (39).

GA's exact mode of action in MS is not completely understood, but extensive research has shown that GA, initially considered to be specific for MBP-related T cell immune responses, affects a variety of immune and non-immune pathways. GA cross-reacts with MBP on the cellular and humoral levels (39) and probably functions as an altered peptide ligand that promotes regulatory T cells instead of stimulating adverse T cell autoreactivity (40). GA's immunomodulatory effects probably stem from strong and indiscriminate binding to MHC class II molecules on APCs, while competing with MBP (41) and probably other myelin antigens (42) for these binding sites. This binding effectively displaces MBP, proteolipid protein (PLP), and MOG-derived peptides from their MHC binding sites (43), resulting in altered T cell responses, as evidenced by the suppression of myelin-reactive T cells by GA (42, 44, 45) and the generation of regulatory Th2 cells recognizing both GA and MBP that can cross the BBB, secrete anti-inflammatory cytokines, and exert bystander suppression of auto-aggressive inflammatory T cells in the CNS (46–48). These GA-specific Th2 cells also secrete large amounts of brain-derived neurotrophic factor (BDNF) that might be neuroprotective (49). Other effects of GA on T cells include T cell receptor (TCR) antagonism via the specific engagement of TCR recognizing MBP through the GA-MHC complex in a manner that results in functional receptor inactivation (50) and induction of regulatory CD4+CD25+ T cells through activation of the transcription factor FoxP3 (51).

GA also modulates macrophages, microglia, and dendritic cells, and drives them into M2 phenotype and anti-inflammatory responses (52–54). Incubation of the human monocytic cell line THP-1 with GA results in down-regulation of the expression of MHC class II and molecules on the cell surface and reduced secretion of TNF-α and cathepsin-B (55). These effects may contribute to the modulation of CNS neuroinflammation (56).

Much attention has recently been drawn to the role of B cells in the pathogenesis of MS, and to the beneficial effects of anti-B cell therapy in both RRMS and PPMS (57). Several recent studies have shown that treatment with GA is associated with reductions in the number of B cells, plasmablasts, and memory B cells, as well as a shift from a pro-inflammatory to an anti-inflammatory B cell phenotype (58). It has been hypothesized that this may be mediated by the cross-reactivity of B cell receptors for GA with antigen (possibly myelin basic protein) expressed in the MS lesion (58).

GA has also been shown to promote repair mechanisms, remyelination, and neurogenesis in the EAE model by augmenting the proliferation, migration, and differentiation of oligodendroglial and neuronal progenitor cells (48, 59).

GA was initially tested on a small number of patients with advanced MS ($n = 4$) or acute disseminated encephalomyelitis ($n = 3$) in Israel (60) and in 16 MS patients in the US (61). No side effects or clinical deterioration were noted, and several patients even improved. These encouraging results prompted a pivotal phase-II clinical trial in 50 RRMS patients who were randomized to receive either daily SC injections of 20 mg GA or matching placebos. A marked reduction in the rate of relapses was noted in the GA group, especially in less-disabled patients (62). However, another 2-center randomized trial in 106 progressive MS patients

TABLE 1 | Brand name as well as data on efficacy, dose, route of administration, adverse events of approved injectables.

DMT	**Interferon β-1b**	**Interferon β-1a**	**Interferon β-1a**	**Peg-Interferon β-1a**	**Glatiramer acetate**
Brand name	**Betaferon®/Betaseron® Extavia®**	**Avonex®**	**Rebif®**	**Plegridy®**	**Copaxone®**
Production process	*E. coli*	Chinese hamster ovary	Chinese hamster ovary	Chinese hamster ovary + Pegylation	Synthetic polymer
Molecular structure	165 AA recombinant Non-glycosylated protein lacking amino acid at position 1, serine substitution for cysteine at position 17	166 AA recombinant glycoprotein Identical to human IFN-β	166 AA recombinant glycoprotein Identical to human IFN-β	166 AA recombinant glycoprotein Identical to human IFN-β + Polyethylene glycol	Random copolymer of glutamate, lysine, alanine, tyrosine
Route	SC	IM	SC	SC	SC
Dose	250 μg	30 μg	22/44 μg	125 μg	20/40 mg
Frequency	Every other day	Weekly	Thrice weekly	Every 2 weeks	Daily/thrice weekly
Study	IFNβ MS Study Group 1993	MSCSG 1996	PRISMS 1998	ADVANCE 2014	Cop1 MSSG 1995/GALA 2013
Relapses Annualized rate	0.84	0.61 (ITT –0.67)	0.91/0.86	0.3	0.59/0.33
Relative RR	**34%**	**32% (ITT –18%)**	**27/33%**	**36%**	**29/34.4%**
Absolute RR	0.43	0.29 (ITT –0.15)	0.37/0.42	0.14	0.25/0.17
NNT	**2.3**	**3.5** (ITT–**6.7**)	**2.7/2.4**	**7**	**4/5.9**
Reduction in disease Progression	29%*	37%	30%	38%	12%*
NNT	**9**	**8**	**8**	**37**	**33**
Reduction in new T2	83%	52%	78%	67%	35/35%
and Gd+ MRI activity	75%	50%	84%	86%	39/45%
Main AE	ISR, flu-like symptoms, increased spasticity and fatigue, depression, migraine headache, menstrual irregularities, leukopenia, LFT abnormalities, Thrombotic microangiopathy (manifest mainly as TTP or HUS)				ISR, IPIR, urticaria lipoatrophy, lymphadenopathy

*AA, amino acids; HUS, haemolytic-uremic syndrome; IM, intramuscular; IPIR, immediate post injection reactions; ISR, injection site reactions; ITT, intention to treat; LFT, liver function tests; μg, microgram; MIU, million international units; MRI, magnetic resonance imaging; ND, not determined; SC, subcutaneous; TTP, thrombotic thrombocytopenic purpura; *Non-significant. Bold values indicate most important outcome parameters and AEs.*

failed to demonstrate a beneficial effect on disability progression resulting from 15 mg of GA injected SC twice daily. Nevertheless, two additional secondary disability endpoints and the primary endpoint in one center were met (63).

A pivotal phase-III clinical trial with GA was conducted in 11 US centers. In this trial, 251 RRMS patients were randomized to receive either 20 mg of GA or a placebo via daily SC injections for 2 years. A significant 29% reduction in the annual relapse rate (ARR) was observed in the GA group compared to the placebo group ($p = 0.007$). Significantly more patients on GA improved on the EDSS score, and significantly fewer patients worsened (64, 65). Unfortunately, no MRI scans were performed in this trial, except for at one center where patients on GA had significantly fewer gadolinium (Gd)-enhancing lesions and reduced brain volume loss compared to patients taking placebo (66). To better appreciate GA's effect on MRI parameters, 239 RRMS patients in Europe and Canada were randomized to daily GA or placebo treatment and had monthly MRI scans for 9 months. GA reduced the number of Gd-enhancing and new T2-weighted lesions (67) and the proportion of new Gd-enhancing lesions evolving into black holes (68). The daily dose of 20 mg of GA had similar efficacy as 40 mg GA administered daily (69) or thrice weekly (70), and both regimens (20 mg qd or 40 mg tiw) are approved for use in RRMS. Similarly to the interferons, GA has not been shown to reduce disability progression in PPMS (71), but is highly effective in delaying clinically definite MS after CIS (72). Long-term follow-up of patients with RRMS shows continuous efficacy with low relapse rates and minimal EDSS progression after 15 years (73).

In comparative trials with available interferons in RRMS, GA was as effective as IFN-β-1b (74) or SC IFN-β-1a (75), and superior to IM IFN-β-1a (76). The latter study also showed that the combination of GA and IM IFN-β-1a was not superior to either therapy alone (76).

GA's good safety profile has been established over many years of clinical use. Its principal side effects include local-injection-site reactions (tenderness, pruritus, erythema, or induration). Regional lymphadenopathy; local lipoatrophy, which may be permanent; allergic reactions and rare injection site skin necrosis may also occur. About 16% of patients experience a rare systemic post injection reaction comprising of various combinations of the following effects: chest tightness, dyspnea, flushing, palpitations, diaphoresis, and anxiety beginning immediately after GA injection and resolving spontaneously within a few minutes without any sequelae. Unlike IFN-β, treatment with GA is not associated with leukopenia, liver, or thyroid abnormalities;

depression; or any additional systemic side effects. It is not associated with any serious AEs seen with other potent newer therapies for MS either, such as opportunistic infections, malignancy, or secondary autoimmunity. Virtually all patients develop binding antibodies, but not NAbs to GA, which do not impair its clinical efficacy (77). GA elicits no adverse effects on fertility, pregnancy, or fetal outcomes (78) and is the only MS drug that is no longer contraindicated during pregnancy in Europe.

Although only moderately effective in reducing disease activity, GA is registered worldwide as a first line platform therapy for patients with RRMS due to its long-term efficacy and safety.

FINGOLIMOD

Therapeutic concepts in MS include the down-regulation or depletion of pro-inflammatory T and B cells, the enhancement of anti-inflammatory immune responses (79, 80), the prevention of encephalitogenic lymphocytes from entering into the CNS, and the retention of auto-reactive lymphocytes within secondary lymphoid organs (as in the case of fingolimod) (81, 82). This recognition was based on the understanding of the interaction between sphingosine-1-phosphate (S1P), a signaling sphingolipid, and its receptors, S1PR1-5, essential for lymphocytes to egress from secondary lymphoid organs into the systemic circulation (83, 84). The search for molecules targeting the S1P pathway resulted in the discovery of the fungal metabolite myriocin, which eventually led to the development of FTY720 (fingolimod), an oral therapy for treating RRMS (85). FTY720, a functional antagonist of S1PR1-3,4,5 (S1PR1 being the dominant receptor in lymphocytes) (10) binds to the receptor, leading to internalization of the S1P/S1PR complex via the β-arrestin-mediated mechanism (86), thereby preventing lymphocytes' egress (10). This effect is primarily observed in the retention of CD4- and CD8-positive naïve lymphocytes and central memory ($CD45RA^-$) T cells in the lymphoid organs. However, effector memory T cells (CD45 $RA^{+/-}$), which primarily use a chemokine-based signaling mechanism, are spared (85, 87). Research dedicated to understanding the effect of fingolimod on lymphocyte subsets additionally identified $CD4^+CD25^+$ regulatory T cell populations as being up-regulated *in-vitro*, which could have implications in down-regulating pro-inflammatory lymphocyte reactivity (88). B lymphocytes are also sequestered in the spleen due to their unique dependence on the S1P pathway, although S1P alone is not sufficient for B cells to exit from the bone marrow (83). S1PRs are expressed at varying levels on endothelial cells, neurons, and CNS glia, however, their function and response to S1PR modulator therapies beyond the immune system are not well-understood (89, 90).

Two landmark, double-blind, randomized trials established the efficacy of fingolimod compared to a placebo or active comparator in treating RRMS. The FREEDOMS trial showed a decrease in the annualized relapse rate (ARR) (0.16 with a regimen of 1.25 mg daily, compared to 0.40 with a placebo), with a relative reduction of ~50% (91). Radiographically, a reduction in both new enhancing and non-enhancing lesions was reported. The results for FREEDOMS II were comparable (92). Subsequently, the TRANSFORMS trial compared two doses of oral fingolimod (0.5 mg daily and 1.25 mg daily) to weekly IM IFN-β-1a for 1 year, which showed a decrease in ARR to 0.16 with 0.5 mg fingolimod, 0.2 with 1.25 mg fingolimod, and 0.33 with IFNβ-1a therapy. Interestingly, this study did not show any difference in the progression of disability assessed using the EDSS (which might be partly explained by the trial design with a short trial duration) (93). The FREEDOMS trial also showed a reduction in the rate of whole-brain atrophy compared to the placebo, suggesting a potential neuro-protective effect of fingolimod (91). However, a recent trial with fingolimod showed no benefit on disability progression compared to placebo when tested for a primary composite endpoint, including EDSS, a 25-foot timed walk test, and a nine-hole peg test in PPMS; although a decrease in radiographic activity has been observed (86). Based on the trial results in RRMS, 0.5 mg daily fingolimod has been approved for the treatment of MS. Fingolimod has been tested in pediatric MS and was associated with a lower rate of relapses and lower accumulation of MRI lesions compared to patients treated with IFN-ß-1a (94). Based on these studies, it has been approved for the treatment of pediatric MS (95)[1].

Fingolimod's most common AEs include bradycardia and less commonly first/second-degree atrioventricular block, likely due to effects on S1PRs in atrial myocytes (85). Notably, these are often asymptomatic, observed during the administration of the first dose, and they also might recur after an interruption of more than 2 weeks[2] (96). Macular edema has been shown to occur in <1% of patients during the first 3 months of treatment and often resolves after treatment is discontinued. Disseminated varicella zoster infection occurred in one patient in previous clinical trials. Elevated liver enzymes (>3× upper limit of normal) were also observed in the FREEDOMS trial, though no cases indicated hepatotoxicity (92). Increased rates of lower respiratory tract infections, cutaneous malignancies (not only basal cell carcinoma, but also squamous cell carcinoma and cutaneous lymphoproliferative disorders), and opportunistic infections including cases of progressive multifocal leukoencephalopathy (PML), varicella-zoster-virus (VZV), and herpes-simplex-virus (HSV) associated encephalitis as well as cryptococcal infections have been reported (5, 97). Retrospective reviews of fingolimod's effects on pregnancy from clinical development trials and additional reports from smaller trials have shown few adverse fetal outcomes. However, the number of adverse outcomes and elective abortion were in the expected range of the general population. Data on fingolimod exposure beyond the first trimester is scarce (38). Since fingolimod exposure causes teratogenicity in rodents, a teratogenic potential cannot be ruled

[1]Commissioner O of the. *FDA Expands Approval of Gilenya to Treat Multiple Sclerosis in Pediatric Patients [Internet]*. FDA (2018). Available online at: http://www.fda.gov/news-events/press-announcements/fda-expands-approval-gilenya-treat-multiple-sclerosis-pediatric-patients (accessed June 13, 2019).

[2]Fingolimod (Gilenya?): bradycardia and heart block [Internet]. GOV.UK. Available online at: https://www.gov.uk/drug-safety-update/fingolimod-gilenya-bradycardia-and-heart-block (accessed May 30, 2019).

out (85). Similarly, since fingolimod can be detected in breast milk, it is also contraindicated in lactating women.

Based on potential untoward effects, screening before initiation of fingolimod treatment comprises baseline laboratory parameters (including a complete blood count, liver-function test, and varicella zoster antibody titers), electrocardiogram, spirometry (in cases of a previous respiratory disease, such as asthma), and an ophthalmologic examination to evaluate for macular edema. Patients are monitored closely for at least 6 h after the first dose (or at re-introduction) in a clinical setting for bradycardia and other cardiac-rhythm abnormalities. Patients with pre-existing cardiac abnormalities, such as conduction block or ischemic heart disease, or those taking medications that interfere with cardiac rhythm and conduction are advised to have a cardiology consultation if clinically indicated (92). Slight and mostly transient hypertension after initial doses of fingolimod also was observed in the FREEDOMS extension study, however, if it did not resolve, it remained stable over the treatment course (91, 98). Increased frequency of basal-cell carcinoma was reported in patients on long-term fingolimod therapy (91). Subsequently, periodic monitoring of blood counts is recommended given lymphopenia's association with fingolimod. The cessation of fingolimod treatment has been associated with cases of severe rebound syndrome leading to severe relapses or high MRI activity. Discontinuing MS treatments needs to be monitored and the sequence of the most suitable treatments needs to be assessed and planned (99).

Recent trials have investigated more receptor-specific agents targeting S1PRsin the hopes of mitigating side effects. Cardiac effects, lymphopenia, elevated liver enzymes, and macular edema still occur with these agents, though a dose-titration strategy was observed to diminish first dose-associated cardiac effects (100). Recently, a remarkable future path for SPMS treatment was revealed in the EXPAND trial, which showed that siponimod (a selective S1P1/S1P5 binding agent) was the first medication of utility in preventing disability progression at 3 months in SPMS (100). It has been approved as Mayzent© by the FDA for CIS, RRMS and active SPMS[3].

Table 2 shows data on all approved oral drugs.

MITOXANTRONE

Mitoxantrone is a synthetic anthracenedione derivate that initially was developed as a cytotoxic treatment for acute myeloid leukemia (101). As a type II topoisomerase inhibitor, the substance has potent anti-inflammatory and, to a lesser extent, immunomodulatory properties (102). The immunosuppressive effect is mediated by effects on proliferating B and T lymphocytes: induction of cell lysis and initiation of programmed cell death (103, 104). Mitoxantrone also demonstrates immunomodulatory effects and preferentially decreases the migratory capacity of monocytes into the CNS and enhances Th2 cytokine production in CD4+T cells (105). *In-vitro*, mitoxantrone interferes with antigen-presenting capabilities of dendritic cells (106).

Mitoxantrone was the first drug that the FDA and several European countries approved to treat worsening relapsing-remitting, secondary-progressive, and progressive-relapsing MS. Research evidence was generated from a phase-III clinical trial in Europe (107) and an earlier phase-II study (108). Both trials confirmed a significant reduction in the relapse rate and worsening of disability. Mitoxantrone is given intravenously (IV) at a dose of 12 mg/m^2 at 3-month intervals. Some healthcare facilities prefer a fixed-dose regimen of mitoxantrone: 20 mg IV monthly together with methylprednisolone (1 g) (108).

Mitoxantrone has myelotoxic effects and reduces leukocyte counts; thus, its administration is not recommended when neutrophil numbers are below 1,500 mm^3 (109). Reversible bone-marrow suppression and nausea are common side effects associated with mitoxantrone infusion (110). Dose adjustment based on leukocyte nadir is mandatory to minimize risks for infections, particularly of the urinary tract. Anemia occurred in 15% of patients (grade $\geq$ 1) (111). Amenorrhea was reported in up to 26% of mitoxantrone-treated women before the age of 45 (112, 113). Liver toxicity and alopecia have also been observed (111).

Severe AEs include therapy-related acute leukemia (TRAL), cardiotoxicity, and colon cancer (114). Acute promyelocytic leukemia (APL) is the most commonly seen TRAL after initiation of mitoxantrone treatment and is characterized by an aggressive, often fulminant disease course due to a life-threatening coagulopathy, e.g., CNS hemorrhages (115). A recent meta-analysis reveals a TRAL risk of ~0.81%, more than 10-fold higher than in previously reported meta-analyses (0.07%) (116). TRAL, in a mitoxantrone setting, has a mortality rate of ~40% (117).

Cardiotoxicity risk increases with cumulative doses of mitoxantrone (118). Therefore, the maximum cumulative dose is restricted to 100–140 mg/m^2, however, cardiotoxicity can develop after doses well below the current maximum recommended levels (111). Re-evaluation by the European Medicine Agency (EMA) concluded that the ordinarily cumulative life-time doses for MS patients should not exceed 72 mg/m^2 [4]. Systolic dysfunction occurs in approximately 12% and congestive heart failure in around 0.4% of treated patients (117). The authors of some studies, therefore, even suggest to limit mitoxantrone treatment to 1 year, or a cumulative dose to <60 mg/m^2, to reduce the risk of TRAL and cardiotoxicity (119).

Treatment with mitoxantrone requires monitoring for possible cardiotoxicity and APL. Cardiac monitoring via regular echocardiography (measurement of left ventricular ejection fraction [LVEF]) is required before treatment begins, prior to each dose, and annually after the discontinuation of therapy (110). Close monitoring of full blood counts in patients with MS before and after mitoxantrone administration needs to be carried out to monitor leukocyte nadir (mostly after 10–14 days)

[3]Commissioner O of the. Press Announcements - FDA approves new oral drug to treat multiple sclerosis [Internet]. Available online at: https://www.fda.gov/NewsEvents/Newsroom/PressAnnouncements/ucm634469.htm (accessed April 7, 2019).

[4]novantrone-article-30-referral-annex-iii_en.pdf [Internet]. Available online at: https://www.ema.europa.eu/en/documents/referral/novantrone-article-30-referral-annex-iii_en.pdf (accessed April 7, 2019).

TABLE 2 | Brand name as well as data on efficacy, dose, route of administration, adverse events of approved oral agents.

	Fingolimod	Teriflunomide	Dimethyl Fumarate	Cladribine	Siponimod⁺
Brand name	**Gilenya®**	**Aubagio®**	**Tecfidera®**	**Mavenclad®**	**Mayzent®**
Year approved	2010	2012	2013	2017	2019
Target	S1P receptors	DHODH	Nrf2	Purines	S1P1,5 receptors
Dose	0.5 mg	14 mg	240 mg	3.5 mg/kg	2 mg
Frequency	Daily	Daily	Twice daily	Yearly course x 2	Daily
Study	FREEDOMS 2010	TEMSO 2011	DEFINE 2012	CLARITY 2010	EXPAND 2018
Relapses					
Annualized rate	0.18	0.37	0.17	0.14	
Relative RR	**54%**	**31%**	**53%**	**57.6%**	**55.5%**
Absolute RR	0.22	0.17	0.19	0.19	
NNT–2y	**4.5**	**5.8**	**5**	**5**	
Disability progression Relative RR	32%	30%	38%	**33%**	**21%**
Absolute RR	0.064	0.071	0.11	0.063	0.055
NNT–2y	**15**	**14**	**9**	**16**	**18**
Reduction in new T2 MRI lesions	74%	67%	85%	73%	79%
Reduction in Gd+ MRI lesions	82%	80%	90%	86%	
Reduction in Brain Volume Loss	36%	25%* (BPF) 37% (SIENA)	NA		23.4%
NEDA-3 vs. comparator	33/13%	23/14%	23/11%	47/17%	
Main AE and AE of interest	Bradycardia, AVB, LFT↑, BP↑, Lymphopenia, macular edema, infections, opportunistic infections (**PML,** cryptococcus), skin malignancies	Diarrhea, BP↑, LFT↑ alopecia, PN, Lymphopenia	flushing, GIT symptoms, LFT↑, UTI, Lymphopenia, **PML**	Infections (herpes), lymphopenia, headache, neoplasms? GIT symptoms	Similar to Fingolimod. Less early bradycardia

*⁺Not approved by the EMA. AVB, atrio-ventricular block; BP, blood pressure; BPF, brain parenchymal fraction; DHODH, dihydroorotate dehydrogenase; GIT, gastrointestinal tract; LFT, liver function tests; NEDA, no evidence of disease activity (NEDA-3); Nrf2, nuclear factor (erythroid-derived 2)-like 2; PML, progressive multifocal leukoencephalopathy; PN, polyneuropathy; S1P, sphingosine-1-phosphate; SIENA, structural image evaluation, using normalization of atrophy; UTI, urinary tract infection; *Non-significant. Bold values indicate most important outcome parameters and AEs.*

and a return to normal levels (~21 days). Clinical vigilance and repeated full blood counts are necessary for 5 years after the termination of treatment (116). Mitoxantrone is contraindicated during pregnancy (38).

In recent years, the use of mitoxantrone has decreased due to the risk of severe AEs and the introduction of novel therapies. The agent should be restricted to selected patients with highly active relapsing multiple sclerosis associated with rapidly evolving disability for whom no alternative treatments are available[5]. In addition, clinical and laboratory vigilance is required both during and after mitoxantrone regimens.

TERIFLUNOMIDE

Teriflunomide is the active metabolite of leflunomide, which has been used in the treatment of rheumatoid arthritis since 1988. Teriflunomide received approval for treating RRMS in 2012 in the US (7 and 14 mg daily) and in 2013 in Europe (14 mg daily) (120). Teriflunomide interferes with *de-novo* pyrimidine synthesis and DNA replication of highly proliferating T and B cells by reversibly inhibiting the mitochondrial enzyme dihydroorotate dehydrogenase (DHODH). Since resting T cells use nucleotides from degrading DNA and RNA and do not need DHODH, the protective immune responses are maintained, while the proliferation of activated T and B cells is reduced; thus, the viability of immune-cells is not affected. In the Teri-DYNAMIC study, a shift to regulatory T cell subtypes and a reduction in clonal diversity in the $CD4^{+}$T cell repertoire were observed (121). An increase in Treg cells in gut associated lymphoid tissue also characterized protection in the autoimmune inflammatory model of MS (122). Teriflunomide crosses the blood-brain barrier (BBB) (121), decreases microglia proliferation, and induces IL-10 production by microglia *in-vitro* (123). Besides the anti-proliferative effect, leflunomide and potentially teriflunomide, inhibit the production of IL-17, TNF-alpha, protein tyrosine kinases, the NF-kB pathway, and the IgG secretion of activated B cells, and interfere with the kynurenine pathway (120, 124, 125).Teriflunomide induces apoptosis of EBV-transformed B cells (126). In a virus-induced animal model of MS, teriflunomide reduced glutamate levels and excitotoxicity (127). Teriflunomide also promotes oligodendrocyte differentiation *in-vitro*, ameliorated axonopathy

[5]ml-concentrate-solution-infusion_de.pdf [Internet]. Available online at: https://www.ema.europa.eu/en/documents/referral/questions-answers-novantrone-associated-names-mitoxantrone-2-mg/ml-concentrate-solution-infusion_de.pdf (accessed April 7, 2019).

by attenuating $CD8^+$ T cell cytotoxicity and supported the proliferation of regulatory $CD8^+$ T cells in the CNS of mice (128, 129). Despite these potent immunomodulatory and cytostatic effects, protective immune responses against foreign antigens are maintained. In the TERIVA study, more than 90% of the MS patients treated with teriflunomide achieved sufficient seroprotection rates when vaccinated against seasonal influenza (130).

Teriflunomide is administered as an oral drug once daily, and a steady-state concentration is reached after ~3 months. After withdrawal, serum levels are maintained above 0.02 µg/mL for 8 months, and in some individuals, up to 2 years, due to enterohepatic recirculation. Accelerated elimination can be achieved by administering 8 g of oral cholestyramine three times daily for 11 days, which can be reduced to 4 g three times daily in cases of intolerance. Alternatively, 50 g of activated charcoal powder every 12 h for 11 days can be used. To confirm proper elimination, the concentration should be below 0.02 µg/mL in two serum samples obtained 14 days apart (131).

Teriflunomide's efficacy and safety have been investigated extensively in one phase-II (132) and four phase-III (TEMSO, TOWER, TENERE, and TOPIC) clinical trials, all with long-term follow-up data involving several thousand patients (133–136). Over 90% of patients in the TEMSO and TOWER trials had RRMS (133, 134). Patients with a first single clinical episode were enrolled in the TOPIC trial (136). In the TENERE trial, teriflunomide was compared to SC IFN-ß-1a (135), whereas the other three phase-III trials were placebo-controlled.

In these clinical trials, teriflunomide showed a consistent effect on disease activity, measured by its impact on relapses, disability worsening, MRI outcomes, and combined measures such as no evidence of disease activity (NEDA). Compared to the placebo, 14 mg of teriflunomide daily reduced the ARR by 31–36% in the pivotal trials (133–136). Disability progression, confirmed after 3 months, was also reduced significantly by 29.8 and 31.5% in the 14 mg trial group in TOWER and TEMSO studies (133, 134). Similar efficacy data have been observed in real-life settings for up to 28 months (137). Comparison of the pooled phase-III trial data from 14 mg of teriflunomide and dimethyl-fumarate (DMF) (TEMSO/TOWER vs. DEFINE/CONFIRM) revealed similar numbers needed to treat (NNT) to prevent one relapse or worsening disability (121, 138). However, in a recent registry-based study, the ARR was ~49% lower in patients treated with DMF, and teriflunomide treatment was associated with an increased risk of first relapse and increased incidence of discontinuation due to disease breakthrough (139). In another recent registry-based study with large patient populations, the ARR was similar between teriflunomide and DMF, and discontinuation rate was also similar; nevertheless, ARR were lower in patients treated with fingolimod compared to both DMF and teriflunomide, while disability accumulation was the same (140). A recent Italian study did not observe differences in discontinuation either during the first 24 months (141). In the TEMSO study, the 14 mg daily dosage reduced the number of Gd-enhancing lesions by 80.4% and the total lesion volume by 67.4%; the effect of a 7 mg daily dose was less but still significant (133). The treatment (14 mg) of patients with a first clinical episode suggestive of MS, i.e., CIS, reduced the risk of conversion to clinically definite MS by 42.6%, however, only 44% of the patients completed the study due to early termination related to changes in MS diagnostic criteria (136).

The long-term outcomes in extension studies indicate that the effect of teriflunomide is maintained (class-III evidence), however, the dropout rates varied, ranging from 40 to 75% (121). The analysis of pooled TEMSO/TOWER long-term data (up to 9 and 5.5 years, respectively) indicated that more than 80% of the 122 patients with progressive relapsing MS did not experience worsening disability (121).

The AEs reported more frequently with teriflunomide than the placebo include hair thinning, ALT increase, nausea, diarrhea, paraesthesia, limb pain, arthralgia, nasopharyngitis, polyneuropathy, and menorrhagia. Hair thinning appeared in 10–14% of patients and led to discontinuation in 1.4–2% of cases in pivotal trials (133, 134, 142). The discontinuation of treatment was most commonly related to ALT elevation driven by the trial protocols. In real life, gastrointestinal AE was the most common cause of discontinuation (143). The pooled analysis of safety data from the phase-II, TEMSO, TOWER, TOPIC, extension of phase-II, and TEMSO (up to 12 years), in addition to the safety data from the TOWER, TOPIC, and TENERE extensions (up to 7 years), consistently supported the long-term beneficial AE profile (121, 143, 144). Deaths were not more common in the active arm compared to placebos in pivotal trials, and two deaths in the extension phases (pulmonary tuberculosis and suicide) were potentially related to treatment (121, 133–136, 143–145). A single case of PML after 3 months of teriflunomide treatment has been reported, but it most likely was carried over from preceding natalizumab therapy (146). During the 2.1 million patient years of leflunomide therapy since 1991, two cases of PML have been reported during monotherapy (120).

Teriflunomide is contraindicated during pregnancy and is classified as category X based on embryo-fetal toxicity and malformations in rats and rabbits (121). However, results from animal studies cannot be transferred unrestrictedly to humans, and among 26 reported live births, by human women taking the drug no abnormalities were present (147). The FDA suggests discontinuing teriflunomide in males who wish to father a child, however, this is not required in Europe. Accelerated elimination is necessary for women taking the drug before pregnancy who wish to become pregnant, and serum concentration must be <0.02 µg/mL in two serum samples obtained 14 days apart.

In summary, extensive and long-term data consistently indicate that teriflunomide's efficacy resembles that of injectables, and that it offers a beneficial AE profile. Its administration is convenient, however, frequent blood tests (blood count and liver transaminases) are required during the first 6 months of treatment.

DIMETHYL FUMARATE (DMF)

DMF has been used to treat psoriasis since 1959 and was approved to treat RRMS in 2013 (148). It is administered as a 240 mg tablet twice daily.

One of the major mechanisms of DMF and its active metabolite mono-methyl fumarate (MMF) is an antioxidant response through activation of the Nrf-2 pathway, which might result in neuroprotective properties besides influencing NF-κB related cellular responses (149, 150). Activation of the Nrf-2 pathway leads to an expansion of FoxP3$^+$ regulatory T cells and CD56^{bright} natural killer cells, as well as to a reduced level of CD8$^+$ T cells and B cells (151). DMF yields profound effects on immune responses *in-vitro* and *in-vivo*: It inhibits NF-κB activation and pro-inflammatory cytokine production by myeloid cells; reduces the generation of encephalitogenic T cells, partially by inhibiting antigen presentation; generates a shift from a Th1/Th17 to a Th2 profile; alters cytokine production by B cells; promotes apoptosis of B and T cells; and elicits an anti-proliferative effect (149, 152–156). In MS patients treated with DMF, the T and B cell subpopulations are reduced, and functional changes are observed in lymphocytes and APCs. Such reductions affect mostly cytotoxic T cells, effector/central memory T cells, Th1 cells, Th17 cells, mucosa-associated lymphoid tissue (MALT) cells follicular T cells with a Tfh1/17 phenotype, antigen experienced and memory B cells, and B cells producing TNF. Immunoregulatory CD56^{bright} NK-cells, naïve T and B cells, Th2 cells, FoxP3$^+$ Tregs, and follicular T cells with a Tfh2 phenotype are increased (151, 153–155, 157–162). Such a pro-tolerogenic shift is associated with NEDA in MS patients (158); higher levels of the NRF2 target gene NAD(P)H quinone dehydrogenase 1 (NQO1) was also associated with NEDA status after 1 year of DMF treatment (151). MMF crosses the BBB, and DMF/MMF alters the function of CNS resident cells *in-vitro*, suppresses inflammatory cytokine production by activated microglia and astrocytes, and increases the number of oligodendrocyte precursor cells (163–165).

DMF's clinical efficacy and safety as an MS drug have been investigated in two randomized placebo-controlled phase-III trials, DEFINE and CONFIRM (166, 167). An active agent, GA, was also included as a reference comparator in the CONFIRM trial. The ARR was reduced by 53% in the DEFINE study and 44% in the CONFIRM study, compared to the placebo (166, 167). The risk of confirmed disability progression sustained for 12 weeks was also reduced by 38% in the DEFINE study and 21% in the CONFIRM study (166, 167). The integrated analysis of the phase-III trials indicated a 32% (29%) risk reduction in 12 (24)-week confirmed disability progression (168). DMF reduced the number of new or enlarging hyperintense lesions on T2-weighted images by 71 and 85%, respectively, and reduced the odds of an increase in the number of Gd-enhancing lesions by 74% and 90% in the CONFIRM and DEFINE study, respectively (166, 167). Compared to the active comparator GA, DMF twice daily also significantly reduced T2-weighted hyperintense lesions in the CONFIRM trial, whereas the other efficacy outcomes were no different (167). The integrated analysis of CONFIRM and DEFINE demonstrated a 38.9% relative reduction in clinical disease activity (relapse and disability progression) over 2 years compared to placebo treated patients (169).

The phase-III trials, integrated analyses, and follow-up studies all indicated DMF's safety and beneficial AE profile. The frequency of AEs and serious AEs was similar to the placebo in the DEFINE and CONFIRM trials (serious AEs 17 and 18% vs. 21 and 22%, respectively) and GA in the CONFIRM study (17%) (166, 167). The most common AEs were flushing (31–38%), diarrhea (13–15%), nausea (11–13%), upper abdominal pain (10%), and vomiting (10%) (166, 167, 170). Increased liver enzymes were detected in 3–6% of patients treated with DMF (171). Overall, the incidence of AEs leading to discontinuation of the study drug was similar across groups. Discontinuations due to flushing and overall gastrointestinal events occurred more frequently in patients who received DMF (166, 167). Compared to the placebo group, at 1 year, the white-cell and lymphocyte counts decreased by ~10 and 28%, respectively (166). Grade 2 or 3 lymphopenia occurred in 4–10% of the patients compared to 1% or less in the placebo group and tends to persist in some patients (166, 167). Infections were common but the incidence was not significantly different between the DMF and placebo or GA groups (50–68%) (171). Although serious and opportunistic infections were not more common among patients treated with DMF, five cases of PML were reported by 2018 (172). Additional 14 cases were related to other DMF formulas used in psoriasis, and 13 out of the 19 cases had grade 3 lymphopenia (173). CD4$^+$ and CD8$^+$ T cell repopulation rates are delayed after switching to other disease modifying therapies (DMT) from DMF, and T cell counts may not recover or even continue to decline if DMF treatment is switched to fingolimod or alemtuzumab (174). Decrease of CD8$^+$ and memory T cells is more likely compared to CD4$^+$ and naïve T cells (156).

In addition to pivotal trials, a few studies have investigated DMF's efficacy and safety in real-life settings, and these recapitulated the findings from the pivotal trials. In two multicenter studies with 1,089 and 735 patients treated for up to 25 and 33 months, the ARR was reduced by 77 and 63% respectively (175, 176), whereas in another multicenter study, the ARR was reduced by 33% (177). NEDA status was achieved in 47.8% of patients after 1 year (176). In the first year, 11–19.5% of patients discontinued treatment, and 30% of patients stopped DMF after 2 years mainly due to poor tolerance (175, 176). Approximately one third of the patients had flushing or gastrointestinal AEs (176). Lymphocytopenia occurred in 16.5 and 18.7% of the patients, respectively (175, 176). Lower baseline lymphocyte counts, female gender and older age (>55 years) were associated with more severe lymphopenia (178). Several recent studies have highlighted the importance of early AE management to improve adherence. In a cohort of 400 patients, 34% stopped treatment within a year and 57% within 2 years (179). The data on treatment with DMF during pregnancy is limited, thus, no final assessment is possible. Generally, it is recommended to stop DMF when planning to conceive (5, 38). Several studies have investigated DMF's efficacy in relation to other DMTs. Fingolimod and DMF were evaluated based on the data from a pivotal study using a matching-adjusted comparison and revealed no significant differences in the effect on clinical parameters between the treatments (180). Similar results were shown in an Italian study based on real-world data. A propensity score-matched study revealed a similar NEDA-3 status for fingolimod (73%) and DMF (70%), however, in patients having switched from other therapeutics, fingolimod was superior to DMF ($p = 0.007$) (181). Another study measuring the indirect effectiveness of fingolimod vs. DMF vs. teriflunomide based on phase-III studies suggested that the probability of achieving NEDA-3 was highest for fingolimod (182). Similarly, a recent study including 3,728 patients from MSBase showed a superior effect of fingolimod on relapse rates and comparable results for disability progression in patients treated with fingolimod, DMF, and teriflunomide (140).

In the STRATEGY study, the risk of relapse after switching from natalizumab was 19.6%, and the ARR was lower in patients with <90 days of a washout period (183). Another study also indicated that DMF can be an option for patients discontinuing natalizumab: After 2 years of DMF treatment, 80% of the patients did not present clinical or MRI evidence of disease activity, and a post natalizumab rebound was observed in 1 out of 39 patients (184).

In summary, the data indicate DMF's efficacy and safety in treating RRMS. Whether its efficacy is higher than teriflunomide's and like fingolimod's is debatable. Sustained lymphopenia after stopping a DMF regimen might complicate the escalation to fingolimod and lymphocyte-depleting therapies. Whereas, pre-treatment with aspirin might mitigate flushing, gastrointestinal side effects are only slighthly mitigated by dose titration and are not worsened by pre-treatment with aspirin (185). Gastrointestinal side effects need early symptomatic treatments which may increase adherence significantly (186).

CLADRIBINE

Cladribine (2-chloro-2′-deoxyadenosine) is a pro-drug that requires intracellular phosphorylation to become an active purine nucleoside analog that interferes with DNA synthesis and repair, and ultimately leads to cell death. The higher ratio of activity between certain enzymes that activate (desoxycytidine kinase) or deactivate (adenosine-monophosphate kinase and nukleoside-diphosphate kinase) the pro-drug explains the preferential and long-lasting depletion of peripheral B and T lymphocytes with a relative sparing of other hematogenic and immune cells. B and T cells are rapidly depleted. The slight recovery of Tregs before B and T cells repopulation might partly explain the long-lasting effects (187). A parenteral formulation of cladribine was first developed for therapy against hairy-cell leukemia, while the oral formulation of cladribine was developed later and tested in RRMS (188, 189).

Oral cladribine was studied in a phase-III trial (CLARITY) (190), a 96-week, placebo-controlled, double-blind, multicenter study. Patients with active RRMS (at least one relapse within 12 months prior to study entry) were included in the trial. Cladribine was administered based on body weight and tested in three groups: 3.5 mg/kg, 5.25 mg/kg, or a placebo. Compared to the placebo, the ARR at week 96 was reduced in both treatment groups by ~57%. The proportion of patients remaining free of relapses at week 96 increased from ~61 to 80%, resulting in an absolute benefit for approximately 19 out of 100 patients treated. In addition, the relative reduction in the risk of a 3-month sustained progression of disability in both cladribine groups, compared to the placebo group, was 31–33%, and patients treated with cladribine had a reduction of 77% in mean active T2 lesions on MRI (190). Furthermore, in patients with a first clinical attack, cladribine was shown to reduce the risk of a second attack, or three-month EDSS progression (191, 192).

The subsequent CLARITY EXTENSION study showed that treatment with cladribine for 2 years followed by 2 years' placebo treatment produced durable clinical benefits similar to 4 years of cladribine treatment, i.e., approximately 75% of patients treated with cladribine 3.5 mg/kg in CLARITY, remained relapse-free when given placebo during the extension (193, 194).

In the CLARITY study, at a dosage of 3.5 mg/kg, CD4+ T cells dropped by 40–45% and CD8+ T cells by 15–30% without significant recovery prior to the next treatment cycle. CD19+ B cells dropped by ~70–90%, slowly recovering to 15–25% of the baseline (195), suggesting a combined T and B cell-mediated mode of action.

Lymphopenia was dose-dependent (nadir at 4 months), with grade 3 lymphopenia (500–200 cells/uL) in ~25% of patients in the 3.5 mg/kg dose group, and grade 4 (<200 cells/uL) in <1% (194). The rate of common infections was similar when comparing placebo- and cladribine-treated patients. The rate of herpes zoster infections per 100 patient years was higher in the 3.5 mg/kg group than the placebo group (0.83 vs. 0.20) and associated with lymphopenia, explaining why patients with grade 4 lymphopenia should receive a prophylactic anti-herpes infection treatment. Furthermore, the incidence of severe infections was generally higher among patients with lymphopenia and who were taking cladribine at a dosage of 3.5 mg/kg compared to the placebo group (194). PML was not reported during an observational period of >8,500 patient years in the MS indication, whereas some PML cases have been observed with parenteral cladribine in lymphoma patients[6]. Three cases of tuberculosis were reported during the clinical trials, of which one case was fatal. Two cases of hepatitis B occurred, and one of those patients died (166).

Thus, not only clinical follow-up and standard laboratory tests, but also screening for HIV infection, active tuberculosis, and hepatitis are mandatory prior to a treatment course of cladribine. The malignancy rates were higher among cladribine-treated patients compared to the placebo cohort (33 vs. 4); these malignancies comprised of solid tumors with no specific patterns typical of tumors commonly seen during immunosuppression. No cases of leukemia, lymphoma, or lymphoproliferative disorders were reported (166). However, this imbalance explained the initial application rejection by the EMA in 2011, when additional safety data were requested. Such

[6]Foechterlen D. oder an das Bundesinstitut für Arzneimittel und Medizinprodukte (BfArM): elektronisch über das Internet www.bfarm.de - Arzneimittel - Pharmakovigilanz - Risiken melden; oder schriftlich an die Postadresse Kurt-Georg-Kiesinger-Allee 3, 53175 Bonn, oder per.

data then were obtained from clinical extension studies, meta-analyses of several other clinical studies with alternative MS drugs, and comparisons with epidemiological data, leading to EU approval in 2017, since the malignancy risk is comparable to other treatment options for MS. However, the EU approved cladribine only for "the treatment of adult patients with highly active relapsing MS as defined by clinical or imaging features"[7], and it was approved by the FDA in 2019[8]. Furthermore, due to potential teratogenic effects, both males and females must use effective contraception during therapy with cladribine, and for 6 months after a treatment cycle.

Overall, the registered dose of 3.5 mg/kg can be applied orally in short treatment cycles, which might lead to a high adherence to therapy, followed by a sustained therapeutic effect, with efficacy confirmed in highly active patients with the registered indication[7]. The downside of cladribine is that lymphopenia can be severe and frequently reaches grade 3, which is associated with a higher risk of infections. Data on lymphopenia in patients with prior immunosuppressive treatment is lacking (due to exclusion criteria in pivotal trials), thus more data needs to be collected. Furthermore, the long-term risks of malignancy and opportunistic infections remains to be established, as well as algorithms on how to treat patients with ongoing disease activity after a 2-year course of therapy. Finally, cladribine interferes with DNA synthesis and repair mechanisms, raising concerns in young adults of child-bearing age until additional safety data become available.

ALEMTUZUMAB

Alemtuzumab is a humanized monoclonal IgG1-antibody that targets CD52, a surface molecule with largely unknown functions predominantly expressed at high levels on B and T cells (196, 197). Lower expression levels are found on monocytes, macrophages, and eosinophils. Mature NK cells, plasma cells, neutrophils, and, most importantly, hematological stem cells show little or no expression (198).

Alemtuzumab leads to a rapid and long-lasting depletion of CD52-positive cells by antibody-dependent, cell-mediated cytolysis (ADCC) and complement dependent cytolysis (CDC) (199), followed by a slow repopulation arising from unaffected hematopoietic precursor cells. Both, quantitative and qualitative changes in the immune-cell repertoire are observed, which might contribute to a rebalancing of autoimmune processes. While the exact mechanisms underlying the reprogramming of the immune system are only vaguely understood, a specific pattern exists to repopulate immune-cell subsets in peripheral blood (200, 201). Monocytes reach baseline levels after 3 months. B cell counts not only return to baseline numbers after 3 months, but also show an excess increase to 124–165% of baseline levels at 12 months. CD8+T lymphocytes are restored after 31 months, whereas CD4+T lymphocytes need ~60 months for complete repopulation. This rapid CD19+ B cell subset repopulation in the absence of effective T cell regulation might explain some of the AEs, e.g., secondary autoimmunities (202). Furthermore, an expansion in CD56bright NK cells also occurs (203). The effects of NK cells on disease progression are unclear, however, it is debated whether they will exhibit immunoregulatory properties (204).

Alemtuzumab's efficacy and safety have been evaluated in treatment naive RRMS patients in phase-II (205) and phase-III trials (206), and in RRMS patients who had an inadequate response (≥1 relapse after ≥6 months of treatment) to prior therapy (207). Due to different inclusion criteria, patients in CARE MS I were younger (mean age was 33.0 vs. 34.7 years), had a lower mean EDSS (2.0 vs. 2.7) and a shorter mean disease duration (2.1 vs. 4.5 years). In the phase-III CARE-MS trials, alemtuzumab demonstrated significantly lower disease activity over 2 years vs. SC IFN-ß-1a administered three times per week (206, 207). In both CARE-MS I and II studies, alemtuzumab significantly reduced the frequency of relapses over 2 years compared to SC IFN-ß-1a (54.9 and 49.4% reduction in relapses in the respective trials); significantly improved MRI outcomes including gd-enhancing lesions and new or enlarging T2 lesions in the alemtuzumab cohort compared to the IFN-ß-1a cohort, and significantly reduced the rate of brain-volume loss. Alemtuzumab also significantly reduced the rate of clinical disease worsening over 36 months in the phase-II CAMMS223 study (205). In CARE-MS II, patients treated with alemtuzumab were more likely to experience 6-month confirmed disability improvement than patients receiving SC IFN-ß-1a treatment (hazard ratio 2.57), whereas this outcome was not significant in CARE-MS I (206, 207).

AEs include infusion-associated reactions (IARs), serious infections, and autoimmune-adverse events, including thyroid disorders and, less frequently, immune thrombocytopenia (ITP) and nephropathies. Malignancies such as thyroid cancer, melanoma, and melanoma-*in-situ* as well as lymphoproliferative disorders have been reported[9].

The IAR rate in the phase-III trials was >90%, mostly mild to moderate in severity and most frequently within the first 3 days of infusion (206, 207). The IARs, which are attributable mainly to cytokine-release syndrome, included headaches, rash, pyrexia, nausea, urticaria, pruritus, flushing, insomnia, fatigue, chills, chest discomfort, and dyspnea. The IARs decrease with successive infusions in a single course and in the second course (206). The clinical trials reported severe IARs ranging from 1 to 3%. Concomitant corticosteroids, antihistamines, and antipyretic drugs are applied with the infusion to avoid IAR. In addition, IARs might be reduced by slowing or temporarily stopping the infusion. Following a safety announcement by the FDA on the rare but serious risks of stroke and blood vessel wall tear (208), Azevedo et al. reported five patients that developed

[7]Commissioner O of the. Press Announcements - FDA approves new oral treatment for multiple sclerosis [Internet]. Available online at: https://www.fda.gov/NewsEvents/Newsroom/PressAnnouncements/ucm634837.htm (accessed April 7, 2019).

[8]WC500234561.pdf [Internet]. Available online at: http://www.ema.europa.eu/docs/en_GB/document_library/EPAR_-_Product_Information/human/004230/WC500234561.pdf (cited September 26, 2018).

[9]LEMTRADA® (alemtuzumab) | Official Healthcare Professional Site [Internet]. Available online at: https://www.lemtradahcp.com/safety-information (accesed June 2, 2019).

intracerebral hemorrhage within a few hours after administration of alemtuzumab (209).

Moreover, in all patients an increase in blood pressure or labile blood pressure was recognized. Labile hemodynamics under alemtuzumab treatment and infusion-associated reactions resulting in an activated immune system involving mast cells, basophils, complement, activation of platelet derived growth factor, and the release of interleukin-6 (Il-6), or tumor necrosis factor α (TNFα) are discussed as possible causes (210).

Infections are mostly mild to moderate and include oral herpes, herpes zoster, nasopharyngitis, urinary-tract infection, upper respiratory-tract infection, sinusitis, influenza, bronchitis, and localized superficial fungal infections. Serious infections were rare, although slightly elevated with alemtuzumab vs. SC IFN-ß-1a (205–207). Since herpes-virus infections increased in clinical trials with alemtuzumab, prophylactic treatment with an oral anti-herpes agent on the first day of alemtuzumab usage and for 1 month of each treatment cycle was introduced in the risk-management plan. Tuberculosis has been reported in patients treated with alemtuzumab; thus, before the initiation of therapy, all patients must be evaluated for both, active and inactive ("latent") tuberculosis infection and treated according to local guidelines if required. Moreover, before receiving treatment with alemtuzumab, patients who have not contracted chickenpox and who have not been vaccinated against VZV should be tested for anti-VZV antibodies. Several cases of opportunistic infections including listeria meningitis, esophageal candidiasis, pyogenic granuloma, spirochetal gingivitis, nocardiosis, and cytomegalovirus were reported.

Listeria infections occur generally within 1 month of infusion. Thus, dietary recommendations require the exclusion of certain foods, such as unpasteurized milk and raw meat, during and for 1 month after treatment with alemtuzumab. Antibacterial treatment may be recommended depending on the different regulatory authorities.

Autoimmune AEs represent the most important risk associated with alemtuzumab treatment. These most commonly affect the thyroid; however, they can include rare cases of ITP and anti-glomerular basement membrane nephropathy. The exact pathomechanism leading to secondary autoimmunity remains to be determined. Currently, it is thought that the different temporal lymphocyte repopulation plays a role in this process (211, 212).

In the 5-year follow-up of CAMMS223, thyroid autoimmune AEs occurred in 39% of patients treated with alemtuzumab 12 mg (213). Onset ranged from 6 to 61 months after the first treatment course (207). Incidence peaked at year 3 and declined in subsequent years. Serious ITP events have been observed in ~1% of patients treated with alemtuzumab in the CARE-MS program, between 14 and 36 months after first exposure to alemtuzumab. The first ITP case, during the phase-II CAMMS223 trial, went unrecognized, and the patient died from intracerebral hemorrhage. Following this index case, a monitoring program was implemented to identify and manage ITP systematically, including education on the signs and symptoms for patients and physicians and monthly blood monitoring (142). Other autoimmune cytopenias such as neutropenia, hemolytic anemia, agranulocytosis, and pancytopenia have been reported in the CARE-MS trials with a lower incidence than ITP (206, 207). One patient experienced a recurrence of pancytopenia, which was associated with a lack of compliance with corticosteroid therapy, resulting in fatal sepsis 20 months after alemtuzumab treatment was completed w.

In pilot studies, two patients developed anti-glomerular basement membrane (anti-GBM) disease that ultimately required a kidney transplant (214). In phase-II and phase-III trials, four cases of glomerulonephritis occurred among 1,486 patients treated with alemtuzumab (0.3%). The onset ranged from 4 to 39 months after the last dose of alemtuzumab. Improvements in renal function were observed in two cases of anti-GBM disease after treatment with plasmapheresis, cyclophosphamide, and glucocorticosteroids, and in two cases of membranous glomerulonephritis after treatment with diuretics and/or lisinopril (215, 216).

Secondary autoimmunity is of special interest, since thyroid autoimmunity might affect almost half of the patients (217). A monitoring program was designed and implemented to facilitate the early detection of autoimmune events to ensure timely and adequate management (218): TSH measurements should be performed at baseline and every 3 months for 48 months following the last course (second or subsequent course) (219), and the patient should be monitored for any drug-induced ITP symptoms. Petechiae are uncommon and are usually observed on the lower limbs of patients with a platelet count $<20 \times 10^9$/L (and often $<10 \times 10^9$/L). Thus, a platelet count should be performed before the initial course of alemtuzumab, followed by monthly testing that should be continued until 48 months after the final course (220). The signs and symptoms of nephropathy often are non-specific. Routine creatinine testing should be performed before treatment, followed by monthly testing during treatment, continuing until 48 months after the last course (second or subsequent course) (221). Since it is given in cycles, there are no continuous levels of alemtuzumab in the blood. It is recommended that contraception should be used for four months after the last dose (221).

Alemtuzumab's high efficacy contrasts its considerable risks; thus, a thorough assessment of the benefits and risks, adherence to long-term monitoring requirements, and pharmacovigilance are mandatory. Long-term monthly monitoring for 48 months after the final alemtuzumab infusion poses a challenge to patient adherence and requires appropriate education of both physicians and patients. Due to the recently reported side effects including immune-mediated conditions and heart and vessels disorders, the EMA started a review on the medication and temporarily restricted it to patients with highly active disease despite treatment with at least two disease-modifying therapies or in cases when other therapies cannot be used (222). Nevertheless, it is a highly effective treatment option with a long-lasting clinical experience. It should be used in the appropriate patients with the appropriate monitoring schemes.

Table 3 shows data on all approved monoclonal antibodies.

TABLE 3 | Brand name as well as data on efficacy, dose, route of administration, adverse events of approved monoclonal antibodies.

	Natalizumab	**Alemtuzumab**	**Ocrelizumab**
Brand name	**Tysabri®**	**Lemtrada®**	**Ocrevus®**
Year approved	2004, 2006	2013	2017
Target	VLA-4	CD52	CD20
Dose	300 mg	12 mg	600 mg
Route	IV	IV	IV
Frequency	Every 4 weeks	Annual course	Every 6 months
Study	AFFIRM 2006	CARE-MS II 2012 (vs. SC IFNβ-1a)	OPERA/ORATORIO (vs. IM IFNβ-1a/placebo)
Relapses			
Annualized rate	0.23	0.26	0.155
Relative RR	**68%**	**50%**	**46%**
Absolute RR	0.5	0.26	0.135
NNT−2y	**2**	**4**	**7.4**
Disability progression			RRMS/PPMS
Relative RR	42%	40%	40/24%
Absolute RR	0.12	0.084	0.054/0.115
NNT−2y	**8**	**12**	**18.5/7**
Reduction in new T2 MRI lesions	83%	32% fewer pt.	80/92%
Reduction in Gd+ MRI lesions	92%	61% fewer pt.	94/95%
Reduction in Brain Volume Loss	NA	23%	19/17.5%
NEDA-3 vs. comparator	37/7%	32/14%	48/27%
Main AE and AE of interest	Infections (**PML,** Herpes), infusion reactions, hepatotoxicity	Infusion reactions, cytopenia, autoimmunity, infections, opportunistic infections, malignancy?	Infusion reactions, Infections

BBB, blood-brain barrier; IAR, infusion associated reactions; IM, intramuscular; IRR, Injection related reactions; IV, intravenous; NEDA, no evidence of disease activity (NEDA-3); NK, natural killer; SC, subcutaneous; VLA-4, very late antigen-4; PML, progressive multifocal leukoencephalopathy. Bold values indicate most important outcome parameters and AEs.

OCRELIZUMAB

Within the past two decades, the pathogenic role of B cells has generated enormous interest in MS research. Traditionally, MS was primarily considered a T cell-mediated inflammatory disorder, although several findings, including, first and foremost, the development of oligoclonal bands (OCB) in the cerebrospinal fluid (CSF), have indicated a role for B cells. Besides being the source of antibody-producing plasma cells, B cells directly contribute to the development and progression of MS. Peripheral and CNS B cells show signs of chronic inflammation, along with a shift toward antigen-experienced memory B cells (223), indicative of an antigen-mediated activation of B cells in MS. Assumedly, as a consequence, MS patients' B cells show an increased expression of major histocompatibility complex (MHC) class II molecules (224), as well as a higher level of co-stimulatory molecules (225, 226), with the potential to promote the pro-inflammatory differentiation of responding T cells (227). Additional roles of B cells in MS pathogenesis are discussed: antigen presentation, driving T cell activation and auto-proliferation, unbalanced cytokine production, and the formation of ectopic lymphoid follicles (TLOs) under the meninges (228, 229).

Predominantly driven by the assumption that immunoglobulins reactive to a yet unknown self-antigen of the CNS are important drivers of MS pathogenesis, the concept of applying B cell-depleting therapies in MS has evolved. Monoclonal antibodies against CD20 deplete immature and mature B cells, but spare plasma cells and hematopoietic stem cells due to their lack of CD20 expression. Rituximab was the first anti-CD20 antibody to be tested in MS trials, and resulted in a rapid decline in the development of new CNS lesions in patients with RRMS (230, 231). In PPMS, a subgroup of young patients with ongoing CNS lesion formation experienced a slowing of disease progression (232). Testing the humanized successor of rituximab, ocrelizumab confirmed a substantial reduction in the frequency of clinical relapses and CNS lesion formation in RRMS (7, 233). Two identical, randomized, double-blind, double-dummy trials comparing IV ocrelizumab to an active comparator, SC IFN-ß-1a, demonstrated a substantially reduced ARR (0.16 vs. 0.29 $p < 0.001$ in both trials) in patients treated with ocrelizumab (7). Furthermore, ocrelizumab was superior to IFN-ß-1a with respect to disability progression confirmed at 12 and 24 weeks. In addition to these highly promising findings in RRMS, a placebo-controlled, phase-III trial in patients with PPMS revealed a significantly decelerated accumulation of disability, particularly in younger patients with MRI findings suggestive of ongoing inflammatory activity (8). Based on these phase-III clinical-trial findings, ocrelizumab has been approved recently for both MS indications: RRMS and PPMS. IARs have been observed, especially during the first administrations. Neoplasms (including breast carcinomas) were more often reported (2.3%) in the ocrelizumab cohort than in those patients receiving placebo (0.8%) in the PPMS trials (8). Long term effects of immunosuppression and B depletion are missing.

The anti-CD20 monoclonal antibodies rituximab and ocrelizumab differ from each other in certain aspects. Rituximab, which has not been brought to a phase-III trial mainly for strategic considerations, is a chimeric antibody and acts predominantly via CDC. Ocrelizumab is more humanized, and its B cell-depleting effector mechanism is mediated more by ADCC. A third anti-CD20 antibody currently tested in phase-III MS trials is ofatumumab (NCT02792231 and NCT02792218), a fully human anti-CD20 antibody (234).

Ocrelizumab is administered IV every 24 weeks at a maintenance dose of 600 mg. Within this interval, the vast majority of patients are continuously depleted of blood B cells. Very little is known about other bodily systems that might be more important immunologically, such as secondary lymphoid organs. In this regard, a recent experimental study revealed that a fraction of $CD20^{+}$B cells in the spleen is resistant to systemic anti-CD20 treatment (235). After cessation of treatment, this population expanded in parallel to *de novo* B cell generation from bone marrow, resulting in an increased frequency of potentially pathogenic B cells in mice containing a B cell-stimulating immunization. This may be enormously important, since in classical autoimmune diseases, such as myasthenia gravis or AQP4-Ab^{+} NMO, the stimulating autoantigen may be present when B cells return after cessation of anti-CD20 treatment. Furthermore, the extinction and recovery of B cells may differ substantially, both quantitatively and qualitatively, when lower doses or other administration routes are used (236). In accordance with this, studies in rheumatoid-arthritis patients revealed that a single administration of 10 mg of ocrelizumab was sufficient to deplete B cells efficiently from blood, whereas B cell recovery started much earlier than with higher doses (237). Along with these lines, investigations have recently suggested that substantially lower doses of SC ofatumumab are sufficient to mediate a virtually complete removal of B cells from the blood (234, 238). Regarding other compartments, such as secondary lymphoid organs, experimental studies have suggested that a SC administration targets B cells most efficiently in draining lymph nodes, whereas the IV application of anti-CD20 exerts a more thorough effect on the removal of splenic B cells (238). These differences might have important clinical implications, since they might substantially impact both the clinical efficacy and safety of anti-CD20 treatment in MS patients. In pivotal trials, 12 patients developed anti-drug antibodies, and two of these were positive for neutralizing antibodies. Due to the low number and low incidence of these antibodies, no final assessment on their incidence and their impact possible[10].

Data on administration of ocrelizumab during pregnancy is scarce, thus no final assessment is possible (239)[10,11]. However, the FDA (the EMA) requires 6 (12) months contraception after the last dose of ocrelizumab.

NATALIZUMAB

A hallmark in the pathogenesis of MS is immune dysregulation, characterized by autoreactive lymphocytes penetrating the BBB, resulting in an inflammatory cascade that leads to demyelination, axonal transection, and neurologic deficits (240). The entry of lymphocytes into the CNS requires transmigration through the inflamed endothelium, and the prevention of this process should provide anti-inflammatory therapy in MS (241). Natalizumab was the first monoclonal antibody approved in 2004 for the treatment of RRMS. It is a humanized recombinant IgG4 monoclonal antibody that inhibits leukocyte extravasation into the CNS and intestinal tract by blocking the α4 subunit of integrin molecules on leukocytes (242). Integrins are cell-surface glycoproteins that facilitate cell-matrix adhesion and mediate leukocyte rolling and adhesion to the endothelium prior to extravasation (243). By inhibiting their interaction with vascular cell-adhesion molecule (VCAM)-1 expressed on endothelial cells, natalizumab prevents T lymphocytes from crossing the BBB, thereby reducing inflammation in the brain-tissue compartment (244). In 1992, a study by Yednock et al. concluded that antibodies against the α4-integrin substantially restricted the accumulation of leukocytes in the CNS and prevented the development of a model mimicking MS in rats known as experimental autoimmune encephalomyelitis (EAE) (245). These findings paved the way for early clinical trials with natalizumab. Perhaps equally important, natalizumab was later shown to sequester T cell and B cell subsets out of the CNS compartment (246–248), providing proof-of-concept evidence that a reduction in adaptive immune-cell access to the CNS benefits RRMS patients.

The efficacy of natalizumab for treating RRMS was shown in two phase-III trials: the AFFIRM and SENTINEL studies (249), In the AFFIRM study, 942 patients with RRMS were enrolled in a 2:1 ratio to receive natalizumab 300 mg every 4 weeks or a placebo. The primary outcomes included the clinical-relapse rate at 1 year and the sustained disability-progression rate at 2 years. The results showed that natalizumab reduced the ARR by 68% and lowered the risk of sustained disability progression at 2 years by 42% (249). The SENTINEL study enrolled 1,171 patients who had at least one relapse whilst on IFNβ-1a therapy in the previous 12 months. They received intramuscular IFNβ-1a in combination with 300 mg of natalizumab or a placebo. The outcome measures were identical to those of the AFFIRM study and showed that combination therapy with natalizumab yielded a 55% reduction in the ARR and a 24% reduction in the risk of sustained disability progression at 2 years (250). Both studies also showed significant reductions in the number of new or enlarging T2 lesions and enhancing lesions on MRI in patients receiving natalizumab. Natalizumab was studied further in patients with SPMS in the phase-III ASCEND trial, which did not meet the primary endpoint of disability progression (251), although its target α4-integrin is highly expressed in active lesions

[10] ocrevus-epar-product-information_en.pdf [Internet]. Available online at: https://www.ema.europa.eu/en/documents/product-information/ocrevus-epar-product-information_en.pdf (accessed June 1, 2019).
[11] OCREVUS safely and effectively, 18.

of patients who died in late secondary progressive MS (252). These results highlight the different disease pathophysiology that drives progressive forms of MS, which is characterized by axonal/neurodegeneration, innate immune responses mediated by CNS resident cells, development of meningeal lymphoid follicles contributing to expanding number of cortical lesions, and compartmentalized inflammation (137, 253).

Shortly after natalizumab was approved in 2004, the drug was withdrawn from the market after three patients developed PML, a life-threatening CNS-demyelinating disease caused by infection of oligodendrocytes with the John Cunningham virus (JCV). Natalizumab associated PML carries an average mortality rate of 23%, and survivors often develop debilitating neurological deficits from the disease and its treatment sequelae (254). In immunocompetent individuals, JCV almost never causes disease and remains latent in more than half of the world's population (255). PML more frequently affects immunosuppressed individuals, such as patients with acquired immune deficiency syndrome (AIDS), however, in patients taking natalizumab who are not systemically immunosuppressed, the disease is thought to be caused by forced migration of cells harboring JCV out of the bone marrow and the upregulation of gene products in B cell maturation that also promote JCV growth (256). For patients with a suspected PML diagnosis, natalizumab must be discontinued, and treatment with plasma exchange or immunoadsorption can help eliminate remaining circulating natalizumab (257). Patients might develop paradoxically worsening neurologic deficits due to an overwhelming inflammatory reaction due to the recovering immune system, a condition known as immune reconstitution inflammatory syndrome (IRIS), for which a corticosteroid can be given to provide modest benefits (258).

In 2006, natalizumab was reintroduced to the market with a black-box warning about PML risks. Prescribers and patients are required to enroll in a program that the FDA developed, known as Tysabri Outreach Unified Commitment to Health (TOUCH), which informs providers and patients about PML risks. The risks of developing PML have been identified in post-marketing analysis and include the presence of anti-JCV antibodies, prior exposure to immunosuppressants, and more than 2 years of natalizumab therapy (259, 260). In the absence of anti-JCV antibodies, the risk for PML is <0.1/1,000, but the risk increases up to 23/1,000 in patients with all three risk factors (261). Testing for JCV serology is recommended every 6 months for patients

TABLE 4 | Overview on supposed modes of action of approved therapeutics in MS and its proposed effects on the immune system.

Substance	Administration	Mode of action	Effects on immune System
IFN-ß	SC, IM	Not elucidated in detail part of the type I interferon class (activation of JAK/STAT pathways)	pro-inflammatory lymphocyte activation ↓; anti-inflammatory lymphocyte activation↑; TH1 → TH2 shift; lymphocyte migration into CNS↓; monocyte activation↓
GA	SC	Not elucidated in detail variety of immunological and non-immunological pathways Competition with myelin antigens for MHC binding site on APCs	T cell autoreactivity to myelin antigens ↓; generation of GA-reactive TH2 cells; TH1 → TH2 shift; Tregs ↑; number of B cells, plasmablasts and memory B cells↓; shift from pro-inflammatory to anti-inflammatory B cell phenotypes
S1P	PO	functional antagonist of S1PR egress of lymphocytes from lymph nodes↓; effects on neuronal and glial cells in CNS	lymphocyte egression ↓; cytotoxicity ↓; regulatory T cells↑
MTX	IV	type II topoisomerase inhibitor induction of cell lysis and initiation of programmed cell death on B cells and T cells	Levels of T cells and B cells↓; effects on innate immune system (macrophage proliferation) ↓; antigen presentation↓; antibody production↓; pro-inflammatory cytokine secretion↓
TERI	PO	Inhibition of DHODH → reduction in de-novo pyrimidine synthesis and DNA replication of highly proliferating T cells and B cells↓	Activated T cell and B cell proliferation ↓; Tregs↑; pro-inflammatory cytokines ↓
DMF	PO	activation of Nrf-2 pathway inhibition of NF-κB pathway activation of HCAR2	Nrf2↑; Tregs and CD56bright NK-cells↑; antioxidant proteins ↑; BBB migration ↓; TH1/TH17→ TH2 shift; pro-inflammatory cytokines ↓; apoptosis of T and B cells↑; Shift from pro-inflammatory to anti-inflammatory microglia
CLAD	PO	Purine nucleoside analog that interferes with DNA synthesis and repair, preferentially in activated lymphocytes	Lymphocytes ↓, relative increase in regulatory T cells
ALT	IV	mAb (IgG1) targeting CD52 predominantly on T cells and B cells, leading to cells lysis via CDC and ADCC	T cells and B cells ↓; CD56bright NK and Tregs↑; remodeling of lymphocytes
OCR	IV	mAb (IgG1) targeting CD20 on immature and mature B cells leading to cells lysis via ADCC > CDC	B cell depletion; regulatory B cells↑
NTZ	IV	mAb (IgG4) targeting and inbiting α4 subunit of integrin molecules on leukocytes;	lymphocyte migration into CNS↓

IFN-ß, interferon beta; GA, glatirameracetate; S1P, sphingosine-1-phosphat receptor modulator (fingolimod, siponimod); MTX, mitoxantrone; TERI, teriflunomide; DMF, dimethylfumarate; CLAD, cladribine; ALT, alemtuzumab; OCR, ocrelizumab; NTZ, natalizumab; IM, intramuscularly; IV, intravenously; PO, orally; SC, subcutaneously; ADCC, antibody-dependent, cell-mediated cytolysis; CDC, complement-dependent cytolysis; DHODH, dihydroorotate dehydrogenase; HCAR2, hydroxycarboxylic acid receptor 2; mAb, monoclonal antibody; MBP, myelin basic protein; MMF, mono-methyl fumarate.

with negative and indeterminate results, given a seroconversion rate of 8.5–10.3% per year in natalizumab treated patients (262). Routine surveillance MRIs also can detect early stages of the disease (263, 264). Since there are no guidelines for quantifying the risk of PML, it is up to the clinician and the patient to be aware of risk factors and consider switching therapies based on the risks and benefits from continuing the drug.

Anti-idiotypic antibodies against natalizumab are known to reduce the clinical efficacy, as well as to increase the likelihood of infusion-related adverse events (265). The presence of anti-natalizumab antibodies may be transient or persistently positive, defined as present on at least two occasions 6 weeks apart (249). In the AFFIRM study, antibodies against natalizumab were detected in 9% of patients on natalizumab (6% persistently positive), and in the SENTINEL study, they were present in 12% of patients on natalizumab and IFNβ-1a (6% persistently positive). It is recommended that patients with ongoing disease activity or persistent adverse infusion reactions be tested for antibodies against natalizumab (265, 266). Natalizumab should not be given during pregnancy. However, available data from reports do not show a significant increase in abnormalities compared to other MS patients, and it might be administered based on the individual case. An individual plan should to be made for each female patient who wishes to conceive (38).

The risk of rebound MS disease activity exists for patients who discontinue natalizumab for reasons such as the increased risk of PML, pregnancy, or the presence of neutralizing antibodies. After cessation of natalizumab, it takes 3 months for serum natalizumab concentrations to fall below the threshold of 1 μg/mL for α4-integrin desaturation (267), and CSF lymphocyte counts remain suppressed for up to 6 months (246). Correlating with these laboratory findings, disease recurrence typically starts from 2 to 6 months after natalizumab discontinuation and peaks at 5–8 months (268). Clinical worsening of MS is seen in 20–30% of patients who stop taking natalizumab, and 50–60% show worsening MRI lesions with either new gadolinium-enhancing lesions or new or enlarging T2-hyperintense lesions (268). Restarting therapy with alternative agents—including GA, IFN-ß, and fingolimod—cannot completely prevent recurrence of disease, however, patients who have switched therapies generally have lower rebound activity (269–275). In addition, shortening the natalizumab washout period and tapering cessation have been shown to reduce the risk of rebound disease further (276–278).

Immunologically, disease reactivation after cessation of natalizumab has been associated with some degree of immune reconstitution in the CNS.

Table 4 summarizes proposed modes of action of all approved MS therapeutics.

CONCLUSION

The widening of the MS treatment landscape over the past few decades mirrors progress in our understanding of MS pathophysiology. Although the mode of action is not known in detail for some of the approved treatments, the known mechanisms for other agents support our current concepts of the pathophysiology of early MS. Moreover, some treatments, such as ocrelizumab, have broadened our perspective on pathogenic MS events (230), highlighting the importance of B cells in treating MS (279).

As stated, the progress that has been achieved over the past few decades regarding MS pharmacotherapies is tremendous, and perhaps unprecedented for any medical subspecialty. In addition to benefitting patients with RRMS and PPMS, many of the agents currently approved for MS patients have informed us about relevant molecular and cellular targets in this disorder. However, challenges remain, including the potentially serious AEs. Long-term safety data is needed to detect rare but serious AEs. Based on these data monitoring must be adapted to decrease the risk of severe or even life-threatening events (as JCV-Abs for PML in patients treated with natalizumab or secondary autoimmunities in alemtuzumab treated patients). Pharmacovigilance and a better understanding of the host factors that lead to these adverse events hopefully will reduce their incidence. MS is a heterogenous disease and the individual disease progression and prognosis is not predictable. Understanding the mode of action of the various treatment options is of utmost importance to (I) foresee side effects, and (II) to define the best possible treatment, especially for patients that have not responded to treatments. Further treatments such as autologous haematopoietic-stem-cell transplantation (aHCST) are assessed in trials (280). aHCST is not approved but shows promising results. Risks and benefits for patients must be balanced, and again the appropriate patient selection is of utmost importance.

Finally, there is no evidence that any of the currently approved agents benefit patients with non-active MS (281). Currently there is no agreement when to stop or de-escalate treatment. Re-activation of disease might be a risk (282, 283). Further studies are ongoing or needed. The definition of active and non-active MS needs to be improved by appropriate biomarkers to prevent patients from being treated with agents that provide no benefit to them yet expose them to potential AEs.

AUTHOR CONTRIBUTIONS

All authors contributed at least one chapter to this review. All authors reviewed for intellectual content.

REFERENCES

1. Feigin VL, Abajobir AA, Abate KH, Abd-Allah F, Abdulle AM, Abera SF, et al. Global, regional, and national burden of neurological disorders during 1990–2015: a systematic analysis for the Global Burden of Disease Study 2015. *Lancet Neurol.* (2017) 16:877–97. doi: 10.1016/S1474-4422(17)30299-5
2. Fredrikson S, Kam-Hansen S. The 150-year anniversary of multiple sclerosis: does its early history give an etiological clue? *Perspect Biol Med.* (1989) 32:237–43. doi: 10.1353/pbm.1989.0000
3. Murray TJ. The history of multiple sclerosis: the changing frame of the disease over the centuries. *J Neurol Sci.* (2009) 277(Suppl. 1):S3–8. doi: 10.1016/S0022-510X(09)70003-6

4. Zettl UK, Hecker M, Aktas O, Wagner T, Rommer PS. Interferon β-1a and β-1b for patients with multiple sclerosis: updates to current knowledge. *Expert Rev Clin Immunol.* (2018) 14:137–53. doi: 10.1080/1744666X.2018.1426462
5. Rommer PS, Zettl UK. Managing the side effects of multiple sclerosis therapy: pharmacotherapy options for patients. *Expert Opin Pharmacother.* (2018) 19:483–98. doi: 10.1080/14656566.2018.1446944
6. Dendrou CA, Fugger L, Friese MA. Immunopathology of multiple sclerosis. *Nat Rev Immunol.* (2015) 15:545–58. doi: 10.1038/nri3871
7. Hauser SL, Bar-Or A, Comi G, Giovannoni G, Hartung H-P, Hemmer B, et al. Ocrelizumab versus interferon Beta-1a in relapsing multiple sclerosis. *N Engl J Med.* (2017) 376:221–34. doi: 10.1056/NEJMoa1601277
8. Montalban X, Hauser SL, Kappos L, Arnold DL, Bar-Or A, Comi G, et al. Ocrelizumab versus placebo in primary progressive multiple sclerosis. *N Engl J Med.* (2017) 376:209–20. doi: 10.1056/NEJMoa1606468
9. Frohman EM, Racke MK, Raine CS. Multiple sclerosis–the plaque and its pathogenesis. *N Engl J Med.* (2006) 354:942–55. doi: 10.1056/NEJMra052130
10. Schwab SR, Cyster JG. Finding a way out: lymphocyte egress from lymphoid organs. *Nat Immunol.* (2007) 8:1295–301. doi: 10.1038/ni1545
11. Ransohoff RM, Engelhardt B. The anatomical and cellular basis of immune surveillance in the central nervous system. *Nat Rev Immunol.* (2012) 12:623–35. doi: 10.1038/nri3265
12. Haji Abdolvahab M, Mofrad MRK, Schellekens H. Interferon beta: from molecular level to therapeutic effects. *Int Rev Cell Mol Biol.* (2016) 326:343–72. doi: 10.1016/bs.ircmb.2016.06.001
13. Madsen C. The innovative development in interferon beta treatments of relapsing-remitting multiple sclerosis. *Brain Behav.* (2017) 7:e00696. doi: 10.1002/brb3.696
14. De Andrea M, Ravera R, Gioia D, Gariglio M, Landolfo S. The interferon system: an overview. *Eur J Paediatr Neurol EJPN Off J Eur Paediatr Neurol Soc.* (2002) 6(Suppl. A):A41–46; discussion: A55–58. doi: 10.1053/ejpn.2002.0573
15. Markowitz CE. Interferon-beta: mechanism of action and dosing issues. *Neurology.* (2007) 68(24 Suppl. 4):S8–11. doi: 10.1212/01.wnl.0000277703.74115.d2
16. Zhang J, Hutton G, Zang Y. A comparison of the mechanisms of action of interferon beta and glatiramer acetate in the treatment of multiple sclerosis. *Clin Ther.* (2002) 24:1998–2021. doi: 10.1016/S0149-2918(02)80094-7
17. Wandinger KP, Stürzebecher CS, Bielekova B, Detore G, Rosenwald A, Staudt LM, et al. Complex immunomodulatory effects of interferon-beta in multiple sclerosis include the upregulation of T helper 1-associated marker genes. *Ann Neurol.* (2001) 50:349–57. doi: 10.1002/ana.1096
18. Schreiner B, Mitsdoerffer M, Kieseier BC, Chen L, Hartung H-P, Weller M, et al. Interferon-β enhances monocyte and dendritic cell expression of B7-H1 (PD-L1), a strong inhibitor of autologous T-cell activation: relevance for the immune modulatory effect in multiple sclerosis. *J Neuroimmunol.* (2004) 155:172–82. doi: 10.1016/j.jneuroim.2004.06.013
19. Yong VW, Chabot S, Stuve O, Williams G. Interferon beta in the treatment of multiple sclerosis: mechanisms of action. *Neurology.* (1998) 51:682–9. doi: 10.1212/WNL.51.3.682
20. Dhib-Jalbut S, Marks S. Interferon-β mechanisms of action in multiple sclerosis. *Neurology.* (2010) 74(Suppl. 1):S17–24. doi: 10.1212/WNL.0b013e3181c97d99
21. Neuhaus O, Kieseier BC, Hartung H-P. Pharmacokinetics and pharmacodynamics of the interferon-betas, glatiramer acetate, and mitoxantrone in multiple sclerosis. *J Neurol Sci.* (2007) 259:27–37. doi: 10.1016/j.jns.2006.05.071
22. *Drug Approval Package: Betaseron Interferon BETA-1B Subcutaneous(Generic Name) NDA # 103471 [Internet].* Available online at: https://www.accessdata.fda.gov/drugsatfda_docs/nda/pre96/103471s0000TOC.cfm (accessed August 8, 2018).
23. *WC500053086.pdf [Internet].* Available online at: http://www.ema.europa.eu/docs/en_GB/document_library/EPAR_-_Summary_for_the_public/human/000081/WC500053086.pdf (accessed August 8, 2018).
24. White JT, Newsome SD, Kieseier BC, Bermel RA, Cui Y, Seddighzadeh A, et al. Incidence, characterization, and clinical impact analysis of peginterferon beta1a immunogenicity in patients with multiple sclerosis in the ADVANCE trial. *Ther Adv Neurol Disord.* (2016) 9:239–49. doi: 10.1177/1756285616633967
25. Interferon beta-1b in the treatment of multiple sclerosis: final outcome of the randomized controlled trial. The IFNB Multiple Sclerosis Study Group and The University of British Columbia MS/MRI Analysis Group. *Neurology.* (1995) 45:1277–85. doi: 10.1212/WNL.45.7.1277
26. Interferon beta-1b is effective in relapsing-remitting multiple sclerosis. I. Clinical results of a multicenter, randomized, double-blind, placebo-controlled trial. The IFNB Multiple Sclerosis Study Group. *Neurology.* (1993) 43:655–61. doi: 10.1212/WNL.43.4.655
27. Vermersch P, de Seze J, Stojkovic T, Hautecoeur P, G-SEP (Groupe Septentrional d'Etudes et de Recherches sur la SEP). Interferon beta1a (Avonex) treatment in multiple sclerosis: similarity of effect on progression of disability in patients with mild and moderate disability. *J Neurol.* (2002) 249:184–7. doi: 10.1007/PL00007862
28. Kappos L, Freedman MS, Polman CH, Edan G, Hartung H-P, Miller DH, et al. Effect of early versus delayed interferon beta-1b treatment on disability after a first clinical event suggestive of multiple sclerosis: a 3-year follow-up analysis of the BENEFIT study. *Lancet.* (2007) 370:389–97. doi: 10.1016/S0140-6736(07)61194-5
29. Comi G, De Stefano N, Freedman MS, Barkhof F, Polman CH, Uitdehaag BMJ, et al. Comparison of two dosing frequencies of subcutaneous interferon beta-1a in patients with a first clinical demyelinating event suggestive of multiple sclerosis (REFLEX): a phase 3 randomised controlled trial. *Lancet Neurol.* (2012) 11:33–41. doi: 10.1016/S1474-4422(11)70262-9
30. Jacobs LD, Beck RW, Simon JH, Kinkel RP, Brownscheidle CM, Murray TJ, et al. Intramuscular interferon beta-1a therapy initiated during a first demyelinating event in multiple sclerosis. CHAMPS Study Group. *N Engl J Med.* (2000) 343:898–904. doi: 10.1056/NEJM200009283431301
31. Placebo-controlled multicentre randomised trial of interferon beta-1b in treatment of secondary progressive multiple sclerosis. European Study Group on interferon beta-1b in secondary progressive MS. *Lancet.* (1998) 352:1491–7. doi: 10.1016/S0140-6736(98)10039-9
32. Panitch H, Miller A, Paty D, Weinshenker B, North American Study Group on Interferon beta-1b in Secondary Progressive MS. Interferon beta-1b in secondary progressive MS: results from a 3-year controlled study. *Neurology.* (2004) 63:1788–95. doi: 10.1212/01.WNL.0000146958.77317.3E
33. Rommer PS, Stüve O. Management of secondary progressive multiple sclerosis: prophylactic treatment-past, present, and future aspects. *Curr Treat Options Neurol.* (2013) 15:241–58. doi: 10.1007/s11940-013-0233-x
34. Trojano M, Pellegrini F, Paolicelli D, Fuiani A, Zimatore GB, Tortorella C, et al. Real-life impact of early interferon beta therapy in relapsing multiple sclerosis. *Ann Neurol.* (2009) 66:513–20. doi: 10.1002/ana.21757
35. Ebers GC, Traboulsee A, Li D, Langdon D, Reder AT, Goodin DS, et al. Analysis of clinical outcomes according to original treatment groups 16 years after the pivotal IFNB-1b trial. *J Neurol Neurosurg Psychiatry.* (2010) 81:907–12. doi: 10.1136/jnnp.2009.204123
36. Hemmer B, Stüve O, Kieseier B, Schellekens H, Hartung H-P. Immune response to immunotherapy: the role of neutralising antibodies to interferon beta in the treatment of multiple sclerosis. *Lancet Neurol.* (2005) 4:403–12. doi: 10.1016/S1474-4422(05)70117-4
37. Link J, Ramanujam R, Auer M, Ryner M, Hässler S, Bachelet D, et al. Clinical practice of analysis of anti-drug antibodies against interferon beta and natalizumab in multiple sclerosis patients in Europe: a descriptive study of test results. *PLoS ONE.* (2017) 12:e0170395. doi: 10.1371/journal.pone.0170395
38. Thöne J, Thiel S, Gold R, Hellwig K. Treatment of multiple sclerosis during pregnancy - safety considerations. *Expert Opin Drug Saf.* (2017) 16:523–34. doi: 10.1080/14740338.2017.1311321
39. Teitelbaum D, Arnon R, Sela M. Copolymer 1: from basic research to clinical application. *Cell Mol Life Sci.* (1997) 53:24–8. doi: 10.1007/PL00000576
40. Dhib-Jalbut S. Mechanisms of action of interferons and glatiramer acetate in multiple sclerosis. *Neurology.* (2002) 58(8 Suppl. 4):S3–9. doi: 10.1212/WNL.58.8_suppl_4.S3
41. Fridkis-Hareli M, Teitelbaum D, Gurevich E, Pecht I, Brautbar C, Kwon OJ, et al. Direct binding of myelin basic protein and synthetic copolymer

1 to class II major histocompatibility complex molecules on living antigen-presenting cells–specificity and promiscuity. *Proc Natl Acad Sci USA.* (1994) 91:4872–6. doi: 10.1073/pnas.91.11.4872
42. Ben-Nun A, Mendel I, Bakimer R, Fridkis-Hareli M, Teitelbaum D, Arnon R, et al. The autoimmune reactivity to myelin oligodendrocyte glycoprotein (MOG) in multiple sclerosis is potentially pathogenic: effect of copolymer 1 on MOG-induced disease. *J Neurol.* (1996) 243(4 Suppl. 1):S14–22. doi: 10.1007/BF00873697
43. Arnon R, Sela M, Teitelbaum D. New insights into the mechanism of action of copolymer 1 in experimental allergic encephalomyelitis and multiple sclerosis. *J Neurol.* (1996) 243(4 Suppl. 1):S8–13. doi: 10.1007/BF00873696
44. Teitelbaum D, Milo R, Arnon R, Sela M. Synthetic copolymer 1 inhibits human T-cell lines specific for myelin basic protein. *Proc Natl Acad Sci USA.* (1992) 89:137–41. doi: 10.1073/pnas.89.1.137
45. Teitelbaum D, Fridkis-Hareli M, Arnon R, Sela M. Copolymer 1 inhibits chronic relapsing experimental allergic encephalomyelitis induced by proteolipid protein (PLP) peptides in mice and interferes with PLP-specific T cell responses. *J Neuroimmunol.* (1996) 64:209–17. doi: 10.1016/0165-5728(95)00180-8
46. Neuhaus O, Farina C, Yassouridis A, Wiendl H, Then Bergh F, Dose T, et al. Multiple sclerosis: comparison of copolymer-1- reactive T cell lines from treated and untreated subjects reveals cytokine shift from T helper 1 to T helper 2 cells. *Proc Natl Acad Sci USA.* (2000) 97:7452–7. doi: 10.1073/pnas.97.13.7452
47. Chen M, Gran B, Costello K, Johnson K, Martin R, Dhib-Jalbut S. Glatiramer acetate induces a Th2-biased response and crossreactivity with myelin basic protein in patients with MS. *Mult Scler.*(2001) 7:209–19. doi: 10.1177/135245850100700401
48. Aharoni R. Immunomodulation neuroprotection and remyelination - the fundamental therapeutic effects of glatiramer acetate: a critical review. *J Autoimmun.* (2014) 54:81–92. doi: 10.1016/j.jaut.2014.05.005
49. Ziemssen T, Kümpfel T, Klinkert WEF, Neuhaus O, Hohlfeld R. Glatiramer acetate-specific T-helper 1- and 2-type cell lines produce BDNF: implications for multiple sclerosis therapy. Brain-derived neurotrophic factor. *Brain J Neurol.* (2002) 125(Pt 11):2381–91. doi: 10.1093/brain/awf252
50. Aharoni R, Teitelbaum D, Arnon R, Sela M. Copolymer 1 acts against the immunodominant epitope 82-100 of myelin basic protein by T cell receptor antagonism in addition to major histocompatibility complex blocking. *Proc Natl Acad Sci USA.* (1999) 96:634–9. doi: 10.1073/pnas.96.2.634
51. Hong J, Li N, Zhang X, Zheng B, Zhang JZ. Induction of CD4+CD25+ regulatory T cells by copolymer-I through activation of transcription factor Foxp3. *Proc Natl Acad Sci USA.* (2005) 102:6449–54. doi: 10.1073/pnas.0502187102
52. Weber MS, Starck M, Wagenpfeil S, Meinl E, Hohlfeld R, Farina C. Multiple sclerosis: glatiramer acetate inhibits monocyte reactivity *in vitro* and *in vivo*. *Brain J Neurol.* (2004) 127(Pt 6):1370–8. doi: 10.1093/brain/awh163
53. Kim HJ, Ifergan I, Antel JP, Seguin R, Duddy M, Lapierre Y, et al. Type 2 monocyte and microglia differentiation mediated by glatiramer acetate therapy in patients with multiple sclerosis. *J Immunol.* (2004) 172:7144–53. doi: 10.4049/jimmunol.172.11.7144
54. Vieira PL, Heystek HC, Wormmeester J, Wierenga EA, Kapsenberg ML. Glatiramer acetate (copolymer-1, copaxone) promotes Th2 cell development and increased IL-10 production through modulation of dendritic cells. *J Immunol.* (2003) 170:4483–8. doi: 10.4049/jimmunol.170.9.4483
55. Li Q, Milo R, Panitch H, Swoveland P, Bever CT. Glatiramer acetate blocks the activation of THP-1 cells by interferon-gamma. *Eur J Pharmacol.* (1998) 342:303–10. doi: 10.1016/S0014-2999(97)01509-4
56. Weber MS, Prod'homme T, Youssef S, Dunn SE, Rundle CD, Lee L, et al. Type II monocytes modulate T cell-mediated central nervous system autoimmune disease. *Nat Med.* (2007) 13:935–43. doi: 10.1038/nm1620
57. Milo R. Therapeutic strategies targeting B-cells in multiple sclerosis. *Autoimmun Rev.* (2016) 15:714–8. doi: 10.1016/j.autrev.2016.03.006
58. Kuerten S, Jackson LJ, Kaye J, Vollmer TL. Impact of glatiramer acetate on B cell-mediated pathogenesis of multiple sclerosis. *CNS Drugs.* (2018) 32:1039–51. doi: 10.1007/s40263-018-0567-8
59. Aharoni R, Arnon R, Eilam R. Neurogenesis and neuroprotection induced by peripheral immunomodulatory treatment of experimental autoimmune encephalomyelitis. *J Neurosci Off J Soc Neurosci.* (2005) 25:8217–28. doi: 10.1523/JNEUROSCI.1859-05.2005
60. Abramsky O, Teitelbaum D, Arnon R. Effect of a synthetic polypeptide (COP 1) on patients with multiple sclerosis and with acute disseminated encephalomeylitis. Preliminary report. *J Neurol Sci.* (1977) 31:433–8. doi: 10.1016/0022-510X(77)90220-9
61. Bornstein MB, Miller AI, Teitelbaum D, Arnon R, Sela M. Multiple sclerosis: trial of a synthetic polypeptide. *Ann Neurol.* (1982) 11:317–9. doi: 10.1002/ana.410110314
62. Bornstein MB, Miller A, Slagle S, Weitzman M, Crystal H, Drexler E, et al. A pilot trial of Cop 1 in exacerbating-remitting multiple sclerosis. *N Engl J Med.* (1987) 317:408–14. doi: 10.1056/NEJM198708133170703
63. Bornstein MB, Miller A, Slagle S, Weitzman M, Drexler E, Keilson M, et al. A placebo-controlled, double-blind, randomized, two-center, pilot trial of Cop 1 in chronic progressive multiple sclerosis. *Neurology.* (1991) 41:533–9. doi: 10.1212/WNL.41.4.533
64. Johnson KP, Brooks BR, Cohen JA, Ford CC, Goldstein J, Lisak RP, et al. Copolymer 1 reduces relapse rate and improves disability in relapsing-remitting multiple sclerosis: results of a phase III multicenter, double-blind placebo-controlled trial. The Copolymer 1 Multiple Sclerosis Study Group. *Neurology.* (1995) 45:1268–76. doi: 10.1212/WNL.45.7.1268
65. Johnson KP, Brooks BR, Cohen JA, Ford CC, Goldstein J, Lisak RP, et al. Extended use of glatiramer acetate (Copaxone) is well tolerated and maintains its clinical effect on multiple sclerosis relapse rate and degree of disability. Copolymer 1 Multiple Sclerosis Study Group. *Neurology.* (1998) 50:701–8. doi: 10.1212/WNL.50.3.701
66. Ge Y, Grossman RI, Udupa JK, Fulton J, Constantinescu CS, Gonzales-Scarano F, et al. Glatiramer acetate (Copaxone) treatment in relapsing-remitting MS: quantitative MR assessment. *Neurology.* (2000) 54:813–7. doi: 10.1212/WNL.54.4.813
67. Comi G, Filippi M, Wolinsky JS. European/Canadian multicenter, double-blind, randomized, placebo-controlled study of the effects of glatiramer acetate on magnetic resonance imaging-measured disease activity and burden in patients with relapsing multiple sclerosis. European/Canadian Glatiramer Acetate Study Group. *Ann Neurol.* (2001) 49:290–7. doi: 10.1002/ana.64
68. Filippi M, Rovaris M, Rocca MA, Sormani MP, Wolinsky JS, Comi G, et al. Glatiramer acetate reduces the proportion of new MS lesions evolving into 'black holes'. *Neurology.* (2001) 57:731–3. doi: 10.1212/WNL.57.4.731
69. Comi G, Cohen JA, Arnold DL, Wynn D, Filippi M, FORTE Study Group. Phase III dose-comparison study of glatiramer acetate for multiple sclerosis. *Ann Neurol.* (2011) 69:75–82. doi: 10.1002/ana.22316
70. Khan O, Rieckmann P, Boyko A, Selmaj K, Zivadinov R, GALA Study Group. Three times weekly glatiramer acetate in relapsing-remitting multiple sclerosis. *Ann Neurol.* (2013) 73:705–13. doi: 10.1002/ana.23938
71. Wolinsky JS, Narayana PA, O'Connor P, Coyle PK, Ford C, Johnson K, et al. Glatiramer acetate in primary progressive multiple sclerosis: results of a multinational, multicenter, double-blind, placebo-controlled trial. *Ann Neurol.* (2007) 61:14–24. doi: 10.1002/ana.21079
72. Comi G, Martinelli V, Rodegher M, Moiola L, Bajenaru O, Carra A, et al. Effect of glatiramer acetate on conversion to clinically definite multiple sclerosis in patients with clinically isolated syndrome (PreCISe study): a randomised, double-blind, placebo-controlled trial. *Lancet.* (2009) 374:1503–11. doi: 10.1016/S0140-6736(09)61259-9
73. Ford C, Goodman AD, Johnson K, Kachuck N, Lindsey JW, Lisak R, et al. Continuous long-term immunomodulatory therapy in relapsing multiple sclerosis: results from the 15-year analysis of the US prospective open-label study of glatiramer acetate. *Mult Scler.* (2010) 16:342–50. doi: 10.1177/1352458509358088
74. O'Connor P, Filippi M, Arnason B, Comi G, Cook S, Goodin D, et al. 250 microg or 500 microg interferon beta-1b versus 20 mg glatiramer acetate in relapsing-remitting multiple sclerosis: a prospective, randomised, multicentre study. *Lancet Neurol.* (2009) 8:889–97. doi: 10.1016/S1474-4422(09)70226-1

75. Mikol DD, Barkhof F, Chang P, Coyle PK, Jeffery DR, Schwid SR, et al. Comparison of subcutaneous interferon beta-1a with glatiramer acetate in patients with relapsing multiple sclerosis (the REbif vs Glatiramer Acetate in Relapsing MS Disease [REGARD] study): a multicentre, randomised, parallel, open-label trial. *Lancet Neurol.* (2008) 7:903–14. doi: 10.1016/S1474-4422(08)70200-X
76. Lublin FD, Cofield SS, Cutter GR, Conwit R, Narayana PA, Nelson F, et al. Randomized study combining interferon and glatiramer acetate in multiple sclerosis. *Ann Neurol.* (2013) 73:327–40. doi: 10.1002/ana.23863
77. Karussis D, Teitelbaum D, Sicsic C, Brenner T, AC001 multi-center Israeli study group. Long-term treatment of multiple sclerosis with glatiramer acetate: natural history of the subtypes of anti-glatiramer acetate antibodies and their correlation with clinical efficacy. *J Neuroimmunol.* (2010) 220:125–30. doi: 10.1016/j.jneuroim.2010.01.009
78. Sandberg-Wollheim M, Neudorfer O, Grinspan A, Weinstock-Guttman B, Haas J, Izquierdo G, et al. Pregnancy outcomes from the branded glatiramer acetate pregnancy database. *Int J MS Care.* (2018) 20:9–14. doi: 10.7224/1537-2073.2016-079
79. Kalinke U, Prinz M. Endogenous, or therapeutically induced, type I interferon responses differentially modulate Th1/Th17-mediated autoimmunity in the CNS. *Immunol Cell Biol.* (2012) 90:505–9. doi: 10.1038/icb.2012.8
80. Lalive PH, Neuhaus O, Benkhoucha M, Burger D, Hohlfeld R, Zamvil SS, et al. Glatiramer acetate in the treatment of multiple sclerosis: emerging concepts regarding its mechanism of action. *CNS Drugs.* (2011) 25:401–14. doi: 10.2165/11588120-000000000-00000
81. Straus Farber R, Harel A, Lublin F. Novel agents for relapsing forms of multiple sclerosis. *Annu Rev Med.* (2016) 67:309–21. doi: 10.1146/annurev-med-052814-023415
82. Chun J, Brinkmann V. A mechanistically novel, first oral therapy for multiple sclerosis: the development of fingolimod (FTY720, Gilenya). *Discov Med.* (2011) 12:213–28.
83. Cyster JG, Schwab SR. Sphingosine-1-phosphate and lymphocyte egress from lymphoid organs. *Annu Rev Immunol.* (2012) 30:69–94. doi: 10.1146/annurev-immunol-020711-075011
84. Matloubian M, Lo CG, Cinamon G, Lesneski MJ, Xu Y, Brinkmann V, et al. Lymphocyte egress from thymus and peripheral lymphoid organs is dependent on S1P receptor 1. *Nature.* (2004) 427:355–60. doi: 10.1038/nature02284
85. Pelletier D, Hafler DA. Fingolimod for multiple sclerosis. *N Engl J Med.* (2012) 366:339–47. doi: 10.1056/NEJMct1101691
86. Reeves PM, Kang Y-L, Kirchhausen T. Endocytosis of ligand-activated sphingosine 1-phosphate receptor 1 mediated by the clathrin-pathway. *Traffic Cph Den.* (2016) 17:40–52. doi: 10.1111/tra.12343
87. Mehling M, Brinkmann V, Antel J, Bar-Or A, Goebels N, Vedrine C, et al. FTY720 therapy exerts differential effects on T cell subsets in multiple sclerosis. *Neurology.* (2008) 71:1261–7. doi: 10.1212/01.wnl.0000327609.57688.ea
88. Zhou PJ, Wang H, Shi GH, Wang XH, Shen ZJ, Xu D. Immunomodulatory drug FTY720 induces regulatory CD4(+)CD25(+) T cells *in vitro*. *Clin Exp Immunol.* (2009) 157:40–7. doi: 10.1111/j.1365-2249.2009.03942.x
89. Yamagata K, Tagami M, Torii Y, Takenaga F, Tsumagari S, Itoh S, et al. Sphingosine 1-phosphate induces the production of glial cell line-derived neurotrophic factor and cellular proliferation in astrocytes. *Glia.* (2003) 41:199–206. doi: 10.1002/glia.10180
90. Edsall LC, Pirianov GG, Spiegel S. Involvement of sphingosine 1-phosphate in nerve growth factor-mediated neuronal survival and differentiation. *J Neurosci Off J Soc Neurosci.* (1997) 17:6952–60. doi: 10.1523/JNEUROSCI.17-18-06952.1997
91. Kappos L, O'Connor P, Radue E-W, Polman C, Hohlfeld R, Selmaj K, et al. Long-term effects of fingolimod in multiple sclerosis: the randomized FREEDOMS extension trial. *Neurology.* (2015) 84:1582–91. doi: 10.1212/WNL.0000000000001462
92. Calabresi PA, Radue E-W, Goodin D, Jeffery D, Rammohan KW, Reder AT, et al. Safety and efficacy of fingolimod in patients with relapsing-remitting multiple sclerosis (FREEDOMS II): a double-blind, randomised, placebo-controlled, phase 3 trial. *Lancet Neurol.* (2014) 13:545–56. doi: 10.1016/S1474-4422(14)70049-3
93. Cohen JA, Barkhof F, Comi G, Hartung H-P, Khatri BO, Montalban X, et al. Oral fingolimod or intramuscular interferon for relapsing multiple sclerosis. *N Engl J Med.* (2010) 362:402–15. doi: 10.1056/NEJMoa0907839
94. Chitnis T, Arnold DL, Banwell B, Brück W, Ghezzi A, Giovannoni G, et al. Trial of fingolimod versus interferon Beta-1a in pediatric multiple sclerosis. *N Engl J Med.* (2018) 379:1017–27. doi: 10.1056/NEJMoa1800149
95. Anonymous. *Gilenya [Internet].* European Medicines Agency (2018). Available online at: https://www.ema.europa.eu/en/medicines/human/EPAR/gilenya (cited June 13, 2019).
96. Meissner A, Limmroth V. Update on the cardiovascular profile of fingolimod in the therapy of relapsing-remitting multiple sclerosis (MS). *Mult Scler Relat Disord.* (2016) 8:19–26. doi: 10.1016/j.msard.2016.04.002
97. Winkelmann A, Loebermann M, Reisinger EC, Hartung H-P, Zettl UK. Disease-modifying therapies and infectious risks in multiple sclerosis. *Nat Rev Neurol.* (2016) 12:217–33. doi: 10.1038/nrneurol.2016.21
98. Druart C, El Sankari S, van Pesch V. Long-term safety and real-world effectiveness of fingolimod in relapsing multiple sclerosis. *Patient Relat Outcome Meas.* (2017) 9:1–10. doi: 10.2147/PROM.S122401
99. Hatcher SE, Waubant E, Nourbakhsh B, Crabtree-Hartman E, Graves JS. Rebound syndrome in patients with multiple sclerosis after cessation of fingolimod treatment. *JAMA Neurol.* (2016) 73:790–4. doi: 10.1001/jamaneurol.2016.0826
100. Kappos L, Bar-Or A, Cree BAC, Fox RJ, Giovannoni G, Gold R, et al. Siponimod versus placebo in secondary progressive multiple sclerosis (EXPAND): a double-blind, randomised, phase 3 study. *Lancet.* (2018) 391:1263–73. doi: 10.1016/S0140-6736(18)30475-6
101. Thomas X, Archimbaud E. Mitoxantrone in the treatment of acute myelogenous leukemia: a review. *Hematol Cell Ther.* (1997) 39:63–74. doi: 10.1007/s00282-997-0163-8
102. Putzki N, Kumar M, Kreuzfelder E, Grosse-Wilde H, Diener HC, Limmroth V. Mitoxantrone does not restore the impaired suppressive function of natural regulatory T cells in patients suffering from multiple sclerosis. A longitudinal *ex vivo* and *in vitro* study. *Eur Neurol.* (2009) 61:27–32. doi: 10.1159/000165346
103. Chan A, Weilbach FX, Toyka KV, Gold R. Mitoxantrone induces cell death in peripheral blood leucocytes of multiple sclerosis patients. *Clin Exp Immunol.* (2005) 139:152–8. doi: 10.1111/j.1365-2249.2005.02653.x
104. Neuhaus O, Wiendl H, Kieseier BC, Archelos JJ, Hemmer B, Stüve O, et al. Multiple sclerosis: mitoxantrone promotes differential effects on immunocompetent cells *in vitro*. *J Neuroimmunol.* (2005) 168:128–37. doi: 10.1016/j.jneuroim.2005.01.024
105. Kopadze T, Dehmel T, Hartung H-P, Stüve O, Kieseier BC. Inhibition by mitoxantrone of *in vitro* migration of immunocompetent cells: a possible mechanism for therapeutic efficacy in the treatment of multiple sclerosis. *Arch Neurol.* (2006) 63:1572–8. doi: 10.1001/archneur.63.11.1572
106. Neuhaus O, Kieseier BC, Hartung H-P. Mechanisms of mitoxantrone in multiple sclerosis–what is known? *J Neurol Sci.* (2004) 223:25–7. doi: 10.1016/j.jns.2004.04.015
107. Hartung H-P, Gonsette R, König N, Kwiecinski H, Guseo A, Morrissey SP, et al. Mitoxantrone in progressive multiple sclerosis: a placebo-controlled, double-blind, randomised, multicentre trial. *Lancet.* (2002) 360:2018–25. doi: 10.1016/S0140-6736(02)12023-X
108. Edan G, Miller D, Clanet M, Confavreux C, Lyon-Caen O, Lubetzki C, et al. Therapeutic effect of mitoxantrone combined with methylprednisolone in multiple sclerosis: a randomised multicentre study of active disease using MRI and clinical criteria. *J Neurol Neurosurg Psychiatry.* (1997) 62:112–8. doi: 10.1136/jnnp.62.2.112
109. Martinelli V, Cocco E, Capra R, Salemi G, Gallo P, Capobianco M, et al. Acute myeloid leukemia in Italian patients with multiple sclerosis treated with mitoxantrone. *Neurology.* (2011) 77:1887–95. doi: 10.1212/WNL.0b013e318238ee00
110. Cocco E, Marrosu MG. The current role of mitoxantrone in the treatment of multiple sclerosis. *Expert Rev Neurother.* (2014) 14:607–16. doi: 10.1586/14737175.2014.915742
111. Kingwell E, Koch M, Leung B, Isserow S, Geddes J, Rieckmann P, et al. Cardiotoxicity and other adverse events associated with mitoxantrone treatment for MS. *Neurology.* (2010) 74:1822–6. doi: 10.1212/WNL.0b013e3181e0f7e6

112. Le Page E, Leray E, Edan G, French Mitoxantrone Safety Group. Long-term safety profile of mitoxantrone in a French cohort of 802 multiple sclerosis patients: a 5-year prospective study. *Mult Scler.*(2011) 17:867–75. doi: 10.1177/1352458511398371
113. Cocco E, Sardu C, Gallo P, Capra R, Amato MP, Trojano M, et al. Frequency and risk factors of mitoxantrone-induced amenorrhea in multiple sclerosis: the FEMIMS study. *Mult Scler.*(2008) 14:1225–33. doi: 10.1177/1352458508094882
114. Wingerchuk DM, Weinshenker BG. Disease modifying therapies for relapsing multiple sclerosis. *BMJ.* (2016) 354:i3518. doi: 10.1136/bmj.i3518
115. Ammatuna E, Montesinos P, Hasan SK, Ramadan SM, Esteve J, Hubmann M, et al. Presenting features and treatment outcome of acute promyelocytic leukemia arising after multiple sclerosis. *Haematologica.* (2011) 96:621–5. doi: 10.3324/haematol.2010.036657
116. Chan A, Lo-Coco F. Mitoxantrone-related acute leukemia in MS: an open or closed book? *Neurology.* (2013) 80:1529–33. doi: 10.1212/WNL.0b013e31828cf891
117. Soelberg Sorensen P. Safety concerns and risk management of multiple sclerosis therapies. *Acta Neurol Scand.* (2017) 136:168–86. doi: 10.1111/ane.12712
118. Fleischer V, Salmen A, Kollar S, Weyer V, Siffrin V, Chan A, et al. Cardiotoxicity of mitoxantrone treatment in a german cohort of 639 multiple sclerosis patients. *J Clin Neurol Seoul Korea.* (2014) 10:289–95. doi: 10.3988/jcn.2014.10.4.289
119. Ellis R, Brown S, Boggild M. Therapy-related acute leukaemia with mitoxantrone: four years on, what is the risk and can it be limited? *Mult Scler.* (2015) 21:642–5. doi: 10.1177/1352458514541508
120. Aly L, Hemmer B, Korn T. From leflunomide to teriflunomide: drug development and immunosuppressive oral drugs in the treatment of multiple sclerosis. *Curr Neuropharmacol.* (2017) 15:874–91. doi: 10.2174/1570159X14666161208151525
121. Miller AE. Oral teriflunomide in the treatment of relapsing forms of multiple sclerosis: clinical evidence and long-term experience. *Ther Adv Neurol Disord.* (2017) 10:381–96. doi: 10.1177/1756285617722500
122. Ochoa-Repáraz J, Colpitts SL, Kircher C, Kasper EJ, Telesford KM, Begum-Haque S, et al. Induction of gut regulatory CD39+ T cells by teriflunomide protects against EAE. *Neurol Neuroimmunol Neuroinflamm.* (2016) 3:e291. doi: 10.1212/NXI.0000000000000291
123. Wostradowski T, Prajeeth CK, Gudi V, Kronenberg J, Witte S, Brieskorn M, et al. *In vitro* evaluation of physiologically relevant concentrations of teriflunomide on activation and proliferation of primary rodent microglia. *J Neuroinflamm.* (2016) 13:250. doi: 10.1186/s12974-016-0715-3
124. Manna SK, Aggarwal BB. Immunosuppressive leflunomide metabolite (A77 1726) blocks TNF-dependent nuclear factor-kappa B activation and gene expression. *J Immunol Baltim.* (1999) 162:2095–102.
125. González-Alvaro I, Ortiz AM, Domínguez-Jiménez C, Aragón-Bodi A, Díaz Sánchez B, Sánchez-Madrid F. Inhibition of tumour necrosis factor and IL-17 production by leflunomide involves the JAK/STAT pathway. *Ann Rheum Dis.* (2009) 68:1644–50. doi: 10.1136/ard.2008.096743
126. Bilger A, Plowshay J, Ma S, Nawandar D, Barlow EA, Romero-Masters JC, et al. Leflunomide/teriflunomide inhibit Epstein-Barr virus (EBV)- induced lymphoproliferative disease and lytic viral replication. *Oncotarget.* (2017) 8:44266–80. doi: 10.18632/oncotarget.17863
127. Modica CM, Schweser F, Sudyn ML, Bertolino N, Preda M, Polak P, et al. Effect of teriflunomide on cortex-basal ganglia-thalamus (CxBGTh) circuit glutamatergic dysregulation in the Theiler's Murine Encephalomyelitis Virus mouse model of multiple sclerosis. *PLoS ONE.* (2017) 12:e0182729. doi: 10.1371/journal.pone.0182729
128. Göttle P, Manousi A, Kremer D, Reiche L, Hartung H-P, Küry P. Teriflunomide promotes oligodendroglial differentiation and myelination. *J Neuroinflamm.* (2018) 15:76. doi: 10.1186/s12974-018-1110-z
129. Groh J, Hörner M, Martini R. Teriflunomide attenuates neuroinflammation-related neural damage in mice carrying human PLP1 mutations. *J Neuroinflamm.* (2018) 15:194. doi: 10.1186/s12974-018-1228-z
130. Bar-Or A, Freedman MS, Kremenchutzky M, Menguy-Vacheron F, Bauer D, Jodl S, et al. Teriflunomide effect on immune response to influenza vaccine in patients with multiple sclerosis. *Neurology.* (2013) 81:552–8. doi: 10.1212/WNL.0b013e31829e6fbf
131. Freedman MS. Teriflunomide in relapsing multiple sclerosis: therapeutic utility. *Ther Adv Chronic Dis.* (2013) 4:192–205. doi: 10.1177/2040622313492810
132. O'Connor PW, Li D, Freedman MS, Bar-Or A, Rice GPA, Confavreux C, et al. A Phase II study of the safety and efficacy of teriflunomide in multiple sclerosis with relapses. *Neurology.* (2006) 66:894–900. doi: 10.1212/01.wnl.0000203121.04509.31
133. O'Connor P, Wolinsky JS, Confavreux C, Comi G, Kappos L, Olsson TP, et al. Randomized trial of oral teriflunomide for relapsing multiple sclerosis. *N Engl J Med.* (2011) 365:1293–303. doi: 10.1056/NEJMoa1014656
134. Confavreux C, O'Connor P, Comi G, Freedman MS, Miller AE, Olsson TP, et al. Oral teriflunomide for patients with relapsing multiple sclerosis (TOWER): a randomised, double-blind, placebo-controlled, phase 3 trial. *Lancet Neurol.* (2014) 13:247–56. doi: 10.1016/S1474-4422(13)70308-9
135. Vermersch P, Czlonkowska A, Grimaldi LME, Confavreux C, Comi G, Kappos L, et al. Teriflunomide versus subcutaneous interferon beta-1a in patients with relapsing multiple sclerosis: a randomised, controlled phase 3 trial. *Mult Scler.* (2014) 20:705–16. doi: 10.1177/1352458513507821
136. Miller AE, Wolinsky JS, Kappos L, Comi G, Freedman MS, Olsson TP, et al. Oral teriflunomide for patients with a first clinical episode suggestive of multiple sclerosis (TOPIC): a randomised, double-blind, placebo-controlled, phase 3 trial. *Lancet Neurol.* (2014) 13:977–86. doi: 10.1016/S1474-4422(14)70191-7
137. Elkjaer ML, Molnar T, Illes Z. Teriflunomide for multiple sclerosis in real-world setting. *Acta Neurol Scand.* (2017) 136:447–53. doi: 10.1111/ane.12755
138. Freedman MS, Montalban X, Miller AE, Dive-Pouletty C, Hass S, Thangavelu K, et al. Comparing outcomes from clinical studies of oral disease-modifying therapies (dimethyl fumarate, fingolimod, and teriflunomide) in relapsing MS: assessing absolute differences using a number needed to treat analysis. *Mult Scler Relat Disord.* (2016) 10:204–12. doi: 10.1016/j.msard.2016.10.010
139. Buron MD, Chalmer TA, Sellebjerg F, Frederiksen J, Góra MK, Illes Z, et al. Comparative effectiveness of teriflunomide and dimethyl fumarate: a nationwide cohort study. *Neurology.* (2019) 92:e1811–20. doi: 10.1212/WNL.0000000000007314
140. Kalincik T, Kubala Havrdova E, Horakova D, Izquierdo G, Prat A, Girard M, et al. Comparison of fingolimod, dimethyl fumarate and teriflunomide for multiple sclerosis. *J Neurol Neurosurg Psychiatry.* (2019) 90:458–68. doi: 10.1136/jnnp-2018-319831
141. D'Amico E, Zanghì A, Sciandra M, Borriello G, Callari G, Gallo A, et al. Discontinuation of teriflunomide and dimethyl fumarate in a large Italian multicentre population: a 24-month real-world experience. *J Neurol.* (2019) 266:411–6. doi: 10.1007/s00415-018-9144-9
142. Rommer PS, Zettl UK, Kieseier B, Hartung H-P, Menge T, Frohman E, et al. Requirement for safety monitoring for approved multiple sclerosis therapies: an overview. *Clin Exp Immunol.* (2014) 175:397–407. doi: 10.1111/cei.12206
143. Comi G, Freedman MS, Kappos L, Olsson TP, Miller AE, Wolinsky JS, et al. Pooled safety and tolerability data from four placebo-controlled teriflunomide studies and extensions. *Mult Scler Relat Disord.* (2016) 5:97–104. doi: 10.1016/j.msard.2015.11.006
144. O'Connor P, Comi G, Freedman MS, Miller AE, Kappos L, Bouchard J-P, et al. Long-term safety and efficacy of teriflunomide: nine-year follow-up of the randomized TEMSO study. *Neurology.* (2016) 86:920–30. doi: 10.1212/WNL.0000000000002441
145. Confavreux C, Li DK, Freedman MS, Truffinet P, Benzerdjeb H, Wang D, et al. Long-term follow-up of a phase 2 study of oral teriflunomide in relapsing multiple sclerosis: safety and efficacy results up to 8.5 years. *Mult Scler.*(2012) 18:1278–89. doi: 10.1177/1352458512436594
146. Lorefice L, Fenu G, Gerevini S, Frau J, Coghe G, Barracciu MA, et al. PML in a person with multiple sclerosis: is teriflunomide the felon? *Neurology.* (2018) 90:83–5. doi: 10.1212/WNL.0000000000004804
147. Kieseier BC, Benamor M. Pregnancy outcomes following maternal and paternal exposure to teriflunomide during treatment for relapsing-remitting multiple sclerosis. *Neurol Ther.* (2014) 3:133–8. doi: 10.1007/s40120-014-0020-y
148. Schweckendiek W. [Treatment of psoriasis vulgaris]. *Med Monatsschr.* (1959) 13:103–4.

149. Dubey D, Kieseier BC, Hartung HP, Hemmer B, Warnke C, Menge T, et al. Dimethyl fumarate in relapsing-remitting multiple sclerosis: rationale, mechanisms of action, pharmacokinetics, efficacy and safety. *Expert Rev Neurother.* (2015) 15:339–46. doi: 10.1586/14737175.2015.1025755
150. Clausen BH, Lundberg L, Yli-Karjanmaa M, Martin NA, Svensson M, Alfsen MZ, et al. Fumarate decreases edema volume and improves functional outcome after experimental stroke. *Exp Neurol.* (2017) 295:144–54. doi: 10.1016/j.expneurol.2017.06.011
151. Hammer A, Waschbisch A, Kuhbandner K, Bayas A, Lee D-H, Duscha A, et al. The NRF2 pathway as potential biomarker for dimethyl fumarate treatment in multiple sclerosis. *Ann Clin Transl Neurol.* (2018) 5:668–76. doi: 10.1002/acn3.553
152. Mills EA, Ogrodnik MA, Plave A, Mao-Draayer Y. Emerging understanding of the mechanism of action for dimethyl fumarate in the treatment of multiple sclerosis. Front Neurol. (2018) 9:5. doi: 10.3389/fneur.2018.00005
153. Holm Hansen R, Højsgaard Chow H, Sellebjerg F, Rode von Essen M. Dimethyl fumarate therapy suppresses B cell responses and follicular helper T cells in relapsing-remitting multiple sclerosis. *Mult Scler.* (2018). doi: 10.1177/1352458518790417. [Epub ahead of print].
154. Smith MD, Martin KA, Calabresi PA, Bhargava P. Dimethyl fumarate alters B-cell memory and cytokine production in MS patients. *Ann Clin Transl Neurol.* (2017) 4:351–5. doi: 10.1002/acn3.411
155. Li R, Rezk A, Ghadiri M, Luessi F, Zipp F, Li H, et al. Dimethyl fumarate treatment mediates an anti-inflammatory shift in B cell subsets of patients with multiple sclerosis. *J Immunol Baltim.* (2017) 198:691–8. doi: 10.4049/jimmunol.1601649
156. Ghadiri M, Rezk A, Li R, Evans A, Luessi F, Zipp F, et al. Dimethyl fumarate-induced lymphopenia in MS due to differential T-cell subset apoptosis. *Neurol Neuroimmunol Neuroinflamm.* (2017) 4:e340. doi: 10.1212/NXI.0000000000000340
157. Wu Q, Wang Q, Mao G, Dowling CA, Lundy SK, Mao-Draayer Y. Dimethyl fumarate selectively reduces memory T cells and shifts the balance between Th1/Th17 and Th2 in multiple sclerosis patients. *J Immunol Baltim.* (2017) 198:3069–80. doi: 10.4049/jimmunol.1601532
158. Medina S, Villarrubia N, Sainz de la Maza S, Lifante J, Costa-Frossard L, Roldán E, et al. Optimal response to dimethyl fumarate associates in MS with a shift from an inflammatory to a tolerogenic blood cell profile. *Mult Scler.* (2018) 24:1317–27. doi: 10.1177/1352458517717088
159. Diebold M, Sievers C, Bantug G, Sanderson N, Kappos L, Kuhle J, et al. Dimethyl fumarate influences innate and adaptive immunity in multiple sclerosis. *J Autoimmun.* (2018) 86:39–50. doi: 10.1016/j.jaut.2017.09.009
160. Smith MD, Calabresi PA, Bhargava P. Dimethyl fumarate treatment alters NK cell function in multiple sclerosis. *Eur J Immunol.* (2018) 48:380–3. doi: 10.1002/eji.201747277
161. Longbrake EE, Cantoni C, Chahin S, Cignarella F, Cross AH, Piccio L. Dimethyl fumarate induces changes in B- and T-lymphocyte function independent of the effects on absolute lymphocyte count. *Mult Scler.* (2018) 24:728–38. doi: 10.1177/1352458517707069
162. Cunill V, Massot M, Clemente A, Calles C, Andreu V, Núñez V, et al. Relapsing-remitting multiple sclerosis is characterized by a T follicular cell pro-inflammatory shift, reverted by dimethyl fumarate treatment. *Front Immunol.* (2018) 9:1097. doi: 10.3389/fimmu.2018.01097
163. Galloway DA, Williams JB, Moore CS. Effects of fumarates on inflammatory human astrocyte responses and oligodendrocyte differentiation. *Ann Clin Transl Neurol.* (2017) 4:381–91. doi: 10.1002/acn3.414
164. Brennan MS, Matos MF, Richter KE, Li B, Scannevin RH. The NRF2 transcriptional target, OSGIN1, contributes to monomethyl fumarate-mediated cytoprotection in human astrocytes. *Sci Rep.* (2017) 7:42054. doi: 10.1038/srep42054
165. Paraiso HC, Kuo P-C, Curfman ET, Moon HJ, Sweazey RD, Yen J-H, et al. Dimethyl fumarate attenuates reactive microglia and long-term memory deficits following systemic immune challenge. *J Neuroinflamm.* (2018) 15:100. doi: 10.1186/s12974-018-1125-5
166. Gold R, Kappos L, Arnold DL, Bar-Or A, Giovannoni G, Selmaj K, et al. Placebo-controlled phase 3 study of oral BG-12 for relapsing multiple sclerosis. *N Engl J Med.* (2012) 367:1098–107. doi: 10.1056/NEJMoa1114287
167. Fox RJ, Miller DH, Phillips JT, Hutchinson M, Havrdova E, Kita M, et al. Placebo-controlled phase 3 study of oral BG-12 or glatiramer in multiple sclerosis. *N Engl J Med.* (2012) 367:1087–97. doi: 10.1056/NEJMoa1206328
168. Viglietta V, Miller D, Bar-Or A, Phillips JT, Arnold DL, Selmaj K, et al. Efficacy of delayed-release dimethyl fumarate in relapsing-remitting multiple sclerosis: integrated analysis of the phase 3 trials. *Ann Clin Transl Neurol.* (2015) 2:103–18. doi: 10.1002/acn3.148
169. Havrdova E, Giovannoni G, Gold R, Fox RJ, Kappos L, Phillips JT, et al. Effect of delayed-release dimethyl fumarate on no evidence of disease activity in relapsing-remitting multiple sclerosis: integrated analysis of the phase III DEFINE and CONFIRM studies. *Eur J Neurol.* (2017) 24:726–33. doi: 10.1111/ene.13272
170. Fernández Ó, Giovannoni G, Fox RJ, Gold R, Phillips JT, Potts J, et al. Efficacy and safety of delayed-release dimethyl fumarate for relapsing-remitting multiple sclerosis in prior interferon users: an integrated analysis of DEFINE and CONFIRM. *Clin Ther.* (2017) 39:1671–9. doi: 10.1016/j.clinthera.2017.06.012
171. Guarnera C, Bramanti P, Mazzon E. Comparison of efficacy and safety of oral agents for the treatment of relapsing-remitting multiple sclerosis. *Drug Des Dev Ther.* (2017) 11:2193–207. doi: 10.2147/DDDT.S137572
172. Mills EA, Mao-Draayer Y. Understanding progressive multifocal leukoencephalopathy risk in multiple sclerosis patients treated with immunomodulatory therapies: a bird's eye view. *Front Immunol.* (2018) 9:138. doi: 10.3389/fimmu.2018.00138
173. Gieselbach R-J, Muller-Hansma AH, Wijburg MT, de Bruin-Weller MS, van Oosten BW, Nieuwkamp DJ, et al. Progressive multifocal leukoencephalopathy in patients treated with fumaric acid esters: a review of 19 cases. *J Neurol.* (2017) 264:1155–64. doi: 10.1007/s00415-017-8509-9
174. Khatri BO, Tarima SS, Essig B, Sesing J, Olapo T. Delayed lymphocyte re-population following discontinuation of dimethyl fumarate and after switching to other disease modifying drug therapies. *Mult Scler Relat Disord.* (2017) 18:60–4. doi: 10.1016/j.msard.2017.09.014
175. Mirabella M, Prosperini L, Lucchini M, Boffa L, Borriello G, Buscarinu MC, et al. Safety and efficacy of dimethyl fumarate in multiple sclerosis: an Italian, multicenter, real-world study. *CNS Drugs.* (2018) 32:963–70. doi: 10.1007/s40263-018-0543-3
176. Mallucci G, Annovazzi P, Miante S, Torri-Clerici V, Matta M, La Gioia S, et al. Two-year real-life efficacy, tolerability and safety of dimethyl fumarate in an Italian multicentre study. *J Neurol.* (2018) 265:1850–9. doi: 10.1007/s00415-018-8916-6
177. Miclea A, Leussink VI, Hartung HP, Gold R, Hoepner R. Safety and efficacy of dimethyl fumarate in multiple sclerosis: a multi-center observational study. *J Neurol.* (2016) 263:1626–32. doi: 10.1007/s00415-016-8175-3
178. Baharnoori M, Gonzalez CT, Chua A, Diaz-Cruz C, Healy BC, Stankiewicz J, et al. Predictors of hematological abnormalities in multiple sclerosis patients treated with fingolimod and dimethyl fumarate and impact of treatment switch on lymphocyte and leukocyte count. *Mult Scler Relat Disord.* (2018) 20:51–7. doi: 10.1016/j.msard.2017.12.003
179. Eriksson I, Cars T, Piehl F, Malmström RE, Wettermark B, von Euler M. Persistence with dimethyl fumarate in relapsing-remitting multiple sclerosis: a population-based cohort study. *Eur J Clin Pharmacol.* (2018) 74:219–26. doi: 10.1007/s00228-017-2366-4
180. Fox RJ, Chan A, Zhang A, Xiao J, Levison D, Lewin JB, et al. Comparative effectiveness using a matching-adjusted indirect comparison between delayed-release dimethyl fumarate and fingolimod for the treatment of multiple sclerosis. *Curr Med Res Opin.* (2017) 33:175–83. doi: 10.1080/03007995.2016.1248380
181. Prosperini L, Lucchini M, Haggiag S, Bellantonio P, Bianco A, Buscarinu MC, et al. Fingolimod vs dimethyl fumarate in multiple sclerosis: a real-world propensity score-matched study. *Neurology.* (2018) 91:e153–61. doi: 10.1212/WNL.0000000000005772
182. Nixon R, Bergvall N, Tomic D, Sfikas N, Cutter G, Giovannoni G. No evidence of disease activity: indirect comparisons of oral therapies for the treatment of relapsing-remitting multiple sclerosis. *Adv Ther.* (2014) 31:1134–54. doi: 10.1007/s12325-014-0167-z
183. Cohan SL, Moses H, Calkwood J, Tornatore C, LaGanke C, Smoot KE, et al. Clinical outcomes in patients with relapsing-remitting multiple sclerosis who switch from natalizumab to delayed-release dimethyl fumarate: a multicenter

retrospective observational study (STRATEGY). *Mult Scler Relat Disord.* (2018) 22:27–34. doi: 10.1016/j.msard.2018.02.028

184. Calabrese M, Pitteri M, Farina G, Bajrami A, Castellaro M, Magliozzi R, et al. Dimethyl fumarate: a possible exit strategy from natalizumab treatment in patients with multiple sclerosis at risk for severe adverse events. *J Neurol Neurosurg Psychiatry.* (2017) 88:1073–8. doi: 10.1136/jnnp-2017-316236
185. O'Gorman J, Russell HK, Li J, Phillips G, Kurukulasuriya NC, Viglietta V. Effect of aspirin pretreatment or slow dose titration on flushing and gastrointestinal events in healthy volunteers receiving delayed-release dimethyl fumarate. *Clin Ther.* (2015) 37:1402–1419.e5. doi: 10.1016/j.clinthera.2015.03.028
186. Sejbaek T, Nybo M, Petersen T, Illes Z. Real-life persistence and tolerability with dimethyl fumarate. *Mult Scler Relat Disord.* (2018) 24:42–6. doi: 10.1016/j.msard.2018.05.007
187. Ceronie B, Jacobs BM, Baker D, Dubuisson N, Mao Z, Ammoscato F, et al. Cladribine treatment of multiple sclerosis is associated with depletion of memory B cells. *J Neurol.* (2018) 265:1199–209. doi: 10.1007/s00415-018-8830-y
188. Warnke C, Leussink VI, Goebels N, Aktas O, Boyko A, Kieseier BC, et al. Cladribine as a therapeutic option in multiple sclerosis. *Clin Immunol.* (2012) 142:68–75. doi: 10.1016/j.clim.2011.05.009
189. Warnke C, Wiendl H, Hartung H-P, Stüve O, Kieseier BC. Identification of targets and new developments in the treatment of multiple sclerosis–focus on cladribine. *Drug Des Devel Ther.* (2010) 4:117–26. doi: 10.2147/DDDT.S6627
190. Giovannoni G, Comi G, Cook S, Rammohan K, Rieckmann P, Soelberg Sørensen P, et al. A placebo-controlled trial of oral cladribine for relapsing multiple sclerosis. *N Engl J Med.* (2010) 362:416–26. doi: 10.1056/NEJMoa0902533
191. Leist TP, Comi G, Cree BAC, Coyle PK, Freedman MS, Hartung H-P, et al. Effect of oral cladribine on time to conversion to clinically definite multiple sclerosis in patients with a first demyelinating event (ORACLE MS): a phase 3 randomised trial. *Lancet Neurol.* (2014) 13:257–67. doi: 10.1016/S1474-4422(14)70005-5
192. Freedman MS, Leist TP, Comi G, Cree BA, Coyle PK, Hartung H-P, et al. The efficacy of cladribine tablets in CIS patients retrospectively assigned the diagnosis of MS using modern criteria: results from the ORACLE-MS study. *Mult Scler J.* (2017) 3:2055217317732802. doi: 10.1177/2055217317732802
193. Comi G, Cook S, Rammohan K, Soelberg Sorensen P, Vermersch P, Adeniji AK, et al. Long-term effects of cladribine tablets on MRI activity outcomes in patients with relapsing-remitting multiple sclerosis: the CLARITY Extension study. *Ther Adv Neurol Disord.* (2018) 11:175628561775(3365). doi: 10.1177/1756285617753365
194. Giovannoni G, Soelberg Sorensen P, Cook S, Rammohan K, Rieckmann P, Comi G, et al. Safety and efficacy of cladribine tablets in patients with relapsing-remitting multiple sclerosis: results from the randomized extension trial of the CLARITY study. *Mult Scler.* (2017) 24:1594–604. doi: 10.1177/1352458517727603
195. Baker D, Herrod SS, Alvarez-Gonzalez C, Zalewski L, Albor C, Schmierer K. Both cladribine and alemtuzumab may effect MS via B-cell depletion. *Neurol Neuroimmunol Neuroinflamm.* (2017) 4:e360. doi: 10.1212/NXI.0000000000000360
196. Ruck T, Bittner S, Wiendl H, Meuth SG. Alemtuzumab in multiple sclerosis: mechanism of action and beyond. *Int J Mol Sci.* (2015) 16:16414–39. doi: 10.3390/ijms160716414
197. Hale G. The CD52 antigen and development of the CAMPATH antibodies. *Cytotherapy.* (2001) 3:137–43. doi: 10.1080/146532401753174098
198. Ginaldi L, De Martinis M, Matutes E, Farahat N, Morilla R, Dyer MJ, et al. Levels of expression of CD52 in normal and leukemic B and T cells: correlation with *in vivo* therapeutic responses to Campath-1H. *Leuk Res.* (1998) 22:185–91. doi: 10.1016/S0145-2126(97)00158-6
199. Rao SP, Sancho J, Campos-Rivera J, Boutin PM, Severy PB, Weeden T, et al. Human peripheral blood mononuclear cells exhibit heterogeneous CD52 expression levels and show differential sensitivity to alemtuzumab mediated cytolysis. *PLoS ONE.* (2012) 7:e39416. doi: 10.1371/journal.pone.0039416
200. Coles AJ, Cox A, Le Page E, Jones J, Trip SA, Deans J, et al. The window of therapeutic opportunity in multiple sclerosis: evidence from monoclonal antibody therapy. *J Neurol.* (2006) 253:98–108. doi: 10.1007/s00415-005-0934-5
201. Thompson SAJ, Jones JL, Cox AL, Compston DAS, Coles AJ. B-cell reconstitution and BAFF after alemtuzumab (Campath-1H) treatment of multiple sclerosis. *J Clin Immunol.* (2010) 30:99–105. doi: 10.1007/s10875-009-9327-3
202. Baker D, Herrod SS, Alvarez-Gonzalez C, Giovannoni G, Schmierer K. Interpreting lymphocyte reconstitution data from the pivotal phase 3 trials of alemtuzumab. *JAMA Neurol.* (2017) 74:961–9. doi: 10.1001/jamaneurol.2017.0676
203. Gross CC, Ahmetspahic D, Ruck T, Schulte-Mecklenbeck A, Schwarte K, Jörgens S, et al. Alemtuzumab treatment alters circulating innate immune cells in multiple sclerosis. *Neurol Neuroimmunol Neuroinflamm.* (2016) 3:e289. doi: 10.1212/NXI.0000000000000289
204. Gross CC, Schulte-Mecklenbeck A, Wiendl H, Marcenaro E, Kerlero de Rosbo N, Uccelli A, et al. Regulatory functions of natural killer cells in multiple sclerosis. *Front Immunol.* (2016) 7:606. doi: 10.3389/fimmu.2016.00606
205. CAMMS223 Trial Investigators, Coles AJ, Compston DAS, Selmaj KW, Lake SL, Moran S, et al. Alemtuzumab vs. interferon beta-1a in early multiple sclerosis. *N Engl J Med.* (2008) 359:1786–801. doi: 10.1056/NEJMoa0802670
206. Cohen JA, Coles AJ, Arnold DL, Confavreux C, Fox EJ, Hartung H-P, et al. Alemtuzumab versus interferon beta 1a as first-line treatment for patients with relapsing-remitting multiple sclerosis: a randomised controlled phase 3 trial. *Lancet.* (2012) 380:1819–28. doi: 10.1016/S0140-6736(12)61769-3
207. Coles AJ, Twyman CL, Arnold DL, Cohen JA, Confavreux C, Fox EJ, et al. Alemtuzumab for patients with relapsing multiple sclerosis after disease-modifying therapy: a randomised controlled phase 3 trial. *Lancet.* (2012) 380:1829–39. doi: 10.1016/S0140-6736(12)61768-1
208. FDA Drug Safety Communication. *FDA Warns About Rare But Serious Risks of Stroke and Blood Vessel Wall Tears With Multiple Sclerosis Drug Lemtrada (alemtuzumab)*. FDA [Internet]. (2019). Available online at: http://www.fda.gov/drugs/drug-safety-and-availability/fda-warns-about-rare-serious-risks-stroke-and-blood-vessel-wall-tears-multiple-sclerosis-drug (accessed June 2, 2019).
209. Azevedo CJ, Kutz C, Dix A, Boster A, Sanossian N, Kaplan J. Intracerebral haemorrhage during alemtuzumab administration. *Lancet Neurol.* (2019) 18:329–31. doi: 10.1016/S1474-4422(19)30076-6
210. Doessegger L, Banholzer ML. Clinical development methodology for infusion-related reactions with monoclonal antibodies. *Clin Transl Immunol.* (2015) 4:e39. doi: 10.1038/cti.2015.14
211. Jones JL, Thompson SAJ, Loh P, Davies JL, Tuohy OC, Curry AJ, et al. Human autoimmunity after lymphocyte depletion is caused by homeostatic T-cell proliferation. *Proc Natl Acad Sci USA.* (2013) 110:20200–5. doi: 10.1073/pnas.1313654110
212. Jones JL, Phuah C-L, Cox AL, Thompson SA, Ban M, Shawcross J, et al. IL-21 drives secondary autoimmunity in patients with multiple sclerosis, following therapeutic lymphocyte depletion with alemtuzumab (Campath-1H). *J Clin Invest.* (2009) 119:2052–61. doi: 10.1172/JCI37878
213. Daniels GH, Vladic A, Brinar V, Zavalishin I, Valente W, Oyuela P, et al. Alemtuzumab-related thyroid dysfunction in a phase 2 trial of patients with relapsing-remitting multiple sclerosis. *J Clin Endocrinol Metab.* (2014) 99:80–9. doi: 10.1210/jc.2013-2201
214. Meyer D, Coles A, Oyuela P, Purvis A, Margolin DH. Case report of anti-glomerular basement membrane disease following alemtuzumab treatment of relapsing-remitting multiple sclerosis. *Mult Scler Relat Disord.* (2013) 2:60–3. doi: 10.1016/j.msard.2012.07.002
215. Cuker A, Coles AJ, Sullivan H, Fox E, Goldberg M, Oyuela P, et al. A distinctive form of immune thrombocytopenia in a phase 2 study of alemtuzumab for the treatment of relapsing-remitting multiple sclerosis. *Blood.* (2011) 118:6299–305. doi: 10.1182/blood-2011-08-371138
216. Clatworthy MR, Wallin EF, Jayne DR. Anti-glomerular basement membrane disease after alemtuzumab. *N Engl J Med.* (2008) 359:768–9. doi: 10.1056/NEJMc0800484
217. Tuohy O, Costelloe L, Hill-Cawthorne G, Bjornson I, Harding K, Robertson N, et al. Alemtuzumab treatment of multiple sclerosis: long-term safety and efficacy. *J Neurol Neurosurg Psychiatry.* (2015) 86:208–15. doi: 10.1136/jnnp-2014-307721

218. Devonshire V, Phillips R, Wass H, Da Roza G, Senior P. Monitoring and management of autoimmunity in multiple sclerosis patients treated with alemtuzumab: practical recommendations. *J Neurol.* (2018) 265:2494-2505. doi: 10.1007/s00415-018-8822-y
219. Decallonne B, Bartholomé E, Delvaux V, D'haeseleer M, El Sankari S, Seeldrayers P, et al. Thyroid disorders in alemtuzumab-treated multiple sclerosis patients: a Belgian consensus on diagnosis and management. *Acta Neurol Belg.* (2018) 118:153–9. doi: 10.1007/s13760-018-0883-2
220. Lambert C, Dubois B, Dive D, Lysandropoulos A, Selleslag D, Vanopdenbosch L, et al. Management of immune thrombocytopenia in multiple sclerosis patients treated with alemtuzumab: a Belgian consensus. *Acta Neurol Belg.* (2018) 118:7–11. doi: 10.1007/s13760-018-0882-3
221. Sprangers B, Decoo D, Dive D, Lysandropoulos A, Vanopdenbosch L, Bovy C. Management of adverse renal events related to alemtuzumab treatment in multiple sclerosis: a Belgian consensus. *Acta Neurol Belg.* (2018) 118:143–51. doi: 10.1007/s13760-017-0864-x
222. FRANCISCO EM. *Lemtrada [Internet].* European Medicines Agency. (2019). Available online at: https://www.ema.europa.eu/en/medicines/human/referrals/lemtrada (cited June 2, 2019).
223. Duddy M, Niino M, Adatia F, Hebert S, Freedman M, Atkins H, et al. Distinct effector cytokine profiles of memory and naive human B cell subsets and implication in multiple sclerosis. *J Immunol.* (2007) 178:6092–9. doi: 10.4049/jimmunol.178.10.6092
224. Mathias A, Perriard G, Canales M, Soneson C, Delorenzi M, Schluep M, et al. Increased *ex vivo* antigen presentation profile of B cells in multiple sclerosis. *Mult Scler.* (2017) 23:802–9. doi: 10.1177/1352458516664210
225. Aung LL, Balashov KE. Decreased Dicer expression is linked to increased expression of co-stimulatory molecule CD80 on B cells in multiple sclerosis. *Mult Scler.* (2015) 21:1131–8. doi: 10.1177/1352458514560923
226. Genç K, Dona DL, Reder AT. Increased CD80(+) B cells in active multiple sclerosis and reversal by interferon beta-1b therapy. *J Clin Invest.* (1997) 99:2664–71. doi: 10.1172/JCI119455
227. Harp CT, Ireland S, Davis LS, Remington G, Cassidy B, Cravens PD, et al. Memory B cells from a subset of treatment-naïve relapsing-remitting multiple sclerosis patients elicit CD4(+) T-cell proliferation and IFN-γ production in response to myelin basic protein and myelin oligodendrocyte glycoprotein. *Eur J Immunol.* (2010) 40:2942–56. doi: 10.1002/eji.201040516
228. Wekerle H. B cells in multiple sclerosis. *Autoimmunity.* (2017) 50:57–60. doi: 10.1080/08916934.2017.1281914
229. Häusser-Kinzel S, Weber MS. The role of B cells and antibodies in multiple sclerosis, neuromyelitis optica, and related disorders. *Front Immunol.* (2019) 10:201. doi: 10.3389/fimmu.2019.00201
230. Hauser SL, Waubant E, Arnold DL, Vollmer T, Antel J, Fox RJ, et al. B-cell depletion with rituximab in relapsing-remitting multiple sclerosis. *N Engl J Med.* (2008) 358:676–88. doi: 10.1056/NEJMoa0706383
231. Bar-Or A, Calabresi PAJ, Arnold D, Arnlod D, Markowitz C, Shafer S, et al. Rituximab in relapsing-remitting multiple sclerosis: a 72-week, open-label, phase I trial. *Ann Neurol.* (2008) 63:395–400. doi: 10.1002/ana.21363
232. Hawker K, O'Connor P, Freedman MS, Calabresi PA, Antel J, Simon J, et al. Rituximab in patients with primary progressive multiple sclerosis: results of a randomized double-blind placebo-controlled multicenter trial. *Ann Neurol.* (2009) 66:460–71. doi: 10.1002/ana.21867
233. Kappos L, Li D, Calabresi PA, O'Connor P, Bar-Or A, Barkhof F, et al. Ocrelizumab in relapsing-remitting multiple sclerosis: a phase 2, randomised, placebo-controlled, multicentre trial. *Lancet.* (2011) 378:1779–87. doi: 10.1016/S0140-6736(11)61649-8
234. Sorensen PS, Lisby S, Grove R, Derosier F, Shackelford S, Havrdova E, et al. Safety and efficacy of ofatumumab in relapsing-remitting multiple sclerosis: a phase 2 study. *Neurology.* (2014) 82:573–81. doi: 10.1212/WNL.0000000000000125
235. Häusler D, Häusser-Kinzel S, Feldmann L, Torke S, Lepennetier G, Bernard CCA, et al. Functional characterization of reappearing B cells after anti-CD20 treatment of CNS autoimmune disease. *Proc Natl Acad Sci USA.* (2018) 115:9773–8. doi: 10.1073/pnas.1810470115
236. Greenberg BM, Graves D, Remington G, Hardeman P, Mann M, Karandikar N, et al. Rituximab dosing and monitoring strategies in neuromyelitis optica patients: creating strategies for therapeutic success. *Mult Scler.* (2012) 18:1022–6. doi: 10.1177/1352458511432896
237. Genovese MC, Kaine JL, Lowenstein MB, Del Giudice J, Baldassare A, Schechtman J, et al. Ocrelizumab, a humanized anti-CD20 monoclonal antibody, in the treatment of patients with rheumatoid arthritis: a phase I/II randomized, blinded, placebo-controlled, dose-ranging study. *Arthritis Rheum.* (2008) 58:2652–61. doi: 10.1002/art.23732
238. Bar-Or A, Grove RA, Austin DJ, Tolson JM, VanMeter SA, Lewis EW, et al. Subcutaneous ofatumumab in patients with relapsing-remitting multiple sclerosis: the MIRROR study. *Neurology.* (2018) 90:e1805–14. doi: 10.1212/WNL.0000000000005516
239. Juanatey A, Blanco-Garcia L, Tellez N. Ocrelizumab: its efficacy and safety in multiple sclerosis. *Rev Neurol.* (2018) 66:423–33. doi: 10.33588/rn.6612.2018132
240. Reich DS, Lucchinetti CF, Calabresi PA. Multiple sclerosis. *N Engl J Med.* (2018) 378:169–80. doi: 10.1056/NEJMra1401483
241. Luster AD, Alon R, von Andrian UH. Immune cell migration in inflammation: present and future therapeutic targets. *Nat Immunol.* (2005) 6:1182–90. doi: 10.1038/ni1275
242. Stüve O, Bennett JL. Pharmacological properties, toxicology and scientific rationale for the use of natalizumab (Tysabri) in inflammatory diseases. *CNS Drug Rev.* (2007) 13:79–95. doi: 10.1111/j.1527-3458.2007.00003.x
243. Sheremata WA, Minagar A, Alexander JS, Vollmer T. The role of alpha-4 integrin in the aetiology of multiple sclerosis: current knowledge and therapeutic implications. *CNS Drugs.* (2005) 19:909–22. doi: 10.2165/00023210-200519110-00002
244. Ali R, Nicholas RSJ, Muraro PA. Drugs in development for relapsing multiple sclerosis. *Drugs.* (2013) 73:625–50. doi: 10.1007/s40265-013-0030-6
245. Yednock TA, Cannon C, Fritz LC, Sanchez-Madrid F, Steinman L, Karin N. Prevention of experimental autoimmune encephalomyelitis by antibodies against alpha 4 beta 1 integrin. *Nature.* (1992) 356:63–6. doi: 10.1038/356063a0
246. Stüve O, Marra CM, Jerome KR, Cook L, Cravens PD, Cepok S, et al. Immune surveillance in multiple sclerosis patients treated with natalizumab. *Ann Neurol.* (2006) 59:743–7. doi: 10.1002/ana.20858
247. Stüve O, Marra CM, Bar-Or A, Niino M, Cravens PD, Cepok S, et al. Altered CD4+/CD8+ T-cell ratios in cerebrospinal fluid of natalizumab-treated patients with multiple sclerosis. *Arch Neurol.* (2006) 63:1383–7. doi: 10.1001/archneur.63.10.1383
248. Stüve O, Cravens PD, Frohman EM, Phillips JT, Remington GM, von Geldern G, et al. Immunologic, clinical, and radiologic status 14 months after cessation of natalizumab therapy. *Neurology.* (2009) 72:396–401. doi: 10.1212/01.wnl.0000327341.89587.76
249. Polman CH, O'Connor PW, Havrdova E, Hutchinson M, Kappos L, Miller DH, et al. A randomized, placebo-controlled trial of natalizumab for relapsing multiple sclerosis. *N Engl J Med.* (2006) 354:899–910. doi: 10.1056/NEJMoa044397
250. Rudick RA, Stuart WH, Calabresi PA, Confavreux C, Galetta SL, Radue E-W, et al. Natalizumab plus interferon beta-1a for relapsing multiple sclerosis. *N Engl J Med.* (2006) 354:911–23. doi: 10.1056/NEJMoa044396
251. Kapoor R, Ho P-R, Campbell N, Chang I, Deykin A, Forrestal F, et al. Effect of natalizumab on disease progression in secondary progressive multiple sclerosis (ASCEND): a phase 3, randomised, double-blind, placebo-controlled trial with an open-label extension. *Lancet Neurol.* (2018) 17:405–15. doi: 10.1016/S1474-4422(18)30069-3
252. Frisch T, Elkjaer ML, Reynolds R, Michel TM, Kacprowski T, Burton M, et al. MS Atlas – A molecular map of brain lesion stages in progressive multiple sclerosis. *bioRxiv [Preprint].* (2019). doi: 10.1101/584920
253. Lassmann H. Pathogenic mechanisms associated with different clinical courses of multiple sclerosis. *Front Immunol.* (2018) 9:3116. doi: 10.3389/fimmu.2018.03116
254. Clerico M, Artusi CA, Di Liberto A, Rolla S, Bardina V, Barbero P, et al. Long-term safety evaluation of natalizumab for the treatment of multiple sclerosis. *Expert Opin Drug Saf.* (2017) 16:963–72. doi: 10.1080/14740338.2017.1346082
255. Berger JR, Khalili K. The pathogenesis of progressive multifocal leukoencephalopathy. *Discov Med.* (2011) 12:495–503.
256. Major EO, Yousry TA, Clifford DB. Pathogenesis of progressive multifocal leukoencephalopathy and risks associated with treatments for multiple

sclerosis: a decade of lessons learned. *Lancet Neurol.* (2018) 17:467–80. doi: 10.1016/S1474-4422(18)30040-1

257. Wenning W, Haghikia A, Laubenberger J, Clifford DB, Behrens PF, Chan A, et al. Treatment of progressive multifocal leukoencephalopathy associated with natalizumab. *N Engl J Med.* (2009) 361:1075–80. doi: 10.1056/NEJMoa0810257
258. Tan IL, McArthur JC, Clifford DB, Major EO, Nath A. Immune reconstitution inflammatory syndrome in natalizumab-associated PML. *Neurology.* (2011) 77:1061–7. doi: 10.1212/WNL.0b013e31822e55e7
259. Bloomgren G, Richman S, Hotermans C, Subramanyam M, Goelz S, Natarajan A, et al. Risk of natalizumab-associated progressive multifocal leukoencephalopathy. *N Engl J Med.* (2012) 366:1870–80. doi: 10.1056/NEJMoa1107829
260. Gorelik L, Lerner M, Bixler S, Crossman M, Schlain B, Simon K, et al. Anti-JC virus antibodies: implications for PML risk stratification. *Ann Neurol.* (2010) 68:295–303. doi: 10.1002/ana.22128
261. Berger JR, Fox RJ. Reassessing the risk of natalizumab-associated PML. *J Neurovirol.* (2016) 22:533–5. doi: 10.1007/s13365-016-0427-6
262. Schwab N, Schneider-Hohendorf T, Pignolet B, Breuer J, Gross CC, Göbel K, et al. Therapy with natalizumab is associated with high JCV seroconversion and rising JCV index values. *Neurol Neuroimmunol Neuroinflamm.* (2016) 3:e195. doi: 10.1212/NXI.0000000000000195
263. Lindå H, von Heijne A, Major EO, Ryschkewitsch C, Berg J, Olsson T, et al. Progressive multifocal leukoencephalopathy after natalizumab monotherapy. *N Engl J Med.* (2009) 361:1081–7. doi: 10.1056/NEJMoa0810316
264. McGuigan C, Craner M, Guadagno J, Kapoor R, Mazibrada G, Molyneux P, et al. Stratification and monitoring of natalizumab-associated progressive multifocal leukoencephalopathy risk: recommendations from an expert group. *J Neurol Neurosurg Psychiatry.* (2016) 87:117–25. doi: 10.1136/jnnp 2015 311100
265. Calabresi PA, Giovannoni G, Confavreux C, Galetta SL, Havrdova E, Hutchinson M, et al. The incidence and significance of anti-natalizumab antibodies: results from AFFIRM and SENTINEL. *Neurology.* (2007) 69:1391–403. doi: 10.1212/01.wnl.0000277457.17420.b5
266. Fox EJ, Vartanian TK, Zamvil SS. The immunogenicity of disease-modifying therapies for multiple sclerosis: clinical implications for neurologists. *Neurologist.* (2007) 13:355–62. doi: 10.1097/NRL.0b013e318148c08e
267. Khatri BO, Man S, Giovannoni G, Koo AP, Lee J-C, Tucky B, et al. Effect of plasma exchange in accelerating natalizumab clearance and restoring leukocyte function. *Neurology.* (2009) 72:402–9. doi: 10.1212/01.wnl.0000341766.59028.9d
268. Rasenack M, Derfuss T. Disease activity return after natalizumab cessation in multiple sclerosis. *Expert Rev Neurother.* (2016) 16:587–94. doi: 10.1586/14737175.2016.1168295
269. Havla J, Gerdes LA, Meinl I, Krumbholz M, Faber H, Weber F, et al. De-escalation from natalizumab in multiple sclerosis: recurrence of disease activity despite switching to glatiramer acetate. *J Neurol.* (2011) 258:1665–9. doi: 10.1007/s00415-011-5996-y
270. Clerico M, Schiavetti I, De Mercanti SF, Piazza F, Gned D, Brescia Morra V, et al. Treatment of relapsing-remitting multiple sclerosis after 24 doses of natalizumab: evidence from an Italian spontaneous, prospective, and observational study (the TY-STOP Study). *JAMA Neurol.* (2014) 71:954–60. doi: 10.1001/jamaneurol.2014.1200
271. Jokubaitis VG, Li V, Kalincik T, Izquierdo G, Hodgkinson S, Alroughani R, et al. Fingolimod after natalizumab and the risk of short-term relapse. *Neurology.* (2014) 82:1204–11. doi: 10.1212/WNL.0000000000000283
272. Rinaldi F, Seppi D, Calabrese M, Perini P, Gallo P. Switching therapy from natalizumab to fingolimod in relapsing-remitting multiple sclerosis: clinical and magnetic resonance imaging findings. *Mult Scler.* (2012) 18:1640–3. doi: 10.1177/1352458512464282
273. Prosperini L, Annovazzi P, Capobianco M, Capra R, Buttari F, Gasperini C, et al. Natalizumab discontinuation in patients with multiple sclerosis: profiling risk and benefits at therapeutic crossroads. *Mult Scler.* (2015) 21:1713–22. doi: 10.1177/1352458515570768
274. Sangalli F, Moiola L, Ferrè L, Radaelli M, Barcella V, Rodegher M, et al. Long-term management of natalizumab discontinuation in a large monocentric cohort of multiple sclerosis patients. *Mult Scler Relat Disord.* (2014) 3:520–6. doi: 10.1016/j.msard.2014.04.003
275. Capobianco M, di Sapio A, Malentacchi M, Malucchi S, Matta M, Sperli F, et al. No impact of current therapeutic strategies on disease reactivation after natalizumab discontinuation: a comparative analysis of different approaches during the first year of natalizumab discontinuation. *Eur J Neurol.* (2015) 22:585–7. doi: 10.1111/ene.12487
276. Kappos L, Radue E-W, Comi G, Montalban X, Butzkueven H, Wiendl H, et al. Switching from natalizumab to fingolimod: a randomized, placebo-controlled study in RRMS. *Neurology.* (2015) 85:29–39. doi: 10.1212/WNL.0000000000001706
277. Cohen M, Maillart E, Tourbah A, De Sèze J, Vukusic S, Brassat D, et al. Switching from natalizumab to fingolimod in multiple sclerosis: a French prospective study. *JAMA Neurol.* (2014) 71:436–41. doi: 10.1001/jamaneurol.2013.6240
278. Weinstock-Guttman B, Hagemeier J, Kavak KS, Saini V, Patrick K, Ramasamy DP, et al. Randomised natalizumab discontinuation study: taper protocol may prevent disease reactivation. *J Neurol Neurosurg Psychiatry.* (2016) 87:937–43. doi: 10.1136/jnnp-2015-312221
279. Li R, Patterson KR, Bar-Or A. Reassessing B cell contributions in multiple sclerosis. *Nat Immunol.* (2018) 19:696–707. doi: 10.1038/s41590-018-0135-x
280. Collins F, Kazmi M, Muraro PA. Progress and prospects for the use and the understanding of the mode of action of autologous hematopoietic stem cell transplantation in the treatment of multiple sclerosis. *Expert Rev Clin Immunol.* (2017) 13:611–22. doi: 10.1080/1744666X.2017.1297232
281. Lublin FD, Reingold SC, Cohen JA, Cutter GR, Sørensen PS, Thompson AJ, et al. Defining the clinical course of multiple sclerosis: the 2013 revisions. *Neurology.* (2014) 83:278–86. doi: 10.1212/WNL.0000000000000560
282. Sellner J, Rommer PS. A review of the evidence for a natalizumab exit strategy for patients with multiple sclerosis. *Autoimmun Rev.* (2019) 18:255–61. doi: 10.1016/j.autrev.2018.09.012
283. Weideman AM, Tapia-Maltos MA, Johnson K, Greenwood M, Bielekova B. Meta-analysis of the age-dependent efficacy of multiple sclerosis treatments. *Front Neurol.* (2017) 8:577. doi: 10.3389/fneur.2017.00577

Permissions

All chapters in this book were first published by Frontiers; hereby published with permission under the Creative Commons Attribution License or equivalent. Every chapter published in this book has been scrutinized by our experts. Their significance has been extensively debated. The topics covered herein carry significant findings which will fuel the growth of the discipline. They may even be implemented as practical applications or may be referred to as a beginning point for another development.

The contributors of this book come from diverse backgrounds, making this book a truly international effort. This book will bring forth new frontiers with its revolutionizing research information and detailed analysis of the nascent developments around the world.

We would like to thank all the contributing authors for lending their expertise to make the book truly unique. They have played a crucial role in the development of this book. Without their invaluable contributions this book wouldn't have been possible. They have made vital efforts to compile up to date information on the varied aspects of this subject to make this book a valuable addition to the collection of many professionals and students.

This book was conceptualized with the vision of imparting up-to-date information and advanced data in this field. To ensure the same, a matchless editorial board was set up. Every individual on the board went through rigorous rounds of assessment to prove their worth. After which they invested a large part of their time researching and compiling the most relevant data for our readers.

The editorial board has been involved in producing this book since its inception. They have spent rigorous hours researching and exploring the diverse topics which have resulted in the successful publishing of this book. They have passed on their knowledge of decades through this book. To expedite this challenging task, the publisher supported the team at every step. A small team of assistant editors was also appointed to further simplify the editing procedure and attain best results for the readers.

Apart from the editorial board, the designing team has also invested a significant amount of their time in understanding the subject and creating the most relevant covers. They scrutinized every image to scout for the most suitable representation of the subject and create an appropriate cover for the book.

The publishing team has been an ardent support to the editorial, designing and production team. Their endless efforts to recruit the best for this project, has resulted in the accomplishment of this book. They are a veteran in the field of academics and their pool of knowledge is as vast as their experience in printing. Their expertise and guidance has proved useful at every step. Their uncompromising quality standards have made this book an exceptional effort. Their encouragement from time to time has been an inspiration for everyone.

The publisher and the editorial board hope that this book will prove to be a valuable piece of knowledge for researchers, students, practitioners and scholars across the globe.

List of Contributors

Silke Häusser-Kinzel
Institute of Neuropathology, University Medical Center, Göttingen, Germany

Martin S. Weber
Institute of Neuropathology, University Medical Center, Göttingen, Germany
Department of Neurology, University Medical Center, Göttingen, Germany

Florian Deisenhammer
Department of Neurology, Innsbruck Medical University, Innsbruck, Austria

Henrik Zetterberg
Department of Psychiatry and Neurochemistry, Institute of Neuroscience and Physiology, The Sahlgrenska Academy at the University of Gothenburg, Mölndal, Sweden
Clinical Neurochemistry Laboratory, Sahlgrenska University Hospital, Mölndal, Sweden
Department of Neurodegenerative Disease, UCL Institute of Neurology, London, United Kingdom
The Fluid Biomarker Laboratory, UK Dementia Research Institute at UCL, London, United Kingdom

Brit Fitzner and Uwe K. Zettl
Division of Neuroimmunology, Department of Neurology, University Medicine Rostock, Rostock, Germany

Xing Li and Yuan Zhang
National Engineering Laboratory for Resource Development of Endangered Crude Drugs in Northwest China, Key Laboratory of the Ministry of Education for Medicinal Resources and Natural Pharmaceutical Chemistry, College of Life Sciences, Shaanxi Normal University, Xi'an, China
Department of Neurology, Thomas Jefferson University, Philadelphia, PA, United States

Li Zhao, Juan-Juan Han, Fei Zhang, Shuai Liu and Zhe-Zhi Wang
National Engineering Laboratory for Resource Development of Endangered Crude Drugs in Northwest China, Key Laboratory of the Ministry of Education for Medicinal Resources and Natural Pharmaceutical Chemistry, College of Life Sciences, Shaanxi Normal University, Xi'an, China

Lin Zhu
Department of Pharmacy, Zhengzhou University, Zhengzhou, China

Guang-Xian Zhang
Department of Neurology, Thomas Jefferson University, Philadelphia, PA, United States

Wolfgang Faigle, Carolina Cruciani, Marco Puthenparampil, Paula Tomas-Ojer, Carla Sellés-Moreno Ivan Jelcic, Mireia Sospedra and Roland Martin
Neuroimmunology and MS Research Section, Neurology Clinic, University Zurich, University Hospital Zurich, Zurich, Switzerland

Witold Wolski and Bernd Roschitzki
Functional Genomics Center Zurich, ETH Zurich & University of Zurich, Zurich, Switzerland

Thomas Zeis and Nicole Schaeren-Wiemers
Neurobiology, Department of Biomedicine, University Hospital Basel, University of Basel, Basel, Switzerland

Mei Fang, Ryo Yamasaki, Guangrui Li, Katsuhisa Masaki, Hiroo Yamaguchi, Atsushi Fujita and Jun-ichi Kira
Department of Neurology, Neurological Institute, Graduate School of Medical Sciences, Kyushu University, Fukuoka, Japan

Noriko Isobe
Department of Neurology, Neurological Institute, Graduate School of Medical Sciences, Kyushu University, Fukuoka, Japan
Department of Neurological Therapeutics, Neurological Institute, Graduate School of Medical Sciences, Kyushu University, Fukuoka, Japan

Franziska Di Pauli and Thomas Berger
Clinical Department of Neurology, Medical University of Innsbruck, Innsbruck, Austria

Nicholas E. Martinez
Department of Microbiology and Immunology, Louisiana State University Health Sciences Center-Shreveport, Shreveport, LA, United States

Ah-Mee Park and Mitsugu Fujita
Department of Microbiology, Kindai University Faculty of Medicine, Osakasayama, Japan

Nikki J. Kennett
Department of Pathology, University of Utah, Salt Lake City, UT, United States

Urška Cvek
Department of Computer Science, Louisiana State University Shreveport, Shreveport, LA, United States

Alireza Minagar
Department of Neurology, Louisiana State University Health Sciences Center-Shreveport, Shreveport, LA, United States

J. Steven Alexander
Department of Neurology, Louisiana State University Health Sciences Center-Shreveport, Shreveport, LA, United States
Department of Molecular and Cellular Physiology, Louisiana State University Health Sciences Center-Shreveport, Shreveport, LA, United States

Ikuo Tsunoda
Department of Microbiology, Kindai University Faculty of Medicine, Osakasayama, Japan
Department of Microbiology and Immunology, Louisiana State University Health Sciences Center-Shreveport, Shreveport, LA, United States
Department of Neurology, Louisiana State University Health Sciences Center-Shreveport, Shreveport, LA, United States

Patrizia LoPresti
Department of Psychology, University of Illinois at Chicago, Chicago, IL, United States

Hans Lassmann
Center for Brain Research, Medical University of Vienna, Vienna, Austria

Nils Venhoff, Jens Thiel, Marta Rizzi, Ana Venhoff, Carolin Hentze, Julian Staniek, Reinhard E. Voll and Ulrich Salzer
Department of Rheumatology and Clinical Immunology, Faculty of Medicine, Medical Center - University of Freiburg, Freiburg im Breisgau, Germany

Sebastian Rauer and Tilman Hottenrott
Department of Neurology and Neurophysiology, Faculty of Medicine, Medical Center - University of Freiburg, Freiburg im Breisgau, Germany

Dominique Endres
Department of Psychiatry and Psychotherapy, Faculty of Medicine, Medical Center - University of Freiburg, Freiburg im Breisgau, Germany

Daniela Huzly
Faculty of Medicine, Institute of Virology, Medical Center - University of Freiburg, Freiburg im Breisgau, Germany

Xiaonan Zhong, Yifan Zhou, Yanyu Chang, Jingqi Wang, Yaqing Shu, Xiaobo Sun, Lisheng Peng and Wei Qiu
Department of Neurology, The Third Affiliated Hospital of Sun Yat-sen University, Guangzhou, China

Alexander Y. Lau
Department of Medicine and Therapeutics, The Chinese University of Hong Kong, Shatin, China

Allan G. Kermode
Department of Neurology, The Third Affiliated Hospital of Sun Yat-sen University, Guangzhou, China
Centre for Neuromuscular and Neurological Disorders, University of Western Australia, Perth, WA, Australia
Department of Neurology, Sir Charles Gairdner Hospital, Queen Elizabeth II Medical Centre, Perth, WA, Australia
Institute of Immunology and Infectious Diseases, Murdoch University, Perth, WA, Australia

Katrin Hanken and Andreas Kastrup
Klinikum Bremen-Ost, Department of Neurology, Bremen, Germany

Carina Sander
Department of Psychology, Carl von Ossietzky Universität Oldenburg, Oldenburg, Germany
Rehabilitationszentrum Oldenburg GmbH, Oldenburg, Germany

Lara Qaiser
Department of Psychology, Carl von Ossietzky Universität Oldenburg, Oldenburg, Germany

Hans-Peter Schlake
Rehabilitationszentrum Oldenburg GmbH, Oldenburg, Germany

Michael Haupts
Augustahospital Anholt, Clinic for Neurology, Anholt, Germany
Department of Neurology, Heinrich-Heine-Uni, Dusseldorf, Germany

Paul Eling
Donders Institute for Brain, Cognition and Behaviour, Radboud University Nijmegen, Nijmegen, Netherlands

Helmut Hildebrandt
Klinikum Bremen-Ost, Department of Neurology, Bremen, Germany
Department of Psychology, Carl von Ossietzky Universität Oldenburg, Oldenburg, Germany

Mehendi Goyal and Manoj Baranwal
Department of Biotechnology, Thapar Institute of Engineering and Technology, Patiala, India

Divya Khanna and Prashant Singh Rana
Department of Computer Science and Engineering, Thapar Institute of Engineering and Technology, Patiala, India

Timur Khaibullin
Republican Clinical Neurological Canter, Republic of Tatarstan, Russian Federation, Kazan, Russia

Ekaterina Martynova and Albert A. Rizvanov
Institute of Fundamental Medicine and Biology, Kazan Federal University, Kazan, Russia

Cory Teuscher
Department of Medicine, University of Vermont, Burlington, VT, United States

Harald Hegen, Gabriel Bsteh, Michael Auer, Sebastian Wurth, Anne Zinganell, Franziska Di Pauli, Florian Deisenhammer and Thomas Berger
Department of Neurology, Medical University of Innsbruck, Innsbruck, Austria

Janette Walde
Department of Statistics, Faculty of Economics and Statistics, University of Innsbruck, Innsbruck, Austria

Tobias Zrzavy and Isabella Wimmer
Department of Neurology, Medical University of Vienna, Vienna, Austria

Herwig Kollaritsch
Institute of Specific Prophylaxis and Tropical Medicine, Medical University of Vienna, Vienna, Austria

Paulus S. Rommer
Department of Neurology, Medical University of Vienna, Vienna, Austria
Department of Neurology, Neuroimmunological Section, University of Rostock, Rostock, Germany

Nina Boxberger
Department of Neurology, Neuroimmunological Section, University of Rostock, Rostock, Germany

Micha Loebermann
Department of Tropical Medicine and Infectious Diseases, University of Rostock, Rostock, Germany

Alexander Winkelmann
Department of Neurology, University of Rostock, Rostock, Germany

Uwe K. Zettl
Department of Neurology, Neuroimmunological Section, University of Rostock, Rostock, Germany
Department of Neurology, University of Rostock, Rostock, Germany

Dimitry N. Krementsov and Mahalia M. McGill
Department of Biomedical and Health Sciences, University of Vermont, Burlington, VT, United States

Svetlana F. Khaiboullina
Institute of Fundamental Medicine and Biology, Kazan Federal University, Kazan, Russia
Department of Microbiology and Immunology, University of Nevada, Reno, NV, United States

Loredana Asarian and Qian Fang
Department of Medicine, University of Vermont, Burlington, VT, United States
Department of Pathology, University of Vermont, Burlington, VT, United States

Johanna Balslev Andersen, Julie Yoon Moberg and Tim Spelman
Danish Multiple Sclerosis Registry, Department of Neurology, Copenhagen University Hospital, Rigshospitalet, Denmark

Melinda Magyari
Danish Multiple Sclerosis Registry, Department of Neurology, Copenhagen University Hospital, Rigshospitalet, Denmark
Department of Neurology, Danish Multiple Sclerosis Center, Copenhagen University Hospital, Rigshospitalet, Denmark

Armando Sena
Centro de Investigação Multidisciplinar Egas Moniz (CiiEM), Instituto Universitário Egas Moniz, Caparica, Portugal
Faculdade de Ciências Médicas, Universidade Nova de Lisboa, Lisbon, Portugal
Departamento de Neurociências, Serviço de Neurologia, Centro Hospitalar de Lisboa-Central, Lisbon, Portugal

Ana Macedo
Keypoint, Consultora Científica, Algés, Portugal
Departamento de Ciências Biomédicas e Medicina (DCBM), Universidade do Algarve, Faro, Portugal

Véronique Ferret-Sena
Centro de Investigação Multidisciplinar Egas Moniz (CiiEM), Instituto Universitário Egas Moniz, Caparica, Portugal

Carlos Capela and Rui Pedrosa
Departamento de Neurociências, Serviço de Neurologia, Centro Hospitalar de Lisboa-Central, Lisbon, Portugal

Majid Ghareghani
CERVO Brain Research Center, Quebec City, QC, Canada
Medicinal Plants Research Center, Yasuj University of Medical Sciences, Yasuj, Iran

Russel J. Reiter
Department of Cell Systems and Anatomy, The University of Texas Health Science Center, San Antonio, TX, United States

Kazem Zibara
PRASE, Biology Department, Faculty of Sciences-I, Lebanese University, Beirut, Lebanon

Naser Farhadi
Cellular and Molecular Research Center, Yasuj University of Medical Sciences, Yasuj, Iran

Paulus S. Rommer
Department of Neurology, Medical University of Vienna, Vienna, Austria

Ron Milo
Department of Neurology, Barzilai University Medical Center, Ashkelon, Israel
Faculty of Health Sciences, Ben-Gurion University of the Negev, Beer-Sheva, Israel

May H. Han and Sammita Satyanarayan
Neuroimmunology Division, Department of Neurology and Neurological Sciences, Stanford University, Stanford, CA, United States

Johann Sellner
Department of Neurology, Christian Doppler Medical Center, Paracelsus Medical University, Salzburg, Austria
Department of Neurology, Klinikum Rechts der Isar, Technische Universität, Munich, Germany

Zsolt Illes
Department of Neurology, Odense University Hospital, Odense, Denmark
Institute of Clinical Research, University of Southern Denmark, Odense, Denmark

Clemens Warnke and Sarah Laurent
Department of Neurology, Medical Faculty, University of Köln, Cologne, Germany

Martin S. Weber
Institute of Neuropathology, University Medical Center, Göttingen, Germany
Department of Neurology, University Medical Center, Göttingen, Germany

Yinan Zhang
Department of Neurology and Neurotherapeutics, University of Texas Southwestern Medical Center, Dallas, TX, United States

Olaf Stuve
Department of Neurology, Klinikum Rechts der Isar, Technische Universität, Munich, Germany
Department of Neurology and Neurotherapeutics, University of Texas Southwestern Medical Center, Dallas, TX, United States
Neurology Section, VA North Texas Health Care System, Medical Service Dallas, VA Medical Center, Dallas, TX, United States

Index